Latinx Mental Health:
From Surviving to Thriving

Edward A. Delgado-Romero
University of Georgia, USA

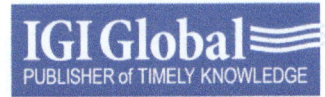

A volume in the Advances in Psychology, Mental Health, and Behavioral Studies (APMHBS) Book Series

Published in the United States of America by
IGI Global
Medical Information Science Reference (an imprint of IGI Global)
701 E. Chocolate Avenue
Hershey PA, USA 17033
Tel: 717-533-8845
Fax: 717-533-8661
E-mail: cust@igi-global.com
Web site: http://www.igi-global.com

Copyright © 2023 by IGI Global. All rights reserved. No part of this publication may be reproduced, stored or distributed in any form or by any means, electronic or mechanical, including photocopying, without written permission from the publisher. Product or company names used in this set are for identification purposes only. Inclusion of the names of the products or companies does not indicate a claim of ownership by IGI Global of the trademark or registered trademark.
    Library of Congress Cataloging-in-Publication Data

Names: Delgado-Romero, Edward A., editor.
Title: Latinx mental health : from surviving to thriving / Edward A.
    Delgado-Romero, editor.
Description: Hershey, PA : Medical Information Science Reference, [2023] |
    Includes bibliographical references and index. | Summary: "This book
    focuses on the way that Latinx issues can be studied and addressed in a
    culturally and linguistically appropriate way and seeks to inspire a new
    generation of mental health researchers and practitioners to engage with
    the Latinx population in a strength-based way"-- Provided by publisher.
Identifiers: LCCN 2022025925 (print) | LCCN 2022025926 (ebook) | ISBN
    9781668449011 (hardcover) | ISBN 9781668449028 (ebook)
Subjects: MESH: Mental Health--ethnology | Hispanic or Latino--psychology |
    Culturally Competent Care | Health Inequities | Social Determinants of
    Health--ethnology | United States
Classification: LCC RC451.5.H57 (print) | LCC RC451.5 H57 (ebook) | NLM
    WA 305 AA1 | DDC 362.2089/68073--dc23/eng/20220727
LC record available at https://lccn.loc.gov/2022025925
LC ebook record available at https://lccn.loc.gov/2022025926

This book is published in the IGI Global book series Advances in Psychology, Mental Health, and Behavioral Studies (APMHBS) (ISSN: 2475-6660; eISSN: 2475-6679)

British Cataloguing in Publication Data
A Cataloguing in Publication record for this book is available from the British Library.

All work contributed to this book is new, previously-unpublished material. The views expressed in this book are those of the authors, but not necessarily of the publisher.

For electronic access to this publication, please contact: eresources@igi-global.com.

Advances in Psychology, Mental Health, and Behavioral Studies (APMHBS) Book Series

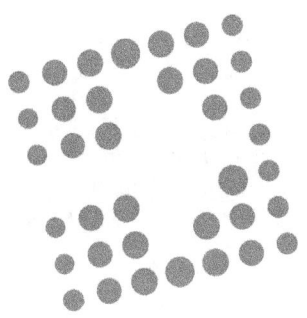

Harish C. Chandan
Argosy University, USA
Bryan Christiansen
Southern New Hampshire University, USA

ISSN:2475-6660
EISSN:2475-6679

Mission

The complexity of the human mind has puzzled researchers and physicians for centuries. While widely studied, the brain still remains largely misunderstood.

The **Advances in Psychology, Mental Health, and Behavioral Studies (APMHBS)** book series presents comprehensive research publications focusing on topics relating to the human psyche, cognition, psychiatric care, mental and developmental disorders, as well as human behavior and interaction. Featuring diverse and innovative research, publications within APMHBS are ideally designed for use by mental health professionals, academicians, researchers, and upper-level students.

Coverage

- Emotional Health
- Human Interaction
- Human Behavior
- Mental Health & Disorders
- Substance Abuse
- Cognition
- Socialization
- Developmental Disorders
- Trauma & Stress
- Personality Disorders

IGI Global is currently accepting manuscripts for publication within this series. To submit a proposal for a volume in this series, please contact our Acquisition Editors at Acquisitions@igi-global.com or visit: http://www.igi-global.com/publish/.

The Advances in Psychology, Mental Health, and Behavioral Studies (APMHBS) Book Series (ISSN 2475-6660) is published by IGI Global, 701 E. Chocolate Avenue, Hershey, PA 17033-1240, USA, www.igi-global.com. This series is composed of titles available for purchase individually; each title is edited to be contextually exclusive from any other title within the series. For pricing and ordering information please visit http://www.igi-global.com/book-series/advances-psychology-mental-health-behavioral/110200. Postmaster: Send all address changes to above address. Copyright © 2023 IGI Global. All rights, including translation in other languages reserved by the publisher. No part of this series may be reproduced or used in any form or by any means – graphics, electronic, or mechanical, including photocopying, recording, taping, or information and retrieval systems – without written permission from the publisher, except for non commercial, educational use, including classroom teaching purposes. The views expressed in this series are those of the authors, but not necessarily of IGI Global.

Titles in this Series

For a list of additional titles in this series, please visit: www.igi-global.com/book-series/advances-psychology-mental-health-behavioral/110200

Handbook of Research on Play Specialism Strategies to Prevent Pediatric Hospitalization Trauma
Giulia Perasso (University of Milano-Bicocca, Italy) and Yagmur Ozturk (University of Trento, Italy)
Medical Information Science Reference • copyright 2023 • 400pp • H/C (ISBN: 9781668450680) • US $425.00 (our price)

The Role of Child Life Specialists in Community Settings
Genevieve Lowry (Bank Street College of Education, USA) Lindsey Murphy (Missouri State University, USA) and Cara Smith (Missouri State University, USA)
Information Science Reference • copyright 2023 • 435pp • H/C (ISBN: 9781668450970) • US $245.00 (our price)

Counseling Strategies for Children and Families Impacted by Incarceration
Kenya Johns (Geneva College, USA)
Medical Information Science Reference • copyright 2022 • 365pp • H/C (ISBN: 9781799892090) • US $295.00 (our price)

The Reproduction and Maintenance of Inequalities in Interpersonal Relationships
Tyler Ross Flockhart (Viterbo University, USA) Abigail Reiter (University of North Carolina at Pembroke, USA) and Matthew R. Hassett (University of North Carolina at Pembroke, USA)
Information Science Reference • copyright 2022 • 332pp • H/C (ISBN: 9781668441282) • US $215.00 (our price)

Applying Mind Genomics to Social Sciences
Howard Moskowitz (Moskowitz Jacobs, Inc., USA) Arthur Kover (Fordham Business Schools, USA) and Petraq Papajorgji (European University of Tirana, Albania)
Information Science Reference • copyright 2022 • 281pp • H/C (ISBN: 9781799884095) • US $215.00 (our price)

Developing, Delivering, and Sustaining School Counseling Practices Through a Culturally Affirming Lens
Sarah N. Brant-Rajahn (Messiah University, USA) Eva M. Gibson (Austin Peay State University, USA) and Mariama Cook Sandifer (Columbus State University, USA)
Information Science Reference • copyright 2022 • 383pp • H/C (ISBN: 9781799895145) • US $215.00 (our price)

The Impact of the COVID-19 Pandemic on Child, Adolescent, and Adult Development
Nava R. Silton (Marymount Manhattan College, USA)
Information Science Reference • copyright 2022 • 262pp • H/C (ISBN: 9781668434840) • US $195.00 (our price)

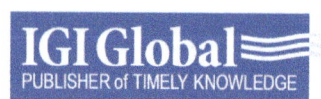

701 East Chocolate Avenue, Hershey, PA 17033, USA
Tel: 717-533-8845 x100 • Fax: 717-533-8661
E-Mail: cust@igi-global.com • www.igi-global.com

Table of Contents

Preface xiv

Acknowledgment xix

Chapter 1
Introduction to Latinx Mental Health 1
    Edward A. Delgado-Romero, University of Georgia, USA
    Ammy E. Sena, University of Georgia, USA
    Cristalís Capielo Rosario, Arizona State University, USA

Chapter 2
La Historia de Afrodescendientes: A Look Into the Surviving and Thriving of Afro-Descent People From Latin America 14
    Ammy Sena, University of Georgia, USA
    Amanda Shannon, University of Georgia, USA

Chapter 3
Dichos for Culturally Responsive Practice: LGBTQ+ Latinxs 37
    Bekah Estevez, Georgia Southern University, USA
    Jennifer N. Merrrifield, Medical College of Georgia, USA

Chapter 4
Creando un Mundo Nuevo (Creating a New World): Campesinos in the United States 57
    Maritza Y. Duran, University of California, Berkeley, USA
    Jason A. Cade, University of Georgia, USA
    Alyssa Marquez, University of California, Los Angeles, USA
    Gisela Cruz, University of Georgia, USA

Chapter 5
Reclamando Lo Que Nos Arrebataron: Spiritual Reclaiming and Reconnection 72
    Ana Carina Ordaz, University of Georgia, USA
    Jocelyn Jimenez-Ruiz, University of Georgia, USA
    Vanessa Placeres, San Diego State University, USA

Chapter 6
Madrinas Paving the Way: Understanding the Development of Latinx Feminism............................ 86
    Kiara Manosalvas, Teachers College, Columbia University, USA
    Brooke Rappaport, Tennessee State University, USA
    Lucia Quezada, University of Georgia, USA
    Grace-Ellen Mahoney, University of Maryland, USA

Chapter 7
Contemporary Views on Latinx Feminism: Applying Our Collective Histories to Create a More Brilliant Future... 103
    Brooke Rappaport, Tennessee State University, USA
    Lucia Quezada, University of Georgia, USA
    Kiara Manosalvas, Teachers College, Columbia University, USA
    Grace-Ellen Mahoney, University of Maryland, USA

Chapter 8
Somos Fuertes Pero También Sufrimos (We Are Strong but We Also Suffer): *La Salud Mental de Hombres Latino* (The Mental Health of Latino Men) 124
    Eckart Werther, Clayton State University, USA
    Bryan O. Rojas-Araúz, In Lak'ech Counseling, Education, and Consulting, USA
    Ruben Atilano, Yale University, USA

Chapter 9
Higher Education: Latinx Individuals Luchando for Higher Education... 165
    Leslie Espinoza, University of Georgia, USA
    Monica Sanchez, University of Georgia, USA
    Alexina Pilo, University of Georgia, USA
    Nancy Muro-Rodriguez, University of Georgia, USA

Chapter 10
Yo Nací Aquí: Maintaining a Connection With One's Country of Origin 182
    Alejandra Martínez Villalba, University of Georgia, USA
    Marta J. González, Latinx Mental Health, USA
    Julia Roncoroni, University of Denver, USA

Chapter 11
Rompiendo Cadenas: Breaking Down Intergenerational Trauma in the Latinx Community............. 196
    Charmaine Mora-Ozuna, University of Georgia, USA
    Inés Rodriguez, Georgia State University, USA
    Marjory Vazquez, Kaiser Permanente, USA
    Jacqueline Fuentes, University of Georgia, USA

Chapter 12
Juntos Resistimos y Sanamos: The Strength of Latinx Families 211
    Jacqueline Fuentes, *University of Georgia, USA*
    Violeta J. Rodriguez, *University of Georgia, USA & Department of Psychiatry and*
        Behavioral Sciences, University of Miami Miller School of Medicine, USA
    Madison L. Rodriguez, *University of Georgia, USA*
    Ana Carina Ordaz, *University of Georgia, USA*

Chapter 13
Un Paso Adelante (A Step Forward): A Family's Migration Testimonino and Recommendations
for Mental Health Providers.. 228
    Elizabeth Cárdenas Bautista, *Cambridge Health Alliance, Harvard Medical School, USA*
    Gabriela Cárdenas, *Independent Researcher, USA*
    Manuela Silvia Bautista Gil, *Independent Researcher, USA*
    Mario Cárdenas Villanueva, *Independent Researcher, USA*

Chapter 14
From Silos to Integration: Healthcare, Politics, and Transformation 248
    Jhokania De Los Santos, *Philips, USA*
    Pierluigi Mancini, *Multicultural Development Institute, Inc., USA*
    Amelia Hoyle Miller, *Best Within You Therapy & Wellness, USA*

Chapter 15
Gaining Access and Treatment Equity (GATE): A Framework for Culturally Responsive Clinical
Care 268
    Ana Julia Bridges, *University of Arkansas, USA*

Chapter 16
From Surviving to Thriving: Future Directions... 281
    Eckart Werther, *Clayton State University, USA*
    Jhokania De Los Santos, *Philips, USA*
    Brooke Rappaport, *Tennessee State University, USA*
    Ammy E. Sena, *University of Georgia, USA*
    Cristalis Capielo Rosario, *Arizona State University, USA*
    Edward A. Delgado-Romero, *University of Georgia, USA*

Compilation of References 293

About the Contributors 340

Index... 351

Detailed Table of Contents

Preface xiv

Acknowledgment xix

Chapter 1
Introduction to Latinx Mental Health 1
    Edward A. Delgado-Romero, University of Georgia, USA
    Ammy E. Sena, University of Georgia, USA
    Cristalís Capielo Rosario, Arizona State University, USA

This chapter provides an overview of what is Latinx mental health. The authors reviewed traditional definitions of mental health and offered a new conceptualization for defining mental health. They defined Latinx mental health as the ability to author a sense of self where one has critically thought about both Latinx cultural and mainstream values, beliefs, and behaviors and selectively constructs an identity that is consistent with one's beliefs and aspirations. They believe that a healthy Latinx mental health identity involves selectively valuing one's cultural and ethnic heritage with pride and valuing the cultural and ethnic heritage of others. They believe that Latinx mental health is ever evolving and involves critical reflection of traditions based in colonization, racism/colorism, prejudice, and internalized hatred and is a continual process not a static event. The associate editors of this book share their journey as Latinx individuals with mental health, psychology, and wellness. This positionality creates the context for the pillars of this book.

Chapter 2
La Historia de Afrodescendientes: A Look Into the Surviving and Thriving of Afro-Descent
People From Latin America 14
    Ammy Sena, University of Georgia, USA
    Amanda Shannon, University of Georgia, USA

The current chapter will explore relevant history of Afrodescendientes, its impact on their psychological wellbeing, and the research and clinical implications. Lastly, this chapter will discuss Afrodescendientes' resistance and the importance of continued liberation. This chapter is an amalgamation of interdisciplinary research, including history, sociology, and psychology, and is intended for the individual who works with Afro-Descent people of Latin America. Specifically, it is for the individual who wants to grow in their understanding of the Afrodescendiente story.

Chapter 3
Dichos for Culturally Responsive Practice: LGBTQ+ Latinxs 37
    Bekah Estevez, Georgia Southern University, USA
    Jennifer N. Merrrifield, Medical College of Georgia, USA

In this chapter, the authors present important concepts, language, and information regarding the lived experiences of Latinx LGBTQ+ individuals (e.g., identity development, sociopolitical impacts on health, resilience processes). They aim to highlight the complexity, nuances, and unique strengths of this community by reviewing relevant research and also interspersing personal anecdotes from our own lives. They offer practitioners and researchers practical advice and take-aways for culturally responsive and relevant practice with and for the Latinx LGBTQ+ community.

Chapter 4
Creando un Mundo Nuevo (Creating a New World): Campesinos in the United States 57
    Maritza Y. Duran, University of California, Berkeley, USA
    Jason A. Cade, University of Georgia, USA
    Alyssa Marquez, University of California, Los Angeles, USA
    Gisela Cruz, University of Georgia, USA

Farm workers have faced additive barriers with the pandemic and environmental issues that are exceedingly making their jobs more difficult. Coupled with the pandemic, farm workers are facing more obstacles in their everyday life. Despite these challenges, farm workers are finding ways to create organizations and advocacy avenues within their communities. Farm workers are also continuing to keep cultural practices alive and are creating communities where they migrate. These factors are resiliency factors that allow farm workers to create lives that feel meaningful and joyful to them.

Chapter 5
Reclamando Lo Que Nos Arrebataron: Spiritual Reclaiming and Reconnection 72
    Ana Carina Ordaz, University of Georgia, USA
    Jocelyn Jimenez-Ruiz, University of Georgia, USA
    Vanessa Placeres, San Diego State University, USA

The terms religion and spirituality are used interchangeably and often shown as symbols of strength, resiliency, and resistance among Latinxs with intersecting identities who are impacted by various forms of oppression in their daily lives. The authors will explore the shifts that have taken place in the Latinx population, moving away from predominantly Catholic practices and returning to practices pre-colonization and more Spiritual practices. The authors will weave intersectionality throughout this chapter, highlighting the diversity that exists within the Latinx community, focusing on cultural strengths, resiliency, and decolonization. The chapter will focus on central aspects of spirituality that include the return to indigenous healing practices, coping, and recommendations and implications focused on training through a multicultural lens and highlighting the strengths and growth areas of available interventions and research.

Chapter 6
Madrinas Paving the Way: Understanding the Development of Latinx Feminism 86
Kiara Manosalvas, Teachers College, Columbia University, USA
Brooke Rappaport, Tennessee State University, USA
Lucia Quezada, University of Georgia, USA
Grace-Ellen Mahoney, University of Maryland, USA

This chapter provides an overview of the history of Latinx feminism. It includes a brief history about Latinx feminist leaders and the development of feminism including womanism, Black feminism, mujerismo, and womanista. The chapter includes ways in which Latina feminism highlights indigenous ways of knowing including mestiza consciousness, borderlands, and nepantla. This chapter sets the groundwork for the authors to explore contemporary perspectives on Latinx feminism including their own feminist identity developments in another chapter.

Chapter 7
Contemporary Views on Latinx Feminism: Applying Our Collective Histories to Create a More Brilliant Future 103
Brooke Rappaport, Tennessee State University, USA
Lucia Quezada, University of Georgia, USA
Kiara Manosalvas, Teachers College, Columbia University, USA
Grace-Ellen Mahoney, University of Maryland, USA

This chapter discusses contemporary perspectives related to Latinx feminism. This chapter builds upon a previous chapter about the history of Latinx feminism. Ways in which feminism and gender identity intersect with other identities are discussed. The authors discuss how Latinx feminism provides avenues to resist oppression. The chapter ends with a discussion of application of feminist concepts discussed and future directions. A combination of third-person research and personal narrative is utilized.

Chapter 8
Somos Fuertes Pero También Sufrimos (We Are Strong but We Also Suffer): *La Salud Mental de Hombres Latino* (The Mental Health of Latino Men) 124
Eckart Werther, Clayton State University, USA
Bryan O. Rojas-Araúz, In Lak'ech Counseling, Education, and Consulting, USA
Ruben Atilano, Yale University, USA

The mental health of men has recently become a topic of interest to social scientists and mental health professionals. The chapter presents a strength-based and culturally informed understanding of the interrelated factors associated with the mental health of Latinx men. Concepts such as masculine ideologies, gender socialization, help-seeking behaviors, as well as relevant trends within higher education and the mental health fields. The authors engage readers in an adapted version of the Latinx oral tradition of testimonios. The authors incorporate personal and professional experiences throughout the chapter that are relevant to the topics and to facilitate a deeper connection and appreciation with the experiences of Latinx men and their mental health.

Chapter 9
Higher Education: Latinx Individuals Luchando for Higher Education 165
    Leslie Espinoza, University of Georgia, USA
    Monica Sanchez, University of Georgia, USA
    Alexina Pilo, University of Georgia, USA
    Nancy Muro-Rodriguez, University of Georgia, USA

This chapter focuses on the history and educational experiences of current and past Latinx students. It helps understand governmental policies and systemic barriers that Latinx students and faculty face in the education system. This chapter provides information regarding higher education by highlighting the different experiences of first-generation college students. Authors help identify multicultural considerations when working with Latinx students both in higher education and in the counseling space. Lastly, the authors focus on future directions and resources to support and better help Latinx students create a pipeline towards higher education.

Chapter 10
Yo Nací Aquí: Maintaining a Connection With One's Country of Origin 182
    Alejandra Martínez Villalba, University of Georgia, USA
    Marta J. González, Latinx Mental Health, USA
    Julia Roncoroni, University of Denver, USA

This chapter will focus on cross-border ties that Latinx immigrants maintain with their countries of origin. The authors discussed factors related to ethnic identity, language, and biculturalism/multiculturalism and explored issues associated with navigating changes faced when returning to their native countries, such as shifts in roles and social identities. The authors also engaged in reflecting about the significance of support and finding symbolic ways for individuals to uphold a connection with their roots. Finally, the chapter ends with a discussion on the importance of representation and advocacy for the Latinx immigrants.

Chapter 11
Rompiendo Cadenas: Breaking Down Intergenerational Trauma in the Latinx Community 196
    Charmaine Mora-Ozuna, University of Georgia, USA
    Inés Rodriguez, Georgia State University, USA
    Marjory Vazquez, Kaiser Permanente, USA
    Jacqueline Fuentes, University of Georgia, USA

Four first-generation Latinxs use their personal lived experiences and the experiences that they bear witness to as mental health practitioners to provide a critical lens on the decolonization of intergenerational trauma (IGT) in the Latinx community. The authors acknowledge that IGT is rooted in systemic oppression and colonization. They explore the systemic, cultural, interpersonal, and intrapersonal bidirectional impact that these areas have on the well-being of Latinxs. They highlight the inherent resistance and resilience skills that Latinxs have to survive and thrive from trauma. The authors share culturally responsive interventions that reclaim the cultural values of Latinxs to promote holistic healing and end the transmission of trauma.

Chapter 12
Juntos Resistimos y Sanamos: The Strength of Latinx Families 211
    Jacqueline Fuentes, University of Georgia, USA
    Violeta J. Rodriguez, University of Georgia, USA & Department of Psychiatry and
        Behavioral Sciences, University of Miami Miller School of Medicine, USA
    Madison L. Rodriguez, University of Georgia, USA
    Ana Carina Ordaz, University of Georgia, USA

The authors seek to provide a more holistic, compassionate, and liberatory understanding of Latinx families. This chapter will highlight the importance of understanding families from a historical, culturally centered manner that honors their layered experiences of contextual factors, intergenerational trauma, and strengths-based approach. This chapter seeks to honor ethnic heterogeneity and cultural strengths and expand the notion of what consists of the family constellation. In doing so, the chapter will focus on central aspects of la familia, including child development, parenting, and recommendations focused on engaging Latinx families and improving the assessment and family interventions.

Chapter 13
Un Paso Adelante (A Step Forward): A Family's Migration Testimonino and Recommendations
for Mental Health Providers.. 228
    Elizabeth Cárdenas Bautista, Cambridge Health Alliance, Harvard Medical School, USA
    Gabriela Cárdenas, Independent Researcher, USA
    Manuela Silvia Bautista Gil, Independent Researcher, USA
    Mario Cárdenas Villanueva, Independent Researcher, USA

This chapter includes powerful testimoninos in Spanish and English of the history and impact of immigration on individual and familial levels. Framed from the perspective of different family members, the authors share their migration experience to the U.S. South between 1980 and 1990. Topics of pre-migration, acculturation, trauma, the impact of post-migration experiences, and psychological growth are addressed from the perspective of first-generation Mexican immigrants and children of immigrants. The chapter also provides recommendations for mental health providers as they assess and conceptualize Latinx immigrant communities in the U.S. South.

Chapter 14
From Silos to Integration: Healthcare, Politics, and Transformation 248
    Jhokania De Los Santos, Philips, USA
    Pierluigi Mancini, Multicultural Development Institute, Inc., USA
    Amelia Hoyle Miller, Best Within You Therapy & Wellness, USA

This chapter introduces integrated behavioral healthcare and why it shows promise to be effective in Latinx populations. While the field is shifting rapidly toward an integrated care model, discussions on cultural factors and how they interplay with integrated care are substantially lacking. This chapter attempts to fill this gap and provide understanding of the current socio-political landscape, outline integrated care application when treating Latinxs with eating disorders, and briefly summarize key strategies to consider when part of an effective IBHC team that promotes patient-centered culturally-responsive care.

Chapter 15
Gaining Access and Treatment Equity (GATE): A Framework for Culturally Responsive Clinical Care 268
> *Ana Julia Bridges, University of Arkansas, USA*

Despite often similar or higher prevalence rates of many psychiatric disorders, Latinxs residing in the continental US are significantly less likely to seek needed clinical care than ethnic majority group members. This inequality creates or exacerbates mental health disparities. Here, the authors provide a framework for understanding barriers Latinxs may face to accessing and receiving culturally-responsive mental healthcare. The gaining access and treatment equity (GATE) model articulates four major barriers: perceived need, internal barriers, external barriers, and clinical/procedural barriers. Increasing mental health equity for Latinxs will require attending to all four levels. The authors articulate how clinics have used the GATE model to expand the reach of services.

Chapter 16
From Surviving to Thriving: Future Directions 281
> *Eckart Werther, Clayton State University, USA*
> *Jhokania De Los Santos, Philips, USA*
> *Brooke Rappaport, Tennessee State University, USA*
> *Ammy E. Sena, University of Georgia, USA*
> *Cristalis Capielo Rosario, Arizona State University, USA*
> *Edward A. Delgado-Romero, University of Georgia, USA*

The authors of this book are part of a diverse network of scholars and practitioners with expertise in various aspects of Latinx psychology and mental health. They share a similar purpose of expanding the pipeline of Latinx counselors and psychologists to collectively create a just and healthy society for all Latinxs. This chapter reflects on the common linkages and underdeveloped areas among the chapters. Future directions for Latinx mental health are presented and include but are not limited to the incorporation of liberatory frameworks and interdisciplinary approaches.

Compilation of References 293

About the Contributors 340

Index 351

Preface

This book is the result of over two decades of clinical work, research, outreach and teaching with the U.S. Latinx community. The authors Latinx people and allies, represent mental health professionals and graduate students who have devoted themselves to advancing the state of Latinx mental health in the U.S. through clinical practice, research, outreach and teaching/training.

The editor of the book, Edward Delgado-Romero, is a first-generation American who was born of two immigrant Colombian parents. His journey as a first-generation American in the U.S. educational system fueled his passion for helping to define and refine Latinx mental health. Delgado-Romero (1999, 2010, 2017) has written extensively about his personal and professional journey towards becoming a recognized authority in Latinx mental health. True to the traditional Latinx cultural value of collectivism and *personalismo* (preference for close personal interactions; Arredondo et al., 2014) Delgado-Romero forged collaborative relationships with colleagues, students and alumni to build the necessary professional infrastructure to diversity the mental health workforce both in terms of personnel and a shift in focus from supposedly universal concepts (in reality based in White middle to upper class values and norms; Guthrie, 2004, White, 1970) towards cultural and linguistic competence.

Ammy Sena, senior associate editor, is an immigrant from Dominican Republic. Although arriving in the U.S. at an early age, she often flew back home for extended periods of time. Navigating the stressors of being a foreign-born Afro-Latina in the United States, while observing the perpetual marginalization of her darker skin family in the Dominican Republic galvanized her to pursue a degree that brought liberatory healing to those with intersecting oppressed identities. Thus, she is pursuing a degree in counseling psychology and is engaged in research and practice that aims to bring justice to those oppressed. At the core of her work is the belief that helpers are uniquely positioned to bear witness to these injustices and thus have the duty to collaborate with and advocate for those most marginalized (Varghese et al., 2019).

This book is based on several foundational tenets which run throughout the book and are interwoven throughout all the chapters. The first tenet is that *Latinx people deserve to be viewed from a strength and resilience perspective rather than from a deficit model*. Traditionally, psychology has defined cultural values, beliefs and behaviors that differed from Eurocentric middle to upper class values, beliefs and behaviors as pathological and tended to view ethnic/racial minority communities from a deficit perspective (Guthrie, 2004). Thus, there was some understanding of the pathology of Latinx people and cultural behaviors were often viewed as deviant and maladjusted. This understanding reinforced prejudiced and stereotypical beliefs about Latinx people and served to underscore the need for rapid assimilation into mainstream U.S. culture. This tension between holding on to cultural beliefs, values and behaviors and embracing mainstream U.S. values, beliefs and behaviors can result in a great deal of (acculturative) stress and internalized racism and xenophobia. We believe that Latinx people deserve

Preface

to have the option to see the beauty and strengths of their culture and make their own decisions about what values, beliefs and behaviors to hold on to or discard. In this regard well-being then also relies upon the collaboration and democratic participation of Latinx people and respecting the diversity that exists among them (Prilleltensky, 2003).

The second tenet is that *Latinx people deserve to be seen (and heard) in their relevant context historically and contemporaneously*. Often in the psychological literature, when the focus was not on pathology, Latinx people were invisible or treated as statistical noise to be controlled or removed. In fact, in the 1990s much psychological research (Delgado-Romero et al., 2005) did not report the race or ethnicity of their participants. This was true for two reasons, the first is that race/ethnicity was thought to be irrelevant. Secondly, the use of predominantly White samples promoted the idea that psychological research was universal. The multicultural revolution in psychology challenged both of these ideas to the point that many modern readers may think that not reporting the race/ethnicity of research participants is absurd. Yet it was common practice in research and currently much research reports race/ethnicity as a categorical variable using broad ethnic categories that offers little insight into the psychological variable which is race/ethnicity. Therefore, in this book we will take care to cite research that provides the relevant context for Latinx people and we will stay away from pan-ethnic categories unless theses are relevant identities. You may have noticed that throughout this book we use the term "Latinx" to refer to those from Latin America living in the United States. However, we urge our readers to be critical of this this term. We invite you to explore the works by Salinas and Lozano (2017) who explores the complexities and history of the "x" amongst descendants of Latin America. As editors, we acknowledge that this term is not perfect and may create further marginalization for certain communities such as *Afrodescendientes*, those who speak Portuguese and French and those who are transgender. As such we recommend using the term most preferred by individuals when working within the Latinx community.

The third tenet is that, given a history of exclusion and misrepresentation, *Latinx people deserve to critically question social science research including the preponderance of quantitative and statistical methods that have used to oppress Latinx people in the past* (Guthrie, 2004). There are two main implications for this tenet. The first is that we will be using critical theories that question the societal structures that oppress Latinx people as they manifest in mainstream research and practice. Although critical theories like Critical Race Theory are currently being targeted by conservative groups in the U.S., we believe that critical theories like Lat Crit (Delgado & Stefancic, 2017), Latinx feminist thought (see Chapters 7 and 8 this volume), Liberation psychology (Martín-Baró, Aron, & Corne, 1994; Duran, Firehammer & Gonzalez, 2008), decolonization (Fanon, 1963, 1967; Freire, 1970) and dismantling Anti-Blackness and heteronormativity can help interrogate oppressive structures and dynamics. The second implication is that while we cite culturally sensitive quantitative research, we believe that qualitative research is particularly compatible with Latinx cultural values (Delgado-Romero et al., 2018) and can provide in depth perspectives that serve as an important counterweight to research that aspires to find broad and generalizable results on average.

A tenet that has guided the authors over two decades is the *imperative for social scientists to give their research, practice, teaching and outreach away*. Rather than viewing mental health research, training and practice as a means to an economic end, we aspire to make mental health research, practice, training/teaching and outreach accessible to everyone. We do this through minimizing the barriers to full participation of the Latinx community in our work. This is done by minimizing jargon, inviting Latinx people to serve as partners in research, not charging for therapy or assessments and by actively participating in the life of the community. This philosophy is evident in the name of our free psychology clinic, *Clinica In LaK'ech*, which translated means: you are my other me. We view ourselves as part of the Latinx community rather than an outside force working on it, therefore we attend community events like festivals and parades. We actively work in the community in which we live since our future is bound together. By viewing our work as part of the community rather than something to be bought or sold, we are directly challenging capitalistic norms regarding the value of money and work. And to be consistent, the proceeds from this book are being donated to U-Lead, a group in our community that works towards fostering and identifying educational opportunities for undocumented youth in our community.

Finally, our last tenet is that *Latinx people deserve culturally and linguistically competent mental health providers*. Achieving cultural and linguistically competent care is not easy and sometimes runs counter to traditional notions of professionalism. I (Ed) have often told my students that their presence and success in higher education is an act of rebellion against a curriculum that was not designed for them or their needs. I note that a culturally and linguistically competent provider does not have to be Latinx themselves. However, a Latinx mental health effort is not complete without a critical and significant number of Latinx providers. The need to diversify the mental health workforce is an ethical imperative but also a matter of demographics. In addition, the ongoing COVID-19 pandemic has clearly illustrated the impact of how health disparities are exacerbated by crisis. In many areas of the U.S. the toll on Latinx people of the pandemic has been severe and there will much grief, trauma and medical issues to process in the years following the pandemic. The needs for culturally and linguistically competent mental health providers has never been clearer. As part of this last point, we note that these chapters are far from exercises in objectivity, rather we sought out people who had first-hand experience with the subjects they were writing about. It was important for us to amplify the voices of both the people we wrote about and the psychologists who want to work with them.

In Chapter 1 we introduce the concept of Latinx Mental Health and explain the framework of the book. We wrestle with the definition of mental health and how Latinx mental health might be distinct from and related to universal notions of mental health. We point out the cultural embeddedness of mental health and the potential to reject a pathology and deficit focus of comparing Latinx people to a default norm of White people.

In Chapter 2 we focus on Afro-descended people from Latin America. Afrodescendientes are usually subjected to the racial dynamic of invisibility in the US, and this is no different within Latinx culture. The authors review the general dynamics of race, racism, and colorism in the Latinx community. We chose to lead with marginalized or invisible groups first in this book in a way to argue for visibility and acknowledgement. Similarly, Chapter 3 highlights research and advocacy around Latinx LGBTQ+ Latinx people. Latinx trans people in particular are both vulnerable to suicide and homicide, and have been woefully under-appreciated and not included in Latinx research, training and practice.

Chapter 4 highlights the psychology of farm workers and related immigration issues. Farm workers were classified as "essential workers" during the COVID-19 pandemic, but failed to gain any ground in terms of permanent recognition of the work they do or a viable path to citizenship (if relevant). The pandemic highlighted the brutality of farm work where workers dealt with the pandemic, pesticides, extreme weather, fires and workplace violence and sexual assault.

Chapter 5 deals with spirituality and the centrality of spiritualty to Latinx life in the US. The authors make clear to differentiate spirituality and religion for Latinx people. Although not all Latinx people practice a faith, the issue of spirituality is key for mental health for many Latinx people. As descents of the both the colonizer and the colonized, Latinx people have a complex inheritance and legacy with regards to spirituality. Key to mental health might be recognizing and reclaiming indigenous spiritual practices.

Preface

Chapters 6 and 7 are an exciting view of the historical and contemporary perspectives of Latinx feminism. The authors review the significant contributions of pioneering Latinx feminists providing details and stories that not often been widely shared. With a thorough grounding of the history of Latinx feminism the authors then delve into contemporary views of Latinx feminism, including research investigating the connection and disconnections to mainstream feminism. With an increasing majority of Latinx mental health providers and faculty being Latinx women, the issue of Latinx feminism increases in importance. With this growing gender disparity in mind, Chapter 8 addresses issues related to Latinx men in psychology and in general. All three chapters focus on the need to break free from restrictive gender roles, and Chapter 8 highlights the need to attend to Latinx men and their unique challenges.

Chapter 9 focuses on Latinx people in the US educational system. Although the US Supreme Court established a right to K-12 education for all people in the US, there was no such right to higher education. Coupled with a constricted pipeline of Latinx faculty and administrators, lack of significant numbers of Latinx people at many universities, and the chronic underfunding of Hispanic Serving Institutions, there are many challenges in higher education. However, true to the theme of the book, there is also excellence, achievement, and hope.

Chapter 10 challenges the binary nature of immigration. Traditionally one was a foreigner or American. Immigrants were expected to assimilate into US culture or preserve their culture in certain enclaves. However, the authors of this chapter share their stories of being in the US and maintaining a strong and vital connection to their home countries. This chapter rejects an "either/or" conceptualization with a "both/and" conceptualization of immigration Latinx identity.

Chapter 11 explores the role of intergenerational trauma in Latinx people and families. Trauma can occur pre-, during and post-immigration to the US and is often complicated by the lack of bilingual and bicultural mental health services in the US which often leads to silence around trauma. However, even without being named, trauma can be transmitted across generations and left unaddressed can continue to harm Latinx mental health. Related to trauma is the strength of Latinx families to serve as buffers, resistance and as source of resilience in spite of trauma. Chapter 12 explores ways in which the Latinx family can be a source of strength and coping. Chapter 13 is a first-hand account of a family's immigration journey in which Elizabeth (soon to be a psychologist) and her family illustrate through their *testimonios* (testimony) many of the issues we have raised in the book in a vivid and powerful way. It's an honor to include their story.

Chapter 14 focuses on ways in which Latinx mental health can be addressed and improved through integrated care. Traditionally health services have worked in isolation from each other without addressing the overlaps and linkages that might provide more effective treatment. The treatment of substance abuse and eating disorders are highlighted as lacking cultural adaptations and integrated approaches to provide better care for Latinx people. Both integrating care and communicating with clients on the how and why of integrated care are cited as factors to address health inequities. Chapter 15 provides a model for equitable and culturally responsive care through the GATES model using the author's clinic and *La Clinica in LaK'ech* as examples of how to apply the model.

Finally, Chapter 16 identifies common linkages, underdeveloped areas, and future directions for Latinx mental health. We have spent two decades advancing Latinx psychology and there is much more to do. The *BIENestar* team and the staff of *La Clinica* have fulfilled their requirements as community members, graduate students, and professionals to ensure that there are more culturally and linguistically competent people to do this much needed work.

Edward A. Delgado-Romero
University of Georgia, USA

REFERENCES

Delgado, R., & Stefancic, J. (2017). *Critical Race Theory: An introduction* (3rd ed.). New York University.

Delgado-Romero, E. A. (1999). The face of racism. *Journal of Counseling and Development, 77*(1), 23–25. doi:10.1002/j.1556-6676.1999.tb02408.x

Delgado-Romero, E. A. (2010). Stepping into the future. In J. Koch, M. Trotter, S. Sanger, & T. Skovholt (Eds.), *Voices from the Field: Defining Moments in Counselor Development* (pp. 188–190). Routledge.

Delgado-Romero, E. A. (2017). *No Parece, pero soy Latino*: The privilege and prejudice inherent in being a light skinned Latino with no accent. In S. K. Anderson & V. A. Middleton (Eds.), *Explorations in oppression, diversity and privilege* (3rd ed.). Oxford University Press.

Delgado-Romero, E. A., Galvan, N., Maschino, P., & Rowland, M. (2005). Race and Ethnicity: Ten years of counseling research. *The Counseling Psychologist, 33*, 419–448. doi:10.1177/0011000004268637

Delgado-Romero, E. A., Singh, A., & De Los Santos, J. (2018). *Cuéntame*: The Promise of Qualitative Research with Latinx Populations. *Journal of Latina/o Psychology, 6*(4), 318–328. doi:10.1037/lat0000123

Duran, E., Firehammer, J., & Gonzalez, J. (2008). Liberation psychology as the path toward healing cultural soul wounds. *Journal of Counseling and Development, 86*(3), 288–295. doi:10.1002/j.1556-6678.2008.tb00511.x

Fanon, F. (1963). *The wretched of the earth* (C. Farrington, Trans.). Grove Press.

Fanon, F. (1967). *Black skin, white masks* (C. L. Markmann, Trans.). Grove Press.

Freire, P. (1970). *Pedagogy of the oppressed*. Herder and Herder.

Guthrie, R. V. (2004). Even the rat was White: A historical view of psychology (2nd ed.). Allyn and Bacon.

Jr, S. (2017). Mapping and recontextualizing the evolution of the term Latinx: An environmental scanning in higher education. *Journal of Latinos and Education, 18*(4), 1–14. doi:10.1080/15348431.2017.1390464

Martín-Baró, I., Aron, A., & Corne, S. (1994). *Writings for a liberation psychology*. Harvard University Press.

Prilleltensky, I. (2003). Understanding, resisting, and overcoming oppression: Toward psychopolitical validity. *American Journal of Community Psychology, 31*(1-2), 195–201. doi:10.1023/A:1023043108210 PMID:12741700

Varghese, F. P., Israel, T., Seymour, G., Becker Herbst, R., Suarez, L. G., & Hargons, C. (2019). Injustice in the Justice System: Reforming Inequities for True "Justice for All.". *The Counseling Psychologist, 47*(5), 682–740. doi:10.1177/0011000019892329

White, J. L. (1970). Toward a Black psychology. *Ebony Magazine, 25*(11), 44–52.

Acknowledgment

One hundred percent of the proceeds from this book will be donated to U-Lead Athens (https://www.uleadathens.org/home). U-Lead is a group with the mission to enable college access for immigrant students and students from immigrant families. We have worked closely with U-Lead and their founders, Betina Kaplan and JoBeth Allen. In particular, JoBeth has been a champion of our team, research and practice.

This book was made possible through the efforts of many dedicated people over a twenty-year span. The group most responsible, however, for making this book a reality was the Senior Associate Editor and the Associate Editors.

Ammy Sena was the Senior Associate Editor and she kept everyone on task and focused. Her project management skills helped bring the book into reality. Ammy was responsible for communicating with authors and editors, as well as generally keeping everyone on task. Ammy is a third year Ph.D. student at UGA, having received her master's degree from Boston College. Ammy embodies the strength and resilience that we talk about in the book, and she is sure to become an influential psychologist.

The associate editors are Ruben Atilano, Cristalis Capielo Rosario, Jhokania De Los Santos, Brooke Rappaport and Eckart Werther. Each one took great care to encourage, mentor and shape the writing of this book and the development of the authors as writers. As they continue with their own career pathways and students, we are fortunate that they shared their time, wisdom, and expertise with the authors of the book.

The research team began in 2005. Initially the team came up with the acronym of BIEN, which stood for Behavioral Interventions in Exercise and Nutrition. As the team developed a focus on psychological services with Latinx populations the acronym lost its' meaning and eventually in 2021 the team changed the name to BIENestar (well-being). Members of the research team included: Eliza Belle, Kimber Shelton, Dominique Broussard, Stephanie Clouse, Allie Smith, Alessandra Urbano, Eckart Werther, Erin Schwartz, Cassaundra Govan, Timika Edwards, Carla Sutton-Moore, Yi-Chen Wu, Krystal Meares, Candice Hargons, Cristalis Capielo Rosario, Bailey Nevels, Carissa Balderas, Erin Unkefer, Alica Brown, Reisha Moxley, Lauren Bigham, Marta Gonzalez, Jennifer Merrifield, Courtney Williams, Brooke Rappaport, Jasmine Jenkins, Stephen Fogelman, Anthony Hansen, Lauren Harper, Amelia Miller, Beth Perlman, Melissa Will, Paloma Ocampo, David Stanley, Marjory Vazquez, Ruben Atilano, Jhokania De Los Santos, Daphne Jones, Marlaine Monroig Garcia, Rebekah-Ann Ingram Estevez, Ana Hill, Maritza Duran, Grace-Ellen Mahoney, Charmaine Mora-Ozuna, Jacqueline Fuentes, Ana Carina Ordaz, Elizabeth, Cardenas Bautista, Shawnteli Pace, Nancy Muro-Rodiriguez, Denise Powers, Ammy Sena, Alexina Pilo, Leslie Espinoza, Jocelyn Jiminez-Ruiz, Lucia Quesada, Maria Alejandra Martinez, Monica Sanchez, Andrea Garcia, Gisela Cruz, Jasmine Murillo, Neda Nickfardjam, Anna McConaghie,

Acknowledgment

Alejandra Calva, Claire Mistretta, Cerenity Robeson, Emily Vargas, Jordan Brown, Dolton Collins, Alex Granados, Julia Pavon, Maria Isabel Ceron, Madison Rodriguez, Violetta Rodriguez, Jasmine McGhee, Amanda Shannon, Lauren Mann, Keishla Sauzo-Padilla, Sandra Gomez, Jungsu Oh, Stephanie Shiffler, Whitney Marks and Cle Savage. Eckart Werther and Geysa Flores served as clinical supervisors for the work of the students.

Edward would like to thank his family. His wife Angie has been a pillar of strength and another mentor for generations of BIEN students. His children J., Isa, Nick, Emery and Gil are a constant inspiration for his work as they represent the next generation. Edward wishes to acknowledge Denise Spangler, Dean of the Mary Frances Early College of Education, for always valuing his work and nominating him for several awards. In addition, Edward has been supported by his family, Isabel Delgado, Eduardo Delgado Polo, Angie Morales, Maria Martin, Julian Delgado, and Judy and Takis Iakovou. Edward is lucky to count among his friends George and Nancy Howard, Jeanett Castellanos, Lisa Flores, Melanie Domenech Rodriguez, Patricia Arredondo, Cynthia Guzman, Annelise Singh, Deb Altschul, John Mitchell, Mike Lau, Carlos Hernandez and Michael Horseman. Without friends and family this work is not possible.

Ammy would like to thank her father Elvis Sena and mother Taina "Davieba" Sena and her brothers Elvis Jaser Sena and Nathaniel Sena who has provided her with unconditional love and support throughout life. She would like to thank her grandparents, especially her great grandmother- Modesta "mama" Aguero who passed away during this book journey. Modesta was her introduction to social justice, healing and faith. Next, she acknowledges other loved ones including Therian Manly Williams, Angelica Mora, Harolyn Sena, Soranica Corrente, Rutdileny Cabrera, Jen Ellis, Kiara Manosalvas and her Boston College family including formerly known group "Race Culture Challengers" for their unwavering support. Lastly, she would like to acknowledge her University of Georgia family- BIEN-estar and Dr. Edward Delgado-Romero "DR" who has provided her with the most exceptional mentorship and has demystified academia for her and many students. Gracias DR!

Chapter 1
Introduction to Latinx Mental Health

Edward A. Delgado-Romero
University of Georgia, USA

Ammy E. Sena
University of Georgia, USA

Cristalís Capielo Rosario
Arizona State University, USA

ABSTRACT

This chapter provides an overview of what is Latinx mental health. The authors reviewed traditional definitions of mental health and offered a new conceptualization for defining mental health. They defined Latinx mental health as the ability to author a sense of self where one has critically thought about both Latinx cultural and mainstream values, beliefs, and behaviors and selectively constructs an identity that is consistent with one's beliefs and aspirations. They believe that a healthy Latinx mental health identity involves selectively valuing one's cultural and ethnic heritage with pride and valuing the cultural and ethnic heritage of others. They believe that Latinx mental health is ever evolving and involves critical reflection of traditions based in colonization, racism/colorism, prejudice, and internalized hatred and is a continual process not a static event. The associate editors of this book share their journey as Latinx individuals with mental health, psychology, and wellness. This positionality creates the context for the pillars of this book.

LATINX MENTAL HEALTH: FROM SURVIVING TO THRIVING

Mental health, like health in general, is much more than the absence of pathology. Mental health is a state of well-being, holistic integration, and wholeness. Although many psychologists have chosen the "self" as the unit of analysis, we believe that the self is imbedded within physical, psychological, spiritual, historical, and cultural contexts that overlap and influence each other. Thus, we believe that people strive

DOI: 10.4018/978-1-6684-4901-1.ch001

to be healthy within the many contexts and intersectional identities they hold. In our work we focus on Latinx mental health as the transformation of contextualized individuals from oppression to freedom, and from surviving to thriving, all while honoring an ever-evolving cultural dynamic. In this chapter we set the stage for the rest of the book and talk about our approach to Latinx mental health.

Before beginning we acknowledge that there are many terms used to describe the people known as Hispanic or Latinx. We choose the term Latinx unless we are referring to specific groups or in specific contexts (e.g., the U.S. Census uses the term Hispanic). We use Latinx because we believe it to be the most inclusive term used in psychology now (see Salinas & Lozano, 2019), while at the same understanding that there is power in naming oneself, both individually and collectively.

The history of psychology is often told from the perspectives of the White male pioneers of the field who are often romanticized as striving to understand the human condition and motivated to cure mental illness and improve humanity. These pioneers were often unaware of their biases, prejudices and their efforts to maintain White supremacy through law, science and education. For example, for decades after its inception, psychology was dedicated to highlighting differences between White and People of Color (POC), not to understand human behavior but to legitimize violent oppression and exploitation of POC (Howard, 1986; Tomicic & Berardi, 2018). For example, Guthrie (2004) discusses several examples in which differences between White and POC across measures of motor, perception and cognitive performance were distorted to support anti-Black, anti-Latinx, and anti-Indigenous racism. Besides fomenting racist ideology and violence, this epistemic violence also helped establish White European values, knowledge, and experiences as the universal standard to understand human behavior and psychology (Gould, 1996; Tomicic & Berardi, 2018). These violent methods rejected all African and Indigenous psychology (Tomicic & Berardi, 2018). In essence early psychologists defined mental health by their own narrow standards and deviance from these standards was deemed as illness. Mental health education, practice and research focused on what Henrich (2020) termed WEIRD people; that is Western, Educated, Industrialized, Rich and Democratic. Despite the cultural, racial and economic context of their work, psychologists continued to believe that they were simply studying human nature.

Mental health in the United States was conceptualized as conformity to the social norms of the time and those people who resisted those norms were thought to be mentally ill or maladjusted. Although often scrubbed from the history books, there was a long tradition of pathologizing the experience of women, LGBTQ+ people, people with disabilities, ethnic/racial minority people and enslaved people in the U.S. For example, Guthrie (2004) wrote about disorders created by physicians to explain why enslaved people who would try to escape their captors! Clearly, mental health professionals were invested in preserving the power and humanity of some racial groups over others. As another example, cultural and religious values in the early 20th century led to the social hygiene movement that resulted in the forced sterilization of people deemed unfit to reproduce (Farreras, 2014). Latina women were particularly targeted by this sterilization campaign (Presser, 1969; Stern, 2005). The chillingly efficient social hygiene movement in the U.S., targeted towards minority or marginalized groups (Guthrie, 2004) served as an inspiration for the Holocaust in Germany during World War II (Lifton, 2000). Thus, notions of mental health and what society should do with people who were deemed ill in U.S. were often time and culture bound. As society shifted demographically, economically and technologically, the issue of mental illness was often redefined.

The early (mostly White) feminists reveled in their maladjustment and challenged society to broaden the definition of mental health as did civil rights activists, Vietnam war protesters, LGBTQ+ activists and the Movement for Black Lives. Societal forces consistently brought forth a re-examination of the definition of what it meant to be mentally healthy. Although there has been progress in broadening what mental health entails, and a recognition of the many differences that people have, there has also been backlash and groups in society that want to return to previous idealized values and definitions of mental health based on White, Christian and heteronormative norms. For example, as we write this book there is a wave of anti-trans legislation that is being passed across the U.S. In Texas where the attorney general has defined gender-affirming medical therapy for minors as "child abuse", there exists a stunning reversal of progress in understanding gender-affirming therapy. Several families with trans children were investigated by the Texas state government. Thus, progress with regards to redefining mental health in diverse and just ways, is often met by backlash by those people who want to stay in power and define what mental health is. Ironically in 2022 there are governmental efforts to address mental health and ensure parity at the same time that anti-trans, anti-gay (Florida's "don't say gay" law) and anti-Black (the outlawing of the teaching Critical Race Theory and "divisive concepts") also are underway. Thus, defining mental health can be a tricky, context-dependent, political and value laden endeavor.

Mental health as it is still currently defined and conceptualized should be understood as a product of power and influence in society to maintain White supremacy. As an example, tattoos and piercings are now ubiquitous in U.S. society and no longer carry the connotations of mental illness (in most places) that they did in the recent past. This shift in thinking about tattoos and piercings occurred when they were adopted by the White middle class.

Over the last decades mental health language has come into vogue and youth in the U.S. commonly talk about self-care and often, therapy openly. Yet while mental health awareness is commonplace, there are still social inequities in access to mental health care, disparities in illness, interpersonal violence, mass shootings and oppression of minority groups in society that directly impact mental health. When individuals and communities affected by these injustices rise up and resist, White-centered conceptualization of mental health and those who endorse such conceptualization, again exert their dominance and power by pathologizing protest and resistance (Shin, 2014).

Therefore, for the purposes of this book, we define mental health as the ability to resist oppression (external and internal) and cope with critical life events in productive ways. We believe that mental health involves an ability to identify and use personal cultural strengths, resistance, and resilience to navigate daily life. Key to our definition of mental health is a growth orientation and striving for the improvement of self, loved ones and one's community.

We believe that a healthy Latinx mental health identity involves selectively valuing one's cultural and ethnic heritage with pride, and valuing the cultural and ethnic heritage of others. We believe that Latinx Mental Health is ever evolving, and involves critical reflection of traditions based in colonization, racism/colorism, prejudice and internalized hatred. Note that we do not specify what values, beliefs and behaviors make up Latinx mental health or identify specific authenticity markers that are often narrowly defined. Some examples include the names one uses, the pronunciation of names, the use of Spanish language (or not), dress, food preferences and the people one chooses to have as friends or family. We believe that attempts to demarcate what constitutes an authentic Latinx identity is often an exercise in enforcing narrow beliefs about identity (the in group versus the out group) as the diversity of Latinx experience is as varied as the 66 million people who are classified in this group in the U.S.

Despite many inter-group differences, Latinx people share a history in the U.S. and may share to some extent some overarching cultural values (see Arredondo et al., 2014). However, the existence of these common values has been difficult to demonstrate empirically. If it is difficult to determine the commonalities of Latinx populations regarding mental health, then why attempt to do it? The answer is that whether Latinx people are different from each other or not, Latinx people are often defined as a monolithic group and compared to other monolithic groups such as Whites, Blacks, Native Americans and Asians. Although the process of identifying unique Latinx values, beliefs and behaviors that are unique and distinctive from other groups is often a challenge, we challenge the process of defining the group monolithically as a goal and defining normality as closeness to Whiteness. We believe that we can identify Latinx cultural/ethnic factors that lead to positive outcomes and that might be superior to dominant norms. This thought is embedded in the notion of the controversial Latino Health Paradox, which states that Latinx people, despite lower income and education, have some health outcomes that are superior to non-Hispanic Whites. In terms of health, are there aspects of Latinx values, beliefs and behaviors that lead to superior outcomes, despite disadvantages? What are the cultural strengths that foster resilience to stress and adversity for Latinx people? And despite some advantages in health, in what ways are Latinx people particularly vulnerable? For example, the COVID 19 pandemic disproportionately killed elderly Latinx people and shortened the Latinx advantage in lifespan, effectively and chillingly resolving the Latinx health paradox.

You might already notice a different tone and emphasis to this book than those commonly found in mental health. First, we do endorse a critical perspective of the relationship of U.S. law to Latinx people, known as LatCrit. LatCrit is derived from Critical Race Theory and began as an examination of how the law serves to protect and advance the material interests of White people over Latinx people, who are often invisible in U.S. society (Valdes, 1999). LatCrit scholarship is influenced by critical feminism and queer approaches and takes a decidedly anti-colonial emphasis. We are explicitly using a strength and resilience perspective and we have many years of research, practice, teaching, and outreach from which to build off. At this point, it might be instructive to learn a little bit more about the authors of this chapter and their journey to this point. As we stated in the preface, we believe that personal stories can be inspirational and instructive and help deepen our understanding of the perspectives we are taking. In this next section Delgado-Romero, Sena and Capielo share their experience with Latinx Mental Health throughout their life in the U.S. and in their countries of heritage.

CHANNELING THE IMMIGRANT SPIRIT

I vividly remember the first time I met a psychologist. My parents had immigrated to the United States in the mid 1960's from Colombia. They settled in Mount Vernon, New York and had three children, but soon grew tired of the cold and moved to the South, stopping in Atlanta, Georgia and deciding to stay there. In the 1970's Atlanta's Latinx population was small and centered around Catholic churches and schools. Latinx people usually gathered together at Spanish mass and at social events. I attended a Catholic school, and although almost all the Latinx people were Catholics, most of the Catholic population were European immigrants. Thus, being Latinx was a bubble identity in the sense that most of us identified as Catholic immigrants unless we were within our Latinx bubble where we were free to identify as simply Latinx or in terms of our specific countries of origin. My friends were Cuban, Mexican and Puerto Rican and we had a pan-ethnic notion of what it meant to be Latinx since no one country of origin dominated unlike in New York, Miami, or Los Angeles.

Mental health was not something we ever talked about. I saw many things growing up like substance abuse, infidelity, and poverty but these behaviors were never linked to mental health. Bad events were just things to tolerate and unfortunately it fell to my mother to have to tolerate and cope with my father's mental health issues. He was an angry man who was verbally abusive, unfaithful, and most likely, depressed. In retrospect, it seems my father struggled with life in the U.S. and his accent often targeted him for ridicule at work. I've since learned that his issues started in Colombia, and he had a history of unstable, violent relationships. Like many immigrants, my father thought he could reinvent himself by moving to the U.S. To some extent he was able to reinvent himself as he lied about his education and was able to get into a nascent computer programmer training program in the late 1960's. But the reality was that his demons came with him and were not left behind in Colombia. Stripped of the comfort of his home country and language, he often struggled in his attempts to assimilate into the U.S. He took out his anger, depression, and rage on his family. No one in family ever thought of my father as mentally ill, they would describe him as difficult, passionate, or angry. Therefore, we never thought about trying to get him any help, we just endured his outbursts.

After many miserable years my father left my mother when I went away to college. He called to inform me that he was leaving right before finals, and I failed every final I took. If it were not for the grace of understanding professors, I would have failed out of college. When I returned home, I was angry and upset, especially since my father had taken my college money and left us destitute. At the time, my family was more concerned about my mother's reaction (shock, depression, panic) than my father's behavior. So, they sought to medicate her in an effort help her make it through the divorce.

Rather than look for help for herself, my mother felt guilty that I was so upset, and she asked her friends if there was a Latinx Psychologist who might help me with my anger. In true Latinx style, my mother came up with a plausible alternate explanation for my meeting the psychologist, since I had just switched my major to psychology, perhaps Dr. Aguilar (not his real name) could give me career advice. I was aware of the ruse, but I decided to go anyhow since I had only ever seen a psychologist on film or TV, and I was curious to meet a Latinx psychologist.

Dr. Aguilar's office was like stepping back in time. He had shelves of books; a large leather couch and his office was decorated with classical statues and an impressive antique wooden globe. His office smelled of cigar smoke and dust. Dr. Aguilar wore a three-piece suit and exuded a deliberate, formal air. On his desk he had a ceramic human head that had the phrenological markings that mapped out the areas of the head that corresponded with supposed psychological attributes such as joy and intention. I remember that in my intro psychology classes they called phrenology a discredited pseudo-science.

Dr. Aguilar began to question me about my career goals, quickly transitioning into questions about my relationship with my mother. He asked if I knew about the story of Oedipus. I grew up reading mythology and I knew about Oedipus, and I knew what he was getting at: he was saying that I was overinvolved with my mom and I should let her figure things out on her own. Dr. Aguilar's approach might have worked had my mother had equal access to lawyers, banks, and an understanding of US culture. My father had kept her from acculturating and was thus able to swindle the house from her, deny her his social security benefits and not pay child support for my youngest sibling. Dr. Aguilar's advice was sexist, irrelevant, outdated and enabled my father to steal from his own family. Although at the time I could not articulate any of these dynamics, I just knew Dr. Aguilar, although he was Latinx, was upholding the values of European White supremacy and other than sharing a personal culture and a language with other Latinx people, was complicit in the oppression of Latinx people, particularly women and children. There wasn't much I could do at 18 years old, but I vowed that I would be a different type of psychologist, although at the time I had no idea of what that might look like.

In my psychology courses at college culture was never addressed. Instead, we learned about human dynamics that were derived from middle to upper class White European male culture and then applied to all human beings. My assistantship in the psychology department was to run the animal lab where I took care of the rats and pigeons that were trained in Skinner boxes to demonstrate operant conditioning principles. As I taught the pigeons and rats to turn in circles, I wondered what relevance this work had for working with people beyond simple and automatic ways of learning.

To be fair, in my private elite college, there were two professors who challenged the dominant paradigm. Dr. Queener taught a course on the psychology of religion and was a committed humanistic psychologist. He required us to read the writings of Viktor Frankl (1962) and in doing so I saw the first tangible mention of the strength and resilience of culture, specifically Jewish culture. Dr. Walton was a feminist in a highly traditional school with respect to gender roles. I remember her challenging the Greek social fraternities and sororities for their sexist and misogynistic behavior and beliefs. She taught us about resistance and redefinition through the lens of gender and active feminism. Both professors taught me that psychology needed to address human beings in all of their complexities and intersectional identities. I felt this need acutely as my college was a predominantly White school nested in a city that was 60% African American. There were very few Latinx students, and I perpetually felt like an outsider amongst wealthy White classmates. When the time came to graduate, despite winning the departmental award as the outstanding psychology student, I had no idea what to do next.

I eventually began work in a variety of settings as a research assistant and then a psychology technician. I also enrolled in a counseling master's course in an effort to find a direction to inspire me. The program did little to motivate me, but I spent weekends in the library going through the psychology and counseling journals hoping to find kindred spirts. I stumbled upon the work of George Howard, Mary Fukuyama and Patricia Arredondo. Each one helped me find and define my career trajectory. Howard (1991) wrote about culture as stories we tell, and he became my doctoral advisor. Fukuyama (Fukuyama & Reid, 1996) wrote an article about using poetry in multicultural counseling, and she became a co-worker, co-author and friend. Arredondo (Arredondo et al., 1996) operationalized multicultural competence in a clear way that made sense to me, and she eventually became my mentor. Each person inspired me by capturing my interest and imagination, and I was lucky enough to work with each one in a career defining capacity. Howard, Fukuyama and Arredondo identified closely as descendants of immigrants and their culture and intersectional identities served as a role model for me as I tried to make sense of my own experience.

In my doctoral program there was limited coursework about multiculturalism or diversity. I sought out opportunities to work with students of color and ended up working closely with Native American and first-generation college students. On internship at Michigan State University, I had my first Latinx supervisor and the diverse staff there helped solidify my interest and participation in multicultural psychology just as the movement was beginning to take shape in the early 2000's.

My first job at the University of Florida was working in the University Counseling Center and specializing in outreach to Latinx populations. During this time, I solidified my professional and personal interest in Latinx psychology, learned a great deal about my heritage by traveling to Colombia and decided that I enjoyed research and teaching more than direct services and decided to take an academic appointment at Indiana University. In parallel to my own development, I helped found the National Latinx Psychological Association (NLPA) and during my presidency raised enough money to start NLPA's journal, the *Journal of Latinx Psychology*. In my stewardship of NLPA and the journal, I learned a great deal about the limits of current Latinx research and the potential for research and professional ethics to reflect the strengths and resiliency of the US Latinx population as a counterpoint to pathologically focused research.

In 2005 I left Indiana University to come to the University of Georgia. This move was motivated by my desire to work more closely on Latinx issues, and I felt that although the support was limited at UGA, there was not resistance to my research agenda. Basically, I was given the freedom to do what I wanted. I set about creating an infrastructure for Latinx mental health through research and training partnerships with doctoral students who wanted to become culturally competent. Left to my own devices I created a research team that began attracting students from around the country who wanted to focus on Latinx work. By the time I'm finished at UGA I will have graduated 58 PhD students, 80% who are people of color and half who are Latinx and bilingual. These students have spread out in the US and are now practicing, teaching, and researching around the country.

This book represents a homecoming of sorts for those alumni and current students to focus on their work and for us to share the work we have completed together. In addition to many completed dissertations and research projects, I also created two popular Latinx courses, one at the undergraduate level and one for both undergraduates and graduate students. But our crowning achievement was the establishment and running of *la Clinica In LaK'ech*, our Spanish language free psychology clinic. Thus, my journey was one where I was socialized in traditional views of mental health and sought through my career to develop alternative approaches to positive Latinx mental health. I didn't always know what I was doing, but I was able to channel the immigrant spirit of my mother and help create an infrastructure in Latinx psychology for those who came after me.

AMMY'S (AH-ME) JOURNEY INTO PSYCHOLOGY

My interest in psychology came from my lived and observed experiences in the United States and the Dominican Republic. Vacillating between these two spaces exposed me to various forms of marginalization and the universal concept of oppression. The first experience I had with oppression occurred when I was very young. This formative moment became one that stayed with me forever.

Confused about why anyone would eat slimy, saucy meat, I had one bite of the sandwich and threw it in the garbage. My teacher reprimanded me by sitting me at a table alone, grabbing the meatball sub from the trash can, and forcing me to finish it. I had never heard of a meatball sub, but when classmates rushed me in the lunch line, I panicked. I was three years old, and I had just entered a predominantly White Catholic preschool. I knew I was different from my classmates; I looked different, spoke a foreign language, and was consistently misunderstood by peers and teachers. I internalized the belief that I was "bad," incompetent and did everything wrong. I believed my teachers saw me as less than human, evidenced by the fact that one of them made me eat a sandwich out of the trash. In retrospect, I now believe this encounter was an example of overt racism. This moment coupled with other experiences I had during my preschool year had damaging effects on my racial and ethnic identity as well as my academic self-efficacy.

Enrolling in a Catholic preschool was my parents' way of providing me with a quality education. Prior to attending school, I was cared for by my great-grandmother, with whom I spent hours watching *Univision*, singing Celia Cruz and Selena songs, and making Dominican sweet *Arepa*. Worried that my lack of English fluency would have detrimental effects on my academic success, my parents enrolled me in this private preschool. Although they could not afford it, they wanted to do everything possible to keep me from experiencing the hardships they faced. My parents grew up in the Dominican Republic in families that struggled with the challenges of systemic oppression. When the opportunity arose to move to the United States, they seized it, arriving in Providence, Rhode Island.

Providence is a small city; however, it is comprised of diverse groups, including immigrants and refugees. There are prominent Dominican, Haitian, Puerto Rican, Cambodian, Laotian, Hmong, Portuguese, Italian, Polish, Cape Verdean, Nigerian, and African American communities. After my preschool year, I attended a public elementary school in Providence, with a strong emphasis on bilingual education and multicultural pride. Upon arriving at kindergarten, I felt right at home; the concept of cultural pride in a school, although foreign to me, became one of great healing in repairing my internalized oppression. This period was the first time I was encouraged to speak Spanish, perfect it, and celebrate my Latinx heritage. For example, one year, we had the president of the Dominican Republic at the time- Hipolito Mejia- visit our school for an assembly. Although all the Dominican kids "booed" him off the stage because we were aware of his corrupt political agenda, it was still affirming to see our history right in our American school. This elementary school experience ingrained in me the importance of an affirming environment in positive identity development for marginalized peoples.

Although I had these experiences, mental health was never explicitly discussed in my family or community. It wasn't until high school that my family became transparent about why my beloved uncle would spend days in the hospital. This was the first time I heard about schizophrenia. My uncle, also a Dominican immigrant, struggled with receiving culturally competent care when hospitalized during a crisis. As a family, we barely received psychoeducation, and we didn't know how to support my uncle, his wife, and his children. At the same time, it was hard for me to see my uncle struggle because when outside of a crisis; he was this man who told the best *chistes*, would do anything for *mangu con los tres golpes*, was a technology nerd, and led Sunday school children's worship at our local church. This feeling of collective helplessness stayed with me and informed my desire for culturally competent psychiatric care.

Although we did not discuss mental health, we did talk about discrimination. My father and I would often converse about the racism we faced, the overall challenges of living in America, and the need for continued resilience. Although the US was hard, he would share that living in America was our way of gaining more economical, educational, and political "freedoms." My father did not just talk about freedom; he lived this value by working third shift at a factory, caring for a family, starting his own business, and increasing his English fluency, all while obtaining an MBA in accounting. His work ethic instilled in me the value and importance of education as a tool for consciousness building, access to power, and social mobility. My father taught me that I had access to economic and educational opportunities that were not readily afforded to those in the Dominican Republic, and thus I had an obligation to obtain a degree.

Simultaneously, I experienced the effects of systemic oppression. There were unique issues marginalized communities faced, such as financial instability and challenges creating generational wealth, stress, substance misuse/abuse, infidelity and subsequent marital distress, gang violence, difficulties completing educational degrees, and death from medical issues such as cancer and heart disease. These problems were present within my community in the United States and to a more severe degree with my darker-skinned family in the Dominican Republic. We used words and phrases in Spanish to describe the effects of these issues and our responses to crisis such as "*le dio el yeyo*", "*se le subio la biribulina*", "*se le metio el diablo*", "*le dio un ataque de nervios*", "*ella aguanto mucho*", and "*estoy cansada*".

Galvanized by the unique experiences of people of color both in the United States and in the Dominican Republic, I decided to declare psychology as a major. I did not entirely understand what a psychology degree entailed; however, I knew it had to do with understanding the human mind and helping people. I had hopes of using my degree to promote healing in my community. I learned a lot through my psychology courses and was very fascinated by the theories. But I often felt they did not wholly explain or relate to our issues. For example, I experienced this lack of connection when learning about Abraham Maslow's hierarchy of needs and the need to fulfill basic needs to self-actualize.

Growing up, we would often travel back to the Dominican Republic, spending weeks in *el barrio* with my grandparents and extended family members. The road that led to *el barrio* was a narrow dirt road, houses on this "main" road mainly were built with cinder blocks; however, rows and rows of one room houses were built in between, either adjacent or in backyards made of mixed materials, including wood, cinder blocks, and steel. Water was brought into *el barrio* on a giant water truck that barely was able to travel down this dirt road, and if there were a week where the truck was not able to come, multiple homes would run out of water. Thus, water was a privilege and was often rationed. Other necessities like electricity and food were also, at times, inconsistent. However, those moments of lack of a "basic" need often facilitated moments of love and belonging, which was not possible according to Maslow. When electricity was out and everything was dark, we would all sit in one room, the grandparents, uncles, cousins, visiting neighbors, and tell *cuentos*. Perched up against my voluptuous *mamibuela's* (my maternal grandmother's nickname) chest, the connection, community, and love were felt tenfold.

I felt disconnected in my psychology courses and often wondered if it would be a useful major. It wasn't until the second year of my undergraduate when I took an educational psychology course that I was exposed to concepts of social justice and equity. This course was taught by Dr. Carmen Veloria, a Puerto Rican professor, the first Latinx educator I ever met. I immediately fell in love with the course and was finally able to see myself in psychology. She quickly became my mentor and pushed me to study issues related to communities of color. My first paper for that class was on the positive effects of bilingualism, which was powerful for me to write as I continued to grow in my racial and ethnic identity development.

Upon completing the course, I knew I needed to supplement my learning. I decided to declare a second major in Latin America and Caribbean Studies with a minor in Educational Studies. Through this second major and minor, I learned about the history of colonialism, Paulo Freire and Frantz Fanon, Marxist ideologies, Liberation theories, art and literature as a form of resistance, the school-to-prison pipeline, and many other concepts. I became cognizant of how an individual's experiences were inseparable from the broader social and historical context. An increased understanding of oppression empowered me to challenge my self-criticism and critically reflect on my internalized oppression. My newfound perception created goals of using research to accurately capture the voices of marginalized people and create healing practices. Although I still had to work on the residual effects of my preschool experience on my academic self-concept, I decided that for me to facilitate the most change for my community, I needed to obtain a graduate degree.

On a whim, I applied to Boston College's masters in mental health counseling. Upon acceptance, I worked with Dr. Janet E. Helms in her lab- the Institute and Study for the Promotion of Race and Culture, where I learned about multicultural theories, including Black racial identity development. This time was one of those influential moments in my life where I again felt seen in my experiences in psychology. My experiences at Boston College with Dr. Helms and her lab led me to apply to doctoral programs in counseling psychology. The process of getting into a doctoral program was not easy, and the resulting stress became the catalyst to engaging in my own personal therapy. My academic self-concept and related anxiety paralyzed me during the application process, especially as I thought about the entrance exam. I am grateful for my Nigerian therapist Margarete who helped me work through some of my academic trauma and introduced me to Eye Movement Desensitization and Reprocessing (EMDR). Margarete, my family, and my community of mentors got me through this process and kept me encouraged even when I could not see this as possible.

I feel privileged to be working with my community in the way that I do, exploring ways to decolonize psychology with some of the leading voices in the field and using liberation as essential to healing marginalized individuals. I feel even more honored to work with Ed, or as his students refer to him- DR- who sets the example of what academia should look like and reminds us that the most radical thing us (his students) can do is to graduate. His mantra removes the pressure of over-compensating for the lack of visibility I felt throughout my life and reminds me of my power. Seeing this book come to fruition with his mentees reminds me of the importance of building a critical mass of people to work on a goal, and I am honored to be a part of this legacy.

CRISTALÍS' STORY: WHY I DECIDED TO WALK AWAY FROM ACCULTURATION RESEARCH

Growing up in Puerto Rico, my family would often argue about which political status would be best for Puerto Rico. About half supported US statehood for Puerto Rico, the other supported *el Estado Libre Asociado* (Commonwealth; current status). Only my mother supported independence. We all seemed to agree however, that our association with the US was beneficial. Ease of migration, military protection, and access to federal funds appeared to be most important to my family. All these beliefs were predicated on the idea that our US citizenship translated to having US rights and protections, and full integration into the US polity upon migration.

In 1998, my family migrated to the US looking for the promise of full integration, and as a result a better quality of life. I describe the period when my family migrated to the US as being the prequel to Puerto Rico's millennial migration (2005 – present). During the millennial migration period, Puerto Rico has lost about 14% of its population to migration (Meléndez & Hinojosa, 2017). The company my dad had worked for 18 years closed after the US unilaterally canceled a 20-year-old tax incentive-driven jobs program. The most significant cause of Puerto Rican millennial migration is the island's persistent economic crisis (Silver & Vélez, 2017). When my parents announced we were migrating to Florida, sadness about the impending family separation was laced with a narrative that praised Puerto Ricans' ability to openly migrate to the US to seek a better life. *No se preocupen que el los estados vamos a estar bien* (Don't worry we are going to be fine in the USA), my mother would remind my sibling and I every time we got upset about having to leave.

Upon arrival, we discovered that my family was defrauded by a contractor who never built the house my parents had paid a down payment on while they still lived in Puerto Rico. We lived in a motel for a month and spent the rest of savings we had. Simultaneously, my parents' accents, race, and language difficulties prevented them from finding employment commensurate with their pre-migration employment. My mother was a teacher and my father was a plumber. Soon thereafter, my sibling and I entered a school system that assumed we were stupid and incapable of succeeding in higher education as long as we remained in the US. While my sibling and I were trying to navigate a hostile school environment, my parents faced frequent racist and xenophobic harassment and violence at work. Even after my parents found jobs that better aligned with their experience in Puerto Rico, we struggled with the barriers of living in what Burgos and colleagues (2017) called *a racialized place of inequality* in Central Florida (Buena Ventura Lakes in Kissimmee). Eventually, my sibling and I acquired enough privilege to leave these circumstances. In my case, it was thanks to my mother who was took the role of being my undergraduate academic advisor that I was able to identify psychology as my career path.

These personal experiences together with the experiences of Latinx immigrant communities in Central and South Florida led me to want to understand the economic and health disparities Latinxs experienced in the US. Specific to my Puerto Rican community, I wanted to understand how post-migration health disparities might be explained by Puerto Rico's political status. During the opportunity to work as a doctoral student with Ed Delgado-Romero at the University of Georgia, I began to examine these questions. Acculturation theory (Berry, 1997) was my first area of focus. Doing this work, I kept concluding that these models were not complex enough to capture the pre- and post-migratory experiences of Puerto Ricans. At that time, another great mentor Melanie Domench-Rodríguez introduced me to the work on colonial mentality by EJR David. This discovery, in turn open the door to further situate the pre- and post-migration experiences of Puerto Ricans within the sociopolitical context in which they took place. I no longer think about Puerto Rican migration as a benefit for the result of expulsion and extraction conditions created by US colonialism in Puerto Rico. This work has also pushed me to unlearn what I thought was effective psychological research, practice, and advocacy, with Latinx immigrant populations. For my community, this means a psychology that: a) disrupts narratives of Puerto Rican mental health and health disparities that ignore the impact of US colonialism on Puerto Rican migration and health, b) demands and facilitates reparation for colonial harm, and c) centers and learns from Puerto Rican resistance to colonialism and *autogestión* [self-management, self-development, and self-functioning].

My journey has also taught me the importance of having mentors and expanding the academic freedom train (Castellanos et al., 2022). As an assistant professor at Arizona State University, I do this work through the PLENA lab (Latinx Psychology in Action). Just like I learned in Delgado-Romero's BIENestar Lab, the students in PLENA are socialized to expect that research activities should be accompanied by advocacy, political, organizational, relational, and spiritual actions on behalf of and as a member of community. Scholarship by members of PLENA is guided by the principle that ALL scientific activity should translate into advantages, protections, resources, rights, and support for the communities we serve and are part of. I look forward to seeing how my student continue to expand this mentoring within and outside of academic settings.

CONCLUSION

Our personal stories intertwine with the history of psychology and as we join the profession of psychology, we try to influence the profession to become more linguistically and culturally sensitive. We seek to influence how our community and culture is represented in the practice, teaching, training, and research of psychology. We are aware of the great privilege that higher education affords us and the way we can share and amplify counter-narratives of strength, resistance and resiliency that have traditionally been silenced or ignored.

We are also aware that we do not only change and influence psychology. In the process of doctoral training, professional practice, and higher education, we also face attempts to change us. Latinx psychologists face enormous pressure to conform and mold our narratives to fit within the dominant narratives of psychology, higher education, and U.S. society in general. In the process of acculturation and enculturation for Latinx psychologists, we mediate and navigate many systems of oppression and privilege. From our privileged positions we can often become both the oppressed and the oppressors. To maintain our cultural humility, we are often reminded of the saying, *In La K'ech*, also the name of our clinic, which means "you are my other me". This saying reminds us that we have a consistent duty to remain connected to those whom we work with and we cannot afford to focus on concepts like objectivity or professional standards that emphasize individuality over collectivism. We are bound together to move the Latinx community from a state of surviving to a state of thriving.

REFERENCES

Arredondo, P., Toporek, R. L., Pack Brown, S., & Jones, J. (1996). Operationalization of the Multicultural Counseling Competencies. *Journal of Multicultural Counseling and Development*, 24(1), 42–78. doi:10.1002/j.2161-1912.1996.tb00288.x

Berry, J. W. (1997). Immigration, acculturation, and adaptation. *Applied Psychology*, 46(1), 5–34. doi:10.1111/j.1464-0597.1997.tb01087.x

Burgos, G., Rivera, F. I., & Garcia, M. A. (2017). Contextualizing the relationship between culture and Puerto Rican health: Towards a place-based framework of minority health disparities. *Centro Journal*, 29(3), 36–73.

Castellanos, J., White, J. L., & Franco, V. (2022). *Riding the academic freedom train: A Culturally responsive, multigenerational mentoring model*. Stylus Publishing.

Farreras, I. G. (2014). Clara Harrison Town and the origins of the first institutional commitment law for the "feebleminded": Psychologists as expert diagnosticians. *History of Psychology*, 17(4), 271–281. doi:10.1037/a0036123 PMID:24885000

Frankl, V. E. (1962). *Man's search for meaning: an introduction to logotherapy*. Beacon Press.

Fukuyama, M. A., & Reid, A. D. (1996). The politics and poetry of multiculturalism. *Journal of Multicultural Counseling and Development*, 24(2), 82–88. doi:10.1002/j.2161-1912.1996.tb00291.x

Gould. (1996). Space, time and the human being. *International Social Science Journal*, 48(150), 449–460. doi:10.1111/j.1468-2451.1996.tb00099.x

Guthrie, R. V. (2004). *Even the rat was White: A historical view of psychology*. Pearson/Allyn and Bacon.

Henrich, J. (2020). *The WEIRDest people in the world: How the West became psychologically peculiar and particularly prosperous*. Farrar, Straus and Giroux.

Howard, G. S. (1986). *Dare we develop a human science?* Academic Publications.

Howard, G. S. (1991). Culture tales. A narrative approach to thinking, cross-cultural psychology, and psychotherapy. *The American Psychologist*, 46(3), 187–197. doi:10.1037/0003-066X.46.3.187 PMID:2035929

Lifton, R. J. (2000). *The Nazi doctors: Medical killing and the psychology of genocide*. Basic Books.

Meléndez, E., & Hinojosa, J. (2017). *Estimates of Post-Hurricane Maria Exodus from Puerto Rico*. Retrieved from https://centropr.hunter.cuny.edu/research/data-center/research-briefs/estimates-post-hurricane-maria-exodus-puerto-rico

Presser. (1969). The role of sterilization in controlling Puerto Rican fertility. *Population Studies, 23*(3), 343–361. doi:10.1080/00324728.1969.10405290

Salinas, C. Jr, & Lozano, A. (2019). Mapping and recontextualizing the evolution of the term Latinx: An environmental scanning in higher education. *Journal of Latinos and Education, 19*(4), 302–315. doi:10.1080/15348431.2017.1390464

Shin, R. Q. (2014). The application of critical consciousness and intersectionality as tools for decolonizing racial/ethnic identity development models in the fields of counseling and psychology. In Decolonizing multicultural counseling through social justice. Springer.

Silver, P., & Vélez, W. (2017). "Let me go check out Florida": Rethinking Puerto Rican diaspora. *Journal of the Center for Puerto Rican Studies, 29*(3), 98–125.

Stern. (2005). Eugenics and Historical Memory in America. *History Compass, 3*(1), 1-11. doi:10.1111/j.1478-0542.2005.00145.x

Tomicic, A., & Berardi, F. (2018). Between past and present: The sociopsychological constructs of colonialism, coloniality and postcolonialism. *Integrative Psychological & Behavioral Science, 52*(1), 152–175. doi:10.100712124-017-9407-5 PMID:29063442

Valdes, F. (1999). Theorizing "OutCrit" Theories: Coalitional Method and Comparative Jurisprudential Experience-RaceCrits, QueerCrits and LatCrits. *U. Miami L. Rev., 53*, 1265–1299.

Chapter 2
La Historia de Afrodescendientes:
A Look Into the Surviving and Thriving of Afro-Descent People From Latin America

Ammy Sena
University of Georgia, USA

Amanda Shannon
University of Georgia, USA

ABSTRACT

The current chapter will explore relevant history of Afrodescendientes, its impact on their psychological wellbeing, and the research and clinical implications. Lastly, this chapter will discuss Afrodescendientes' resistance and the importance of continued liberation. This chapter is an amalgamation of interdisciplinary research, including history, sociology, and psychology, and is intended for the individual who works with Afro-Descent people of Latin America. Specifically, it is for the individual who wants to grow in their understanding of the Afrodescendiente story.

AN INTRODUCTION TO AFRO-DESCENT PEOPLE FROM LATIN AMERICA

"Las caras lindas

De mi gente negra

Son un desfile

De melaza en flor

Que cuando pasan

DOI: 10.4018/978-1-6684-4901-1.ch002

La Historia de Afrodescendientes

Frente a mi se alegra

De su negrura todo el corazón

Las caras lindas

De mi raza prieta

Tienen de llanto

De pena y dolor

Son las verdades

Que la vida reta

Pero que llevan

Dentro mucho amor"- Susana Baca, Caras Negras[1]

The story of *Afrodescendientes*[2] is one that is rooted in a history of forced extraction, displacement, colonization, and capitalism (Morner, 1967; Jimenez Roman & Flores, 2010). History has informed and maintained current-day socio-cultural norms for these people, including invisibility and anti-Blackness within the Latinx community. The consequences of a history of oppression have led to unique psychological and health disparities for Afrodescendientes. However, amidst their tragic history, many Afrodescendientes held on to their African roots and engaged in resistance. The current chapter will explore the relevant history of Afrodescendientes, its impact on their psychological wellbeing, and the research and clinical implications. Lastly, this chapter will discuss Afrodescendientes' resistance and the importance of continued liberation. This chapter is an amalgamation of interdisciplinary research including history, sociology, and psychology, and is intended for the individual who works with Afro-Descent people of Latin America and wants to grow in their understanding of their story.

The authors of this chapter are representative of the diversity of the African diaspora. Ammy Sena is an immigrant from the Dominican Republic, raised in Providence, Rhode Island. She identifies as an aspiring psychologist, researcher, *hermana grande*[3], and outdoors fanatic. She grew up vacillating between American, Dominican, and the greater Latinx spaces. She identifies as a Black Latina of light skin privilege. Given the complex history of race in Latin America, precisely that of the Dominican Republic which has maintain anti-Black sentiment (Mayes, 2014), Ammy has challenged herself to grow in her Black racial identity development. This awareness has galvanized her to pursue a career that centers on the wellness and cultural strengths of Afrodescendientes.

Amanda Shannon was raised throughout most of her childhood in Montana and North Dakota, spending her adolescent and young adult years in North Carolina. Since then, she has lived in the southern region of the United States. She has also spent a significant amount of time throughout her life in Illinois, where she has close family ties. Amanda identifies as a Black Multiracial woman of African American, Indigenous Native American, and French European ancestry. The 8th and youngest child in a nuclear family of 10, she was raised with a large, close-knit, culturally diverse immediate and extended family. Throughout her life, she has been heavily influenced by growing up immersed in African American, Indigenous, and Latinx cultures. These experiences fostered a passion for advocating for health equity and celebrating the diversity of Afrodescendientes.

It is through these lenses that we both navigate the world and encourage us to make visible the counter-narratives of the African Diaspora. Our social identities are foundational in this chapter and provide the unique understandings needed to write this text. We have limitations as we assess the diversity of Afro-Descent people in Latin America and the United States (U.S.) as we do not embody all identities and thus may have unintentionally overlooked related topics. However, we hope this chapter provides you with the tools needed to understand and work *with* Afrodescendientes.

HISTORY AND INVISIBILITY OF AFRODESCENDIENTES

Rarely are people in the U.S. taught the historical accounts of Indigenous and African people. This is especially true of Indigenous and African civilizations prior to colonialism, rendering invisible the historical achievements of these peoples. But how would work with the Latinx community change if we knew more about Indigenous and African history? What if we knew more about their legacy before colonization and independently of European conquerors? To truly understand the experiences of Afrodescendientes and how to support them, we must be cognizant of all aspects of their history- pre-colonial, colonial, and post-colonial (Chapman-Hilliard & Adam-Bass, 2016). For mental health practitioners, collective group histories are just as essential as personal histories to accurately understand a client's presentation (Adames & Chavez-Dueñas, 2017). Thus, we highlight some historical events that have informed the lives of Afrodescendientes, beginning with a brief history of the Indigenous communities of Latin American and African communities, followed by a brief Iberian history as it relates to Latin America and a discussion on U.S. migration. It is important to note that it is impossible to consolidate hundreds of years of history into a single section of a chapter; thus, readers will need to further their understanding by exploring additional resources- some of which are provided at the end of this chapter

Prior to the arrival of the Spanish and before *Maafa*[4], there existed thriving Indigenous and African civilizations in Latin America and Africa. Indigenous and African societies had made significant medical, technological, and scientific advances, created organized social structures, and had complex spiritual beliefs and traditions. Adames and Chavez-Dueñas (2017), in their book *Cultural Foundations and Interventions in Latino/a Mental Health*, outline some of the pre-colonial histories of four main Indigenous groups of Latin America: Aztecs, Mayans, Inkas, and Tainos/Caribs. For example, they shared that the Aztecs had excellent knowledge and appreciation for agriculture, built *chinampas* or small artificial islands where crops were grown in a muddy environment and had extensive knowledge of the medicinal properties of plants and herbs. Additionally, they were one of the first civilizations to have mandatory education for everyone. The Tainos/Caribs were hardworking and joyful people with advanced nautical knowledge, which helped predict hurricanes and tsunamis (Adames & Chavez-Dueñas, 2017).

Documents and artifacts from many Indigenous communities in Latin America were destroyed by the Spanish, erasing critical historical and cultural information such as the Aztec codices, which held information regarding the origins of Aztec people (Duran, 1967; Adames & Chavez-Dueñas, 2017). However, Indigenous civilizations have influenced present-day Latin American society. For example, Indigenous words permeate present-day culture, such as *casabe*[5] and *Quisqueya*[6]. Additionally, spiritual

La Historia de Afrodescendientes

beliefs and traditions that have their roots in Indigenous societies are seen today such as Day of the Dead (a celebration with Aztec origins) or beliefs on deceased relatives, and our ability to feel and even see them has its roots in the Taino people (Adames & Chavez-Dueñas, 2017).

When exploring African civilizations before Maafa, we also see notable accomplishments. In particular, West Africa (where most enslaved Africans originated from) had diverse kingdoms, developed city-states, complex political structures, and were key participants in international trading and transoceanic travel (National Museums Liverpool, 2022). In his book *West Africa Before the Colonial Era: A History to 1850,* Basil Davidson discusses the precolonial civilizations and legacies of West Africa, arguing for its influence on present-day society (2014). For example, Davidson shares the importance of spirituality and concepts of moral good and evil. He highlights the centrality of spirituality in West African life, discussing its' role in things such as agriculture and ceremonial life events. Additionally, he shares that many technological advances (e.g., ironwork) influenced agriculture, allowing for greater human control over the ever-changing elements. As communities evolved and populations grew, the development of government ordinance occurred as well as the development of specialized skills (e.g., craftsman or spiritual leaders). This development was seen in Yoruba, a region of West Africa. Strong intercommunication amongst West African towns, the Mediterranean, and greater Europe, also took place, not just in the form of oral exchange but in the arts and writing, facilitating things such as trade and commerce (Davidson, 2014).

Despite the accomplishments of Indigenous and African people, colonialism dramatically impacted their lives, and their legacy was erased through violence. Exploring this history of colonialism is vital in understanding the lives of Afrodescendientes and how it led to their invisibility and dominant discourse on anti-Blackness. Colonialism led to the racial mixing of Indigenous, Iberian, and African peoples. The indigenous population of Latin America is said to have comprised more than 123 linguistic families and almost 260 languages in Mexico and Guatemala alone (Morner, 1967). The exact pre-colonial population number of Indigenous persons in Latin America varies across the literature; however, one estimate suggests that at least 8 million people died due to diseases, burning and destruction of cities, war/genocide, and harsh labor conditions under colonial rule (Morner, 1967; Adames & Chavez-Dueñas, 2017).

The colonizers that arrived in Latin America were initially Spanish and Portuguese, also known as the Iberians. The Iberian population was not ethnically homogeneous, and a history of racial mixing precedes that of the colonization of the Americas. This history is embedded in conquest, religious freedoms, and politics. Specifically, the Moors- a predominantly Black Muslim group- ruled over parts of Spain and Portugal for over 500 years and were considered culturally and politically superior to the Spaniards (Morner, 1967). However, Christian Europeans saw themselves as superior to Indigenous, Moorish, and Jewish people, and their socio-political standing was tied to purity of Christian blood (Nieto-Phillips, 2004). Nieto-Philips, in his book *The language of blood: The making of Spanish-American identity in New Mexico, the 1880s-1930s,* states:

"...containment and preservation of blood were signs of power, honor, fortitude and prestige...[in] the Iberian Peninsula, blood was believed to capture the essence of one's spiritual purity and nobility." (Nieto-Phillips, 2004, pg. 17)

Conflicts arose as Christian Europeans reclaimed the Iberian Peninsula and propagated anti-Muslim and anti-Jew sentiments. They persecuted, discriminated against, and tried to forcibly convert Muslims and Jews. Some Moors and Jews converted to Christianity creating two identity groups: the converts and the *Cristianos viejos*[7]. However, proving who was a Cristiano viejo became difficult; thus, the church and the crown created elaborate systems for naming, credentialing and regulating persons based on their supposed religious and racial bloodlines, which was termed the *casta* (Nieto-Phillips, 2004). Documentation to prove blood purity was expensive, and some people who were not a Cristiano viejo or even an Iberian could obtain this documentation (Nieto-Phillips, 2004; Jimenez Roman & Flores, 2010). This situation was the start of Spanish identity politics which caused years of conflict between converts and Cristianos viejos. In 1492, the expulsion of the Moors from Spain coincided with the "discovery" of the "new world" (Nieto-Phillips, 2004). Those who were not "pure of blood" were not allowed to travel to the new world, but some Moors like conquistador Juan Garrido[8] did. However, anti-Black and anti-Muslimism rhetoric came with the colonizers, and the remnants of anti-Moor, anti-Black sentiment penetrated the sociopolitical climate of Latin America (Martinez, 2008).

As the Indigenous population of Latin America rapidly declined, enslaved Africans were forced to meet the demand for work and were subjected to inhumane labor conditions in the Spanish colonies (Adames & Chavez-Dueñas, 2017). It is estimated that around 12.5 million Africans were forcefully removed and displaced to Latin America in the sixteenth and nineteenth centuries (Gates & Pollack, 2011). Unfortunately, of those 12.5 million enslaved Africans, only 10.7 million survived the brutal travel conditions (Morner, 1967; Gates & Pollack, 2011). Contrary to popular belief, only a small number of enslaved Africans arrived in the U.S.- 388,000 - most were brought to Latin America and the Caribbean (Gates & Pollack, 2011).

Since arriving in Latin America, Africans were treated as inferior to the Spanish. As the mixing of Spanish, Indigenous, and African people occurred, the *casta* or the *system of stratification* was further developed, which maintained social, political, and economic control for the Spanish and oppression of African and Indigenous peoples (Adames & Chavez-Dueñas, 2017; Nieto-Phillips, 2004). Skin color and phenotypes were at the core of this system; Spaniards were at the top, and Africans were at the bottom. As other European countries traveled to the "new world," similar structures were placed to oppress Africans and support White superiority (Adames & Chavez-Dueñas, 2017). For example, the French created the 1685 code noir, which regulated the fundamental rights of enslaved persons, mandated conversion to Catholicism, outlined punishments, and prohibited formerly enslaved people from obtaining property in the Caribbean islands (Jimenez Roman & Flores, 2010).

As political and economic changes occurred, migration became an essential factor in the survival of Afrodescendientes. Migration of Afrodescendientes occurred throughout Latin American countries and North America. The earliest Afrodescendientes migrants in North America predate English settlement and the "founding" of the United States. Early Afrodescendientes migrants sought relief from Latin America's economic and social restrictions (Jimenez Roman & Flores, 2010). Jimenez Roman and Flores (2010) present various historical accounts of Afrodescendientes migration and influence in the United States. For example, Afrodescendientes were the first to settle in St. Augustine, Florida, in 1565 and were vital in the Spanish conquest and settlements in North America (the Southwest United States, present-day Arizona, California, New Mexico, and Texas). However, the arrival of the British and the founding of the United States introduced violently racist attitudes affecting the beliefs and treatment of Afrodescendientes. In California, for example, racially mixed individuals began to disconnect from their mixed ancestral past, making the existence of their African ancestry invisible to gain social acceptance. Other accounts of migration to the United States includes the arrival of Cubans to the Key West and later Tampa, Florida, from 1869-1880s for cigar manufacturing, 15% of which were Black (Jimenez

Roman & Flores, 2010). It is also noted that around 10,000 Afrodescendientes from Haiti migrated to New Orleans by 1809 after the Haitian revolution (Lewis, 2020).

In the modern day, 25% of people in Latin America identify as Afrodescendientes, residing all over the continent (The World Bank, 2018). When examining the Afrodescendiente population in the U.S., there are roughly 6 million self-identifying Afrodescendiente adults, making up 2% of the overall adult population and 12% of the adult Latinx population (Pew Research Center, 2022). Afrodescendientes are a significant part of the Latinx population yet have been made invisible. The historical treatment of the Afrodescendientes has had severe impacts on their wellness. History, socio-political climates, religion, socialization, and phenotypic traits are some of the many factors that influence the experiences of modern-day Afrodescendientes in Latin America and the U.S. This history has led to the lack of Afrodescendiente visibility and has had significant psychological implications for Afrodescendientes, such as issues regarding racial self-identification and subsequent racial identity development. The following section will expound upon these themes.

AFRODESCENDIENTE INVISIBILITY, RACIAL SELF-IDENTIFICATION, AND RACIAL IDENTITY DEVELOPMENT

One of the manifestations of a history of oppression is the general dynamic of invisibility and hypervisibility of Afrodescendientes. Invisibility refers to society's inability (and unwillingness) to see and value the issues and the excellence of persons or groups of people. Hypervisibility refers to society's heightened scrutiny of individuals for their "otherness" or deviance from the norm (Settles et al., 2019). Both invisibility and hypervisibility are connected to biases created by dominant group members and thus relate to power (Lewis & Simpson, 2010; Settles et al., 2019). Invisibility and hypervisibility are not mutually exclusive, and individuals from marginalized groups can experience both (Settles et al., 2019). Invisibility and hypervisibility of communities are so pervasive and damaging in society that in 1948 the Universal Declaration for Human Rights was created. This document by the United Nations outlines a common standard of achievement for peoples of all nations, centering on the core value of human dignity and legitimacy (United Nations, 1948). Although a document like the Universal Declaration exists, human rights are perpetually violated; this is especially true for Afrodescendientes.

More concretely, invisibility is seen in the disparities that exist for Afrodescendientes. In a report by The World Bank (2018), disparities amongst Afrodescendientes living in Latin America were highlighted. Afrodescendientes are overrepresented among the impoverished as they are 2.5 times more likely to live in chronic poverty and, as a result, experience social mobility difficulty. For example, Afro-Brazilians are twice as likely than White Brazilians to be impoverished. Similarly, Afro-Uruguayans are three times as likely to be impoverished than White Uruguayans. Even when accounting for factors like marital status, gender, educational attainment, sector of work, and household characteristics, Afrodescendientes earn 16% less in Brazil, 11% less in Ecuador, and 6.5% less in Peru, often experiencing glass ceilings in their work. Afrodescendientes in Latin America have a higher likelihood of not completing formal education and are more likely to drop out of secondary education, only accounting for 12% of those with tertiary education. Disparities no doubt are due to the insidious racist systems of Latin America- a product of colonialism (The World Bank, 2018).

Invisibility is also seen intersectionally through misogyny, classism, and heterosexism and impacts things such as land rights, further marginalizing the Afrodescendiente. For example, it was not until the

1990s that Afrodescendientes in Colombia was recognized as an autonomous ethnic group, challenging the dominant discourse on Colombian identity (Adames & Chavez-Dueñas, 2017). Lack of acknowledgment of Afrodescendientes in Colombia impacted their ability to obtain land ownership, but when they were able to acquire land, it was often neglected land by the government (Adames & Chavez-Dueñas, 2017). Another example is seen in the media and entertainment industry. Afrodescendientes are less likely to be cast for leading roles or play roles outside Black stereotypes (Negron-Muntaner et al., 2014; Chow, 2020). Amara la Negra, a Dominican artist born and raised in Miami, brought to attention this dynamic as it relates to gender by sharing her experiences of being cast for roles such as a maid or a sex worker, stating the lack of inclusion of Afrodescendientes in Latinx novelas, movies, commercials, and editorials (The Breakfast Club, 2018). Regarding music, the invisibility of Afrodescendientes is seen as it intersects with skin color and class when looking at the most popular *reggaetoneros*[9]. However, a Puerto Rican genre with African roots created by the impoverished Afrodescendientes, the most well-known and decorated reggaeton artists are light-skinned who have asserted that they are not Afrodescendiente, such as Daddy Yankee, Pitbull, or J. Balvin (River-Rideau, 2015; Deaderick, 2022).

In the U.S., Afrodescendientes from Latin America experience racial discrimination and disparities similar to those of Afro-Descendant people from the U.S. However, experiences with oppression for the Afrodescendientes are invisible in research; this is primarily due to the lack of intersectional research on both race and ethnicity; research often compares Latinx participants to Black participants (Flores & Jimenez Roman, 2009; Fuentes et al., 2021). However, some research highlights the disparities often experienced between Afrodescendientes and other groups in Latin America. For example, one study found that Afrodescendientes are at greater risk for hypertension (Borrell, 2009). Another study found that darker-skinned Latinx persons reported more discriminatory experiences than lighter-skinned ones (Pew Research Center, 2021).

Hypervisibility for Afrodescendientes from Latin America is similar to those experienced by Afro-Descendants from the U.S. Racial profiling, and police brutality play a key role in the injustices faced by all Afro-descent people. For example, in the U.S., when remembering the wrongful convictions of the Central Park Five, one of the members was Afrodescendiente -Ray Santana- he was further marginalized as his primary Spanish-speaking grandmother's limited English language fluency placed him at a disadvantage when navigating the judicial system (Hordge-Freeman & Loblack, 2021). In Latin America, police brutality has been seen to disproportionally impact darker-skinned Latinx people. The wrongful murders of Beto Freitas in Brazil and Anderson Arboleda in Colombia at the hands of police highlight this disparity (Pousadela, 2021). Additionally, in Puerto Rico, Abadia-Rexach (2021) discusses the murder of Adolfina Villanueva Osorio, a mother of six, in 1980, demonstrating this disproportionality of violence directed to Afro-descendant women. For Adolfina, the Catholic church desired her property, and the state demanded that she leave her home, giving her an eviction notice; after Adolfina refused to leave her home, police murdered Adolfina with 16 bullets. No one was charged for her death (Abadia-Rexach, 2021). The example of Adolfina entails both hypervisibility (she was murdered for her resistance) and invisibility (her murders were never charged for her death).

INVISIBILITY SYNDROME

The lack of visibility of Afrodescendiente inequities has been couched within the romanticized notions of Mestizo Racial Ideologies (MRI) and Racial Democracies (Adames et al., 2020; World Bank, 2018).

La Historia de Afrodescendientes

Although some political leaders in Latin American countries are *mestizo*, and *mestizaje*[10] is celebrated as seen in Vasconcelos' *La Raza Cosmica* (1925), it does not mean that equity exists amongst all races in Latin America. Adherence to MRI instead maintains oppression for Afrodescendientes in Latin America as it provides a color-blind approach to social issues perpetuating social exclusion (Adames et al., 2020). Social exclusion keeping Afrodescendientes from living a good life (Prilleltensky, 1997).

Invisibility has damaging effects on the psychological wellbeing of Afrodescendientes. Frantz Fanon (1967) highlights the invisibility of Black people, stating that Black people cannot be seen past their flesh and thus states "a feeling of inferiority? No, a feeling of not existing" (pg. 118). This dynamic limits a Black person's ability to be seen as unique, whole, and able to create their own identity. Thus, Afrodescendientes who have struggled to be seen in society are at increased risk of experiencing the Invisibility Syndrome, a term coined by Franklin (1999). This term describes the intrapsychic process and outcomes of invisibility, stating that repeated racial slights can create within an individual the belief that they are not a worthy person (Franklin & Boyd-Franklin, 2000). Invisibility Syndrome is a subjective sense of psychological invisibility where Afrodescendientes believe their talents and abilities are not valued by others, including society at large, because of racism (Franklin & Boyd-Franklin, 2000). Although originally coined to describe the experiences of African Americans (particularly men), the Invisibility Syndrome can be used to describe the intrapsychic process of Afro-Descent people of Latin America.

For the advancement of Latinx people to occur, society must explicitly and intentionally consider the issues of Afrodescendientes, centering on their visibility. Visibility refers to being seen by others in the plurality of human existence, including expression of emotions, thoughts and passions (Lollar, 2015). Visibility also centers agency or the idea that an individual has control over what others see and hold power in our society (Lollar, 2015). However, social identities and related biases created by dominant White-European ideals have plagued Afro-Descent people from being fully seen and made them either invisible or hypervisible.

Progress needs to happen to bring more recognition, dignity, legitimacy, and authority to Afrodescendientes.

AFRODESCENDIENTE RACIAL SELF-IDENTIFICATION

Racial Identity is a term for how a person racially identifies based on their racial ancestry. While Racial Identification is how a person is racially perceived by others (Franco, 2019). For Afrodescendientes, various terms are used to identify with their African heritage. However, given the sociopolitical histories across Latin America and the U.S., defining those who are Afrodescendiente can be challenging. Traditionally, the racial origins of Latinx people in the Americas have been veiled with racial ambiguity (Rodriguez, 2014). Racial ambiguity can be observed when an individual's race is not clearly identifiable by others. Therefore, racial ambiguity is directly related to racial identification, which is how a person is racially perceived. Racial ambiguity is related to racial identity, acting as a disrupting factor that challenges the binary concept of race that has reigned for generations within the U.S. (Rodriguez, 2014).

Disruption in identification can be seen in the U.S. Census. For Latinx people, about 50% of individuals classified as "Hispanic" by the U.S. Census choose to self-identify based on the country of origin of their family, 23% use pan-ethnic labels, and 23% use the term "American" (Salinas & Lozano, 2021). However, the U.S. Census Bureau acknowledges those who identify as "Hispanic" origin as identified with a separate racial identity. Therefore, in the eye of U.S. governmental data collection policy, "Hispanic" origin and race are separate concepts of identity from race. For example, in the U.S. Census, "Black Hispanics" are represented in both the number of "Hispanics" and the number of "Blacks" within the U.S. The U.S. Census Bureau recognizes that this cross-tabulation can be confusing, especially because this allows for the total number of the population to be inconsistent with the actual number of individuals within the population of the U.S. In this instance, the individual is counted twice, once in each group, creating the phenomenon of overlapping racial-ethnic groups (U.S. Census Bureau, 2021b).

The U.S. census is a primary example of how race, especially for Afro-Descent people, has been represented in U.S. history (US Census Bureau, 2021b). The system of Latinx classification often creates the ability for Latinx persons that are racially ambiguous to assimilate in the direction of Blackness or Whiteness to gain any number of advantages that comes along with this steering of self-identity (Rodriguez, 2014). However, depending on socio-economic status, language abilities, and even skin color, the identity of an Afro-Descent person that is not racially ambiguous is not privileged with the opportunity to self-identify because they are often automatically categorized in one of the ethnic-racial binaries (Rodriguez, 2014). This racial phenomenon highlights the advantages and disadvantages of racial ambiguity in reference to the racial identification and racial identity of Afrodescendientes. This issue also highlights the weight discrimination and institutionalized racism can have on racial identity.

As mentioned earlier in the chapter, the rich history of Latinx people can be traced back to African, Indigenous, and Iberian groups that experienced considerable racial mixing during colonization; resulting in physical characteristics that include a broad range of variations in phenotype including nose width, hair texture, and skin color (Adames et al., 2021). However, simultaneously the Spaniards were diligently creating racial inequity by institutionalizing a hierarchical social system that placed White and lighter-skinned persons at the top and Black and darker-skinned persons at the bottom (Adames et al., 2021). Thus, this definition stratified and ranked individuals into superior and inferior groups based on physical characteristics (Adames et al., 2021). Afrodescendientes continue to experience being positioned at the bottom of the racial hierarchy. These experiences of privilege and stigma based on racial classification, phenotype, and skin color expose advantages and disadvantages that have a direct influence on the overall health outcomes of Afro-Descent individuals, often resulting in higher rates of discrimination leading to increased adverse socioeconomic and psychological outcomes (Sanchez, 2021).

To better grasp the complexities of the racial discrimination that Afrodescendientes often face, we must explore Latinx identification with a clear understanding of *identity incongruent discrimination*. Identity incongruent discrimination is defined as discrimination that is directed at an individual's perceived racial identity that does not match that individual's racial self-identity (Franco, 2019). The question then becomes, for Afrodescendientes, is it easier to contend with identity incongruent discrimination or traditional discrimination? Franco's research concludes that it is easier to cope with incongruent identity discrimination, which allows the person to distance themselves from the discrimination (Franco, 2019). Specifically, it becomes a protective factor against discrimination, allowing the person to shield the identity that they hold dear (Franco, 2019). However, this dynamic is not without psychological impact.

Like traditional discrimination, incongruent discrimination can lead to poorer mental health outcomes. Additionally, research findings show that traditional discrimination comes with already curated coping strategies because there is a community of others within that group that are dealing with the same discrimination. However, for those who experience incongruent discrimination, that built-in support system is nonexistent because the identity is misperceived. Identity incongruent discrimination calls us to pay more attention to the complexities of racial discrimination and how it shows up in a person's life (Franco, 2019).

For those who migrate to the U.S., choosing referents can become even more complex. The concept of the triple consciousness embodies the experience of those who migrate, where race, nationality, and ethnicity all interplay. Triple consciousness recognizes the implications of being Black, American, and Latinx and gives insight into the experiences of Afrodescendientes and the flawed traditional view that tells them and the rest of the world that being Black, American, and Latinx are mutually exclusive. This limited view of identity impedes social inclusion within groups and invalidates the intersecting Afrodescendiente identities that have shaped a person's being (Rodriguez, 2014). In some cases, Afrodescendientes may reject terms that closely associate them to Black and choose referents that minimize their proximity to Africa/Blackness. Self-referents for Afro-Descent people of Latin America are a very individual experience. This dynamic sheds light on the rationale of the selection process of referents, illuminating the ways in which Afrodescendientes negotiate their identities by balancing both their inherent and public selves. This process of identity development will be further explored in the next section.

AFRODESCENDIENTE RACIAL IDENTITY DEVELOPMENT

Racial identity development theory can be defined as the process of developing a notion of ones' race. More specifically, members of various socio-racial groups overcome the version of internalized racism that typifies their group and move towards achieving a more self-affirming and realistic collective identity (Helms & Cook, 1999). This developmental process is essential because society differentially rewards and punishes members of ascribed racial groups (Helms & Cook, 1999). Originated in Black psychology, Black Racial Identity Development (BRID) theories have been crucial in articulating the psychological experiences of Black persons, but few are specifically geared towards Afrodescendientes.

William E. Cross Jr. published a seminal article in 1971 titled *Toward a Psychology of Black Liberation: The Negro-to-Black Conversion Experience*. This article introduced BRID, describing it in stages and coining it the Nigrescence scale. In this work, stages can be discussed in three parts- pro-white/anti-black, anti-white/pro-black, and humanist where Black individuals move from self-degradation to pride (Adames & Chavez-Dueñas, 2017). The initial theory consisted of 5 stages: pre-encounter, encounter, immersion-emersion, internalization, and internalization-commitment. Since this publication, however, the scales have been revised and expanded and are currently called the Cross Racial Identity Scale (CRIS; Vandiver et al., 2000). Helms further developed Dr. Cross's model, considering each stage's psychological and cognitive process and emphasizing that each stage is a distinct worldview (Helms, 1990; Adames & Chavez-Dueñas, 2017). Additionally, Helms considered each stage to be a dynamic process calling it instead *ego statuses*, allowing scholars to see racial identity development as workable and not a fixed inherent state (Helms, 1990; Adames & Chavez-Dueñas, 2017)

More recent adaptations of BRID incorporated other identities, including ethnicity. The CRIS is now called the Cross Ethnic-Racial Identity Scale-Adults, and the authors have developed an assessment tool for measurement (CERIS-A; Worrell et al., 2016; Worrell et al., 2019). Another way to conceptualize BRID was posited by Sellers and his colleagues (1998). Rooted in identity theory, the Multidimensional Model of Racial Identity (MMRI) states that behaviors are connected to identity salience (Sellers et al., 1998). The authors of this model argued that African Americans have several hierarchically ordered identities, not just race, and thus a great deal of diversity exists in the African American experience (Sellers et al., 1998). This model considers the historical and cultural significance of race and states that African Americans define themselves, their attitudes, and beliefs influencing behaviors (Sellers et al.,

1998). This model has four dimensions: identity salience, the centrality of identity, ideology associated with identity, and lastly, African American regard.

When contemplating the Latinx experience, one model explicitly addresses both ethnic and racial identity development. Adames and Chavez-Dueñas (2017) developed the Centering Racial-Ethnic Identity for Latinx framework (C-REIL). The C-REIL model explicitly discusses the damaging effects of MRIs, stating that Latinx socialization has maintained denial, deflection, and minimization of skin-color hierarchies (Adames & Chavez-Dueñas, 2017). This framework accounts for the various intersectional factors that influence the racial and ethnic identity of Latinx people. This model has four major parts- (1) ethnic identity & racial identity within an individual context and its interplay with other social identities; (2) factors that contribute to the development of ethnic identity development; (3) factors that contribute to racial identity development; (4) skin color and phenotype. Although this framework does not present identity in stages or discuss the process of development, it does explore the various factors that contribute to identity formation centering on race and ethnicity and calling for a more accurate and nuanced understanding of the Latinx experiences (Adames & Chavez-Dueñas, 2017).

In part 1, the context allows us to see that Latinx experiences are not universal and instead are influenced by congruence or acceptance within their ethnic identity and the meaning persons ascribe to their racial group (Adames & Chavez-Dueñas, 2017). Specially, a Latinx self-identification and view of others may be impacted by the community they grew up in and the sociohistorical and political climate that either generates and/or maintains oppressions. According to Adames and Chavez-Dueñas (2017), part 2 or ethnic identity development is influenced by socialization which often comes from family; social mirroring, or how a group is portrayed in society; and the individual's context, which moderates people's awareness of ethnic group membership and connection. In part 3 of the C-REIL model, they state that racial identity development is impacted by history or the meaning a Latinx person attributes to their racial group membership based on race history; MRI's and their agreeance to it; the preference an individual has in identifying with their nationality when asked about race and lastly internalized racism. As discussed earlier in this chapter, given the complex history of race in Latin America and the remnants of the *castas* on present-day racial hierarchy, it is imperative that the Latinx person see themselves as a racial being regardless of the context (Adames & Chavez-Dueñas, 2017). Lastly, part 4 of the model highlights the saliency of a Latinx person's skin color and phenotypes, underscoring the importance of colorism, which has detrimental effects on the Afrodescendiente (Adames & Chavez-Dueñas, 2017). This framework may be helpful when working with Afrodescendientes, understanding the complexity of identity, and assisting individuals in developing a healthier, more affirming identity. Additionally, it is useful in understanding the insidious effects of history on the Latinx experience and how systems of oppression may be maintained.

TOWARDS THE FUTURE OF THRIVING:

Afrodescendiente Inclusion, Resiliency and Liberation

The information in this chapter invites the reader to look towards the future as people continue to support the thriving and liberation of Afrodescendientes. The following section will explore implications for research and clinical work for those working with Afro-Descent people. This section culminates with a discussion on Afrodescendiente resiliency and the importance of liberatory practices.

RESEARCH CONSIDERATIONS: STRUCTURAL RACISM AND SKIN COLOR

"Given the relevance of skin color and colorism in Latinx communities, it is important to understand how often we are measuring it, how we are measuring it, and if there is a viable, reliable, and economical option for measuring it effectively." – (Fuentes et al., 2021)

The term "race" has many different definitions. This was true even before the invention of genetics, and evolutionary biology, which proved separating humans into race taxonomies has no scientific basis. Racial categories are based on social constructs, and racial taxonomies are utilized openly in healthcare for teaching, practice, and research, oftentimes being detrimental to Afro-descent people (Witzig, 1996). Human diversity is taught in healthcare programs and presented in healthcare texts inconsistently and erratically, perpetuating the falsehood that they are necessary to properly diagnose and treat disease processes in humans (Witzig, 1996). The concept of 'race" from its inception has fueled racism and institutional oppression based on the belief that one group of people is racially superior to another (Adames et al., 2021).

Black identity, for example, is typically presented in empirical studies, theorizing about the negative effects of slavery and presenting Black identity as synonymous with psychopathology (Cross, 2016). There is, however, a counter-narrative that positions Black identity and Black self-esteem as ordinary and normal. Although not often appreciated historically in psychological research, Black people have maintained an astonishing record of adjustment, patience, acculturation, religiosity, and compromise (Cross, 2016). This counter-narrative challenges the propensity to immediately place Black people in this category that does not even allow them to present as normal (Cross, 2016).

Research often lumps Latinx subgroups together for the purpose of national and international clinical trials data. Subsequently characterizing an expected response from those within this generalized Latinx group (Ruiz, 2000). Researchers often include demographic measures that have race and ethnicity categories as open-ended questions, attempting to better understand cultural group differences and identity (Fuentes et al., 2021). Nearly four decades of data show that in reference to Latinx populations, the reporting of demographic information of race and ethnicity in research is negligible (Mazzula & Sanchez, 2021). Particularly, studies are limited to self-reported race and the inconsistent use of skin color measurements and pan-ethnic labeling practices to identify Latinx populations (Mazzula & Sanchez, 2021).

Recently, research has begun to explore Latinx people, specifically those with African ancestry, with more vigor. This is due to increased interest in diaspora studies that provide new insight into Latinx history, culture, heritage, and the recent "Latinization" of many communities throughout the U.S. The relationship between psychological adjustment and skin color satisfaction for Afrodescendientes suggests that skin color satisfaction is a predictor of psychological adjustment and has even been linked to anxiety and depression (Fuentes et al., 2021). For Latinx persons with dark-skin tones that face discrimination, worse health status was reported over Latinx people of lighter skin tones (Cuevas et al., 2016). Overall, it can be concluded from the emerging research literature that skin color appears to negatively impact those with a darker skin tone (Fuentes et al., 2021). This effect is not due to any innate flaw in any person of darker skin tone. Rather it illustrates the impact and manifestation of institutionalized racism faced by individuals with darker skin tones.

Identifying the ethnicity, race, and even skin color of an individual may provide generalizable information about that individual, but none of these categories should be considered in isolation (Flanagan, 2021; Fuentes et al., 2021). It is evident that colorism and skin color are relevant and salient factors that impact the Latinx community in the U.S., the Caribbean, Latin America, and worldwide. By acknowledging these constructs, a better understanding and effort can be made to eradicate these ideals rooted in colonization and White privilege (Fuentes et al., 2021). The authors of this chapter propose that although skin color is a salient factor that impacts the Latinx community, skin color measurement can be detrimental. Skin color measurement has historically been used to dehumanize people of color. Guthrie gives an extensive historical account of skin color measurement in *Even the Rat Was White: A Historical View of Psychology* and the subsequent tools that mirror present-day skin color measurement practices. Shedding light on the racist pseudoscientific practices of skin color measurement under the guise of science, these Eurocentric investigations, observations, and systematic categorizations of race often lead to conclusions based on racial superiority and inferiority (Guthrie, 2004). Understanding the salience of skin color on Latinx identity and impact in Latinx communities is necessary without focusing on skin color measurement as a primary way to address inequality. Instead, we must consider the individual's unique experiences with discrimination, being cautious not to repeat a history that has repeatedly led to the systemic oppression of Afro-Descent people by setting a focused gaze on skin color measurement. Which may inadvertently perpetuate the contrived fallacy that lighter skin is better and that darker skin individuals only exist in comparison to lighter or White persons.

Jayawardene and McDougal (2017) provide insight into this obsession with skin color measurement with their review of the Cress Theory of Color Confrontation (CTCC). Welsing, a Black psychiatrist and medical professor, advanced this controversial theory addressing global White supremacy. She was most interested in the primary motivation of racism itself, stating anyone that who is truly interested in promoting social change must have a firm grasp on racism and White supremacy, which are both rooted in a war against all persons that are classified as non-White (Jayawardene & McDougal, 2017). Welsing postulated that White supremacy is based on genetic and numeric deficiencies that are innate in White people and that the psychological response to these deficiencies is conscious and unconscious in nature. This process stems from individuals that identify as White being the genetic minority on a global scale. Individuals that are non-White or have increased potential to produce varying degrees of skin color, are the genetic majority on a global scale. Wesling uses this information to explain the motivation for the force behind the evolution of the patterns of White supremacist behavior. She argues that Black people are the most significant threat to White people because Black people have the most skin color producing potential of all the races on a global scale, threatening the genetic survival of the White race. This scenario prompts the expression of psychological defense maneuvers in response to their genetic and numerical inadequacies in the form of hostility and aggression toward Black people (Jayawardene & McDougal, 2017). Welsing was insightful in her interpretation of racism, and while much of this theory has understandably been heavily debated, the foundation of Welsing's argument, that racism is pathological in nature, is undeniably astute.

CLINICAL CONSIDERATIONS: RACE, ETHNICITY, AND HEALTH EQUITY

"The vast majority of Black people are ordinary in their psychological make-up...In the end such personal victories over oppression are embodied, resulting in high blood pressure and the premature breakdown of the body, because the ultimate healthy adjustment requires that racism be eliminated." - (Cross, 2016).

The concept of present-day race is connected to racism, eugenics movements, and the idea of racial superiority and inferiority. Even though modern-day terms for race can vary in meaning slightly, the same three to six racial classifications still appear in medical literature. Human diversity has essentially been medicalized, promoting the idea that the cause of certain diseases is inherently from being Black, placing blame on race and, ultimately, the patient due to their race (Witzig, 1996; Smith & Spodak, 2021). Race correction is being used to legitimize the use of these categories for their use in healthcare literature and practice creating negative consequences for individual patient outcomes (Smith & Spodak, 2021). The healthcare system has attempted to consider these factors in many ways but has unfortunately missed the mark. Race correction is an example of this attempt. *Race correction* is a tool that tries to account for the previously mentioned racial and ethnic disparities amongst people and the subsequent clinical considerations. It utilizes a patient's race within a scientific equation that ultimately influences how they are treated. These tools that predict risk and diagnostic algorithms are correcting for or adjusting the results based on the patient's race. When we look at this process, it can be determined that racism is built into these very algorithms.

For example, *Heaton norms,* a form of race correction, also known as race norming, has been used in Neuropsychology assessment for decades to adjust for race. The primary purpose of Heaton norms is solely to adjust for the cognitive functioning of a Black person, with the assumption that Black people have lower baseline cognitive functioning than their White counterparts. This algorithm is based on lower cognitive scores in studies that failed to consider the social factors, socioeconomic status, and education, etc., of the Black people they are assessing. Heaton norms also failed to consider that there are no biological differences in the brain of a Black and White person reducing individuals to mathematical equations (Smith & Spodak, 2021). This process does not consider the unique identities and intersectionality of Black individuals, which has a negative impact on them (Smith & Spodak, 2021).

Race correcting equations are not just used in one area of healthcare; they are used across the board, from Neuropsychology to Obstetrics. Essentially this is propagating race-based healthcare practice, creating an environment that exacerbates health disparities in Afro-Decent communities, directing the much-needed attention and resources to their White counterparts (Vyas et al., 2020; Smith & Spodak, 2021). An eye-opening result of these practices embedded in the healthcare system is represented in a research study where researchers questioned White medical residents and students about several alleged differences between Black and White physical bodies (Hoffman & Trawalter, 2016). 25% of residents and 40% of first-year medical students reported that they believe that Black people have thicker skin than their White counterparts. Additionally, 7% of the residents and students reported that they believe Black people have less sensitive nerve endings than their White counterparts. To be clear, these are myths that the medical doctors in training believe to be true, based on their training and social-cultural exposure to racist ideologies. Due to these beliefs, trainees were less likely to prescribe sufficient pain medication to Black patients (Hoffman & Trawalter, 2016; Smith & Spodak, 2021).

Inherently, race-based measures could significantly bias clinicians' reports in determining treatment plans for Black and Afro-Descent patients. Furthermore, the use of race-based measures perpetuates the belief that there are innate biological racial differences, which has been exposed as a problem in healthcare practice. Health care providers must acknowledge the impact of race-based corrections on health disparities, especially for Black people (Anderson, 2021). In general, within the healthcare system, Black people receive suboptimal treatment or simply have limited access. A significant number of studies show that Black people are either treated inappropriately or under-treated (The World Bank, 2018). Research has even revealed that Black people have more adverse consequences to medication because, across all diagnostic categories, they often receive higher doses of medication. Research also points to the significance of a patient's cultural and ethnic background in determining how the clinician labels and conceptualizes a patient's problems, ultimately determining the therapeutic intervention (Ruiz, 2000). For example, in one study, ethnic minority groups were given more severe diagnoses in case vignette studies even when all other characteristics were identical except for race. There is significant support to show that variables like clinician bias largely account for differential diagnosis patterns instead of the patient's actual presenting clinical condition (Ruiz, 2000).

On the other hand, ethnicity incorporates many other variables, including diet, linguistics, social and religious factors. Therefore, ethnicity can add to the clinical clues to be more informed in diagnosing and treating the diverse Afrodescendientes. Ethnicity is an example of the dynamic approach that must be taken into consideration as we approach variables that can be truly clinically useful (Witzig, 1996). For example, an Afrodescendiente could be a first-generation Dominican American, monolingual English speaking, and in the U.S., may be perceived as African American solely based on their phenotypic presentation. When a doctor glances at this patient's skin color and presumes their ancestry, this can be very dangerous and misleading (Smith & Spodak, 2021). Instead, it is important to assess other factors, such as if the patient is a first, second, or third-generation immigrant, and if so, from where is crucial. This context will allow the clinician to be cognizant of culture-bound factors that may be salient (Ruiz, 2000; Smith & Spodak, 2021; Adames & Chavez-Dueñas, 2017). Clinicians should enter treatment alliances with patients acknowledging that the bulk of healthcare knowledge in the U.S. is based on colonized practices (Ruiz, 2000).

Afrodescendientes constantly negotiate their racial and ethnic identity. For example, with those who may embrace their racial identity, we may see negation of their ethnic identity (Hordge-Freeman & Loblack, 2021). This is in line with the sentiments around canceling Latinidad due to its perpetuation of racism and invisibility (Flores, 2021). Thus, considering the C-REIL model developed by Adames and Chavez-Dueñas may be critical in the conceptualization of client experiences (2017).

RESILIENCY AND LIBERATION: EMBRACING AFRO-CULTURE AND POWER

"assimilated? que assimilated,

brother, yo soy asimilao...

but the sound LAO was too black

for LATED, LAO could not be

translated, assimilated,

no, asimilao, melao,

it became a black spanish word...

deles gracias a los prietos

La Historia de Afrodescendientes

que cambiaron asimilado al popular asimilao." - Tato Laviera, Asimilao

While the oppression of Afrodescendientes should not be ignored or minimized, neither should their resilience. Cross states, the "history of the social sciences reveals that it is easier to portray Black people as damaged and defeated than to come to terms with their stubborn-resilient humanity" (2016, p18). Thus, it is important to remember that Afrodescendientes have many strengths, have held on to their Afro roots, developed strategies to survive, cope and resist (Adames & Chavez-Dueñas, 2017). This is observed in how they speak; they tend to remove the *s* and *r* sounds or incorporate the *ao* sound at the end of Spanish words. This is also seen in the way they have held onto words from Africa, such as *guineo, chevere,* or *mayimbe*[11]. African cultural remnants and resistance is also seen in music. For example, when examining the popular music genre salsa, the sound of the clave, an instrument used in salsa, mimics African rhythms, preserving African traditions (Gates & Pollack, 2011). Additionally, salsa facilitated the integration of Afrodescendientes allowing for their inclusion in social and intellectual circles (Berrios-Miranda, 2004). At times, salsa lyrics have highlighted the social inequalities of Afrodescendientes, building the consciousness of mainstream society[12]. The documentary *Black in Latin America,* written and presented by Henry Louis Gates, expounds upon these themes discussing the ways African heritage and resistance is seen in things such as food, dance, religious practices, art, etc. Afrodescendientes teach, worship, dress, heal, cook, eat, and sing differently (Gates & Pollack, 2011). African influence in Latin America is undeniable.

Afro-Descent people of Latin America are not weak nor incapable of success. Throughout history, this fact has been clear. They have played a vital role in the liberation of peoples against colonial forces. For example, they revolted in places like Haiti to establish the first Black nation in the Western Hemisphere. Another example can be seen in the rebellion of Gaspar Yanga and other enslaved Africans, who later founded Mexico's first free city- Yanga- 200 years before Mexico won independence from Spain (Carillo, 2021). The activism of Mama Tingo serves yet as another example as she fought for farmworker rights in the Dominican Republic. In the U.S., the work of Arturo Schomburg, a Puerto Rican historian who advocated for African diaspora history and literature, was a key influencer in the Harlem Renaissance. As a result of the revolutionary work of our ancestors, Afro-Descent peoples are now able to move from survival to thriving, tending towards self-preservation as "an act of political warfare" (Lorde, 1988). More recently, this is seen in Puerto Rican Afrodescendientes' resistance against colonial *racecraft* or the production of racial identities embedded in colonialism (Godreau & Bonilla, 2021). We are still revolting, organizing, and aiming to preserve our histories, our culture, our power, and our souls.

Times are changing in Latin America, and the U.S. and Afrodescendientes are being acknowledged and embraced. The World Bank states that one way we have seen this embrace in Latin America is by including ethno-racial variables in national statistics and developing affirmative action policies (The World Bank, 2018). Pride in being of African heritage is primarily due to social movements, organizing of people, access to knowledge, and community leadership. Some of the shifts in Afrodescendiente visibility and pride may be due to multiple reasons; however, one theory is what Juan Flores (2009) calls cultural remittances. Cultural remittances refer to the cultural influence that emigrants have on the values and subsequent practices of their ancestral land when traveling to and fro. Emigrants, through cultural remittance, have radically challenged identity in Latin America, which has begun to demarginalize Afrodescendientes.

As Afro pride arises, so does diasporic consciousness and Afrodescendiente identification with the Black racial group. This developmental process is seen in the U.S., where increased diasporic consciousness for Afrodescendientes means increased stakeholder commitment to the Black Lives Matter movement (Hordge-Freeman & Loblack, 2021). This consciousness raising may be facilitated through learning African/Black history, which can positively influence the wellness and identity development of Afrodescendientes, fostering psychological liberation (Chapman-Hilliard & Adam-Bass, 2016). Thus, incorporating a strengths-based Black history of Afrodescendientes should be foundational in working with this community.

Afro Pride in Latin America and the U.S. is seen through the embracement of natural hair. Historically referred to as *pelo malo*[13]. Afro-Descent people are embracing their natural hair texture and pattern as a form of resistance. Dr. Afiya Mibilishaka has explored the interconnections of hair, heritage, and health for Afro-Descent people. In one qualitative study on Afro-Cuban women, Dr. Afiya and colleagues (2020) found that these women experienced racism and discrimination based on their hair and socialization regarding their natural hair affected participant emotions. However, when socialization was positive regarding hair and heritage, participants experienced strong racial identity and self-acceptance (Mibilishaka et al., 2020). Natural hair in this study was embraced as a form of resistance against anti-Black Cuban sentiment (Mibilishaka et al., 2020).

Healing from the colonial effects for Afrodescendientes must include liberation. Liberation is necessary as we assist Afrodescendientes in dismantling their colonial mentality or the internalization of oppression (Comas-Diaz, 2020). Considering frameworks with liberatory perspectives like the Radical Healing model is essential when working with Afrodescendientes (French et al., 2020). Created by French and colleagues (2020), this framework is grounded in liberation psychology, Black psychology, ethnopolitical psychology, and intersectional perspectives, embracing healing and action. The Radical Healing framework recognizes that persons can sit in the dialect of both resisting oppression and engaging in action. The five components of this model are: critical consciousness or building a person's awareness of systems of oppression; collectivism, or incorporation of a robust support system and engagement in activism in community; radical hope or holding on to hope even in the face of devastating news; strength and resilience which reinforces radical hope; and lastly cultural authenticity and self-knowledge, living fully and without shame in all your identities and increasing knowledge of yourself (French et al., 2020).

Comas-Diaz shares a similar perspective on healing, stating one major factor in healing for marginalized people is solidarity in racial equity (2020). Additionally, she states that for Afro-Descent people, spirituality should be used to facilitate healing and resistance as colonization attempted to suppress Afrodescendiente knowledge and spirituality. Using spirituality helps Afrodescendientes "perceive themselves as part of a larger force within an interrelated spiritual universe" and can help with affirmation, connection, hope, and agency (Comas-Diaz, 2020).

CHAPTER TAKEAWAYS

The fight against oppression is an act of love, and only the oppressed can liberate themselves and the oppressor in this fight (Freire, 2000). As a review of this chapter, here are the major takeaways we hope you bring into your work. Additionally, the authors of this chapter provide some additional resources to further your understanding of Afrodescendientes.

- Afrodescendiente experiences matter and should be accounted for as legitimate Latinx issues
- Racism further marginalizes Afrodescendientes; anti-Black rhetoric is as present today as ever.

- There remains a need to create visibility of Afro-descendant strengths.
- Consider the complexities of self-referents and how that impacts the individuals you work with.
- Challenge yourself to know Afro history to better understand the experiences of Afrodescendientes.
- Check your own identity and biases of Afrodescendientes.

FURTHER YOUR UNDERSTANDING

- Black in Latin America (PBS Documentary)
- When Worlds Collides (PBS Documentary)
- The Afro-Latin@ Reader: History and Culture in the United States by Miriam Jimenez Roman & Juan Flores (Book)
- Overcoming Invisibility: https://www.apa.org/monitor/sep04/overcoming
- Afro-descendants in Latin America: Toward a framework of Inclusion (World Bank): https://openknowledge.worldbank.org/handle/10986/30201

REFERENCES

Abadía-Rexach, B. I. (2021). Adolfina Villanueva Osorio, Presente. *NACLA Report on the Americas*, *53*(2), 174–180. doi:10.1080/10714839.2021.1923222

Adames, H.Y., Chavez-Dueñas, N.Y., & Jernigan, M.M. (2021). The fallacy of a raceless Latinidad: Action guidelines for centering Blackness in Latinx psychology. *Journal of Latina/o Psychology*, *9*(1), 1–19.

Adames, H. Y., & Chavez-Dueñas, N. Y. (2017). *Cultural foundations and interventions in Latino/a mental health: History, theory, and within-group differences*. Routledge.

Anderson, M. A., Malhotra, A., & Non, A. L. (2021). Could routine race-adjustment of spirometers exacerbate racial disparities in COVID-19 recovery? *The Lancet. Respiratory Medicine*, *9*(2), 124–125. doi:10.1016/S2213-2600(20)30571-3 PMID:33308418

Berrios-Miranda, M. (2004). Salsa music as expressive liberation. *Centro Journal*, *16*(2), 158–173.

Borrell, L. N. (2009). Race, ethnicity, and self-reported hypertension: Analysis of data from the national health interview survey, 1997-2005. *American Journal of Public Health*, *99*(2), 313–320. doi:10.2105/AJPH.2007.123364 PMID:19059869

Carillo, K. J. (2021). Mexico's first liberated city commemorates its founding. *Jstor Daily*. https://daily.jstor.org/mexicos-yanga-commenorates-founding/

Chapman-Hilliard, C., & Adam-Bass, V. (2016). A conceptual framework for utilizing Black history knowledge as a path to psychological liberation for Black youth. *The Journal of Black Psychology*, *42*(6), 479–507. doi:10.1177/0095798415597840

Chow, A. R. (2020). These Afro-Latino actors are pushing back against erasure in Hollywood. *Time*. https://time.com/5889072/afro-latino-actors-roundtable/

Comas-Diaz, L. (2020). Afro-Latinxs: Decolonization, healing and liberation. *Journal of Latina/o Psychology*, *9*(1), 65–75. doi:10.1037/lat0000164

Cross, W. E. (1971). Toward a psychology of black liberation: The negro-to-black conversion experience. *Black World*, *20*, 13–27.

Cross, W. E. (2016). *Disjunctive: Social Injustice, black identity, and the normality of black people. In The Oxford Handbook of Social Psychology and Social Justice*. Oxford University Press.

Cross, W. E. Jr, & Vandiver, B. J. (2001). Nigrescence theory and measurement: Introducing the Cross Racial Identity Scale (CRIS). In J. G. Ponterotto, J. M. Casas, L. A. Suzuki, & C. M. Alexander (Eds.), *Handbook of multicultural counseling* (pp. 371–393). Sage Publishers.

Davidson, B. (2014). *West Africa before the colonial era: A history to 1850*. Routledge. doi:10.4324/9781315840369

Deaderick, L. (2022). A White reggaeton artist was named 'Afro-Latino artist of the year' and that's a problem. *The San Diego Union-Tribune*. https://www.sandiegouniontribune.com/columnists/story/2022-01-09/a-white-reggaeton-

Duran, D. (1967). *Historia de las Indias de la Nueva España e Islas de la Tierra Firme* [History of the Indies of New Spain and the Islands of Tierra Firme]. Porrua.

Fanon, F. (1967). *Black skins, White masks*. Grove.

Flanagin, A., Frey, T., Christiansen, S. L., & Bauchner, H. (2021). The reporting of race and ethnicity in medical and science journals: Comments invited. *Journal of the American Medical Association*, *325*(11), 1049–1052.

Flores, J. (2009). *The diaspora strikes back: Caribeno tales of learning and turning*. Routledge.

Flores, J., & Jimenez Roman, M. (2009). Triple-consciousness? Approaches to Afro-Latino culture in the United States. *Latin American and Caribbean Ethnic Studies*, *4*(3), 319–328.

Flores, T. (2021). "Latinidad is canceled": Confronting an anti-Black construct. *Latin American and Latinx Visual Culture*, *3*(3), 58–79.

Franco, M. (2019). *What Racial Discrimination Will Look Like in 2060*. https://blogs.scientificamerican.com/voices/what-racial-discrimination-will-look-like-in-2060/

Franklin, A. J. (1999). Invisibility syndrome, and racial identity development in psychotherapy, and counseling African American men. *The Counseling Psychologist*, *27*(6), 761–793.

Franklin, A. J., & Boyd-Franklin, N. (2000). Invisibility syndrome: A clinical model of the effects of racism on African-American males. *Journal of Orthopsychiatry*, *70*(1), 33–41.

Freire, P. (2000). *Pedagogy of the oppressed* (30th ed.). Continuum.

French, B. H., Lewis, J. A., Mosley, D. V., Adames, H. Y., Chavez-Duenas, N. Y., Chen, G. A., & Neville, H. A. (2020). Toward a psychological framework of radical healing in communities of color. *The Counseling Psychologist*, *48*(1), 14–46.

Fuentes, M. A., Reyes-Portillo, J. A., Tineo, P., Gonzalez, K., & Butt, M. (2021). Skin color matters in the Latinx community: A call for action in research, training, and practice. *Hispanic Journal of Behavioral Sciences, 43*, 32–58.

Gates, H.L. (Presenter, Writer) & Pollack, R. (Director, Producer). (2011). *Black in Latin America* [Film Series]. PBS Distribution.

Godreau, I., & Bonilla, Y. (2021). Nonsovereign racecraft: How colonialism, debt, and disaster are transforming Puerto Rican racial subjectivities. *American Anthropologist, 123*, 509–525. doi:10.1111/aman.13601

Guthrie, R. V. (2004). *Even the rat was white: A historical view of psychology* (2nd ed.). Pearson/Allyn & Bacon.

Helms, J. E. (1990). *Black and white racial identity: Theory research, and practice.* Greenwood Press.

Helms, J. E., & Cook, D. A. (1999). *Using race and culture in counseling and psychotherapy: Theory and process.* Allyn and Bacon.

Hoffman, K. M., Trawalter, S., Axt, J. R., & Oliver, M. N. (2016). Racial bias in pain assessment and treatment recommendations, and false beliefs about biological differences between blacks and whites. *Proceedings of the National Academy of Sciences, 113*(16), 4296-4301.

Hordge-Freeman, E. & Loblack, A. (2021). "Cops only see the brown skin, they could care less where it originated": Afro-Latinx perceptions of the #BlackLivesMatter movement. *Sociological Perspectives, 64*(4), 518-535. doi: 107.171/077/30173112124124020996611135

Jayawardene, S. M., & McDougal, S. III. (2017). Francis Cress Welsing's contributions to Africana studies epistemology. *Journal of Black Studies, 48*(1), 43–56.

Jimenez Roman, M., & Flores, J. (2010). *The Afro-Latin@ reader: History and culture in the United States.* Duke University Press.

Lewis, A. (2020). *Krewe Du Kanaval honors the Haitian roots of New Orleans.* NPR. https://www.npr.org/sections/world-cafe/2020/02/12/804873908/krewe-du-kanaval-honors-the-haitian-roots-of-new-orleans

Lewis, P., & Simpson, R. (2010). *Introduction: Theoretical insights into the practices of revealing and concealing gender within organizations.* Academic Press.

Lollar, K. (2015). Strategic Invisibility: Resisting the Inhospitable Dwelling Place. *The Review of Communication, 15*(4), 298–315. https://doi.org/10.1080/15358593.2015.1116592

Lorde, A. (1988). *A burst of light.* Firebrand Books.

Martinez, M. E. (2008). *Genealogical fictions: Limpieza de sangre, religion and gender in colonial Mexico.* Stanford University Press.

Mayes, A. (2014). *The mulatto republic: Class, race and Dominican national identity.* University Press of Florida.

Mazzula, S. L., & Sanchez, D. (2021). The state of Afrolatinxs in Latinx psychological research: Findings from a content analysis from 2009 to 2020. *Journal of Latina/o Psychology*, *9*(1), 8–25.

Mibilishaka, A., Ray, M., Hall, J., & Wilson, I. P. (2020). 'No toques mi pelo' (don't touch my hair): Decoding Afro-Cuban identity politics through hair. *African and Black Diaspora: An International Journal*, *13*(1), 114–126.

Morner, M. (1967). *Race mixture in the history of Latin America*. Little Brown and Company.

National Museum Liverpool. (2022). *West Africa*. https://www.liverpoolmuseums.org.uk/history-of-slavery/west-africa

Negron-Muntaner, F., Abbas, C., Figueroa, L., & Robson, S. (2014). *The Latino media gap: A report on the state of Latinos in U.S. media*. The Center for the Study of Ethnicity and Race Columbia University.

Nieto-Phillips, J. M. (2004). *The language of blood: The making of Spanish-American identity in New Mexico*. The University of New Mexico Press.

Pew Research Center. (2021). *Majority Latinos say skin color impacts opportunity in America and shapes daily life*. https://www.pewresearch.org/hispanic/2021/11/04/majority-of-latinos-say-skin-color-impacts-opportunity-in-america-and-shapes-daily-life/

Pew Research Center. (2022). *About 6 million U.S. adults identify as Afro-Latino*. https://www.pewresearch.org/fact-tank/2022/05/02/about-6-million-u-s-adults-identify-as-afro-latino/

Pousadela, I. (2021). *#BLM beyond the US: Anti-racist struggles in Latin America*. Open Democracy. https://www.opendemocracy.net/en/democraciaabierta/blm-beyond-the-us-anti-racist-struggles-in-latin-america/

Prilleltensky, I. (1997). Values, assumptions, and practices: Assessing the moral implications of psychological discourse and action. *The American Psychologist*, *52*(5), 517–535.

Rivera-Rideau, P. (2015). *Remixing reggaeton: The cultural politics of race in Puerto Rico*. Duke University Press.

Rochin, R. I. (2016). Latinos and Afro-Latino legacy in the United States: History, culture, and issues of identity. *Professional Agricultural Workers Journal*, *3*(2).

Rodriguez, Y. (2014). The triple double: Racially ambiguous Afro-Latino identities in America. *Master of Arts in American Studies Capstones*. Paper 1.

Ruiz, P. (2000). *Ethnicity and psychopharmacology* (1st ed.). American Psychiatric Press.

Salinas, C., & Lozano, A. (2021). History and evolution of the term Latinx. In E. G. Murillo, D. Delgado Bernal, S. Morales, L. Urrieta, E. Ruiz Bybee, J. Sánchez Muñoz, V. B. Saenz, D. Villanueva, M. Machado-Casas, & K. Espinoza (Eds.), *Handbook of Latinos and Education* (2nd ed., pp. 249–263). Rutledge.

Sanchez, D. (2021). Introduction to special issue on AfroLatinidad: Theory, research, and practice. *Journal of Latina/o Psychology*, *9*(1), 1–7.

Sellers, R. M., Smith, M. A., Shelton, J. N., Rowley, S. A., & Chavous, T. M. (1998). Multidimensional model of racial identity: A reconceptualization of African American racial identity. *Personality and Social Psychology Review*, *2*, 18–39.

Settles, I. H., Buchanan, N. T., & Dotson, K. (2019). Scrutinized but not recognized: (In)visibility and hypervisibility experiences of faculty of color. *Journal of Vocational Behavior*, *113*, 62–74. https://doi.org/10.1016/j.jvb.2018.06.003

Simpson. (Eds.). (n.d.). *Revealing and concealing gender: Issues of visibility in organizations*. Palgrave Macmillan.

Smith, J., & Spodak, C. (2021). *Black or 'Other'? Doctors may be relying on race to make decisions about your health.* https://www.cnn.com/2021/04/25/health/race-correction-in-medicine-history-refocused/index.html

The Breakfast Club. (2018, January 22). *Amara La Negra discusses being Afro-Latina & the standards of beauty in the entertainment industry* [Radio Broadcast]. Power 105.1FM. https://www.youtube.com/watch?v=0yAiI3Hs-p4

The World Bank. (2018). *Afro-descendants in Latin America: Towards a framework of inclusion*. https://openknowledge.worldbank.org/handle/10986/30201

United Nations. (1948). *The universal declaration for human rights*. https://www.un.org/sites/un2.un.org/files/udhr.pdf

U.S. Census Bureau. (2002). *Measuring America: The Decennial Census from 1790 to 2000*. https://www.census.gov/history/pdf/measuringamerica.pdf

U.S. Census Bureau. (2021a). *Decennial Census of Population and Housing by Decades Origin Data.* https://www.census.gov/programs-surveys/decennial-census/decade.2010.html

U.S. Census Bureau. (2021b). *Guidance on the Presentation and Comparison of Race and Hispanic Origin Data.* https://www.census.gov/topics/population/hispanic-origin/about/comparing-race-and-hispanic-origin.html

Vandiver, B., Cross, W.E., Jr., Fhagen-Smith, P.E., Worrell, F., Swim, J., & Caldwell, L. (2000). *The cross-racial identity scale*. Unpublished scale.

Vasconcelos, J. (1925). *La raza cósmica. Agencia Mundial de Librería* [The Cosmic Race. World Book Agency]. Retrieved from www.filosofia.org/aut/001/razacos.htm

Vyas, D. A., Eisenstein, L. G., & Jones, D. S. (2020). Hidden in plain sight— Reconsidering the use of race correction in clinical algorithms. *The New England Journal of Medicine*, *383*(9), 874–882.

Witzig, R. (1996). The medicalization of race: Scientific legitimization of a flawed social construct. *Annals of Internal Medicine*, *125*(8), 675–679.

Worrell, F. C., Mendoza-Denton, R., & Wang, A. (2019). Introducing a new assessment tool for measuring ethnic-racial identity: The Cross ethnic-racial identity scale–adult (CERIS-A). *Assessment*, *26*(3), 404–418. https://doi.org/10.1177/1073191117698756

Worrell, F. C., Vandiver, B. J., Cross, W. E., & Fhagen, P. E. (2016). *The Cross Ethnic-Racial Identity Scale–Adult (CERIS-A)*. University of California.

Chapter 3
Dichos for Culturally Responsive Practice:
LGBTQ+ Latinxs

Bekah Estevez
Georgia Southern University, USA

Jennifer N. Merrrifield
Medical College of Georgia, USA

ABSTRACT

In this chapter, the authors present important concepts, language, and information regarding the lived experiences of Latinx LGBTQ+ individuals (e.g., identity development, sociopolitical impacts on health, resilience processes). They aim to highlight the complexity, nuances, and unique strengths of this community by reviewing relevant research and also interspersing personal anecdotes from our own lives. They offer practitioners and researchers practical advice and take-aways for culturally responsive and relevant practice with and for the Latinx LGBTQ+ community.

PART I

Author Subjectivities and Experiences

As Counseling Psychologists informed by qualitative and social justice-oriented approaches to our work (Delgado-Romero et al., 2012; Delgado-Romero et al., 2018), we, the authors of this chapter, feel strongly that our author positionality matters in the construction of knowledge and sharing of information. To this end, each of us will share information pertaining to our identities and experiences working with the Latinx LGBTQ+ community and will also infuse personal anecdotes pertaining to the information shared below. The personal is powerful, and can often bring concepts and theories to life.

Dr. Rebekah "Bekah" Estevez: I am a white, non-Latinx cisgender woman with a queer sexual orientation who is married to a 3rd generation Latinx (Puerto Rican and Cuban) trans man. Therefore, I am an outsider-insider (Dwyer & Buckle, 2009) in my relationship to the Latinx LGBTQ+ community. My experiences and understandings of Latinx LGBTQ+ identities are shaped by and filtered through my relationship with my husband, his family, as well as the broader majority white LGBTQ+ community and the Latinx LGBTQ+ community. My clinical, advocacy, and research work is focused on the trans and nonbinary (TNB) community, particularly focused on TNB people living in rural areas as well as the Latinx TNB community's unique experiences and needs.

Dr. Jennifer Merrifield: I am a bisexual, cisgender, third-generation Chicana/Mexican American woman living and practicing in the Southern United States. I was born in San Juaquin Valley, California and was raised by married, heterosexual parents. Central to my identity development was my experience of becoming keenly aware of my bicultural and bisexual identities. Moving from California to the Southern United States during my pre-teen years was the catalyst to my self-exploration and understanding of cultural differences and "otherness." This became paramount in my journey of growth both culturally and sexually. My clinical work is predominately in trauma recovery with military service members and Veterans. I have had the honor of serving in an appointed position in the Veterans Health Administration as the Lesbian, Gay, Bisexual, Transgender and Queer (LGBTQ+) Veteran Care Coordinator at two large facilities in the South. In this role, I serve as the hospital's expert consultant on all LGBTQ+ issues and care; spearhead all training and programming for LGBTQ+ Veterans; write, review, and enact anti-discriminatory hospital policies; and ensure equitable delivery of care to all Veterans who served regardless of their LGBTQ+ identities. My personal lived experiences have shaped my research interests and work on social justice and advocacy, as well as Latinx's experiences of discrimination, intimate partner violence, acculturation, and immigration.

PART II

Setting the Frame - Essential Concepts

Language and Terms

While we will use the term Latinx throughout this chapter, it is important to note that in some personal narratives interspersed in this chapter, we will use "Latina" as this term fits the author's lived experience and personal preference. Additionally, we use the term LGBTQ+ to denote individuals with sexual orientations that reflect diverse sexual and/or romantic attractions (e.g., lesbian, bisexual, queer). We also use the term "trans and nonbinary" or "TNB" as an umbrella term to refer to individuals whose gender identities do not align with their sex assigned at birth, and/or do not align with the Western conceptualization of the gender binary (e.g., man, woman; APA, 2015). This umbrella term subsumes identity labels that TNB community members use for themselves, such as trans man, trans woman, genderqueer, and agender. The term "cisgender" is used to denote individuals whose sex assigned at birth aligns with their gender identity (e.g., cisgender woman, cisgender man; APA, 2015).

Other terms of importance for describing concepts and considerations regarding the Latinx LGBTQ+ community in a culturally responsive manner are cisgenderism, anti-trans prejudice, and heterosexism. Anti-trans prejudice is a type of prejudice enacted against TNB individuals due to cisgenderism, or the belief system that there are two genders (man, woman) defined by socially agreed-upon biological markers (e.g., sex chromosomes, secondary sex characteristics; APA, 2015; Tebbe & Moradi, 2017). Similarly, heterosexism refers to the type of prejudice enacted against individuals who are attracted to the same gender due to the societal belief that sexual and romantic attraction should be between "opposite" gender individuals (APA, 2021). Finally, we define "resilience" within the framework put forth by scholars and community organizers focusing on resistance and wellbeing in TNB communities (e.g., Chang et al., 2018; Matsuno & Israel, 2018; Singh et al., 2011). Thus, resilience in this chapter refers to the ability to resist, challenge, and persist in the face of ongoing chronic, social level oppressive experiences that are experienced within the interpersonal and intrapersonal realms (Chang et al., 2018; Estevez, 2022; Matsuno & Israel, 2018; Singh et al., 2011; Singh, 2013).

Theories and Frameworks

As previously discussed in this volume, the Latinx diaspora is a diverse community of individuals representing various ethnicities, gender identities, sexual orientations, relationships to class, and ability statuses. These identities and their subsequent relationship to systems of power, privilege, and oppression impact the ways in which Latinx people experience their own identity, as well as how they are treated from both the majority white culture and from within the Latinx culture (Noyola et al., 2020). In order to fully understand the Latinx LGBTQ+ community, there are certain theoretical lenses we will use in this chapter that are essential to gain understanding into the complexity of Latinx LGBTQ+ individuals.

First, intersectionality theory (Collins, 1989; Crenshaw, 1991; Cross, 1991) was created by Black feminist scholars to illustrate the ways in which various systems of oppression (e.g., racism, heteronormativity, classism, ableism) operate in interlocking manners to create unique experiences of oppression and social inequity. Instead of thinking about and focusing on individual's identities, intersectionality theory directs us to consider the ways in which identities are connected to systems of power and oppression and thus impact the mental and physical wellbeing of minoritized individuals and communities (Moradi & Grzanka, 2017). For example, a Latina trans woman who immigrated to the United States from Mexico lives at the intersection of Latinx-specific racism, xenophobia, and transprejudice. Living at this intersection of these systems of oppression produces specific and unique experiences of prejudice manifesting in ways such as intimate partner violence, high rates of police surveillance and brutality, and job discrimination (James & Salcedo, 2017; Meza Lazaro & Bacio, 2021). Similarly, living at this unique intersection of oppression and risks to wellbeing means that there are unique ways Latina trans women immigrants cultivate resilience. While we will discuss this in further detail later in this chapter, some resilience processes can include cultivating hope for the future, embracing spirituality and personal definitions of the Divine, and creating strong social networks that confer tangible (e.g., clothing, safe housing) and intangible (e.g., emotional support) resources (Abreu et al. 2021; Cerezo et al. 2014; Estevez, 2022; Hwahng et al. 2018).

The minority stress model (Meyer, 1995; 2015) is an extension of stress theory that helps scholars make sense of the disparate rates of negative physical and mental health inequities observed in the lesbian, gay, and bisexual, or LGB, community. Briefly, this model states that both stress and prejudice through distal (e.g., hearing microaggressions or facing housing discrimination) and proximal (e.g., internalized negative beliefs about LGB people) sources are uniquely experienced by LGB individuals and contribute to negative outcomes of stress (Meyer 2003; Meyer 2015). The minority stress model has been expanded to include the unique ways that transprejudice and cisnormativity negatively impact the health and wellbeing of trans and nonbinary, or TNB individuals (Hendricks & Testa 2012; Matsuno & Israel 2018; Testa et al., 2015). Gender minority stress includes unique distal (e.g., lack of access to safe public spaces like restrooms) and proximal (e.g., expectations of misgendering and/or interpersonal rejection) stressors distinctive to TNB individuals' experiences (Matsuno & Israel 2018; Testa et al. 2015).

Similar to intersectionality, the minority stress model highlights ways that identities tied to social systems negatively impact the Latinx LGBTQ+ community. However, the minority stress model also points to sites of resilience and resistance cultivated by the Latinx LGBTQ+ community. For instance, we can understand the actions of Latinx LGBTQ+ individuals of educating themselves about queer and trans identities, fostering and connecting with community, exploring and defining their own racialized gender identity, and navigating familial relationships in culturally-congruent ways as means by which Latinx LGBTQ+ individuals are consciously responding to and resisting the impact of minority stress (Abreu et al. 2021; Estevez, 2022; Schmitz et al. 2020).

Latinx Cultural Values and Traditional Gender Roles

A brief discussion of gender is warranted here because gender and sexuality are related yet distinct constructs that impact one another. As an individual moves through the world, they begin to obtain and encode information about gender from social cues, environmental influences, religion, cultural norms, media etc. It is through the process of learning and conditioning that schemas then develop from a combination of the information gathered from external sources. People then enact their learned schematic themes of gender through behaviors. Gender roles are then repeated and reinforced pattern of learned gendered behaviors, attitudes and outside appearances that are culturally adopted. As a result, each person then develops their unique gender identity (Miville & Ferguson, 2014). Gender roles have become a popular area of interest in modern psychology. The literature clearly demonstrates that constructs of gender, particularly learned gender roles influence behaviors (Miville et al., 2017).

Given the connectedness of culture and gender roles, it is important to acknowledge that *Latinx culture refers to a collective ethnic heterogeneous group of individuals from various regions* (Arredondo et al., 2014). Thus, we examine gender roles and values shared by the majority of Latinx ethnic regions, but it is imperative to remember that there are subtle nuances and differences that may exist within subgroups of Latinx culture. It is equally important to refrain from attributing stereotypical views of gender roles to Latinx individuals and one must remain in tuned with any personal reactions elicited when discussing Latinx gender roles and identity (Arredondo et al., 2014). Further, it is important to bear in mind that the way many current pan-ethnic Latinx gender norms and roles are experienced are a result of colonization by European conquistadors (e.g., Hardin, 2002). Thus, while Latinx cultures once embraced more fluid understandings of gender identity and sexuality, colonizers' beliefs of two gender identities (men and women) and heteronormative romantic/sexual pairings, driven largely by the Christian Church, became interwoven with Latinx cultural norms and values (Hardin, 2002; Mendoza-Álvarez & Espino-Armendáriz, 2018; Mirandé, 2011).

PART III

Lived Experiences of the LGBTQ+ Latinx Community

This section will introduce you to some of the larger concepts and experiences central to the lives of Latinx LGBTQ+ community members.

Latinx LGBTQ+ Identity Development

Cultural identity development is a process that occurs as an individual interacts with their sociocultural environment and learns about the self in relation to their identities and connections to systems of oppression and privilege (Comas-Diaz, 2012). In general, cultural identity development models detail the process through which an individual comes to an awareness of, learns to value, and finally integrate, their minoritized identity into their overall understanding of themselves (Comas-Diaz, 2012). As a note, since research focusing on Latinx LGBTQ+ community members' lived experiences is scarce (Cerezo, 2020; Cerezo et al., 2020), below we review research focusing on Black, Indigenous, and People of Color or BIPOC LGBTQ+ individuals that include Latinx LGBTQ+ participants.

Multicultural-focused research has emphasized the importance of understanding identity using an intersectional lens, meaning that one identity cannot be separated from another (e.g., Bowleg, 2008). As an example, this means that one does not develop their "Latinx + lesbian" identity, but rather their identity as a Latinx lesbian person is developed over time. However, some research has shown that the *processes* through which one develops their ethnic/racial LGBTQ+ identity may differ in important ways. For instance, many identity development models track milestones, or critical experiences across the lifespan that mark important developmental events. Examples of milestones include awareness of the self as an ethnic/racial minority, experiencing same-gender attraction, experiencing gender affirmation of one's TNB identity within community contexts, and coming out to friends or family (Bockting & Coleman, 2016; D'Augelli, 1994; Jamil et al., 2009; Kuper et al., 2018).

Jamil and colleagues' (2009) study of gay, bisexual, and questioning (GBQ) Black and Latinx men found that while their participants' identity development in regards to sexual orientation and ethnic/racial identity occurred at the same time (early/late teen years), ethnic/racial identity development was enacted through interactions with close, easily accessible familial and community resources (e.g., neighborhood contexts) that helped participants develop a sense of understanding and pride in their ethnic/racial identity. However, participants in this study reported having to be more proactive and search for positive interactions with the broader LGBTQ+ community (e.g., use of the Internet) in order to understand and develop their sexual minority identity. The authors of this study propose that these divergent pathways or processes in exploration and development of identities is due to observed and documented heterosexism within ethnic/racial communities, and racism within the broader LGBTQ+ community (Jamil et al., 2009).

Hidden - Jen's Story

I never really "came out" but every day I continue to come out. Like that of my cultural and ethnic identity, I have always been able to "pass" my hidden identities. My skin tone is light enough that most people assume I default to majority White culture. If I claim to be White, my Whiteness is almost never questioned. However, I am frequently met with disbelief from other White individuals when I do disclose that I am Mexican or bicultural. This has served me well when navigating predominately White spaces, especially in spaces I find unsafe. In the same way, society assumes my default sexuality to be heteronormative. It is not unless I choose to correct this assumption that one would ever find out. In fact, I never "came out" because that concept always seemed odd to me and it never felt necessary, which I acknowledge is a privileged stance that I am lucky to have. The process to disclose my identities always weighs heavy on my heart. I constantly vacillate and weigh my options to disclose or not disclose, both my ethnicity and my sexuality. With both identities, I am afforded the luxury of deliberating whether I am safe, comfortable, or empowered to disclose. I acknowledge that this is a privilege and is unique to my lived experience. I mention this internal struggle because I experience shame and guilt either way, with whatever self-disclosure decision I ultimately make. Either I deny my authentic self and feel more empowered in less safe spaces, or I claim my real identity and risk facing judgment or potential discriminatory treatment. This has become more salient as I progress in my career and serve in leadership positions with authority. I first noticed this phenomenon play out in therapeutic relationships. As therapists, we are constantly faced with quick deliberations to self-disclose or not. I have found my authentic self-disclosures of my marginalized identities to be an extremely powerful tool in challenging biases and maladaptive belief systems held by clients. However, it is with extreme caution that I choose to use self-disclosure and one must ensure that a strong therapeutic rapport has been built.

Similarly, a recent study by Bishop and colleagues (2021) found significant differences in milestone attainment in their sample of Black, white, and Latinx sexual minority individuals while also considering cohort (generation) and sociocultural contexts (e.g., passage of same-sex marriage in the U.S. in 2015). Briefly, this study found that Black and Latinx participants experienced same-gender attraction at younger ages, as well as self-identification as a sexual minority, than white participants (Bishop et al., 2021). The authors postulate that since Black and Latinx individuals already hold a minoritized racial/ethnic identity, these communities may be more adept at integrating their sexual minority identity at earlier phases of life (Bishop et al., 2021). Additionally, Balsam and colleagues' (2015) study of identity development and mental health outcomes in sexual minority women of color contributes to our understanding that, while BIPOC sexual minority communities experience heightened levels of oppression and prejudice than their white counterparts, BIPOC sexual minority individuals demonstrate resilience and the ability to understand and integrate their minoritized identities at advanced rates than white folks. This has been hypothesized as likely being due to BIPOC individuals' socialization into their racial/ethnic communities at young ages, which required an earlier understanding of oppression and prejudice and thus an earlier resilience-building process (Balsam et al., 2015; Bishop et al., 2021).

While little research has examined the unique experiences of intersectional Latinx TNB identity development, Cerezo and colleagues (2020) point the field in the direction of future study examining the impact of the intersection of race and gender on identity development. This study of Latinx and Black gender expansive women found that participants formed their racialized gender identities through a process of resisting cultural/familial beliefs regarding gender and sexual orientation (e.g., pressure to hide their identity for the sake of the family's social status), encountering spaces and places that were encouraging and allowing of identity exploration (e.g., going to college and distancing oneself from familial expectations), and continually navigating minoritized experiences in different life domains (e.g., ethnic/racial community, LGBTQ+ community, family of origin; Cerezo et al., 2020). The authors of this study likewise found that the experience of identity integration, described by participants as experiencing positive sense of self as a Black or Latinx gender expansive woman, was borne of resistance and personal inner work to push back against negative social and familial messages experienced throughout the lifespan (Cerezo et al., 2020).

Similarly, in a study by Estevez (2022) which examined the unique resilience strategies of Latinx TNB individuals, participants described a deeply personal process of navigating Latinx cultural values and relationships with family that was intrinsic to both their identity development and resilience. For instance, participants in this study described an unwillingness to "give up" or "cut off" their family of origin, instead finding ways to maintain relationships such as tolerating misgendering and/or dead-naming in order to preserve familial ties (Estevez, 2022). Participants also described exploring their own sense of what it meant to be a Latinx TNB person through a process of deconstructing and reinterpreting their Latinx cultural values to fit with their gender identity (e.g., becoming more spiritually aligned with the Christian God vs. enacting religious behaviors or adhering to dogma; recovering historical memory of fluid gender identities in Latinx cultures pre-colonization). These intentional practices reportedly helped participants synthesize and integrate two cultures that, at the outset of their identity development and resilience building experiences, seemed to negate one another (Estevez, 2022).

Together, these studies suggest that Latinx TNB identity development might entail a process of awareness, unlearning negative social and cultural messages through community connection and internal exploration, and actively reinterpreting and rebuilding an understanding of one's separate identities to synthesize them in an integrative, intersectional fashion.

Well, What Does That Mean for Me and for Us? Devan and Bekah's Story

Note: I (Bekah) obtained consent from Devan to write about our story and his experiences for this chapter.

As a white cisgender queer woman married to a Latinx (3rd generation Puerto Rican and Cuban) trans man, I am an outsider-insider, occupying a 'space between' in my relationship to the Latinx LGBTQ+ community. Discussing and describing my now-husband and my relationship and our subsequent identity development processes is complicated. I met my now-husband before he came into his identity as a trans man, around the age of 19. As a note, the language we use to describe this time of his life is "when he was living AFAB," meaning assigned female at birth. When we met, Devan was closed off to his romantic and sexual attraction to women, as well as his identity as a trans man. Steeped in Latinx cultural values and gender norms, Devan didn't have the space and freedom to question, explore, and further understand himself. In our conversations, Devan points to the role of the Christian faith, familismo, and traditional gender norms and expectations within his Latinx family as barriers to this self-exploration as a young child and teen. It took until Devan attended college to finally have space and thus the opportunity to explore. Likewise, having access to the broader LGBTQ+ community and the language and terminology of what it meant to be trans was pivotal for Devan's self-understanding to grow. He first came into his identity as being attracted to women, identifying as gay but never lesbian. As he continued to deepen his learning and self-understanding, he became more aware of his own internal sense of gender. I will never forget the day I received the phone call letting me know that, after a class on working with trans and nonbinary clients while in his master's in counseling program, Devan had learned what it meant to be trans and felt a deep and settling sense of "oh, there I am". The process of de-constructing and reinterpreting his identity as a Latinx trans man has involved many layers of unlearning and relearning, questioning, and affirming.

Devan and I met at a time when I was likewise closed off to my own sexual orientation as a queer person, having only experienced attraction and sexual/romantic experiences with cisgender men. Meeting Devan when he was living AFAB and continuing to fall and be in love throughout his transition meant that my own sexual orientation was called into question, opening my eyes to my attraction to people of all gender identities. As he enacted traditional masculine roles congruent with Latinx caballerismo gender roles and norms, I found myself enacting roles in line with femininity defined by both my white culture and his Latinx culture. Over a period of several years, we explored and questioned ourselves and our relationship, held together by a deep abiding love for one another and commitment to helping one another inhabit our truest, most authentic selves. Thus, through a reciprocal and ever-evolving exploration process, Devan helped me find myself, and I helped him find himself.

Culturally Congruent Disclosure of Identities

Continuing our conversation around identity development, disclosure of one's minoritized sexual orientation and/or gender identity is a commonly identified "milestone" in identity development models (Villicana et al., 2016). In most research, disclosure is viewed as an essential component of identity integration, which in turn is often viewed as the culmination of the identity development process (Gattamorta & Quidley-Rodriguez, 2018). However, several criticisms have arisen from scholars working at the intersections of race, gender, and sexual orientation. For instance, the majority of foundational research on identity development and disclosure has been centered around white, cisgender, gay men and women, calling into question prevailing understandings' applicability to BIPOC and/or TNB community experiences (Boe et al., 2018; Garvey et al., 2019; Villicana et al., 2016). Additionally, disclosure of identity is often not a one-time event, and is instead a life-long process that is navigated through across several considerations, such as the quality of one's relationships with others, cultural and/or religious background, familial and social (mis)understandings of LGBTQ+ identities, and beliefs about what might occur once the person has divulged their identities (Caba et al., 2022; Gattamorta & Quidley-Rodriguez, 2018). Importantly, most research focuses on LGBQ identities, leaving a dearth of research examining the unique experiences of TNB individuals' experiences of coming out (Brumbaugh-Johnson & Hull, 2019). Subsequently, as we know very little about Latinx TNB communities in general (Abreu et al., 2020a; Abreu et al., 2020b), we know even less about Latinx TNB individuals' unique, culturally informed experiences of the decision to disclose their identities (Garvey et al., 2019).

Currently, there are mixed findings regarding the health benefits of coming out and being out for LGBTQ+ individuals, especially LGBTQ+ BIPOC individuals. Scholars have noted that disclosing one's minoritized sexual orientation and/or gender identity can sometimes confer benefits such as overall positive psychosocial adjustment and experiencing a sense of identity integration and authenticity in daily life (Budge et al., 2017; Huang & Chan, 2022; Russell et al., 2014). However, being verbally out can also carry with it negative impacts such as increased exposure to harassment/abuse from peers, familial-based rejection, and increased rates of negative mental health symptoms such as depression and suicidality (Baams et al., 2015; Rimes et al., 2019). The health benefits of being verbally out are also more precarious for LGBTQ+ BIPOC communities due to the ongoing necessity to simultaneously navigate racial/ethnic community beliefs that might be at odds with an LGBTQ+ identity, as well as the larger majority white cultural beliefs, regarding holding a LGBTQ+ identity (e.g., Eaton & Rios, 2017). This is because being verbally out can limit LGBTQ+ BIPOC individuals' access to social support and resources from their racial/ethnic community and family of origin that acts as a buffer to the negative impact of racism on health and well-being if coming out in this way leads to familial/community strife and rejection (Boe et al., 2018). Likewise, due to racism within the majority white LGBTQ+ community, LGBTQ+ BIPOC individuals may not experience the full impact of social support and affirmation conferred to their white LGBTQ+ peers (Parmenter et al., 2021). Taken together, navigating the intersection of identities tied to multiple systems of oppression can complicate the coming out process, as well as the often-assumed benefits of identity disclosure, for LGBTQ+ BIPOC individuals.

Importantly, scholars taking a multicultural (Hall et al., 2016) approach to understanding the lived experiences of Latinx LGBTQ+ communities have begun to call into question the idea that "coming out" verbally or in direct ways is indeed an important milestone for Latinx LGBTQ+ individuals. For instance, Boe and colleagues (2018) applied a decolonizing ideological lens to the experience of Latinx queer youth navigating disclosure of identity and offer important considerations for clinicians and researchers. They purport that the concept of the "closet" was created in the 1960s by white, cisgender, gay men to help this group position themselves as a minoritized community (Boe et al., 2018). Subsequently, understandings regarding the role of being "out and proud" have been shaped by white, Western norms and values which often center around individuality and autonomy, which can often differ in significant ways from more collectivistic cultural norms and values. Thus, since most research regarding LGBTQ+ identities has been conducted by and for white LGBTQ+ communities, the notion of being "out" has become synonymous with health and authenticity. Thus, scholars (e.g., Boe et al., 2018; Deluicio et al., 2020) contend that the "closet" and being "out" may not, in fact, be an important milestone achievement for Latinx LGBTQ+ individuals identity development and well-being.

A series of recent articles researching the differing coming out experiences of white and Latinx gay, cisgender men reinforce this contention. Villicana and colleagues (2016) explored tacit, or nonverbal, disclosure of sexual orientation among Latinx gay men. Tacit disclosure, they argue, can help Latinx gay cisgender men align themselves with Latinx cultural values of *respeto* and *familismo*, or respecting elders and the family in order to avoid conflict and the central importance of the family and maintaining unity, respectively. These behavioral disclosures took the shape of bringing a partner to family events, being vocal about supporting LGBTQ+ rights, and engaging in public affection with their same-gender partners. The findings of this study confirmed that Latinx gay men came out in more tacit vs. verbal ways compared to their white gay male counterparts, and that verbal disclosure was associated with better overall well-being only for the white gay men in their sample, not for the Latinx gay men in their sample (Villlicana et al., 2016).

The researchers (Villicana et al., 2016) interpreted their findings by purporting that tacit disclosure is not the same as concealment, which has been linked to negative mental health symptomologies. Additionally, Villicana and colleagues' (2016) study explored the potential mediating factors of intrinsic self-exploration (a similar construct to authenticity) and relational self-construal (or forming a sense of connectedness with others via verbal disclosure and receiving positive feedback), and found these variables were associated with verbal disclosure for White gay men but not for Latinx gay men.

Similarly, Delucio and colleagues (2022) examined the relationship between verbal identity disclosure of Latinx and White gay cisgender men and found that high rates of verbal disclosure predicted improved mental health in gay White men, but not in gay Latinx men. In this study, Delucio and colleagues (2022) examined the potential mediating variables of internalized shame and guilt and found that only in white gay men did verbal disclosure predict lower levels of shame and guilt. They contend that this finding could be due to Latinx gay men's racial/ethnic identity being more central to sense of self than one's gay identity. Taken together, this line of inquiry calls into question the centrality of verbal disclosure for well-being in Latinx LGBTQ+ individuals.

Finally, it is important to consider that the identity development and subsequent coming out/disclosure process varies in important ways for TNB and LGBQ+ individuals. While there is a dearth of literature focusing on these differences, existing scholarship explains that because of the role of social perception on gender identity and expression, some TNB people do not have a choice whether or not to disclose their trans identity depending on their decision to engage in medical and/or social transition, and wherein this process the person finds themselves at any given time (Hendricks & Testa, 2012; Testa et al., 2015). Additionally, some trans individuals may not desire to disclose or declare their gender identity as trans after undergoing social and/or medical transition processes (Chang, et al., 2018).

Due to transprejudice and cisgenderism which intersect with racism in the lives of Latinx TNB individuals, the choice to not disclose one's identity as a Latinx TNB person may be due to various reasons to include legitimate safety concerns, socioeconomic preservation, or nondisclosure in order to maintain and protect important social relationships that confer needed social support as is seen with Latinx LGB individuals (e.g., Delucio et al., 2020). Interestingly, a study by Brumbaugh-Johnson and Hull (2019) of TNB individuals navigating identity disclosure processes found that none of their participants' narratives discussed a relationship between self-acceptance and identity disclosure; instead, these participants described the importance of flexible, nuanced navigation of interactions with others that depended on changing contexts and social impacts. Additionally, in a study of TNB resilience processes against cissexism and racism, a sample of 15 Latinx TNB individuals emphasized the internal navigation and synthesis of their Latinx TNB identity as monumental to their resilience and well-being over identity disclosure to others in their life (Estevez, 2022). Taken together, it appears important for scholars to bring a nuanced, intersectional, flexible approach to understanding and working with Latinx TNB community members navigating their identity development and disclosure, accounting for the impact of cultural values and social expectations that may or may not be applicable to this community.

Navigating Disclosure: Devan and Bekah's Story

Devan and I got together at the ages of 18 and 19 as freshmen in college. At the time, Devan was living AFAB and had not yet come into his trans identity as a trans man. Coming from a family that valued traditional Latinx gender norms and imbued with traditional, conservative Christian values, Devan and I did not disclose our relationship to any family, and only disclosed to very close friends who both were and were not members of the LGBTQ+ community. This was an active choice on Devan's end due to his desire to not create a rupture in his relationships with his parents, siblings, and aunts, all of whom he was very close. I decided to conceal my relationship with Devan from my family due to my own family's conservative Christian faith and values. Over time, I became a close, intimate part of Devan's family. From attending family vacations, returning to Devan's family home over weekend breaks, to babysitting Devan's niece and nephew for extended periods of time, I became an integrated and celebrated part of the family, explained to others as a "close family friend" and "Devan's roommate." As Devan transitioned medically and socially and our lives took us through undergrad and into graduate school, Devan and I married in a small, "chosen-family" only attended ceremony. Only my sister was a "blood relative" in attendance, and the marriage was not disclosed outside of our chosen family circle until Devan and I were married for 5 years, together for 12. Today, Devan's family still does not know that Devan is a trans man, which has caused some necessary distancing due to the physical changes Devan has undergone due to medical transition. This has been aided by Devan's familial move to a different state, which has helped explain away the less frequent visits. Devan and I are not accepted or viewed by the family as married, and certain rules are in place for visits (e.g., we can't spend the night in the same home as the family, many of whom live together in one home). However, the family continues to both verbally and tacitly extend and express their love to both Devan and me. From comments like "I can't agree with your "choice," but I love you still," to allowing me to be brought along on visits, to frequent phone calls and FaceTime sessions with extended family members who are more accepting and understanding, to offering help moving us into our new home, Devan and I continue to experience love and support. One difference worth mentioning is my experience as a white non-Latinx cis woman. In our conversations together, Devan continuously expresses his frustration in talking with friends who urge him to cut off his family or "stand up for himself" and come out as trans and/or "defend" his marriage to me. Devan tells me that for him, his parents know who he is, and choose to love him in the best way they can given their cultural and religious beliefs. Being misgendered, not directly talking about his wedding or marriage to me, and not verbally disclosing that he is a trans man to his family does not feel to Devan like he is "in hiding" or being "inauthentic." Instead, Devan describes these experiences as being respectful and necessary for keeping family bonds in-tact. For me, not being accepted and recognized as a daughter or sister-in-law is emotionally painful. Coming from a white, Western cultural background where "outness" is frequently associated with pride in one's identity and "living authentically," the more tacit and covert expressions of love and support are harder for me to accept and be okay with experiencing.

It's Not Either-or: Cultural Impacts on Discrimination and Resilience From Within and Outside the Latinx Community

So far in our discussion on Latinx LGBTQ+ individuals lived experiences, we have pointed to the ways that intersectional perspectives of Latinx LGBTQ+ identities are essential for understanding this community in a culturally responsive way. This is of paramount importance when considering the discrimination and resilience experiences of Latinx LGBTQ+ individuals from within and outside the Latinx community. Without such a lens, it can be easy to fall into the conventional trap of believing that the Latinx culture is more heteronormative and cisnormative than the white majority culture. While there are certainly cultural values and norms that can sometimes serve as boundaries to acceptance for Latinx LGBTQ+ individuals, research taking a more nuanced approach to asking questions about acceptance, integration within families and communities, and lived experiences of Latinx LGBTQ+ individuals has begun to push back on this narrative (Abreu & Gonzalez, 2020).

As noted previously, the values of *familismo*, Christian religiosity, and traditional Latinx gender norms of *machismo* and *marianismo*, are all salient within-cultural impacts on the risk and resilience experiences of Latinx LGBTQ+ individuals. While still vastly under-studied in the extant literature, perhaps one of the biggest cultural impacts on Latinx LGBTQ+ health and well-being is the role of *familismo* in instigating and mitigating LGBTQ+ minority stress (Pastrana, 2015). In their meta-analysis of the extant literature, Przeworski and Piedra (2020) reviewed research studies documenting how *familismo* and the desire to put the needs of, and preserve in-tact harmony of, the familial unit ahead of the individual self-led to participants concealing their identities. This often led to difficulty for participants to achieve integration of their sexual minority and Latinx identities (Przeworski & Piedra, 2020). Additionally, this meta-analysis reviewed research which found that *familismo* motivated participants to stay in potentially harmful relational situations where they experienced ongoing verbal microaggressions and physical abuse (Przeworski & Piedra, 2020). Further, the authors of this meta-analysis reviewed research reporting that LGBTQ+ Latinx individuals expended psychological energy engaging in code-switching behaviors, such as changing their mannerisms, ways of speaking, and dress to "pass" or "blend" as straight and aligned with Latinx cultural gender norms of *machismo* and *marianismo* (Przeworski & Piedra, 2020). However, other research has found similar behaviors (e.g., maintaining awareness of one's context; switching ways of interacting and presenting oneself; psychological distancing through minimization of negative comments) to be described as important modes of coping for Latinx LGBTQ+ community members (e.g., Noyola et al., 2020).

Both Noyola and colleagues' (2020) and Estevez's (2022) participants described *choosing* to navigate difficult familial relationships in this way out of love, respect, and an unwillingness to lose familial ties due to the central importance of the family. Instead of positioning these choices in a negative light, participants in both studies described finding peace and acceptance in their choices. Similarly, Abreu and colleagues (2020) worked with Latinx parents of LGBTQ young adults to examine the acceptance process for these families. Their findings too suggest that the value of *familismo* and subsequent emphasis on family loyalty, solidarity, and support for one's children motivated parents to move through their own internal acceptance processes to affirm and accept their children, as well as navigate extended family members' varied reactions to their child's LGBTQ+ identity (Abreu et al., 2020).

In addition to *familismo*, Latinx cultural gender norms and expectations, inclusive of *machismo* and *marianismo*, have important implications for risk and resilience in the lives of Latinx LGBTQ+ individuals. For instance, *machismo* and *marianismo* can be experienced by Latinx LGBTQ+ individuals and their families as restrictive and antithetical to LGBTQ+ identities and expressions (e.g., Gray et al., 2015). Additionally, religiosity, specifically Catholicism, has also been identified as a salient cultural value that impacts experiences of risk to well-being within the Latinx LGBTQ+ community due to the Church's teachings on sex and gender that are heteronormative and cisnormative (e.g., Morales, 2013). However, as research continues to unearth nuanced impacts of these cultural values on Latinx LGBTQ+ well-being, some studies have underscored the ways Latinx LGBTQ+ individuals deconstruct and re-integrate these values to be sources of strength and resilience. From continuing to engage in religious practices like prayer and attending affirming churches (Schmitz et al., 2020) to redefining and exploring one's own spiritually based beliefs and connection to the Divine (Estevez, 2022), Latinx LGBTQ+ individuals report unlearning and disconnecting harmful messages from their faith traditions and leaning on them for sources of strength. Importantly, such practices and active deconstruction reportedly help Latinx LGBTQ+ individuals remain connected to their Latinx cultural heritage, which in turn can help improve and bolster pride in one's ethnic identity (Estevez, 2022).

Similarly, through the identity development and integration process, Latinx LGBTQ+ individuals have the opportunity to explore, reject, deconstruct, and synthesize *machismo* and *marianismo* gender roles into their own interpretations and understandings that align with their gender and sexuality. Reportedly, an important pathway to this work is recovering historical memory and increasing critical consciousness, achieved through learning about Latinx pan-ethnic cultural understandings of gender and sexuality pre-European and Spanish colonization (e.g., Estevez, 2022). Participants in Estevez's (2022) study of the resilience of Latinx TNB individuals found that participants were sharply aware of the impact of intersecting systems of oppression operating in their lives and leaned into learning more about these systems as a part of their exploration of themselves and connection to the Latinx LGBTQ+ community. Learning more about the historical fluidity of gender identities and expressions, as well as sexual orientations and practices, pre-colonization helped participants of this study meld and rebuild their own personal understanding of what it means to be a Latinx LGBTQ+ person and was described as an act of resilience and resistance (Estevez, 2022).

Finally, it has been well-established that social support is vital for the general LGBTQ+ community's health and well-being (Moe, 2016). However, Latinx LGBTQ+ individuals often experience rejection, stigma, and misunderstanding from within the wider, majority white LGBTQ+ community (McConnell et al., 2018; Parmenter et al., 2021). Additionally, Latinx TNB individuals face the impact of the intersection of racism and cisnormativity within the majority white, cisgender LGBTQ+ community, further alienating them from this important source of support (Balsam et al., 2011; Estevez, 2022). Taken together, these findings present a nuanced, complicated understanding of how Latinx cultural values can be both a risk to well-being and manifest as aspects of resilience for Latinx LGBTQ+ community members.

PART IV

Latinx LGBTQ+ Resilience and Resistance

While understanding the salient factors from within and outside the Latinx community that negatively impact Latinx LGBTQ+ individuals across life domains is important, so too is shining a light on the unique ways this vibrant and strong community resists and enacts resilience. As the great Latinx scholar and healer Patricia Arredondo reminds us, "In practice, [the Latinx people] have led lives of adaptation and resiliency for centuries" (Arredondo et al., 2014, p. 18). This extends to all members of the Latinx culture, inclusive of LGBTQ+ individuals.

Resilience Processes for Latinx LGBTQ+ People

As we have stated throughout this chapter, there is a dearth of literature regarding strengths-based approaches to understanding the unique experiences and needs of Latinx LGBTQ+ individuals (Abreu et al., 2020; Quintero et al., 2015; Velez et al., 2015). However, emerging research (e.g., Abreu et al., 2021; Singh, 2013) has begun to focus on the coping and resilience of BIPOC LGBTQ+ communities, inclusive of the Latinx LGBTQ+ community. Therefore, we will review findings of such research that includes Latinx LGBTQ+ individuals in samples, as well as Latinx LGBTQ+ specific research. Also, returning to our definition of resilience in the beginning of this chapter, it is important to remember that resilience includes *both* internal and community-based contributions and processes (Matsuno & Israel, 2018; Meyer, 2015; Singh, 2013). Especially for collectivistic cultures, resilience is purposeful, active, process-oriented, and rooted in a cyclical relationship between community connectedness and internal undertakings - not merely a set of traits that one is born with or without (Estevez, 2022; Meyer, 2015; Singh, 2013).

Salient sources of resilience among in the lives of LGBTQ+ BIPOC individuals includes affirming neighborhoods, LGBTQ+ organizations, social support via peers, friends, partners, and chosen family members, connecting with the LGBTQ+ racial/ethnic community, and engaging in personal spirituality and connection with the Divine (Abreu et al., 2021; Cerezo et al., 2014; Hwahng et al., 2018; Loza et al., 2017; Singh et al., 2011). Through an iterative cycle of interacting with, as well as contributing to, these sources of resilience, LGBTQ+ BIPOC individuals, inclusive of Latinx LGBTQ+ community members, cultivate the ability to survive and thrive in the face of adversity. Research has examined the actions taken by individuals to build their resilience. Common activities include taking part in activism and social justice efforts to change the sociopolitical climate to be affirming of racial/ethnic minorities and/or LGBTQ+ groups, offering a helping hand to fellow LGBTQ+ Latinx community members through offering housing or helping others access resources and financial security, and educating loved ones in their lives regarding their expressed prejudice and beliefs that are harmful to themselves and their community (Bockting et al., 2020; Hwahng et al., 2018; Schmitz et al., 2020; Singh, 2013). Importantly some studies have shown mixed findings regarding the impact of engaging in activism and social justice efforts, as doing so can bring Latinx LGBTQ+ individuals into heightened contact with prejudice and discriminatory views, as well as add to feelings of overwhelm and burden (Bockting et al., 2020; Breslow et al., 2015).

Considering the Latinx cultural values of *familismo, collectivismo*, and *personalismo*, it makes sense that some of the strongest sources of resilience for Latinx LBGTQ+ individuals are community, friends, and when possible, family of origin. Recent research has taken a closer look at the role of community and social support, finding that "microcommunities" of individuals who hold the same or similar identities (e.g., Latinx and trans) confer more authentic and powerful experiences of belongingness, which can strengthen individuals' pride in their intersectional identities (Abreu et al., 2021; Gray et al., 2015; Koech et al., 2022). In investigating the experiences of immigrant trans Latinx individuals, it appears that the formation of such "microcommunities" is even more important due to the unique difficulties and stigma associated with immigration and documented status (Abreu et al., 2021). In a study by Stone and colleagues (2020), white TNB individuals reported that the broader LGBTQ+ community was a salient source of social support and were able to use their white racialized social groups to leverage connection in ways Latinx and Black TNB individuals could not. Within these "microcommunities," Latinx LGBTQ+ individuals experience support, affirmation, and love, while also giving these intangible resources back to others (Abreu et al., 2021; Stone et al., 2020). This cyclical experience of giving and receiving support has been identified as especially helpful for Latinx TNB individuals (Abreu et al., 2021; Estevez, 2022). Additionally, LGBTQ+ BIPOC individuals report that seeking and being role models for others is a salient source of resilience (Koech et al., 2022; Ruff et al., 2019). Through these connections with others, LGBTQ+ BIPOC community members, inclusive of Latinx LGBTQ+ people, nurture hope and belief in a better future, find the courage to build lives worth living in the face of adversity, and strengthen a sense of self-worth, self-esteem, and self-compassion (Bockting et al., 2020; Cerezo et al., 2014, Ruff et al., 2019; Singh et al., 2011).

CONCLUSION

The Latinx LGBTQ+ community is one of complexity, nuance, love, sorrow, joy, and struggle. Far from monolithic, each Latinx LGBTQ+ person has their own personal experience and understanding of their Latinx LGBTQ+ identity. For some, their identity as a person of Latinx descent might feel more salient, leading to following traditional roles and customs that might seem strange for white practitioners (e.g., tacit or non-verbal disclosure of LGBTQ+ identity). For others, integrating acculturated understandings of their Latinx identity into their overall Latinx LGBTQ+ identity will be important. We hope that you take away from this chapter the knowledge that the Latinx culture is not necessarily more heteronormative or cisnormative than other cultures, that Latinx LGBTQ+ individuals can and do live full, happy lives even in the face of adversity, and the importance of attending to cultural impacts on all facets of health and well-being. For the researchers, we hope that you will take up the charge to further the program of study regarding the Latinx LGBTQ+ community from a strengths-based perspective. We desperately need research on topics such as the lived experiences, needs, and resilience of Latinx trans men and nonbinary people; the impact of Latinx gender norms on bisexual individuals' identity development; interventions for interrupting internalized racialized cis/heteronormativity; and the processes through which Latinx families come to accept and affirm their Latinx LGBTQ+ loved one in light of, not in spite of, traditional norms and values. Whether it be through clinical practice, research, teaching, and/or advocacy, all of us have a role to play in changing our society so that it is salutogenic for Latinx LGBTQ+ communities. Working with, not for, communities from a strengths-based, resilience and liberation focus, we can take strides towards ameliorating health inequities based in racism, transprejudice, and cisnormativity.

REFERENCES

Abreu, R. L., & Gonzalez, K. A. (2020). Redefining collectivism: Family and community among sexual and gender diverse people of color and indigenous people: Introduction to the special issue. *Journal of GLBT Family Studies*, *16*(2), 107–110. doi:10.1080/1550428X.2020.1736038

Abreu, R. L., Gonzalez, K. A., Capielo Rosario, C., Lockett, G. M., Lindley, L., & Lane, S. (2021). "We are our own community": Immigrant Latinx transgender people community experiences. *Journal of Counseling Psychology*, *68*(4), 390–403. Advance online publication. doi:10.1037/cou0000546 PMID:33983757

Abreu, R. L., Gonzalez, K. A., Capielo Rosario, C., Pulice-Farrow, L., & Rodríguez, M. M. D. (2020). "Latinos have a stronger attachment to the family": Latinx fathers' acceptance of their sexual minority children. *Journal of GLBT Family Studies*, *16*(2), 192–210. doi:10.1080/1550428X.2019.1672232

American Psychological Association. (2015). Guidelines for psychological practice with transgender and gender nonconforming people. *The American Psychologist*, *70*(9), 832–864. doi:10.1037/a0039906 PMID:26653312

American Psychological Association. (2021). *Guidelines for psychological practice with sexual minority persons*. Retrieved from www.apa.org/about/policy/psychological-practice-sexual-minority-persons.pdf

Arredondo, P., Gallardo-Cooper, M., Delgado-Romero, E. A., & Zapata, A. L. (2014). *Culturally responsive counseling with Latinas/os*. John Wiley & Sons.

Baams, L., Grossman, A. H., & Russell, S. T. (2015). Minority stress and mechanisms of risk for depression and suicidal ideation among lesbian, gay, and bisexual youth. *Developmental Psychology*, *51*(5), 688–696. doi:10.1037/a0038994 PMID:25751098

Balsam, K. F., Molina, Y., Beadnell, B., Simoni, J., & Walters, K. (2011). Measuring multiple minority stress: The LGBTQ+ People of Color Microaggressions Scale. *Cultural Diversity & Ethnic Minority Psychology*, *17*(2), 163–174. doi:10.1037/a0023244 PMID:21604840

Balsam, K. F., Molina, Y., Blayney, J. A., Dillworth, T., Zimmerman, L., & Kaysen, D. (2015). Racial/ethnic differences in identity and mental health outcomes among young sexual minority women. *Cultural Diversity & Ethnic Minority Psychology*, *21*(3), 380–390. doi:10.1037/a0038680 PMID:25642782

Bishop, M., Mallory, A. B., Gessner, M. K., Frost, D. M., & Russell, S. T. (2021). School-based sexuality education experiences across three generations of sexual minority people. *Journal of Sex Research*, *58*(5), 648–658. doi:10.1080/00224499.2020.1767024 PMID:32486928

Bockting, W., Barucco, R., LeBlanc, A., Singh, A., Mellman, W., Dolezal, C., & Ehrhardt, A. (2020). Sociopolitical change and transgender people's perceptions of vulnerability and resilience. *Sexuality Research & Social Policy*, *17*(1), 162–174. doi:10.100713178-019-00381-5 PMID:32742526

Bockting, W., & Coleman, E. (2016). Developmental stages of the transgender coming-out process: Toward an integrated identity. In R. Ettner, S. Monstrey, & E. Coleman (Eds.), Principles of transgender medicine and surgery (2nd ed., pp. 137–158). Routledge/Taylor & Francis Group.

Boe, J. L., Maxey, V. A., & Bermudez, J. M. (2018). Is the closet a closet? Decolonizing the coming out process with Latin@ adolescents and families. *Journal of Feminist Family Therapy*, *30*(2), 90–108. doi:10.1080/08952833.2018.1427931

Bowleg, L. (2008). When Black+ lesbian+ woman¹ Black lesbian woman: The methodological challenges of qualitative and quantitative intersectionality research. *Sex Roles*, *59*(5-6), 312–325. doi:10.100711199-008-9400-z

Breslow, A. S., Brewster, M. E., Velez, B. L., Wong, S., Geiger, E., & Soderstrom, B. (2015). Resilience and collective action: Exploring buffers against minority stress for transgender individuals. *Psychology of Sexual Orientation and Gender Diversity*, *2*(3), 253–265. doi:10.1037gd0000117

Brumbaugh-Johnson, S. M., & Hull, K. E. (2019). Coming out as transgender: Navigating the social implications of a transgender identity. *Journal of Homosexuality*, *66*(8), 1148–1177. doi:10.1080/00918369.2018.1493253 PMID:30052497

Budge, S. L., Chin, M. Y., & Minero, L. P. (2017). Trans individuals' facilitative coping: An analysis of internal and external processes. *Journal of Counseling Psychology*, *64*(1), 12–25. doi:10.1037/cou0000178 PMID:28068128

Caba, M., Mallory, A. B., Simon, K. A., Rathus, T., & Watson, R. J. (2022). Complex Outness Patterns Among Sexual Minority Youth: A Latent Class Analysis. *Journal of Youth and Adolescence*, *51*(4), 746–765. doi:10.100710964-022-01580-x PMID:35150376

Cerezo, A. (2020). Expanding the reach of Latinx psychology: Honoring the lived experiences of sexual and gender diverse Latinxs. *Journal of Latina/o Psychology*, *8*(1), 1–6. doi:10.1037/lat0000144

Cerezo, A., Cummings, M., Holmes, M., & Williams, C. (2020). Identity as resistance: Identity formation at the intersection of race, gender identity, and sexual orientation. *Psychology of Women Quarterly*, *44*(1), 67–83. doi:10.1177/0361684319875977 PMID:32194296

Cerezo, A., Morales, A., Quintero, D., & Rothman, S. (2014). Trans migrations: Exploring life at the intersection of transgender identity and immigration. *Psychology of Sexual Orientation and Gender Diversity*, *1*(2), 170–180. doi:10.1037gd0000031

Chang, S. C., Singh, A. A., & Dickey, L. m. (2018). *A Clinician's Guide to Gender-Affirming Care: Working with Transgender and Gender Nonconforming Clients*. New Harbinger Publications.

Collins, P. H. (1989). The Social Construction of Black Feminist Thought. *Signs (Chicago, Ill.)*, *14*(4), 745–773. doi:10.1086/494543

Comas-Díaz, L. (2012). *Multicultural care: A clinician's guide to cultural competence*. American Psychological Association. doi:10.1037/13491-000

Crenshaw, K. (1991). Mapping the margins: Intersectionality, identity politics and violence against women of color. *Stanford Law Review*, *43*(6), 1241–1299. doi:10.2307/1229039

Cross, W. E., Jr., Parham, T. A., & Helms, J. E. (1991). The stages of Black identity development: Nigrescence models. Black Psychology, 3, 319–338.

D'Augelli, A. R. (1994). Identity development and sexual orientation: Toward a model of lesbian, gay, and bisexual development. *Human Diversity: Perspectives on People in Context.*, *486*, 312–333.

Delgado-Romero, E. A., Lau, M. Y., & Shullman, S. L. (2012). The Society of Counseling Psychology: Historical values, themes, and patterns viewed from the American Psychological Association presidential podium. In N. A. Fouad (Ed.), APA handbook of counseling psychology (Vol. 1, pp. 3–29). American Psychological Association.

Delgado-Romero, E. A., Singh, A. A., & De Los Santos, J. (2018). Cuéntame: The promise of qualitative research with Latinx populations. *Journal of Latina/o Psychology*, *6*(4), 318–328. doi:10.1037/lat0000123

Delucio, K., Morgan-Consoli, M. L., & Israel, T. (2020). Lo que se ve no se pregunta: Exploring nonverbal gay identity disclosure among Mexican American gay men. *Journal of Latina/o Psychology*, *8*(1), 21–40. doi:10.1037/lat0000139

Delucio, K., Villicana, A. J., & Biernat, M. (2022). Verbal disclosure and mental health among gay Latino and gay white men. *The Counseling Psychologist*, *50*(2), 241–274. doi:10.1177/00110000211051325

Dwyer, S. C., & Buckle, J. L. (2009). The space between: On being an insider-outsider in qualitative research. *International Journal of Qualitative Methods*, *8*(1), 54–63. doi:10.1177/160940690900800105

Eaton, A. A., & Rios, D. (2017). Social challenges faced by queer Latino college men: Navigating negative responses to coming out in a double minority sample of emerging adults. *Cultural Diversity & Ethnic Minority Psychology*, *23*(4), 457–467. doi:10.1037/cdp0000134 PMID:28252982

Estevez, R. (2022). *"Talk about resilient: We just don't give up": The risk and resilience experiences of Latinx trans and nonbinary individuals* [Dissertation, University of Georgia]. ProQuest Dissertations and Theses Global.

Garvey, M., Mobley, S. D. Jr, Summerville, K. S., & Moore, G. T. (2019). Queer and Trans Students of Color: Navigating Identity Disclosure and College Contexts. *The Journal of Higher Education (Columbus)*, *90*(1), 150–178. doi:10.1080/00221546.2018.1449081

Gattamorta, K., & Quidley-Rodriguez, N. (2018). Coming out experiences of Hispanic sexual minority young adults in South Florida. *Journal of Homosexuality*, *65*(6), 741–765. doi:10.1080/00918369.2017.1364111 PMID:28771094

Gray, N. N., Mendelsohn, D. M., & Omoto, A. M. (2015). Community connectedness, challenges, and resilience among gay Latino immigrants. *American Journal of Community Psychology*, *55*(1-2), 202–214. doi:10.100710464-014-9697-4 PMID:25576015

Hall, G. C. N., Yip, T., & Zárate, M. A. (2016). On becoming multicultural in a monocultural research world: A conceptual approach to studying ethnocultural diversity. *The American Psychologist, 71*(1), 40–51. doi:10.1037/a0039734 PMID:26766764

Hardin, M. (2002). Altering masculinities: The Spanish conquest and the evolution of the Latin American machismo. *International Journal of Sexuality and Gender Studies, 7*(1), 1–22. doi:10.1023/A:1013050829597

Hendricks, M. L., & Testa, R. J. (2012). A conceptual framework for clinical work with transgender and gender nonconforming clients: An adaptation of the Minority Stress Model. *Professional Psychology, Research and Practice, 43*(5), 460–467. doi:10.1037/a0029597

Huang, Y. T., & Chan, R. C. (2022). Effects of sexual orientation concealment on well-being among sexual minorities: How and when does concealment hurt? *Journal of Counseling Psychology, 69*(5), 630–641. Advance online publication. doi:10.1037/cou0000623 PMID:35696152

Hwahng, S. J., Allen, B., Zadoretzky, C., Barber, H., McKnight, C., & Des Jarlais, D. (2018). Alternative kinship structures, resilience and social support among immigrant trans Latinas in the USA. *Culture, Health & Sexuality, 21*(1), 1–15. doi:10.1080/13691058.2018.1440323 PMID:29658825

James, S. E., & Salcedo, B. (2017). 2015 U.S. Transgender Survey: Report on the Experiences of Latino/a Respondents. National Center for Transgender Equality and TransLatin@ Coalition.

Jamil, O. B., Harper, G. W., & Fernandez, M. I. (2009). Sexual and ethnic identity development among gay–bisexual–questioning (GBQ) male ethnic minority adolescents. *Cultural Diversity & Ethnic Minority Psychology, 15*(3), 203–214. doi:10.1037/a0014795 PMID:19594249

Koech, J. M., Sostre, J. P., Lockett, G. M., Gonzalez, K. A., & Abreu, R. L. (2022). Resisting by Existing: Trans Latinx Mental Health, Well-Being, and Resilience in the United States. In *Latinx Queer Psychology* (pp. 43–67). Springer. doi:10.1007/978-3-030-82250-7_4

Kuper, L. E., Wright, L., & Mustanski, B. (2018). Gender identity development among transgender and gender nonconforming emerging adults: An intersectional approach. *International Journal of Transgenderism, 19*(4), 436–455. doi:10.1080/15532739.2018.1443869

Loza, O., Beltran, O., & Mangadu, T. (2017). A qualitative exploratory study on gender identity and the health risks and barriers to care for transgender women living in a US–Mexico border city. *International Journal of Transgenderism, 18*(1), 104–118. doi:10.1080/15532739.2016.1255868

Matsuno, E., & Israel, T. (2018). Psychological interventions promoting resilience among transgender individuals: Transgender resilience intervention model (TRIM). *The Counseling Psychologist, 46*(5), 632–655. doi:10.1177/0011000018787261

McConnell, E. A., Janulis, P., Phillips, I., Truong, R., & Birkett, M. (2018). Multiple minority stress and LGBTQ+ community resilience among sexual minority men. *Psychology of Sexual Orientation and Gender Diversity, 5*(1), 1–12. doi:10.1037gd0000265 PMID:29546228

Mendoza-Álvarez, C., & Espino-Armendáriz, S. (2018). A critical approach to gender identities in the "Muxe" case. *Humanities and Social Sciences, 6*(4), 130–136. doi:10.11648/j.hss.20180604.16

Meyer, I. H. (1995). Minority stress and mental health in gay men. *Journal of Health and Social Behavior*, *36*(1), 38–56. doi:10.2307/2137286 PMID:7738327

Meyer, I. H. (2003). Prejudice, social stress, and mental health in lesbian, gay, and bisexual populations: Conceptual issues and research evidence. *Psychological Bulletin*, *129*(5), 674–697. doi:10.1037/0033-2909.129.5.674 PMID:12956539

Meyer, I. H. (2015). Resilience in the study of minority stress and health of sexual and gender minorities. *Psychology of Sexual Orientation and Gender Diversity*, *2*(3), 209–213. doi:10.1037gd0000132

Meza Lazaro, Y., & Bacio, G. A. (2021). Determinants of mental health outcomes among transgender Latinas: Minority stress and resilience processes. *Psychology of Sexual Orientation and Gender Diversity*. Advance online publication. doi:10.1037gd0000545

Mirandé, A. (2011). The Muxes of Juchitan: A preliminary look at transgender identity and acceptance. *Cal. W. Int'l LJ*, *42*(2), 509–540.

Miville, M. L., & Ferguson, A. D. (2014). Intersections of race-ethnicity and gender on identity development and social roles. In M. L. Miville & A. D. Ferguson (Eds.), *Handbook of race-ethnicity and gender in psychology*. Springer. doi:10.1007/978-1-4614-8860-6_1

Miville, M. L., Mendez, N., & Louie, M. (2017). Latina/o Gender Roles: A content analysis of empirical research from 1982 to 2013. *Journal of Latina/o Psychology*, *5*(3), 173–194. doi:10.1037/lat0000072

Moe, J. L. (2016). Wellness and distress in LGBTQ populations: A meta-analysis. *Journal of LGBT Issues in Counseling*, *10*(2), 112–129. doi:10.1080/15538605.2016.1163520

Moradi, B., & Grzanka, P. R. (2017). Using intersectionality responsibly: Toward critical epistemology, structural analysis, and social justice activism. *Journal of Counseling Psychology*, *64*(5), 500–513. doi:10.1037/cou0000203 PMID:29048196

Morales, E. (2013). Latino lesbian, gay, bisexual, and transgender immigrants in the United States. *Journal of LGBT Issues in Counseling*, *7*(2), 172–184. doi:10.1080/15538605.2013.785467

Noyola, N., Sánchez, M., & Cardemil, E. V. (2020). Minority stress and coping among sexual diverse Latinxs. *Journal of Latina/o Psychology*, *8*(1), 58–82. doi:10.1037/lat0000143

Parmenter, J. G., Galliher, R. V., Wong, E., & Perez, D. (2021). An intersectional approach to understanding LGBTQ+ people of color's access to LGBTQ+ community resilience. *Journal of Counseling Psychology*, *68*(6), 629–641. doi:10.1037/cou0000578 PMID:34398620

Pastrana, A. J. Jr. (2015). Being out to others: The relative importance of family support, identity and religion for LGBT Latina/os. *Latino Studies*, *13*(1), 88–112. doi:10.1057/lst.2014.69

Przeworski, A., & Piedra, A. (2020). The role of the family for sexual minority Latinx individuals: A systematic review and recommendations for clinical practice. *Journal of GLBT Family Studies*, *16*(2), 211–240. doi:10.1080/1550428X.2020.1724109

Quintero, D., Cerezo, A., Morales, A., & Rothman, S. (2015). Supporting transgender immigrant Latinas: The case of Erika. In *Gendered journeys: Women, migration and feminist psychology* (pp. 190–205). Springer. doi:10.1057/9781137521477_9

Rimes, K. A., Shivakumar, S., Ussher, G., Baker, D., Rahman, Q., & West, E. (2019). Psychosocial factors associated with suicide attempts, ideation, and future risk in lesbian, gay, and bisexual youth: The youth chances study. *Crisis*, *40*(2), 83–92. doi:10.1027/0227-5910/a000527 PMID:29932021

Ruff, N., Smoyer, A. B., & Breny, J. (2019). Hope, courage, and resilience in the lives of transgender women of color. *Qualitative Report*, *24*(8), 1990–2008. doi:10.46743/2160-3715/2019.3729

Russell, S. T., Toomey, R. B., Ryan, C., & Diaz, R. M. (2014). Being out at school: The implications for school victimization and young adult adjustment. *The American Journal of Orthopsychiatry*, *84*(6), 635–643. doi:10.1037/ort0000037 PMID:25545431

Schmitz, R. M., Robinson, B. A., Tabler, J., Welch, B., & Rafaqut, S. (2020). LGBTQ+ Latino/a young people's interpretations of stigma and mental health: An intersectional minority stress perspective. *Society and Mental Health*, *10*(2), 163–179. doi:10.1177/2156869319847248

Singh, A. (2013). Transgender youth of color and resilience: Negotiating oppression and finding support. *Sex Roles*, *68*(11-12), 690–702. doi:10.100711199-012-0149-z

Singh, A. A., Hays, D. G., & Watson, L. S. (2011). Strength in the face of adversity: Resilience strategies of transgender individuals. *Journal of Counseling and Development*, *89*(1), 20–27. doi:10.1002/j.1556-6678.2011.tb00057.x

Singh, A. A., & McKleroy, V. S. (2011). "Just getting out of bed is a revolutionary act" The resilience of transgender people of color who have survived traumatic life events. *Traumatology*, *17*(2), 34–44. doi:10.1177/1534765610369261

Stone, A. L., Nimmons, E. A., Salcido, R. Jr, & Schnarrs, P. W. (2020). Multiplicity, race, and resilience: Transgender and non-binary people building community. *Sociological Inquiry*, *90*(2), 226–248. doi:10.1111oin.12341

Tebbe, E. N., & Moradi, B. (2012). Anti-transgender prejudice: A structural equation model of associated constructs. *Journal of Counseling Psychology*, *59*(2), 251–261. doi:10.1037/a0026990 PMID:22329343

Testa, R. J., Habarth, J., Peta, J., Balsam, K., & Bockting, W. (2015). Development of the gender minority stress and resilience measure. *Psychology of Sexual Orientation and Gender Diversity*, *2*(1), 65–77. doi:10.1037gd0000081

Velez, B. L., Moradi, B., & DeBlaere, C. (2015). Multiple oppressions and the mental health of sexual minority Latina/o individuals. *The Counseling Psychologist*, *43*(1), 7–38. doi:10.1177/0011000014542836

Villicana, A. J., Delucio, K., & Biernat, M. (2016). "Coming out" among gay Latino and gay White men: Implications of verbal disclosure for well-being. *Self and Identity*, *15*(4), 468–487. doi:10.1080/15298868.2016.1156568

Chapter 4
Creando un Mundo Nuevo (Creating a New World):
Campesinos in the United States

Maritza Y. Duran
University of California, Berkeley, USA

Jason A. Cade
University of Georgia, USA

Alyssa Marquez
University of California, Los Angeles, USA

Gisela Cruz
University of Georgia, USA

ABSTRACT

Farm workers have faced additive barriers with the pandemic and environmental issues that are exceedingly making their jobs more difficult. Coupled with the pandemic, farm workers are facing more obstacles in their everyday life. Despite these challenges, farm workers are finding ways to create organizations and advocacy avenues within their communities. Farm workers are also continuing to keep cultural practices alive and are creating communities where they migrate. These factors are resiliency factors that allow farm workers to create lives that feel meaningful and joyful to them.

INTRODUCTION

Farmworkers have been the main source for sustenance since humans first walked the earth. For instance, indigenous groups in the Americas from pre-Hispanic times developed elaborate farming techniques, many which are still in use today (Adames & Chavez-Duenas, 2017). Thousands of years later, African people were forcibly brought to the Americas, as a result of colonization and their enslavement, where

DOI: 10.4018/978-1-6684-4901-1.ch004

they farmed to produce food for slave-owning families and exports to Europe and the other parts of the Americas (Adames & Chaves-Duenas, 2017). Over time, many factors have transformed farm labor in the United States (U.S.), but one interest, other than the need for sustenance, that has remained constant is keeping an accessible supply of exploitable workers to keep labor costs as cheap as possible. This chapter focuses on the experiences of the farmworker work force today, which is majority Latinx and undocumented. In particular, we call attention to the deep community networks that farmworkers have created to survive and thrive within rural communities, despite the exploitative and racist structures they face.

U.S. farmworkers are often rendered invisible in academic and media discourse. Yet, farmworkers, like the food they produce, are visible to anyone willing to pay attention. When driving through California's Central Valley on State Route 99 or in the rural U.S., generally, traces of their lives can be seen through the open umbrellas, tractors, parked cars, and towns so small that you can miss them if you blink. Their presence in this country can also be understood and felt through the fruits and vegetables they produce, which appear on kitchen tables across the country. As one author of this chapter has previously documented, the *campesinas* in the Central Valley are not so much silent or invisible as they are historically not listened to and ignored by most of U.S. society (Duran, 2022). Systems of exploitation, dating back to colonization and slavery, continue to suppress farmworkers despite their importance to every household in the U.S. (Xiuhtecutli & Shattuck, 2021).

Historic collective advocacy efforts have improved farmworkers' rights and protections. One such effort known as the Delano Grape strike in Delano, California in 1965 brought Mexican and Filipino farmworkers together and led to farmworker access to bathrooms, rest and lunch breaks, and pesticide regulations (Jordan, 2020). Despite these gains, systemic challenges for farmworkers persist. For instance, while many farmworkers have work authorization through the U.S.'s H-2A nonimmigrant visa program, others lack such authorization and are undocumented. Further, while undocumented workers are often better positioned to benefit from community support and information-sharing networks than those temporarily present through the visa program because of their long-term residence, they still face systemic barriers (Yoshikawa, 2011). Nevertheless, both groups experience structural racism and exploitative working conditions, particularly in new-destination areas, where influxes of migrant workers in recent decades have stoked anti-immigrant sentiments (Southern Poverty Law Center, 2021).

While the pandemic replicated past exploitative working conditions, it allowed opportunities for a greater measure of visibility and community-building than ever before. People working on farms quickly became recognized as essential workers in the U.S. as the pandemic caused labor shortages and supply-chain issues. Farmworkers were now seen, and widely reported, as a central and integral part of the U.S. workforce. In turn, this elevated attention highlighted the labor exploitation that farmworkers in the U.S. experience (Sengupta, 2020). Elsewhere, the pandemic revealed–and exacerbated–the lack of accessibility to resources and benefits for farmworkers and their families in the U.S., especially for those who are undocumented. In response, farmworkers have organized for rights throughout the pandemic.

The rural nature of farm working communities, however, has resulted in their experiences of exploitation being understudied. Consequently, not much is known about community networks that farmworkers create to survive and thrive in rural communities to counter the exploitative and racist structures they face. Advocates working in any capacity to support farmworkers should understand and encourage these networks and other forms of resiliency, coping mechanisms, and creation of homes and communities within farm working rural communities (Duran, 2022). Reliance and development of community ties can provide critical support in helping farmworkers and their families navigate structural systems such as the medical and U.S. bureaucratic systems.

Historical Context

The historical account of farmworkers in the U.S. typically begins with the *Bracero* program, a program that began in 1942 because of the labor shortages caused by World War II (Mize & Swords, 2011). This program, based on a partnership between the U.S. and Mexico, facilitated the recruitment of temporary agricultural laborers, most of whom were from rural Mexico (although many were already working in the U.S.). Around four and five million Mexican workers were processed through the Bracero program until it officially ended in 1964.

Although the statutes authorizing the Bracero program sought to ensure humane living and working conditions, along with a minimum wage, government enforcement and oversight over the program was weak; thus, the Braceros faced widespread exploitation, deplorable housing, and racial discrimination (Calavita, 2010). The workers were treated as expendable, and those who protested their working conditions risked losing their job and deportation. (Ngai, 2004; Manzello, 2018). The Bracero program altered migration, and immigration patterns between the U.S. and Mexico. For instance, it altered communities in Mexico and created enclaves in the U.S. It is important to recognize that not all farmworkers are Mexican and are not the only Latinx group affected by U.S. colonialism. In Western New York, Puerto Rican farmworkers organized for their rights in 1966 (Garcia-Colon, 2008). When the U.S. experienced labor shortage, laborers from Puerto Rico were recruited to become farmworkers through labor agents. Therefore, Puerto Rican farmworkers immigrated to the U.S. after the Great Depression and after World War II to aid with labor shortages (Garcia-Colon, 2008). The role of recruitment of labor in Latin America by the U.S. affirms the colonial nature of

Today's farmworkers are still experiencing the legacy of the Bracero program. By the time Congress allowed the program to lapse, the cyclical migration patterns that it had fostered were deeply set and continued for decades (Calavita, 2010). But without even the nominal protections previously provided for by the Bracero program's statutory authority, employers in the post-Bracero era were free to treat noncitizen agricultural laborers as second class and disposable (Manzello, 2018). The current H2A visa guest worker program, and, arguably, discretionary removal forbearance programs like Deferred Action for Childhood Arrivals (DACA), perpetuate government-sanctioned labor colonization within the U.S. (Manzella, 2018; Xiuhtecutli & Shattuck, 2021). In turn, however, the Bracero program and its aftermath were pivotal in leading worker activists and advocates to create the United Farm Workers Association to combat subjugation and exploitation within the farm work industry.

Current Context

Today, there are an estimated 2.4 to 3 million farmworkers in the U.S. (Arcury & Quandt, 2020; Guild & Figueroa, 2018). Data regarding farmworkers in the U.S. is scarce, due in large part to their transient nature and vulnerable experiences (Guild & Figueroa, 2018). These factors present a challenge in ascertaining accurate demographics of farmworkers.

Farmworkers in the U.S. are predominantly of Mexican origin. Some data suggest that 63% of farmworkers in the U.S. are Mexican-born, while 30% were born in Puerto Rico or the U.S (NASW, 2022). In California specifically, roughly 90% of farmworkers were born in Mexico (COVID-19 Farmworker Study (COFS), 2020). New destinations for migrant labor have precipitated significant demographic shifts in the U.S. (Arcury and Quandt, 2020). Arcury and Quandt (2020) indicate that in the Eastern part of the U.S. farmworkers are overwhelmingly Latinx. In the Southeast, 65% of farmworkers are Latinx and 62% of farmworkers in the Southeast region are foreign born (Georgia FarmWorker Health Program Needs Assessment, 2020).

One salient distinction among agricultural laborers concerns migrant farmworkers and seasonal farmworkers. Migrant farmworkers follow crops throughout the country, making them transient workers (Arcury & Quandt, 2020). They further state that seasonal/settled farmworkers only work the season in the area where they live. For the purpose of this chapter, we will generally be discussing farmworkers which encompasses both migrant and seasonal farmworkers. It is important that the reader be aware of the distinction that exists.

The National Agricultural Workers Survey NAWS (2016) estimates that the percentage of farmworkers who are seasonal farmworkers versus migrant farmworkers has grown from 58% in 2002 to 84% in 2013-2014. According to the NAWS, "eighty-seven percent of farmworkers were settled workers, and thirteen percent were migrants" (2018). The NAWS (2018) indicates that settled workers are people who do not follow the crops based on seasons and generally reside 75 miles from their place of work. This suggests that most farmworkers live in a single place for work and do not migrate based on the crop season in the U.S. Some farmworkers work in cold storages, packing houses or receive unemployment if eligible.

The decreased numbers of migrants occupying the temporary agricultural positions in the U.S. can be attributed to multiple factors. Increased militarization of the border, enhanced criminalization and prosecution of unauthorized migration, and close linkages between local law enforcement and federal immigration authorities, all of which dramatically increase the risks for Latinx workers to travel to or within the U.S. (Cade, 2013; 2020; Garcia-Hernandez, 2018; Eagly, 2010; Sreenivasan et al., 2021). The militarization of the U.S.-Mexico border in particular has limited immigrants' abilities to return to their country of birth, drastically curtailing the cyclical migration patterns that characterized the twentieth century.

Despite the fact that more farmworkers tend to live more or less permanently in the locations where they work, only about twenty-one percent are estimated to be legal permanent residents (Guild & Figueroa, 2018). Per the United States Department of Agriculture, 48% of farmworkers in the U.S. currently do not have any work authorization to work in the U.S., while half of farmworkers lacked legal immigration status in the years 2014-2016 (2022). Given the rise of anti-immigrant sentiment in the U.S., the lack of access to resources due to documentation, the rural nature of farm work, and language barriers, undocumented farmworkers are exceptionally vulnerable to exploitation. In areas of the Southeast for example, where there has been a large influx of new migrants in recent decades, many laborers and their families often encounter anti-immigrant sentiment.

Another significant demographic shift that researchers have documented across the country over the last 30 years is the feminization of farm labor in the U.S. and the growing number of women engaging in farm work. Meierotto and Castellano's (2019) pilot research indicates that notwithstanding national demographic data indicating that 66% of farmworkers are male, an estimated half of the farmworker force are female. This demographic shift is mirrored in NAWS (2022), which indicated that 34% of farmworkers identified as female. Meierotto and Castellano (2019) indicated a shift in demographics that will disproportionately impact farm working women's workload within their homes and places of work. They indicate the feminization of the farmworker results from elevated border enforcement and more stringent immigration policies in the U.S.

Farm work is considered one of the most dangerous occupations in the country (Guild & Figueroa, 2018). Some of the dangers include heat stroke, health issues due to pesticide exposure and chronic backbreaking labor, work accidents, and dehydration are some of the few dangers that are often common.

It also provides limited benefits and does not provide stable employment throughout the year due to the seasonal nature of farm work. These features make farmworkers especially vulnerable to occupational exploitation and poverty within their workspaces (Bonner Prado et al., 2018). Despite the incredibly hard labor that farmworkers engage in, they continue to earn minimum wage in the U.S. A recent study of farmworkers in California found that they had a median age of 38 and earned an average of $18,000 per year (COVID-19 Farmworker Study (COFS), 2020). This indicates that most farmworkers live below the poverty threshold. Furthermore, such numbers may not include the full amount of persons that each farmworker is sustaining with their income, within their household or otherwise. Climate dangers, pesticide exposure, and lack of immigration status all contribute to this reality.

Additionally, farmworkers are at high risk of Acute Occupational Pesticide-Related Illness (AOPI) (Bonner Prado et al., 2018). Symptoms related to Acute Occupational Pesticide-Related Illness include teary eyes, runny noses, skin rashes, nausea, and headaches due to pesticide exposure (Arcury & Quandt, 2020). Long-term effects of Acute Occupational Pesticide-Related Illness (AOPI) have included cancer, respiratory problems, neurocognitive decline, reproductive health issues, increased risk of depression, and suicide (May & Arcury, 2020; Agricultural Health Study, 2019). Long-term effects are due to long term and repetitive exposure and impact communities that are chronically exposed to pesticides. Long-term effects without treatment can lead to cancer, neurocognitive decline, depression, and death.

An estimated 88% of AOPI cases are unreported to public health authorities, which makes it challenging to document, treat and rectify when they occur. Lack of reporting often occurs due to the lack of knowledge within communities related to pesticide-induced illness within farm work (Bonner Prado et al., 2018). Because the majority of harmful pesticide exposure and sickness goes unreported, it is difficult to fully appreciate the harmful effects of pesticide exposure among farmworkers. The lack of accurate AOPI reporting also undermines urgency to mitigate pesticide exposure and related illness, as it is not identified as an issue of concern for farmworkers.

Farmworkers also face occupational concerns such as heat stroke and other extreme exposure to inclement weather. Farmworkers in some states have benefited after these states implemented heat standards for farmworkers who work outdoors (Arcury & Quandt, 2020). However, farmworkers in 47 states of the country do not have regulations in regard to inclement weather such as extreme heat despite hot climate conditions being known to cause death within the farm working professions. There are no national regulations protecting farmworkers from heatstroke; the states with regulations include California, Minnesota and Washington (Arcury & Quandt, 2020). Heat stroke deaths can be mis-represented due to comorbidity. California's Office of Environmental Health Hazard (2019) indicates that heat stroke is often mis-diagnosed and preventable, but it is notable that heat stroke associated deaths increase during heat waves. Furthermore, California's office of Environmental Health Hazard (2019) posits that death due to heat stroke is completely preventable with the appropriate precautions such as having shade, drinking water and ensuring that people are not working during excessive heat waves. The authors posit the disproportionate impact climate change will have on farmworkers, and even more so on farmworkers in states where inclement weather regulations do not exist at this time. Furthermore, national regulations for farmworkers is urgently needed as the U.S. is experiencing climate related shifts that will disproportionately impact the health and wellness of farmworkers.

ACTIVISM ON BEHALF OF FARMWORKERS IN THE U.S.

For many decades, researchers and activists have documented the unjust working conditions that farmworkers experience and the broader discrimination and injustices that Mexican and other Latinx immigrants experience in their daily lives. There has been a continuous struggle to protect and advance their rights. In 1950's to 1960's, for example, a farmworker named Cesar Chavez, who himself had experienced these injustices, began advocating for Mexican immigrants. His efforts focused on registering Chicanos to vote; helping those who were eligible to obtain U.S citizenship and pensions; and fighting against both police brutality and the 'urban removal' of Spanish-speaking residents (Hammerback & Jensen, 1998, p. 20). Following the lead of Larry Itliong and Filipino farmworkers, Cesar Chavez also helped organize the Delano grape strike (Grimm, 2009). In 1962, Chavez founded the National Farm Workers Association (NFWA), later known as the United Farm Workers (UFW) with the support of Dolores Huerta and other farmworkers (Grimm, 2009, p. 56). The NFWA was a union that served as a multiracial movement that would result in the creation of UFW and the first contracts for farmworkers in the state of California (Garcia, 2022). The union organized social protests and the most successful consumer boycott in the history of the US, allowing contributions from groups of different ethnic and racial backgrounds (Garcia, 2022). Out of the farmworker movement, Dolores Huerta has continued to organize for migrant farmworkers to register to vote; legalizing one million farmworkers; and the legislation that was passed to get drivers licenses in people's ethnic language (Avalos, 2011). Huerta's work was the prime example of dismantling colonization and fighting for the rights of *la gente y la comunidad*.[1]

Despite years of activism and important historical advances for the justice and health of farmworkers, they currently remain vulnerable to exploitation, oppression, racism, and environmental issues. More recently, during the COVID-19 pandemic, despite being considered essential workers and receiving permission to travel to workplaces during the state's stay-at-home order, farmworkers were still at risk for deportation, exploitative working conditions, and increased exposure to COVID-19 (Xiuhtecutli & Shattuck, 2021). Xiuhtecutli and Shattuck (2021) documented famworkers organizing to fight the lack of protections provided to them. They indicated that many farmworkers who were being exposed to the coronavirus were not being informed about the exposure by their employers, and in some places farmworkers were not being offered any personal protective equipment. Moreover, these types of working conditions and treatment during the pandemic influenced strikes among pistachio plant farmworkers in Wasco, California, and seven fruit packing plants in Yakima Valley. Overall, Xiuhtecutli & Shattuck (2021) express that the farmworkers demanded for basic health and safety protections, as well as hazard pay increase.

Strikes due to Covid-19 and historical strikes specifically highlight farmworker's ability to organize, and utilize their collective power and voices to advocate for themselves. Historically, farmworkers have created change for themselves and their communities. Through their advocacy, they have obtained rights, have been given some protections and have been listened to by society in the past. It is important to note the farmworker advocacy efforts of the past and present have been engineered and ran by farmworkers. Therefore, as practitioners, providers and helpers, it is imperative that we practice listening to farmworkers. As has been posited earlier in this chapter, farmworkers are not silent nor invisible; they have just been unacknowledged by broader U.S. society. Capitalistic practices have served to ignore and render the colonization, oppression and exploitation of these workers as invisible. Through this book chapter, it is imperative to reflect the ways farmworkers are present in and out everyday lives and support for their advocacy efforts that are happening today. On August 3rd, 2022, farmworkers began a march from

Delano, CA to Sacramento, CA to advocate for a union voter rights bill for farmworkers. Bill AB, the Agricultural Labor Relations Voting Choice Act to protect farmworkers in voting.

THE H-2A TEMPORARY WORKER PROGRAM AND UNAUTHORIZED WORKERS

The current Congressionally authorized worker program designed to facilitate temporary work in the agricultural industry is the H-2A program. This program was first enacted in 1986. The use of this program has grown significantly in recent years, with over 204,000 H-2A visas issued in FY 2019 (Arcury & Quandt, 2020). For a time, most H-2A workers were employed in the Southeast, while states in the Southwest continued to rely primarily on undocumented laborers. Currently, usage of the program is widespread throughout the country, although certain states occupy the lion's share of H-2A visas.

The H-2A program sets forth statutory and regulatory protections concerning wages, work conditions, transportation, housing and meals, and workers compensation insurance for foreign born agricultural laborers, which are generally unavailable to undocumented workers. In reality, the Department of Labor's enforcement and oversight of worker protections has fluctuated wildly with changing administrations, and H-2A laborers frequently encounter abuses in their workplaces. Despite this varying level of actual enforcement of worker protections, researchers have found that farmworkers with H-2A visas do typically experience better working and living conditions than those who are undocumented (Arcury & Quandt, 2020). This is congruent with other research on undocumented people's health, work, and living outcomes in comparison to documented people in the U.S. (Asad & Clair, 2017). This distinction is important for advocates working with farm working communities, as documentation status can further impact health outcomes.

Indeed, the large volume of undocumented farmworkers in the country raises acute legal implications. Such workers are typically ineligible for health-related benefits, such as the Supplemental Nutrition Assistance Program (food stamps), health care, disability benefits, and unemployment insurance. Further, in most states they are ineligible for drivers' licenses, which is a key access gateway to many other social determinants of health for workers and their families, particularly in rural areas. A driver's license provides access to employment opportunities, schools, hospitals, churches, grocery stores, parks, and more.

Covid-19 Implications for H-2A Farmworkers and Undocumented Farmworkers

Farmworkers have been disproportionately affected during the Covid-19 pandemic due to multiple factors such as multigenerational households, lack of PPE, and lack of accessibility to resources. For example, in Monterey County, California, the University of California, Berkeley conducted a study that indicated that farmworkers were 4 times as likely to contract COVID-19 between the months of June and November of 2020 (Mora et al., 2021). This study additionally found that agricultural and food workers had a thirty-nine percent increase in risk of death between March-October of 2020.

During the Trump administration, the government initially sought to weaken protections for H-2A workers, and proposed regulations in 2019 that would have set lower wage thresholds. However, when the implications of the COVID-19 pandemic became clearer for the U.S. economy, H-2A laborers were designated as essential workers, and that program continued even as almost all other visa admissions were frozen. Because they were designated as essential, farmworkers were able to keep earning money, but they also faced increased exposure to the coronavirus as they could not work from home. Ultimately, the pandemic has highlighted their vulnerability and lack of infrastructure to sustain their health.

During the pandemic, the federal government implemented two new temporary paid leave programs, emergency Family and Medical Leave Act (FMLA), which was for Covid-19 related needs. The Coronavirus Aid, Relief, and Economic Security Act (CARES) aimed to support U.S. workers during the shut-down that occurred as a direct result of the Covid-19 pandemic (Beatty & et al., 2020). The federal government further created Pandemic Unemployment Assistant (PUA), Pandemic Emergency Unemployment Compensation (PEUC) and Federal Pandemic Unemployment Compensation (FPUC), which unauthorized people were not eligible to access (Kolker, 2020). These relevant aspects of the CARES Act thus excluded undocumented individuals, further excluding unauthorized farmworkers in the U.S. from accessing highly needed services if they became sick or were unable to work during the pandemic. The lack of infrastructure and ability to support farmworkers as they became sick, despite their critical (and officially recognized) value during the pandemic, presents a significant social justice issue.

Farmworkers and Undocumented Farmworkers Mental Health and Strength-Based Factors

As described above, Latinx farmworkers experience multiple systemic issues, including barriers and lack of access to healthcare and support from our society. This section discusses different strength-based factors, including coping mechanisms, protective and resilience factors, that Latinx farmworkers use to navigate these systemic issues that often go unnoticed by researchers and health care providers. Furthermore, the authors suggest using *The Seven Psychological Strengths* when working with Latinx farmworking communities (Adames & Chavez-Duenas 2017, p. 29).

Latinx farmworkers use coping mechanisms to navigate difficult lives and work experiences. We discuss two ways scholarship has shown this to be true. First, Arcury and Quandt (2020) argue that farmworkers often have a fatalistic view of their work, placing their wellness and livelihood in God's hands. This sentiment aligns with Latinx value of *fatalismo* or fatalism. *Fatalismo* is the belief that God is in control and one is to entrust the future to His will. From an outside perspective, fatalism seems like a lack of individual control or surrender. With the Latinx culture fatalism involves surrendering control to God and allows farmworkers to engage in their work in a manner that feels hopeful and entrusting in God's will. This is a strong sentiment that can often be found in the *testimonios* of farm-working women (Duran, 2022).

Second, farmworkers have developed an attitude of *aguantando*, enduring or pushing through a situation so that one can accomplish their responsibility to provide for their families (Arcury & Quandt, 2020). This attitude has allowed farmworkers to cultivate their resiliency and love for their families and community to provide for them. Farmworkers additionally utilize their networks to organize when appropriate and are resourceful. For instance, many switch jobs, or pick and choose what type of farm work they prefer to do such as choosing to either harvest grapes in the summer or working in packing houses or doing other outside work, enduring harsh and dangerous conditions for the good of the family.

Separately, familial and community relationships can be a protective factor for mental health outcomes (Furgurson & Quandt, 2020). Elevated familial stress can be an indicator of higher depression incidence (Roblyer et al., 2016). Family separation among farmworkers can create stress and impact relationships (Furgurson & Quandt, 2020). Research on farmworker stressors have found that family separation and absence of family members leads to higher stress levels and less access to coping mechanisms (Arcury et al., 2016; Grzywacz et al., 2010). These findings indicate that family separation due to the need to do farm work can contribute negatively to health outcomes. Yet, research has found that positive familial relationships and community relationships could mitigate mental health outcomes (Furgurson & Quandt, 2020). Families and communities can also serve as protective factors that mitigate symptoms when it comes to their mental health (Grzywacz et al., 2006). These factors include community building, traveling as a family, and maintaining strong positive relationships in their lives (Grzywacz et al., 2006; Duran, 2022). Marriage can also be a protective factor for farmworkers (Arcury et al., 2016). In sum, these findings enforce the importance of family and community building as protective factors within farm working communities.

Another example of protective factors in practice includes the creation of "rites" (riy-tehs or carpools) within farm working communities. Farmworkers organize "rites" to work, especially if they have to travel long distances. This communal way of approaching work is more economical for farmworkers and helps many who do not own a car get to their job sites. Farmworkers are also mindful of their peers' documentation status or access to a driver's license. Often, those who have access to a car and a driver's license will volunteer to drive others who do not to their job site. This is particularly important for people who live in states that criminalize driving without a driver's license like Georgia. Of course, arrests due to lack of access to a driver's license can lead to arrest and deportation if local law enforcement entities actively work with the U.S. Immigration Customs and Enforcement. This enforcement varies state by state and even within local jurisdictions within those states. Thus, not only do farmworkers carpool to work to save money but they do so to provide each other multiple protective factors. These factors include protections from being pulled over without a license, detained, and being possibly deported. It is important to note that this network of rides exposed farmworkers to a greater risk of contracting COVID-19 because "rites" require, at times, multiple households to share cars. This situation was especially true for those who have worked as essential workers throughout the pandemic. In summary, this type of approach to farm work is part of collective community care that highlights the various forms of farmworker resiliency. In places where driving without a driver's license is criminalized, offering a "rite" is a radical act of community care.

Additionally, Latinx farmworkers are resilient. Resiliency is framed as one's ability to overcome adversity, or difficulty in their everyday lives (Rolnick, 2019). Resiliency can also be posited as someone's ability to manage distress (Rolnick, 2019). In spite of the oppressive experiences that continue to follow from colonization of land and people, farmworkers find creative ways to resist, exist, and build new communities within the U.S. It is important for advocates to understand, draw on, and further develop the coping mechanisms and resistance measures that farmworkers employ. Knowledge of Latinx farmworkers' strengths will allow providers in the U.S. to better serve and address their needs.

In Vermont, Latinx dairy farmers and residents created the nonprofit advocacy organization, Migrant Justice, to address the problems that migrant farmworkers were experiencing in the U.S. dairy farms, especially after the death of Santiz Cruz. Thompson states, "after the death of Santiz Cruz, both migrant farmworkers and Vermonters began to build the foundations of collective agency rooted in a "new collective identity" (p. 134, 2021). The Migrant Justice foundation focused on creating consciousness by informing the community about immigrant farmworkers on Vermont dairy farms and their working conditions. The education provided by the program began collective movements to fight the injustice and expand Migrant Justice's campaigns and programs, such as political campaigns to give drivers' licenses regardless of legal statuses or a Spanish hotline called Teleayuda to assist with labor or human rights violations. Migrant Justice was possible by generating consciousness about Latinx farmworkers' realities and their legitimate rights, such as mobility, health care, better wages and labor conditions, and better housing conditions (Thompson, 2021).

Across the country, in California, a family of indigenous farmworkers created a translating organization for indigenous farmworkers within their hospital and medical system. The creation of this organization was born out of the need for translators within the Central Coast farm working community. Community members identified the language barriers indigenous farmworkers experience in the Central Coast of California (*Herencia Indigena*, 2020). This effort was a community-based solution by the free labor of bilingual community members who were often called upon to translate in medical settings because translating services did not offer translation for some indigenous languages. This organization has created models to compensate indigenous people who are translating to ensure compensation for their skills. The name of this organization is *Herencia Indigena* (2020) and their aim is to address the inequities and inaccessibility to health care services that affect indigenous farmworkers and community members. The Sanchez family created this organization with the help of their eldest daughter who was able to gather data in the community to create a contract with healthcare organizations and integrated health settings in the area. The family was able to identify community needs and apply for grant funding that supported the establishment of bicultural and bilingual translation services to farmworkers from the California Central Coast. More efforts such as this are important in listening to community members needs and appropriately providing linguistic and bicultural healthcare services to community members.

The example of Herencia Indigena is one in which systems listened to grassroots services that were being offered in the area and appropriately responded to community needs. This effort, led by the Sanchez family, shows how resiliency, advocacy, and responsiveness can transform the lives of the community. This example further shows the importance of listening and utilizing existing ways of being to compensate and address needs (*Herencia Indigena*, 2020).

The authors conclude by discussing Adames and Chavez-Duenas's (2017) *The Seven Psychological Strengths of Latinos/as*. We argue that using the seven psychological strengths identified by Adames and Chavez-Duenas can help transform the health treatment of farmworkers. Adames and Chavez-Duenas outline the development of the psychological strengths used by the Latinx community over time, encompassing the dynamic nature and cultures of Latinx people. In doing so, they identify "Determination," "Esperanza," "Adaptability," "Strong Work Ethic," "Connectedness to Others," "Collective Emotional Expression," and "Resistance" as a framework to discuss Latinx people's psychological strengths (2017, p. 29). "The Seven Psychological Strengths" provide a useful approach for working with farm working communities to highlight and build upon existing strength-based mental health treatment.

It is imperative that mental health providers for Latinx farmworkers keep in mind the psychological strengths discussed above. Doing so is important when considering, as this chapter does above, the type of community network developed and relied upon by farmworkers to cope with their mental health while navigating the systemic barriers they confront in their lives and in their work. Accordingly, the authors recommend that practitioners working with farm working people: 1) encourage farmworkers to identify their own resilient and resourceful factors 2) create empowerment by naming the ways that farmworkers are resilient and utilize existing social networks to support their mental health, and 3) create systems that resist existing racist and exploitative structures.

LIMITATIONS OF LITERATURE ON FARMWORKERS AND FUTURE DIRECTIONS

Arcury and Quandt (2020) have found that the demographics of indigenous farmworkers in the U.S. is growing exponentially. A combination of border enforcement, U.S.-Mexico relationships and poverty have been identified as possible contributors to increased demographics of indigenous farmworkers. Therefore, highlighting the additive barriers that some indigenous communities may face as they migrate to the U.S. The indigenous farm working community faces additional barriers such as barriers to care due to language barriers, and colorism. Being indigenous and speaking an indigenous language further limits farmworkers' access to health care or other social services (Arcury & Quandt, 2020). These additive barriers can have great impacts on farmworking indigenous communities in the U.S. An important future direction for research and insight for providers to hold is the lack of research conducted on the experiences, health outcomes, and general information on working with indigenous people who are migrating from other countries to the U.S.

Future directions for care and research with farm working communities is further research on identifying and creating therapeutic interventions and models that address mental health outcomes utilizing farm working communities' resilience factors and psychological strengths (Adames & Chavez-Duenas, 2017). Specifically, more qualitative studies in which the voices of farm working communities are centered through a mental health lens. Additionally, qualitative research in the SouthEast and midwest are additionally important as they are placed in areas of the U.S. that lack protections for farmworkers. Additionally, mental health practitioners knowledge of the law is important in ensuring that practitioners are aware of the laws in place in order to advocate and provide education on farmworkers rights in the U.S.

Furthermore, places like the Southeast and the Midwest do not have standing heat-protective laws. Currently, there is limited research that captures how farmworkers are coping with the lack of protections in these areas. In spite of the lack of protections Arcury and Quandt (2020) indicate that Eastern states do have advocacy groups that are pushing for such protections.

CONCLUSION

This chapter highlighted the intersectional experiences of farmworkers and the exploitation, oppression, and dangers they face in their daily lives. It also focused on resiliency and the creation of communal and systematic systems to overcome these obstacles, urging providers and advocates to understand and build upon these resiliencies and communities.

It is important to distinguish the need to develop resilience in the face of colonialization that farmworkers have experienced. The authors posit that resiliency is a positive coping mechanism that have been developed by Latinx people over centuries of exploitation (Adames & Chavez-Duenas, 2017). It is important to note that despite resiliency factors, farmworkers should not rely on a meritocracy framework to be humanized as people who have been exploited for generations.

Furthermore, as history and current events demonstrate, farmworkers are not silent nor passively accepting of their oppression, although they are infrequently listened to or acknowledged by U.S. society. Their critical role as essential workers in the U.S. economy and food supply during the COVID-19 pandemic provides an important opportunity to focus broader attention on the systems of exploitation and harm that they encounter and must contend with. Providers must find and advocate for solutions that provide a humane path forward for the individuals, families, and communities that provide the food we put on our tables.

REFERENCES

Adames, H., & Chavez-Duenas, N. (2017). *Cultural foundations and interventions in latino/a mental health history, theory and within group differences.* Taylor & Francis.

Agricultural Health Study. (2019). https://aghealth.nih.gov/about/

Arcury, T. A., Laurienti, P. J., Chen, H., Howard, T. D., Barr, D. B., Mora, D. C., Summers, P., & Quandt, S. A. (2016). Organophosphate pesticide urinary metabolites among Latino immigrants: North Carolina farmworkers and fon-farmworkers compared. *Journal of Occupational and Environmental Medicine*, 58(11), 1079–1086. doi:10.1097/JOM.0000000000000875 PMID:27820757

Arcury, T. A., & Quandt, S. A. (2020). *Latinx farmworkers in the eastern united states: Health, safety, and justice.* Springer International Publishing. doi:10.1007/978-3-030-36643-8

Asad, A., & Clair, M. (2017). Racialized legal status as a social determinant of health. *Social Science & Medicine*, 199, 19–28. doi:10.1016/j.socscimed.2017.03.010 PMID:28359580

Avalos, R. (2011). *Lost leader in history: The transforming and empowering partnership of Dolores Huerta & César Chávez.* https://csulb-dspace.calstate.edu/bitstream/handle/10211.14/3/Rebecca%20Avalos.pdf?sequence=1

Beatty, T., Hill, A., Martin, P., & Rutledge, Z. (2020). Covid-19 and farm workers: Challenges facing. *California Agriculture*, 23(5), 2–4.

Bonner-Prado, J., Mulay, P. R., Kasner, E. J., Bojes, H. K., & Calvert, G. M. (2018). Acute pesticide-related illness among farmworkers: Barriers to reporting to public health authorities. *Journal of Agromedicine*, 22(4), 395–405. doi:10.1080/1059924X.2017.1353936 PMID:28762882

Cade, J. (2013). Policing the immigration police: ICE prosecutorial discretion and the fourth amendment. *Columbia Law Review Sidebar*, 113, 182–183.

Cade, J. (2020). "Water is life!" (and speech!): Death dissent, and democracy in the borderlands. *Indiana Law Journal (Indianapolis, Ind.)*, 96(1), 267–272.

Calavita, K. (2010). *Inside the state: The bracero program, immigration, and the I.N.S.* Academic Press.

California office of environmental health hazard assessment. (2019). *Heat-Related Mortality and Morbidity.* https://oehha.ca.gov/epic/impacts-biological-systems/heat-related-mortality-and-morbidity

COVID-19 Farmworker Study (COFS). (2020). *Preliminary Data Brief.* https://cirsinc.org/wp-content/uploads/2021/08/EN-COFS-Preliminary-Data-Brief_FINAL.pdf

Duran, M.Y. (2022). *"Las luchonas" that feed you: Campesinas in the central valley of California.* Academic Press.

Eagly, I. (2010). Prosecuting immigration. *Northwestern University Law Review, 104*(4).

Furgurson, K. F., & Quandt, S. A. (2020). Stress and distress:Mental health among Latinx farmworkers in the eastern United States. In *Latinx farmworkers in the eastern United States: Health, safety and justice* (pp. 83-107). Springer. doi:10.1007/978-3-030-36643-8

Garcia, E. (2021). Blending the gender binary: The machismo-marianismo dyad as a coping mechanism. *Honors Project, 23.*

Garcia, M. (2016). Cesar Chavez and the united farm workers movement. *Oxford Research Encyclopedia of American History.* https://oxfordre.com/americanhistory/view/10.1093/acrefore/9780199329175.001.0001/acrefore-9780199329175-e-217

Garcia-Colon, I. (2008). *Calining equality: Puerto Rican farmworkers in western New York.* CUNY Academic Works.

Georgia Farmworker Health Program. (2019). *Georgia farmworker health program needs assessment. Center for Public Health Practice and Research.* Georgia Southern University.

Grimm, R. T. (2002). *Notable American philanthropists: Biographies of giving and volunteering.* Greenwood Publishing Group.

Grzywacz, J. G., Hovey, J. D., Seligman, L. D., Arcury, T. A., & Quandt, S. A. (2006). Evaluating short-form versions of the CES-D for measuring depressive symptoms among immigrants from Mexico. *Hispanic Journal of Behavioral Sciences.* doi:10.1177/0739986306290645

Guild, A., & Figueroa, I. (2018). The neighbors who feed us: Farmworkers and government policy- challenges and solutions. *Policy Review, 13,* 31.

Guzmán, J. R., & Medeiros, M. A. (2020). Damned if you drive, damned if you don't: Meso-level policy and im/migrant farmworker tactics under a regime of Immobility. *Human Organization, 79*(2), 130–139. https://doi.org/10.17730/1938-3525.79.2.130

Hammerback, J. C., & Jensen, R. J. (1998). *The rhetorical career of Cesar Chavez.* Texas A&M University Press.

IndígenaH. (2020). https://www.herenciaindigena.com/

Jordan, M. (2020). *Farmworkers, mostly undocumented, become 'essential' during pandemic.* https://www.nytimes.com/2020/04/02/us/coronavirus-undocumented-immigrant-farmworkers-agriculture.html

Justice, F. (2013). *Exposed and ignored: How pesticides are endangering our nation's farmworkers.* https://kresge.org/sites/default/files/Exposed-and-ignored-Farmworker-Justice-KF.pdf

Kolker, A. F. (2020). *Unauthorized immigrants' eligibility for COVID-19 relief benefits: In brief.* https://www.everycrsreport.com/files/20200507_R46339_881c6255f6f0c398207472c97e2846375e3a7505.pdf

May, J. J., & Arcuryy, A. (2020). Occupational injury and illness in farmworkers in the eastern united states. In *Latinx Farmworkers in the Eastern United States.* Spring Nature Switzerland AG. doi:10.1007/978-3-030-36643-8

McCurdy, S. A., Stoecklin-Marois, M. T., Tancredi, D. J., Hennessy-Burt, T. E., & Schenker, M. B. (2015). Region of birth, sex, and reproductive health in rural immigrant latino farmworkers: The MI-CASA study: Reproductive health in Latino farmworkers. *The Journal of Rural Health, 31*(2), 165–175. https://doi.org/10.1111/jrh.12083

Meierotto, L., & Som Castellano, R. L. (2019). A case study of transitions in farming and farm labor in southwestern Idaho. *Journal of Agriculture, Food Systems, and Community Development, 8*(4), 111–123. doi:10.5304/jafscd.2019.084.008

Mize, R. L., & Swords, A. C. S. (2011). *Consuming Mexican labor from the bracero program to NAFTA.* University of Toronto Press.

Mora, A. M., Lewnard, J. A., Kogut, K., Rauch, S. A., Hernandez, S., Wong, M. P., Huen, K., Chang, C., Jewell, N. P., Holland, N., Harris, E., Cuevas, M., Eskenazi, B., Camacho, J., Casillas, G., Castro, C., de Vere, M. J., Flores, L., ... Zepeda, L. (2021). Risk factors associated with SARS-CoV-2 infection among farmworkers in Monterey County, California. *JAMA Network Open, 4*(9). doi:10.1001/jamanetworkopen.2021.24116

National Agricultural Worker Survey. (2018). https://www.dol.gov/sites/dolgov/files/ETA/naws/pdfs/NAWS_Research_Report_13.pdf

National Agricultural Worker Survey. (2022). https://www.dol.gov/sites/dolgov/files/ETA/naws/pdfs/NAWS%20Research%20Report%2016.pdf

National Employment Law Project, National Immigration Law Center, & OSH Law Project. (2020). *FAQ: Immigrant workers' rights and COVID-19 -- a resource for Workers and Their Advocates.* https://s27147.pcdn.co/wp-content/uploads/FAQ-immigrant-workers-rights-COVID-19-resource-v-2020-04-10.pdf

Ngai, M. M. (2004). *Impossible subjects: Illegal aliens and the making of modern america.* Princeton University Press.

Ornelas, I., Fung, W., Gabbard, S., & Carroll, D. (2021). *Findings from the national agricultural workers survey (NAWS) 2017–2018: A demographic and employment profile of United States farmworkers.* The U.S. Department of Labor. https://wdr.doleta.gov/research/FullText_Documents/ETAOP2021-22%20NAWS%20Research%20Report%2014%20(2017-2018)_508%20Compliant.pdf

Pinto, K. M., & Coltrane, S. (2013). Understanding structure and culture in the division of household labor for Mexican immigrant families. In S. S. Chuang & C. S. Tamis-LeMonda (Eds.), Gender Roles in Immigrant Families (pp. 43–62). Springer New York. https://doi.org/10.1007/978-1-4614-6735-9_4.

Prado, J. B., Mulay, P. R., Kasner, E. J., Bojes, H. K., & Calvert, G. M. (2017). Acute pesticide-related illness among farmworkers: Barriers to reporting to public health authorities. *Journal of Agromedicine, 22*(4), 395–405.

Roblyer, M. I., Grzywacz, J. G., Suerken, C. K., Trejo, G., Ip, E. H., & Arcury, T. A. (2016). Interpersonal and social correlates of depressive symptoms amoung Latinas in farmworker families living in North Carolina. *Women & Health. Vol., 56*(2), 177–193. doi:10.1080/03630242.2015.108664646

Rolnick, A. C. (2019). Resilience and Native girls: A critique. *BYU L. Rev., 1407*. https://digitalcommons.law.byu.edu/lawreview/vol2018/iss6/8/

Sengupta, S. (2020). Heat, smoke and covid are battering the workers who feed America. *New York Times*. https://www.nytimes.com/2020/08/25/climate/california-farm-workers-climate-change.html

Southern Poverty Law Center. (2021). *Anti-Immigrant*. https://www.splcenter.org/fighting-hate/extremist-files/ideology/anti-immigrant

Sreenivasan, P., Cade, J., & Shahshahani, A. (2021). *Escalating jailhouse immigration enforcement: A report on detainers issued by ICE against persons held by local law enforcement agencies in Georgia, North Carolina, and South Carolina from 2016-2018*. https://www.projectsouth.org/wp-content/uploads/2021/12/120621_Escalating-Jailhouse-Immigration-Enforcement-Report.pdf

Thompson, D. (2021). Building and transforming collective agency and collective identity to address Latinx farmworkers' needs and challenges in rural Vermont. *Agriculture and Human Values, 38*(1), 129–143. https://doi.org/10.1007/s10460-020-10140-7

United States Department of Agriculture. (2022). *Farm Labor*. https://www.ers.usda.gov/topics/farm-economy/farm-labor/#:~:text=In2014-16%2C27percent,ofworkerswhoareU.S.

Xiuhtecutli, N., & Shattuck, A. (2021). Crisis politics and US farm labor: Health justice and Florida farmworkers amid a pandemic. *The Journal of Peasant Studies, 48*(1), 73–98. doi:10.1080/03066150.2020.1856089

Yoshikawa, H. (2011). *Immigrants raising citizens: Undocumented parents and their young children*. Academic Press.

ENDNOTE

[1] "*La gente y la comunidad*" is Spanish for "for the people and community."

Chapter 5
Reclamando Lo Que Nos Arrebataron:
Spiritual Reclaiming and Reconnection

Ana Carina Ordaz
University of Georgia, USA

Jocelyn Jimenez-Ruiz
University of Georgia, USA

Vanessa Placeres
San Diego State University, USA

ABSTRACT

The terms religion and spirituality are used interchangeably and often shown as symbols of strength, resiliency, and resistance among Latinxs with intersecting identities who are impacted by various forms of oppression in their daily lives. The authors will explore the shifts that have taken place in the Latinx population, moving away from predominantly Catholic practices and returning to practices pre-colonization and more Spiritual practices. The authors will weave intersectionality throughout this chapter, highlighting the diversity that exists within the Latinx community, focusing on cultural strengths, resiliency, and decolonization. The chapter will focus on central aspects of spirituality that include the return to indigenous healing practices, coping, and recommendations and implications focused on training through a multicultural lens and highlighting the strengths and growth areas of available interventions and research.

INTRODUCTION

As three Latinas descendants of Nicaragua and Mexico, we use our narratives and understanding of spirituality's significant role in the Latinx community in this chapter. Specifically, we use our lived experiences and those we have witnessed through praxis as healers, mental health therapists, school

DOI: 10.4018/978-1-6684-4901-1.ch005

counselors, professors, and *hijas y nietas de inmigrantes*. Through our bicultural experiences, we highlight the resiliency within the Latinx community. More specifically, we focus on the strengths of these communities, which have served them to survive through slavery, racism, transphobia, homophobia, ableism, genocide, xenophobia, and other experiences of oppression *en lo cotidiano* (Isasi-Díaz, 2002). Latinx communities are returning to indigenous forms of healing, exploring spirituality outside of Catholicism and Christianity, all while newly connecting and strengthening traditional forms of healing that have been in the shadows or completely erased due to colonization and patriarchy (Chavez-Dueñas et al., 2022; Medina & Gonzales, 2019). Mental health professionals must reimagine what incorporating spirituality will look like in practice.

Ana Carina is a first-generation Mexican-American, daughter of immigrants, Georgian and Catholic raised. These salient intersecting identities, along with *Mujerista* Theologies and spiritual *mestizaje*, have informed her spiritual journey. Growing up in a Mexican mixed-status household with "*el Espiritu inmigrante*" (the immigrant spirit), it was a norm to always "*encomendarnos a Dios*" (entrust ourselves to God) to protect us from a roadblock that could lead to deportation and separation of a family system. It was the push to navigate systems fearlessly as a way of resistance and survival. In her family, spirituality and religion allowed them to believe in the ancestral spirits, *Los Santos* (saints) and *el rezo* (prayer), which functioned as a veil to protect the individual, family, and, more importantly, the collective community. Ana Carina's journey through education also made her voice louder, making room for expression that moved away from traditional thinking. Her spiritual journey has unfolded, allowing her to express herself more freely while welcoming this kind of liberating experience in therapeutic spaces.

Jocelyn identifies as a Latina, Nicaraguan-American, and first-generation daughter of immigrant parents. Her spiritual journey was shaped by navigating many systems at home, school, and the Catholic church. Growing up, she frequently heard phrases like "*si Dios lo permite*" or "*Gracias a Dios*" from her mother, grandma, and all *las tías*. Spirituality and "la *relación con Dios*" served as a strong coping and support tool for her and her family when facing adversity, individually or as a whole. Catholic school, youth group, church retreats, and *misa* every Sunday became a staple of her childhood, which allowed her to find her path and create her unique relationship with spirituality.

Vanessa's identity as a Mexican-American is strongly influenced by the polarity in her experiences living in the suburbs of California in a predominately White neighborhood while simultaneously staying connected to her culture through her grandparents lived experiences immigrating from Guadalajara, Mexico and rooting themselves in the United States. Having been raised Catholic but never truly identifying with the practice, most connections to a higher power were through her grandma's spiritual practices like providing the "*bendición*" before leaving the house to protect the family and provide a safe return to the community. Growing up participating in *Posada's,* building *ofrendas* in celebration and remembrance of loved ones, and the habitual practice of the *bendición* created connection to her community and fed her spiritual soul in ways she could not explain while occupying predominately white spaces at home and school. Vanessa's connection to her community and spiritual practices influenced her desire to move away from a Eurocentric way of counseling and changed her conceptualization of healing.

THE CULTURAL SHIFT: HONORING INDIGENOUS SPIRITUAL KNOWLEDGE

There has been an evident cultural shift among Latinxs, as new generations honor Indigenous spiritual knowledge centering in on practices that have been utilized for years. Spirituality is a practice not situated within religious traditions but can be both tangible in ceremonial rituals and abstract as it is influenced by worldviews and attitudes (Hoogasian & Gloria, 2015). It yields an open playing field for more liberating and meaning-making practices that allow the individual and collective to keep the pieces of their spiritual and religious upbringings that make sense for them in their current state. Some people may describe themselves as religious and spiritual. In contrast, others may identify themselves as spiritual but not religious. This is seen in more significant percentages in the Latinx community, where individuals are moving away from Catholicism (i.e., dogmatic practices) and reconnecting to historically marginalized and oppressed religions and spiritual practices (e.g., *Santeria*, Afro-descendant healing practices, Islam, *Espiritismo*) (Pew Research Center, 2014).

Reclamando lo que nos arrebataron (reclaiming what was taken from us) reminds us that the strength and resiliency among Latinxs have always been present, although not without pain. The role of spirituality and religion within the Latinx community plays a significant part in cultural identity, resistance, coping methods, healing, and connection (Bryant Davis & Comas-Diaz, 2016,; Comas-Díaz, 2021; Lee, 2019; NLPA, 2018). Indigenous spiritual practices such as *limpias (*el huevo, sage, palo santo), *danza* (creative prayer through movement of the body), prayer, *remedios*, rituals, *ofrendas*, and *canto* are not new, but decolonized forms of creative expression that are being brought back to life through the awakening of new generations (Medina & Gonzales, 2019). Spirituality among Latinxs also serves a reparative function, allowing the individuals and the collective to connect with sources of healing once deemed abnormal to repress history and erase cultural and ancestral practices (Comas-Diaz, 2021).

We will journey through the various ways that spirituality contributes to the daily lives of Latinxs in the United States. Keep in mind that while the goal is to elucidate how spirituality strengthens the Latinx community, historically, it has also served to oppress already marginalized communities and populations (e.g., LGBTQ+ and women). First, we delve into *a* couple of Indigenous spiritual practices that, through colonization have been syncretized. More specifically, focus on three of the largest syncretized spiritual practices: *Curanderismo, Santeria*, and *Espiritismo*. We also look at the influence of religion on spiritual practice in marginalized communities and how spirituality gives way to acts of resistance, sources of strength, and coping. Lastly, we provide recommendations from the literature on how healers, advocates, and helpers across disciplines can support individuals and communities as they strengthen their connection to spiritual indigenous healing practices.

Indigenous Healing and Practices

Moving away from the imposed Eurocentric values of healing and towards indigenous and spiritual practices is an act of cultural resistance and reconstruction which moves communities towards liberation and decolonized practices. Hoogasian and Gloria (2015) posit *Curanderismo, Santeria*, and *Espiritismo* as the three largest syncretized spiritual practices. *Santeria* and *Espiritismo* are the primary spiritual traditions practiced among Puerto Ricans, Dominicans, and Cubans in the United States (Zerrate et al., 2022). On the other hand, *Curanderismo* is primarily practiced among Mexican communities (Hoogasian & Gloria, 2015; Torres & Hicks, 2016).

Santeria

Santeria, a healing practice based on the West African religion, *Ifa* is a syncretization of Catholic beliefs and African spiritism (Baez & Hernandez, 2001; Hoogasian & Gloria, 2015; Zerrate et al., 2022). Santeria tells a story of cultural resistance, as those enslaved in the Caribbean, newly introduced to Catholicism found ways to keep their deities present by the use Catholic saint names and Catholic religious symbols which allowed them to continue practicing their spiritual practices without fear of punishment or persecution (Baez & Hernandez, 2001; Hoogasian & Gloria, 2015; Zerrate et al., 2022).

Espiritismo

Espiritismo, on the other hand, is not rooted in any religion. Like *Santeria*, the ability to communicate with spirits and *ancestros* for guidance is a shared practice (Baez & Hernandez, 2001; Zerrate et al., 2022). Espiritismo's salient beliefs include *pruebas*, protective spirits that guide one through life. *Brujeria* is sometimes a result of a spell causing good or harm. Spiritualists and practitioners of *Espiritismo* perceive spirits and communicate with them through prayer and group healing (Baez & Hernandez, 2001).

Curanderismo

Curanderismo spiritual practices center on the need to physically, mentally, emotionally, and spiritually balance the self. *Curanderismo* takes on a holistic approach, which offers various specialties that tend to the multi-level needs of a person (e.g., *sobador, huesero, partera, hierbero*). Curanderos also treat non-traditional diagnoses falling into supernatural categories (e.g., *mal ojo, maleficio,* and *enoco*) (Torres & Hicks, 2016).

INFLUENCE OF RELIGION ON SPIRITUAL PRACTICE IN MARGINALIZED COMMUNITIES

Marianismo and Machismo

In most existing literature on Marianismo, Marianismo is defined as an "intertwine of Roman Catholicism and Latino culture, where the Virgin Mary is seen as the absolute role model for adult Latinas and young girls. Specifically, Latinas are expected to be passive, self-sacrificing, and remain pure until marriage" (Morales & Rojas Pérez, 2020). The definition of *Marianismo* goes in hand with the ideology that the female gender role should follow the example laid by the Virgin Mary. Under these expected gender roles, "women are for at home, men are to be out in the streets…women are queens of the home and the incarnation of the values associated with the intimacy of affection and group loyalty. The man, their complementary opposite, must protect from the sacred sanctuary of their family and provide support" (Fuller, 1995, p.1). The traditional gender role involves women being submissive, chaste, selfless, and hyperfeminine. Men have traditional gender roles, ranging from leadership (cabellerismo) to toxic masculinity (machismo). Research has demonstrated that when reinforcing these expected gender roles heavily associated with Marianismo, adverse mental-health outcomes, gender-based violence, and risky sexual behaviors occur more frequently (Morales & Rojas Pérez, 2020). The interplay between traditional gender roles is also rooted in colonialism and excludes feminists, gender non-conformists, LGB people, and trans people.

Despite the common association of Marianismo with Machismo, it is also essential to reflect on the duality of Marianismo itself. More specifically, the Virgin Mary and her dual symbolism. Belief in *Marianismo* can produce mixed results for Latinas. On one end, this ideology can be damaging to Latina women. It is illustrated as if a woman's primary purpose is to fulfill their expected role of mother and wife. This reinforces a sexist lifestyle for young Latina women by restricting them from engaging in sexual behaviors before marriage, willingness to practice more traditional gender roles, remaining pure until marriage, and being in charge of their offspring (Morales & Rojas Pérez, 2020). By following traditional gender roles, young Latina women are limited from going beyond their expected role as a woman instead of being in control of their narrative.

On the other hand, the Virgin Mary can also pose as an image of support and *fortaleza*. Instead of the Virgin Mary's image only representing submissiveness or the "ideal female role," *La Virgen* can also symbolize strength and female empowerment. An example would be the use of marianismo in the fight against Machismo and femicide in all Latin American countries. *Femicide* is defined as killing a girl or woman based on gender (Wright, 2022). To protest, La Virgen is used in activism movements to bring attention to the deaths of numerous women and build empathy. An example of these movements is that of the #NiUnaMenos. Although the #NiUnaMenos movement began in Argentina, it has trickled into many other Latin American countries, especially in the countries with the highest femicide rates, which include Mexico, Brazil, Honduras, El Salvador, the Dominican Republic, and Bolivia (Wright, 2022). By utilizing the image and symbolism of the Virgin Mary as a grieving mother, all Latina women are empowered to go against traditional gender roles and stand in solidarity and the hierarchies of machismo.

LGBTQ+ Communities

Going in hand with aspects of Marianismo and Machismo, it is important to also shed light on how these ideologies can impact other specific populations within the Latinx community. One specific community is that of the LGBTQ+, who are not recognized with a strict traditional gender binary. LGBTQ+ individuals are often viewed as sinners or impure since they go against *lo que Dios manda*. This rejection then leads to a lack of queer representation and lack of acceptance, understanding, and overall support, especially when considering possible negative family opinions on LGBTQ+. This dynamic significantly impacts those who still hold on to their religious or spiritual belief through such sayings as "Love the sinner, hate the sin" which provides judgment and condemnation of LGBTQ+ while in the guise of "loving" them. Within-community microaggressions can further affect any form of closeness and trust felt, or lack of, within existing relationships and can, in turn, impact the ability to seek and accept social support outside of those relationships and among families (Lomash et al., 2018).

Many LGBTQ+ individuals may have been raised with a very strong upbringing around spirituality, which became a vital source of coping and support. This source of support may have also facilitated the individual in learning to accept their true identities and embracing themselves. For many, spirituality paved how they learn to adapt their sense of spirituality, despite what their religion may dictate for/against the LGBTQ+ community. Instead of feeling the need to follow all elements of their faith, one can choose to incorporate whichever element they wish. One has the liberty to follow whichever path of spirituality they most identify with and is more salient to them. In paving their definition of spirituality, one can reconcile their sexuality, religion, and culture without putting any mind to what others dictate as "the norm."

First- Generation

Following the idea that every individual should be free to practice spirituality by their definition, it is also essential to discuss the generational shifts around spirituality and its practices. Triana and colleagues note that although many college students have increasingly identified as more spiritually oriented, they also express less engagement in religious activities (2020). For many first-generation Latinx college students, this may hold true. I resonated with the statement made by Triana and her colleagues because of my (Jocelyn) undergraduate experience and how I navigated through my spiritual journey. I remember feeling overwhelmed with the number of liberties that came with being a college student living on campus away from her parents. I would whisper a prayer to myself before exams, homework, and even leaving my dorm room. I also researched which church I could attend on Sundays to maintain cultural traditions away from home. Despite my efforts, the academic workload increased, my free time disappeared, and my relationship with religion began changing. Despite these changes, I still found myself *rezando* all the prayers my mom had taught me. "*Cuando usted se sienta con miedo, nervio, o que no puede mas... usted dice Que la sangre de Cristo me protega y me ayude*". These *oraciones* were my mom's words that lived in my mind and heart and became prayers I returned to during the most challenging of times. My mom's *oraciones* continue to fill me with peace, calmness, and familial reassurance that everything will be okay. Spirituality was a primary coping skill during my academic career, especially as a woman of color at a predominantly white institution.

Fatalismo

For this chapter, *fatalismo* is defined as a multi-dimensional, culturally based belief in the Latinx community that revolves around predetermination and luck, precisely the idea that our life is out of the control of mortal men (Donner, 2021). More specifically, it is a cultural understanding that our lives, decisions, and destinies are all under the control of God (Arredondo et al., 2014). Even within the Spanish language, anything we manifest, share, or speak into existence includes recognition of God's influence.

Within the Latinx community, it is common to hear cultural references to God, regardless of an individual's religious or spiritual identification, especially within Spanish-speaking communities (Placeres & Ordaz, 2021). This spiritually enriched language represents a historical blend of the Catholic church, indigenous roots, and African religions in Latin America (Delgado-Romero et al., 2021). Common cultural idioms include "*si Dios lo permite*" and "*primero Dios*." Growing up, my mom and grandma reminded me that no day was guaranteed and stressed the importance of God's will or *voluntad*. I (Jocelyn) was so intrigued by God's will and influence in my life and never wanted to test the wrath of God. As an adult, I now recognize how common these cultural idioms and sayings are used in everyday language amongst the Latinx community. The sayings referencing God are predominantly present during life's trials and tribulations (i.e., *eso le pasó por no andar de la mano de Dios*) and if one does not pray or *no lo encomendamos a Dios*, there are commonly fears of punishment or damnation. Despite the fears associated with such cultural practices, using fatalistic language reflects strong values of hope and perseverance within the Latinx community and exemplifies the deeply enrooted relationship with spirituality. The practice of psychospirituality provides protection and strength for many Latinx individuals, especially when facing adversity as members of a marginalized population in the United States.

CULTURAL RESISTANCE AND RECONSTRUCTION: SPIRITUALITY AS A SOURCE OF STRENGTH

When discussing spirituality as a source of strength in the Latinx community, we also make room for protest, resistance, and r/evolution; the Latinx community is growing past survival (Comas-Diaz, 2008). Paloma and Szelenyi (2019) discuss *coloniality of knowledge* as the act of using deceit to impose cultural imperialism as a pathway towards the erasure of cultural and ancestral practices (as cited in Comas-Diaz, 2021). When we discuss spirituality in the Latinx community, we must also name the erasure and colonization of Latinx spirituality rooted in Afro-descendant and Indigenous practices, such as *Santeria, Espiritismo,* and *Curandeirismo* (Baez & Hernandez, 2001). These factors have evolved and been masked and syncretized to fit the mold of acceptability in westernized, white culture in ways that challenge set notions of good and evil. Latinx have always utilized their creative acts of resistance to continue their spiritual practices.

Anzaldua's *La Facultad* is also central as we discuss Latinxs' survival, resistance, resiliency, and *sobresaliendo*. Spirituality serves as a buffer to see the possibility (*Fe, Esperanza*) in situations where the colonizer wanted to see individuals fail and succumb to westernized spiritual practices that center the needs of white supremacy out of instilled fear and pain (Anzaldúa, 2007; Comas-Diaz, 2008). It serves as a source of strength inside and outside of structured institutions. Latinx culture has a deep spiritual base interwoven with symbols and language connected to the various religions practiced throughout. For this reason, the distinction between spirituality from religion continues to be a challenge. While connected to religion, *Que sea lo que Dios quiera* has allowed individuals to take a path of the unknown. At times while seeking ancestral wisdom connected to saints and prayer.

Spirituality as a source of strength can come about in many forms. To illustrate, in a small southeastern immigrant community, spiritual activism and communal solidarity (Bryant Davis & Comas-Diaz, 2016) have transcended religious institutions where many immigrants cannot travel back home when a loved one passes away; the staggering grief of not being able to obtain closure and travel back to their hometown is one beyond the control of the collective community, and to provide some financial relief they engage in a *ceermes*, this usually consists of a community food sale. It is not only a food sale, but a *convivio*, in which meals, tears, prayers, *bendiciones*, and words of motivation are shared. *"Hoy por ellos, manana por nosotros" today for them, tomorrow for us* sends the message that we are okay today, but tomorrow is not promised, encouraging community solidarity during difficult times. The inability to travel back home due to status does not overshadow the ability to *sobresalir*. The cultivations of hope and *fuerza* in the Latinx community can be represented through mindful prayer, building *altares*, and connection to spirits and ancestors, among other spiritual ceremonies. Additionally, making *altares* for loved ones who have passed has been seen throughout the Latinx community in higher numbers creating a window into ancestral knowledge and keeping the spirits of loved ones alive to receive guidance and remain connected (Bermúdez & Bermúdez, 2002).

Furthermore, spirituality allows for liberation and reclaims historical roots (Comas-Diaz, 2008). Comas-Diaz (2008) coined the term *Spirita*, the spirit of liberation among women of color, which promotes gender empowerment, strength, and resiliency, moving away from patriarchal religions that continue to perpetuate oppressive behaviors toward women (Comas-Diaz, 2008). *Spirita* goes beyond women's liberation and is centered on the liberation of all marginalized and oppressed communities. Henceforward, helpers and healers across disciplines must understand how they can continue cultivating sanctuary spaces that welcome all forms of spiritual expression for individuals who decide to step out of their collective communities to seek support.

Spirituality in Healing Spaces

Coping Through Spirituality

Spirituality has evolved as a source of coping and healing for many Latinx people. This is especially true when discussing coping with significant life and traumatic events, Latinxs using spirituality or some aspect of spirituality to heal. Comas-Diaz states, "religious coping is a salient factor for Latinx wellness, longevity, and psychological well-being" (2008). Given that "religious coping" is a salient factor for the Latinx community, it would be beneficial to integrate this coping when discussing the various forms of practicing healing in therapy as clinicians. Spirituality serves as a cultural response to oppression and a way to oppose adversity within the Latinx community (Comas-Diaz, 2008). As described by Comas-Diaz, this cultural response to oppression reinforces the union between spirituality and therapy, which is then better known as psychospirituality. In utilizing psychospirituality, a clinician can provide a healing approach for Latinx clients by integrating Latinx values and existential, liberating, and cultural dimensions into psychotherapy (2008).

One way of integrating Latinx values is through the use of spirituality by incorporating *la Oración*. I, (Jocelyn), recall multiple instances in which my mother told me to *piderle a Diosito que me ayude y illumine en todo lo que necesite*. Spirituality, for many, represents cultural resilience, rescues cultural values, strengthens identity, and ensures historical continuity (Comas-Diaz, 2008). Whenever I faced struggles, felt sad, or wanted extra luck, I would recite a quick prayer or *persignarme*. This practice would give me a sense of comfort and reassurance that someone or something was looking out for me, like a guardian angel. Through the same use of *las oraciones*, I would also reflect on all the *dichos religiosos* my family would use in their everyday language. Even the use of "*primero Dios*", "*sea la voluntad de Dios*", or "*pidele a Papachu*" in all those conversations with my mom, *tía*, or abuelita gave me a sense of hope, comfort, and determination when I was feeling the most down. As we discuss the importance of coping through spirituality and highlight the salient messages received in times of need, it is the healer's responsibility to actively reflect on ways that they can create space that welcome this type of coping.

Healers and Spirituality

As healers, we can contribute to and honor clients' use of spirituality in their daily coping. We will not know everything; therefore, we have a responsibility to go beyond intellectual knowledge and engage actively in ongoing learning experiences. Chavez-Dueñas and colleagues (2022) emphasize the importance of taking historical wounds into account when a healer is engaging with an individual or collective trying to return to their ancestral roots. They discuss it to reach an anti-colonial future yet provide resources that healers and providers across disciplines can use to guide them in this journey with people, not only in the sense of spirituality but in the broader sense of approaching the problem from the root. Furthermore, Captari and colleagues (2018) explained that there are missed opportunities on the psychotherapists' side to explore religion and spirituality, dismissing their critical roles in mental and physical well-being. As a result of this marginalization, clients leave salient identities outside of the therapy room that could cause potential misdiagnosis or a deficit approach to treatment planning.

To fully develop awareness and provide adequate services to clients, the therapist must engage in a reflective process to challenge their notions of spirituality. Individuals across disciplines providing mental health services in the Latinx community, therefore, need to be sensitive to their own experiences as well as seek to understand the following:

1. Internalized anti-Blackness and how this hinders their ability to create sanctuary spaces for clients to practice Afro-descendant spiritual and healing practices.
2. Spiritual and healing practices pre-colonization.
3. The value of spirituality and healing practices within the Latinx community as it fosters mental well-being.

Hoogasian and Gloria (2015) posit the critical need to build psychologist competence in spirituality regardless of how they identify. The authors conducted a study in which they interviewed clinicians of Latina/o descent working with Latino clients to explore how they (1) understand and utilize spirituality in psychotherapy and (2) assess their own experiences, cultural backgrounds, and theoretical orientations within their therapeutic work. The clinicians discussed navigating spirituality and ceremony integration challenges within the therapy room. Additionally, they discussed their concerns about spirituality, social justice, and multicultural competence, as many have noticed the gaps in training to meet the needs of Latinx clients, more specifically concerning spirituality. Lastly, they discuss their use and exploration of spirituality as healers and how this fosters their self-care and clinical work with their clients. Through their learning and unlearning, helpers and healers can either open doors or keep specific communities outside of healing spaces due to lack of training.

Expression of spirituality within Latinxs is woven with diversity. Every client will enter sanctuary spaces at different levels of awareness regarding their spiritual or non-spiritual journey. Understanding and making sanctuary spaces (Chavez-Dueñas et al., 2019) that welcome modalities such as *testimonios*, *cuentos*, rezos, proverbs, greetings, and farewells is vital. Furthermore, healers need to be reflective about their barriers in providing services to welcome the integration of saints, spirits, deities, ancestors, and energies for clients. This is important in their healing journeys (Bryant Davis & Comas-Diaz, 2016). As healers, space must be made for the rediscovery of ancient traditions and beliefs and their exploration of past spiritual traditions. Reclaiming colonized practices can lead to a state of empowerment and liberation. As helpers begin infusing spirituality into their practice, we have several recommendations to aid in the transition to more inclusive healing spaces.

RECOMMENDATIONS FOR INCORPORATING SPIRITUALITY INTO MENTAL HEALTH WITH LATINX CLIENTS

There are several recommendations and clinical implications to consider when infusing spirituality into clinical work and research when working alongside Latinx clients. Spiritual practices are infused into day-to-day practices within the Latinx community, from language to forms of healing and coping with everyday stressors. We believe training is essential to creating a more inclusive and culturally responsive space for Latinx clients. Mental health programs need to move away from relying solely on multicultural counseling competencies and begin approaching training through cultural democracy and promoting preferred forms of healing over Eurocentric counseling models. Cultural democracy centers on localized culture and the cultural diversity of a community and finds ways to engage in cultural expression (Conrad, 2015).

Additionally, training programs should embed the tenets of cultural humility by stressing the significance of taking an other-oriented approach where cultural diversity is centered in therapeutic work (Placeres & Ordaz, 2021). Taking an other-oriented approach will help provide trainees with tools to broach conversations about how spirituality shows up in a client's life. Centering cultural humility will provide trainees with language and tools to explore its significance and provide space for preferred forms of healing in psychotherapy (Hook et al., 2019).

Our clinical recommendations stem from our experiences providing psychotherapy in the Latinx community and literature that documents the lack of spirituality in treatment as a barrier to seeking services (Turner & Llamas, 2017). In my first year as a counselor after graduate school, I (Vanessa) realized many of the counseling techniques learned were not serving the community I was working with. Asking questions using academic jargon like "what can you do to cope with emotional distress and triggers" served as a barrier between my clients and me. I was operating from a Eurocentric lens and relied on what was taught in the classroom versus my lived experience as a Latina and what I knew about healing. I quickly realized I was the issue and that my training did not prepare me to prioritize preferred forms of healing like prayer. I had to unlearn and relearn what it meant to be a helper within the Latinx community and believe doing so served as an act of rebellion against a system and curriculum not designed to educate or serve people like me, a Mexican American first-generation student attempting to do counseling from a Eurocentric lens.

Our primary clinical recommendation is that Latinx people deserve a culturally and linguistically responsive mental health provider. While cultural matching is important, it is not necessary to provide culturally responsive care (Placeres & Ordaz, 2021), especially considering psychotherapy is still a White-dominated profession, with 61% identifying as White (Non-Hispanic) (DataUSA, 2017). Using the multicultural orientation framework (MCO) can help providers operate from a culturally responsive space. The MCO framework has three central tenets (cultural humility, cultural opportunity, and cultural comfort) (Owen et al., 2017). Cultural humility can be defined as taking an other-oriented approach to cultural dialogue and remaining curious about the client's lived experiences. Cultural opportunities address the clinician's willingness and ability to lean into conversations about culture and create space to explore spirituality and the intersection of other identities the client holds. Finally, cultural comfort addresses the level of comfort or discomfort experienced during the exploration of cultural opportunities in session (Owen et al., 2017). Taken together, the variables in the MCO framework provide clinicians with action steps to navigate cultural dialogue and a foundation to operate from a more culturally responsive place.

Receiving culturally responsive supervision is also recommended when working with Latinx clients. Clinical supervisors are responsible for the personal and professional development of their supervisees' which makes their job addressing spirituality in supervision especially significant to professional growth (Perry & Sias, 2018). Regarding language in supervision and cultural idioms, it is important to understand that not all Latinx clients speak Spanish, and linguistic adaptations should be considered when working with a bilingual supervisee (Cotter & Jones, 2020). Although language matching may not always be possible, it is important to have a knowledge and understanding of spiritual and cultural idioms used in session (e.g., "*ataque de nervios*") and the mental processing required for supervisees' to provide services in one language and seek consultation in another (Perry & Sias, 2018). With the noted increase in spiritual issues in session, supervisors need to be intentional about addressing spirituality in supervision (Polanski, 2003). Supervisors need to have a working understanding of the client's clinical needs in relation to the clinician's knowledge and skill and the supervisees' professional development (Polanski, 2003). To achieve these goals of supervision, we recommend that supervisors provide a space for supervisees to reflect on their personal values and belief systems as they attend to their client's spiritual needs (Polanski, 2003).

Additionally, Latinx participants are significantly underrepresented in mental health literature (Cheng & Sue, 2014). The studies that do include Latinx participants use the term Latinx/Hispanic interchangeably. This has led to the homogenization of different ethnicities and the generalization of findings despite participants identifying with only a few of the many ethnicities (e.g., Mexican, Dominican, Cuban) within the Latinx/Hispanic community (Lombana, 2021). One recommendation is to include underrepresented groups within the Latinx population in the research process. It is also important to note the history of the empirical process, the oppressive nature of research, and how it has impacted trust within the Latinx community and the health care system, including the mental health profession (Proulx et al., 2018). We believe the Latinx community deserves the right to question the intent of social science research and believe it is the job of the researcher to earn trust and dismantle barriers and access to mental health services.

Another important recommendation is clearly defining and distinguishing the difference between religion and spirituality within the literature. It is essential to note the shifts that have taken place within the Latinx community as it relates to spiritual practices and create space for all preferred forms of healing in research. In recent years many Latinx individuals have moved away from Catholicism and returned to pre-colonization practices (Calvillo & Bailey, 2015). However, in taking stock of the current literature, many scholars use religion and spirituality interchangeably despite their differences and do not provide open-ended questions to address participants' spiritual or religious affiliations (Zinnbauer et al., 2015). Scholars must be intentional in capturing the variability of spiritual identification. This specificity will help determine what forms of spirituality are used as coping mechanisms and for what populations. Scholars must explore the variability in spirituality as an individual construct related to mental health, coping, and healing to avoid further homogenization of research within the Latinx community.

CONCLUSION

In this chapter, we discussed the importance of recognizing the difference between religion and spirituality and the journey back to indigenous forms of healing within the Latinx community. It is important to note that when incorporating spirituality into mental health services treatment is not a one-size fits all approach as the Latinx population is not a monolith. As clinicians and scholars begin infusing more spiritual practices into psychotherapy, it is necessary to continue unlearning and relearning ways to provide care and conduct research that is not rooted in westernized white norms. The dominant culture has set the standard for healing, and like other authors, we believe it is essential and necessary to reimagine the therapeutic space (Lombana, 2021). We believe prioritizing preferred forms of healing and including spiritual practices in psychotherapy will help increase access and utilization of mental health services amongst the Latinx community and create more inclusive healing spaces.

REFERENCES

Anzaldúa, G. (2007). *Borderlands : the new mestiza = La frontera* (3rd ed.). Aunt Lute Books.

Arredondo, P., Gallardo-Cooper, M., Delgado-Romero, E. A., & Zapata, A. L. (2014). *Culturally responsive counseling with Latinas/os*. American Counseling Association.

Baez, A., & Hernandez, D. (2001). Complementary spiritual beliefs in the Latino community: The interface with psychotherapy. *The American Journal of Orthopsychiatry, 71*(4), 408–415. doi:10.1037/0002-9432.71.4.408 PMID:11822213

Bermúdez, J. M., & Bermúdez, S. (2002). Altar-making with Latino families: A narrative therapy perspective. *Journal of Family Psychotherapy, 13*(3/4), 329–347. doi:10.1300/J085v13n03_06

Bryant-Davis, T., & Comas-Díaz, L. (2016). Womanist and mujerista psychologies: Voices of fire, acts of courage (T. Bryant-Davis & L. Comas-Díaz, Eds.). American Psychological Association. doi:10.1037/14937-000

Calvillo, J. E., & Bailey, S. R. (2015). Latino religious affiliation and ethnic identity. *Journal for the Scientific Study of Religion, 54*(1), 57–78. doi:10.1111/jssr.12164

Captari, L. E., Hook, J. N., Hoyt, W., Davis, D. E., McElroy, H. S. E., & Worthington, E. L. (2018). Integrating clients' religion and spirituality within psychotherapy: A comprehensive meta-analysis. *Journal of Clinical Psychology, 74*(11), 1938–1951. doi:10.1002/jclp.22681 PMID:30221353

Chavez-Duenas, N. Y., Adames, H. Y., & Perez-Chavez, J. G. (2022). Anti-colonial futures: Indigenous Latinx women healing from the wounds of racial-gendered colonialism. *Women & Therapy, 45*(2-3), 191–206. Advance online publication. doi:10.1080/02703149.2022.2097593

Chavez-Dueñas, N. Y., Adames, H. Y., Perez-Chavez, J. G., & Salas, S. P. (2019). Healing ethno-racial trauma in Latinx immigrant communities: Cultivating hope, resistance, and action. *The American Psychologist, 74*(1), 49–62. doi:10.1037/amp0000289 PMID:30652899

Cheng, J. K. Y., & Sue, S. (2014). Addressing cultural and ethnic minority issues in the acceptance and mindfulness movement. In A. Masuda (Ed.), *Mindfulness and acceptance in multicultural competency: A contextual approach to sociocultural diversity in theory and practice* (pp. 21–37). New Harbinger Publications, Inc.

Comas-Diaz, L. (2008). 2007 Carolyn Sherif award address: Spirita: Reclaiming womanist sacredness into feminism. *Psychology of Women Quarterly, 32*(1), 13–21. doi:10.1111/j.1471-6402.2007.00403.x

Comas-Díaz, L. (2008). Latino psychospitituality. In K. J. Schneider (Ed.), Existential-integrative psychotherapy: Guideposts to the core of practice (pp. 100–109). Routledge/Taylor & Francis Group.

Comas-Diaz, L. (2021). Afro-Latinxs: Decolonization, healing, and liberation. *Journal of Latina/o Psychology, 9*(1), 65–75. doi:10.1037/lat0000164

Conrad, D. (2015). Education and social innovation: The youth uncensored project—A case study of youth participatory research and cultural democracy in action. *Canadian Journal of Education/Revue Canadienne de L'éducation, 38*(1), 1-25.

Cotter, E. W., & Jones, N. (2020). A review of Latino/Latinx participants in mindfulness-based intervention research. *Mindfulness, 3*(3), 529–553. doi:10.100712671-019-01266-9

DataUSA. (2017). *DataUSA: Counselors*. https://datausa.io/profile/soc/211010/#demographics

Delgado-Romero, E. A., Mahoney, G.-E., Muro-Rodriguez, N. J., Atilano, R., Cárdenas Bautista, E., De Los Santos, J., Durán, M. Y., Espinoza, L., Fuentes, J., Gomez, S. N., Ingram Estevez, R. E., Jimenez-Ruiz, J., Monroig Garcia, M. M., Mora-Ozuna, C. J., Ordaz, A. C., Rappaport, B., Suazo-Padilla, K., & Vazquez, M. (2021). La Clinica In LaK'ech : Establishing a practicum site integrating practice, advocacy, and research with Latinx clients. *The Counseling Psychologist, 49*(7), 987–1012. doi:10.1177/00110000211025270

Donner, P. (2021, August). *Fatalismo beliefs as a oderator of the relationship between financial stress, depression, anxiety, and life satisfaction among Latinx college students*. Texas Tech University Libraries. https://ttu-ir.tdl.org/handle/2346/87843

Fuller, N. (1995). *Acerca de la polaridad marianismo machismo. Lo femenino y lo masculino: Estudios sociales sobre las identidades de género en América Latina*. Third World Editions & Ediciones Uniandes.

Hoogasian, R. O., & Gloria, A. M. (2015). The healing powers of a patron espiritual: Latina/o clinicians' understanding and use of spirituality and ceremony in psychotherapy. *Journal of Latina/o Psychology, 3*(3), 177–192. doi:10.1037/lat0000045

Hook, J. N., Captari, L. E., Hoyt, W., Davis, D. E., McElroy, S. E., & Worthington, E. L. Jr. (2019). Religion and spirituality. In J. C. Norcross & B. E. Wampold (Eds.), *Psychotherapy relationships that work: Evidence-based therapist responsiveness* (pp. 212–263). Oxford University Press. doi:10.1093/med-psych/9780190843960.003.0008

Isasi-Diáz, A. M. (2002). Lo cotidiano: A key element of mujerista theology. *Journal of Hispanic/Latino Theology, 10*(1), 5–17.

Lee, C. C. (2019). *Multicultural issues in counseling : new approaches to diversity* (5th ed.). American Counseling Association.

Lomash, E. F., Brown, T. D., & Galupo, M. P. (2018). "A whole bunch of love the sinner hate the sin": LGBTQ microaggressions experienced in religious and spiritual context. *Journal of Homosexuality, 66*(10), 1495–1511. doi:10.1080/00918369.2018.1542204 PMID:30475163

Lombana, Y. (2021). Possibilities and challenges in providing psychotherapeutic interventions to meet the needs of the Latinx population in the United States. *Genealogy, 5*(1), 12. doi:10.3390/genealogy5010012

Medina, L., & Gonzales, M. R. (Eds.). (2019). *Voices from the Ancestors: Xicanx and Latinx spiritual expressions and healing practices*. University of Arizona Press. doi:10.2307/j.ctvq4c07x

Morales, A., & Pérez, O. F. R. (2020). Marianismo. The Wiley Encyclopedia of Personality and Individual Differences: Clinical, Applied, and Cross-Cultural Research, 247-251.

NLPA. (2018). *Ethical guidelines national Latina/o psychological association*. https://www.nlpa.ws/assets/docs/ethical%20guidelines%20nlpa_adopted%20jan%201st.pdf

Owen, J., Drinane, J., Tao, K. W., Adelson, J. L., Hook, J. N., Davis, D., & Fookune, N. (2017). Racial/ethnic disparities in client unilateral termination: The role of therapists' cultural comfort. *Psychotherapy Research, 27*(1), 102–111. doi:10.1080/10503307.2015.1078517 PMID:26390171

Perry, V. M., & Sias, S. M. (2018). Ethical concerns when supervising Spanish-English bilingual counselors: Suggestions for practice. *The Journal of Counselor Preparation and Supervisor*, *11*(1), 10.

Pew Research Center. (2014, May 7). *The Shifting Religious Identity of Latinos in the United States*. Pew Research Center. https://www.pewresearch.org/religion/2014/05/07/the-shifting-religious-identity-of-latinos-in-the-united-states/

Placeres, V., & Ordaz, A. C. (2021). Religion and spiritual concerns to consider when using mindfulness interventions with Latinx/Hispanic clients. *Journal of Psychology and Christianity*, *40*(2), 143–150.

Polanski, P. J. (2003). Spirituality in supervision. *Counseling and Values*, *47*(2), 131–141. doi:10.1002/j.2161-007X.2003.tb00230.x

Proulx, J., Croff, R., Oken, B., Aldwin, C. M., Fleming, C., Bergen-Cico, D., & Noorani, M. (2018). Considerations for research and development of culturally relevant mindfulness interventions in American minority communities. *Mindfulness*, *9*(2), 361–370. doi:10.100712671-017-0785-z PMID:29892321

Torres, N., & Hicks, J.F. (2016). Cultural awareness: Understanding Curanderismo. *Ideas and Research You Can Use: VISTAS 2016*.

Triana, C., Gloria, A. M., & Castellanos, J. (2020). Cultivating success for Latinx undergraduates: Integrating cultural spirituality within higher education. *About Campus: Enriching the Student Learning Experience*, *24*(6), 4–9. doi:10.1177/1086482219896793

Turner, E. A., & Llamas, J. D. (2017). The role of therapy fears, ethnic identity, and spirituality on access to mental health treatment among Latino college students. *Psychological Services*, *14*(4), 524–530. doi:10.1037er0000146 PMID:29120210

Wright, A. (2022). Femicide in Latin America: Reimagining Catholic symbolism in the pursuit of justice. *The Theology Journal of Boston College*, *1*(2), 125–139.

Zerrate, M. C., VanBronkhorst, S. B., Klotz, J., Caraballo, A. A., Canino, G., Bird, H. R., & Duarte, C. S. (2022). Espiritismo and Santeria: A gateway to child mental health services among Puerto Rican families? *Child and Adolescent Psychiatry and Mental Health*, *16*(1), 1–10. doi:10.118613034-022-00439-0 PMID:35016702

Zinnbauer, B. J., Pargament, K. I., Cole, B., Rye, M. S., Butfer, E. M., Belavich, T. G., Hipp, K., Scott, A. B., & Kadar, J. L. (2015). Religion and spirituality: Unfuzzying the fuzzy. *Journal for the Scientific Study of Religion*, *36*(4), 549–564. doi:10.2307/1387689

Chapter 6
Madrinas Paving the Way:
Understanding the Development of Latinx Feminism

Kiara Manosalvas
Teachers College, Columbia University, USA

Brooke Rappaport
Tennessee State University, USA

Lucia Quezada
 https://orcid.org/0000-0002-7305-7070
University of Georgia, USA

Grace-Ellen Mahoney
University of Maryland, USA

ABSTRACT

This chapter provides an overview of the history of Latinx feminism. It includes a brief history about Latinx feminist leaders and the development of feminism including womanism, Black feminism, mujerismo, and womanista. The chapter includes ways in which Latina feminism highlights indigenous ways of knowing including mestiza consciousness, borderlands, and nepantla. This chapter sets the groundwork for the authors to explore contemporary perspectives on Latinx feminism including their own feminist identity developments in another chapter.

"Racism in Latin America is sophisticated enough to keep Blacks and Indians in the subordinate condition within the most exploited class, because its most effective form of ideology: the ideology of whitening, so well analyzed by Brazilian scientists. Transmitted by means of communication and the traditional ideological systems, it reproduces and perpetuates the belief that the ratings and values of white West-

DOI: 10.4018/978-1-6684-4901-1.ch006

ern culture are the only true and universal. Once established, the myth of white superiority proves its efficiency and the effects of violent disintegration, fragmentation of ethnic identity produced by him, the desire to whiten ("cleaning the blood" as they say in Brazil), is internalized with the consequent denial of their own race and own culture." (Lèila Gonzalez, 1988, p. 15, translated from Portuguese)

BRIEF HISTORY

History is filled with many examples of Latinx leaders whose activism contributed to the rise of a new, more radical feminism – a feminism that honored and centered the unique experiences of women of color. Latinx feminists such as Gloria Anzaldúa, Dolores Huerta, Cherríe Moraga, Florinda Soriana Muñoz, Yolanda Guzmán, Ana Livia Cordero, Lèila Gonzalez, and several others had a profound impact on future generations of Latinx people. Through story-telling, political activism, and artistry, these influential Latinx feminists began spreading an important message and opened the door for future Latinx feminists (Charleswell, 2014; The Latina Feminist Group, 2001).

Unfortunately, the influence of these powerful women is often minimized when Latinx history is taught. This suppression of history and knowledge is not accidental; instead, it is a systemic suppression of history used to manipulate marginalized communities into participating in their own oppression (Chavez-Dueñas & Adames, 2021). For example, in contemporary Latinx culture, *marianismo* refers to the gender-role expectations placed on Latinx women and the associated behaviors, norms, and guidelines that they are then expected to fulfill. Specifically, marianismo emphasizes self-sacrifice, self-denial, subjugation, honor, nurturance, humility, and chastity (Comas-Diaz, 1988; Ginorio et al., 1995; Gil & Vasquez, 1996). Marianismo has become an incredibly powerful tool of gender oppression amongst Latinas that reinforces a strict binary socialization of gender identity (i.e., male vs. female) and sexual orientation (i.e., heterosexuality; Chavez-Duenas & Adames, 2021). However, marianismo as a gender ideology did not even exist within Latinx culture until the Spanish colonized the Americas. The Spanish enforced these ideas of marianismo (and later institutionalized these beliefs via oppressive, misogynist laws) as a tool of colonization to silence and disempower Latinx women. One of the most insidious ways the Spanish did this was by socializing Latinx women to develop a profound reverence for the Virgin Mary. The Virgin Mary was described as "the worker in the home, the self-sacrificing woman, the balance of motherhood and purity" (Baldwin & DeSouza, 2001, p. 10). Consequently, Latinx women were socialized to believe that being a "good woman" meant behaving just as Virgin Mary would. And so, began the erasure of the powerful, revered Latinx woman.

Understanding the impact of colonization and gendered racism on Latinx women is critical, but what is just as important (yet often dismissed) is a discussion of how Latinx and Indigenous women were regarded prior to Spanish imperialism. Pre-colonial accounts of women in Latin America demonstrate that they were revered and seen as powerful, with many women serving in high leadership positions (Chavez-Duenas & Adames, 2021). For example, Aztec culture enforced laws that ensured that both women and men received equal shares in economic inheritance. Andean culture reinforced that women had rights to all inherited and acquired goods and property, regardless of marital status. Unfortunately, the Spanish could not tolerate the political, religious, and economic power that Latinx women held in society, and thus began the gendered-racism that diminished and silenced women. This gendered-racism was later institutionalized via laws that prevented women from obtaining their own property. Under these same laws imposed by the Spanish, all married women were classified as legal minors, meaning a married woman could not engage in any kind of financial transaction (e.g., earning their own assets) without their husband's permission (Chavez-Duenas & Adames, 2021).

Latinas are descendants of brilliant, strong, and powerful women, yet the erasure of their stories from our history creates a "myopic and inaccurate historical account of traditional Latinx culture as requiring women to be quiet, self-sacrificial, and submissive" (Chavez-Dueñas & Adames, 2021, p. 97). Understanding history – the unedited version – allows individuals to learn about themselves and their group's past while contextualizing this history with present-day strengths, challenges, and realities. We cannot understand the present if we do not study the past.

AFRO-LATINX FEMINISM

Florinda Soriano Muñoz

Florinda Soriana Muñoz (1921-1974), affectionately known in her community as Mamá Tingó, was an Afro-Latina activist who fought for farmer's rights in the Dominican Republic.

Muñoz grew up in a farming community with no opportunity for formal education. When she turned 30, she married another farmer and was gifted a small piece of land by her father-in-law for her to do her own farming in the Hato Viejo region of the Dominican Republic. In 1974, Muñoz learned that several families in her community, including her own, were losing their generational land through illegal land seizures due to the greed of major landowner Pablo Diaz Hernandez. Unwilling to let Hernandez take advantage of her community, Muñoz joined the Christian Agriculture Leagues and quickly became a prominent leader within the organization, organizing large farmer protest rallies and rising against established power (Vaughan, 2020)

The Dominican government felt threatened by Muñoz's influence and leadership and went on to deem these protests illegal. In order to discredit Muñoz's leadership, they began calling her an uneducated, radical, dark-skinned Dominican. Despite these barriers, she continued to fight for farmer's rights and her community continued to stand beside her at protests. Recognizing Muñoz's influence, the government decided to grant her a court hearing to listen to her land complaints. However, on the same day of the court hearing, Hernandez – the greedy landowner Muñoz was fighting back against – hired an assassin who killed Muñoz in her own home (Vaughan, 2020).

Devastated and angered by the death of this revolutionary woman, Muñoz's community went to the streets to protest her death. The public outcry forced the Dominican government to return the stolen land that Hernandez had taken from over 300 impoverished farmers. Muñoz may not have been alive to witness the impact of her activism, but she is honored with a statue in Monte Plata in the Dominican Republic and remembered as a fierce resistance leader (Vaughan, 2020).

Yolanda Guzmán

Yolanda Guzmán (1943-1965) was a young Afro-Latina activist in the Dominican Republic who worked for the Bosch administration, a political party that had been democratically elected after the assassination of vicious dictator Rafael Trujillo. Both of Guzmán's parents were fierce anti-Trujillistas and she eagerly followed in their footsteps. Documentation of her activist work is limited due to the repressive nature of Trujillo-era politics (activists often faced the threat of torture, imprisonment, or death), but it is known that she worked in the women's division within the Bosch administration where she likely helped with weapons training, cared for the wounded, managed funds and food going in and out of the capital, buried the dead, and instructed other combatants.

She was tragically killed at the young age of 21 during the U.S. invasion of the Dominican Republic in 1965. Many Dominicans believe that Guzman was assassinated by the *Centro de Enseñanza de las Fuerzas Armadas* (the federal branch of military education under the dictatorship). She was one of several Black women who engaged in armed combat for the struggle against imperialism and is remembered as a martyr in the fight for Dominican independence (Maiorana, 2021).

Ana Livia Cordero

Ana Livia Cordero, M.D. (1931-1992) was a Puerto Rican physicist and anti-imperialist activist who was committed to Puerto Rican independence. After graduating from Columbia University Medical School in 1953, she returned to her homeland Puerto Rico to advocate for rural communities on the island. Upon her return to Puerto Rico, she conducted a study on how to provide adequate medical services to poor rural communities (Cordero, 1979).

In 1967, she organized the Proyecto Piloto de Trabajo con el Pueblo (Pilot Project of Work with the People), a political organizing initiative that dedicated itself to bringing liberation to Puerto Rico's most exploited and marginalized communities. Cordero was critical in her activism, making explicit the link between racism and colonialism in the development of capitalism. Her activism eventually caught the attention of the Puerto Rican government; one year later, in 1968, Cordero was arrested by Puerto Rican police and accused of attempting to incite a revolution. She continued to fight for Puerto Rican independence but as a result of her arrest, she was forced to limit her public activism to underground work. However, Cordero continued to stay involved in several Caribbean and international efforts to support the Central African revolution during the 1980s (Placido, 2017).

Lèila Gonzalez

Lèila Gonzalez, Ph.D. (1935-1994) was one of the most celebrated Black feminist-activists in Brazil. She was a prolific writer whose work is often compared to Angela Davis and is known for being one of the first Black women to earn a Ph.D. in Anthropology. She traveled extensively throughout the Americas giving lectures about the struggles and resiliency of Black Brazilians. In one of her most famous essays, "The Black Woman: A Portrait (1979)," she uses her own experience as a poor Black woman living in Rio de Janeiro to illustrate how gender oppression and classism contributed to racial inequality. She goes on to criticize the inadequate education systems for Brazil's most marginalized youth, the inhumane treatment within medical institutions, as well as the precarity of Black urban life (de Sant'Anna Machado & Perry, 2021).

One of the most salient themes within *The Black Woman: A Portrait* speaks to the struggles faced by mothers as they navigate life unemployed or making low-wages. Gonzalez highlights the lack of labor rights that existed for Black women and how this lack of legal protection often led to exploitation or sexual violence as they attempted to find work. Given the Brazilian government's negligence towards Black women, Gonzalez shares how these women had no choice but to create a new kind of social system, one that allowed them to feel protected and cared for. She asserts that Black women in Brazil created a system built off of favors and kindness, a system meant to obscure the violence that existed outside of their community of women. While translating Gonzalez's essay, Sant'Anna Machado and Perry (2021) assert that the key question Gonzalez is asking her readers throughout her writing is, "Who is caring for Black women and ensuring their survival individually and collectively?" (p. 41). It is this unapologetic demand that we must protect the livelihood of Black women that makes Gonzalez a legacy.

CHICANX FEMINISM

Gloria Anzaldúa

Gloria Anzaldúa (1942-2004) was a self-described "chicana dyke-feminist, tejana patlache poet, writer, and cultural theorist" (Keating & Anzaldúa, 1993, p. 105) who transformed how a generation thought about issues of identity, history, culture, and sexuality. Anzaldúa was born to sharecropper/fieldworker parents in the South Texas Rio Grande Valley. Her family eventually moved to Hargill, Texas, a city near the Mexico/Texas border. She has written extensively about navigating the racial discrimination and violence Mexican Americans often encountered in her home state. She loosely based her best-known book, *Borderlands/La Frontera: The New Mestiza* (1987), on growing up on the Mexico–Texas border. Anzaldúa was a talented writer for many reasons, but one major reason why her writing is so loved is because she never shied away from incorporating her lifelong experiences of social and cultural marginalization into her work. Her writing showed readers that the personal is indeed political and that there is tremendous strength in using our personal narratives to create social change. For example, her experience of attending segregated schools as a child in Texas deeply impacted her racial identity and it was integrated as a major topic of focus in her book (Anzaldúa, 1987). *Borderlands* has been cited by numerous Latinx feminists, especially in the field of psychology, as being the most influential work in their own feminist identity development (Delgado-Romero & Romero-Shih, 2016).

In *Borderlands* (1987), Anzaldúa discussed the concept of *mestizaje,* the exchange of cultural ideals from one group to another, the navigation of "the borderlands" between two cultures, and the development of *la conciencia de la mestiza* (Anzaldúa, 2007; Martinez, 2000; The Latina Feminist Group, 2001). The concepts of *mestizaje* and the borderlands accounts for various intersecting identities such as social class, race, gender, indigenous heritage, and national origin that influences one's Latina and feminist identity development (Gillman, 2010).

Moreover, Anzaldúa switches between English and Spanish throughout the text in *Borderlands (1987)*. By doing this, she intentionally makes it difficult for non-bilinguals to read; as a child, Anzaldúa had to learn English once she started school and felt the barriers experienced by people who do not speak English. She wanted her readers to feel the frustration of not being able to understand what was happening around them due to language barriers. While Anzaldúa eventually gained fluency in English, she never allowed herself to lose her Spanish fluency. As her writing demonstrates, her connection to her culture through language was essential in exploring her racial/ethnic identity development.

Anzaldúa is also well-known for co-editing *This Bridge Called My Back: Writings by Radical Women of Color (1981)* with Cherríe Moraga, a groundbreaking publication that uses personal essays, criticism, interviews, testimonials, poetry, and visual art to explore the hopes, fears, and accomplishments of women of color. This anthology illuminates the racism and classism found at this time in feminist thinking and empowers women of color to create a new kind of feminism that centered their unique experiences. The collection is also noteworthy for fully embracing lesbian voices and concerns and making a clear case that feminism should be inclusionary.

Cherríe Moraga

Cherríe Moraga (1952–) is a Chicana writer, feminist activist, poet, essayist, and playwright. She is regarded as one of the few writers who introduced the world to the theory of Chicana lesbianism. With Gloria Anzaldúa, she co-edited *This Bridge Called My Back: Writings by Radical Women of Color* (Moraga & Anzaldúa, 1981). Moraga's writing disrupts the traditional narratives of race, gender, sexuality, and feminism in the United States. For example, Moraga (1983) noted that feminists of color "have been actively involved in reproductive rights, especially sterilization abuse, battered women's shelters, rape crisis centers, welfare advocacy" (p. 106), issues that were not centralized within the mainstream feminism movement.

Moraga's memoir, *Native Country of the Heart* (Moraga, 2019), explores what it was like for her to gain consciousness of being Mexican in the United States, of the diaspora's Indigenous roots, as well as what it was like for her to discover her lesbian identity. Additionally, in one of her most well-known essays, "La Guera," Moraga compares the discrimination she faced as a lesbian to her mother's experiences being a poor, uneducated woman. She writes, "My lesbianism is the avenue through which I have learned the most about silence and oppression, and it continues to be the most tactile reminder to me that we are not free human beings" (Moraga, 1997, p. 29).

Dolores Huerta

Dolores Huerta is one of the most influential labor activists of the 20th century and a leader of the Chicano civil rights movement. In 1955, she began her career as an activist, where she co-founded the Stockton chapter of the Community Service Organization (CSO). Here, Huerta led voter registration drives and fought for economic improvements for Hispanics. A CSO colleague eventually introduced her to César Chávez, and together, Huerta and Chávez founded the National Farm Workers Association (which later became known as the United Farm Workers (UFW). Throughout her work with the UFW, Huerta organized workers, negotiated contracts, and advocated for safer working conditions, including eliminating harmful pesticides (Sowards, 2019).

The first testament to her lobbying and negotiating talents were demonstrated after she successfully secured Aid For Dependent Families (AFDC) and disability insurance for farmworkers in California in 1963, an unparalleled feat at the time. Additionally, despite ethnic and gender bias, Huerta was the driving force behind the 1965 Delano strike of 5,000 grape workers and was the lead negotiator in the workers' contract that followed. Her activism and support of agricultural workers led to a successful union contract by 1970. She was also instrumental in enacting the Agricultural Labor Relations Act (ALRA) of 1975, the first law of its kind in the United States. The ALRA granted farm workers in California the right to collectively organize and bargain for better wages and working conditions (Doak, 2008). Throughout the 1970s and '80s, Huerta worked as a lobbyist to improve workers' legislative representation. During the 1990s and 2000s, she worked to elect more Latinos and women to political office and has championed women's issues (Doak, 2008).

THE YOUNG LORDS OF PUERTO RICO

The Young Lords rose to political influence in 1969 with a mission to radically transform society. They were a group of poor and working-class Puerto Rican radicals who believed that the health, basic needs, and dignity of the oppressed needed to be prioritized above capitalistic profit. Fighting back against the stereotypical image of Puerto Ricans as "junkies, knife-wielding thugs, and welfare dependents" (Fernández, 2020, p. 2), the Young Lords worked to create a counter-narrative of Puerto Ricans as a resilient and powerful people. Through community-based campaigns and political propaganda, the Young Lords advocated for the end of colonial rule in Puerto Rico and everywhere, self-determination for all Puerto Ricans and all marginalized people on the mainland, and a socialist society where basic human needs - water, food, health, community, clothing, housing, work, and community – all took priority over profit (Fernández, 2020).

Afro-Puerto Rican Representation in the Young Lords

It is estimated that Afro-descendants make up 20% of the population in Puerto Rico, yet Puerto Rican society often diminished the influence of Black identity and Black culture. Colorism was deeply woven into the island's social fabric. The Young Lords, however, were intentional in denouncing racism and colorism within their membership. The Young Lords not only empowered its Afro-Latinx members to identify as such, but they also taught its members that Puerto Ricans and Black people shared a common experience of racism, colonialism, oppression, poverty, and working-class exploitation; they asserted that a revolution was only possible through cross-ethnic solidarity. The Young Lords were much more explicit than other Puerto Rican activist groups in addressing anti-blackness within their organization. For example, they required their members to examine their own ideologies around race, to study the origins of racial ideology in Puerto Rico and Latin America, and they elected Afro-Latinx members into its highest ranks. In doing this, the Young Lords demonstrated their organizational commitment to building a culture intolerant of racism (Fernández, 2020).

One influential member of the Young Lords was Iris Morales, a Puerto Rican activist who was quick to call out the way racism existed on the island. In one edition of *Palante*, the bilingual newspaper published by the party, she writes, "Puerto Ricans don't like to talk about racism or admit that it exists among Puerto Ricans. Boricuas talk of an island that is free from racism, or they say that the amerikkkan brought it in. Although the amerikkkan did make it worse, racism in Puerto Rico began with the Spanish" (Fernandez, 2020, p. 246). Much of this solidarity with Black people is due to the Young Lord's respect for the Black Power movement. The Young Lords had affiliated itself as a sister organization to the Black Panthers and spoke often of the lessons learned from one of the most influential expressions of organized Black resistance (Fernández, 2020).

Women of the Young Lords

Despite the progressiveness and socialist agenda of the Young Lords, the organization was not immune to oppression existing amongst its members. Specifically, women in the Young Lords forced the membership to pay attention to how racism, sexism, and homophobia appeared within their organization – referred to as the revolution within the revolution. Much is documented on the Young Lords, but limited information is available on how women shaped the party. Nonetheless, the impact of the women in the

Young Lords – Connie Cruz, Luisa Capetillo, Denise Oliver, and Bianca Canales, to name a few – was significant (Fernández, 2020).

To address claims of sexism within the organization, the Young Lords edited its position and platform to reject sexism explicitly. They appointed Denise Oliver to its formal leadership, and they formed men's and women's caucuses to discuss gender oppression internally within their party (Fernández, 2020). The Young Lords worked to ensure that the women in their ranks felt heard, that the men within the party respected their leadership, and that the demands put forth by women were met (Fernández, 2020).

The Young Lords had several other measures of accountability in place to address sexism within the organization. Half of the Young Lords newspaper, *Palante*, had to focus on women's issues. A men's caucus was formed to deal with machismo. A women's union was established with a publication called La Luchadora. The Young Lords operated on a military structure, and therefore, orders from women leaders had to be followed, regardless of men's thoughts on a woman's ability to lead. If male members did not follow orders from women leaders, it would be addressed in the party's open criticism sessions, a practice that forced members to deal with the issues within their organization (Gonzalez, 2009).

Women's Caucus. In January 1970, the women of the Young Lords began to meet informally on Sundays, independently of men, to get to know each other better, discuss their frustration in the organization and society, and build sisterhood. They called these meetings the women's caucus. They were embracing a practice popularized by the predominately white second-wave feminist movement—the women's consciousness-raising circle —in which women gathered to analyze and explore how structures of gender oppression played out in their personal lives (Fernández, 2020).

The caucus created a space for grievances, big and small. It addressed how machismo manifested within the organization, such as through its division of labor between men and women, interpersonal relationships, and through the use of political power by men in the organization to sleep with women. Women began to share stories of feeling humiliated and demeaned by some men in the Young Lords. As Fernández (2020) notes, the male members often objectified and sought out potential female recruits whom they'd later sexually proposition, a behavior they came to denounce as "sexual fascism" (p. 255).

In addition to holding the men accountable for sexist behavior, the women in these meetings would also challenge each other to unlearn dominant gender roles. They helped women recognize how the fight for feminism was not a white woman's struggle and inspired each other to become leaders. For example, conversations took place with young Puerto Rican women who were often socialized in Catholic homes where their bodies were heavily policed. As a result of this, these young Puerto Rican women often came to associate their sexuality with shame. The Women's Caucus would facilitate discussions to deepen women's understanding of oppression and their analysis of power so that each woman felt empowered to explore their sexuality and femininity without shame. This proved to be incredibly liberating (Fernández, 2020).

UNDERSTANDING THE DEVELOPMENT OF FEMINISM

The history of feminism is often described as occurring in waves. Some view these waves as occurring chronologically, whereas others view the waves more thematically (Scholz, 2012). Regardless of the way in which one views the trajectory of the feminist movement in the United States, it is important to be knowledgeable of the history of the movement to be able to understand contemporary feminism.

Waves of Feminism

The first wave of feminism occurred between 1848 to 1920 and it marked the first time the West engaged in a sustained political movement dedicated to the political equity of women. The primary focus of the first wave of feminism was White women gaining equality as human beings with full rights: civil, intellectual, social, economic, and legal (Scholz, 2012). The second wave of feminism focused on activism that examined various sources of oppression facing women. However, this view of various oppressions was quite narrow and assumed that all women had the same experiences of gender, class, and race (Eagly et al., 2012; Scholz, 2012)

The third wave of feminism began to challenge the language and thought previously associated with feminism. Additionally, the third wave of feminism advocated for women's agency in their own creation of a feminist identity (Scholz, 2012). Anzaldúa's (2007) work emerged during the third wave of feminism, offering a new perspective of Chicana and Third World feminism for those who did not identify with the mainstream. The fourth wave of feminism is contested to exist (some feminists argue that we are still in the third wave), but a noticeable shift has occurred. Feminists who argue for a fourth wave assert that this is the point in history where society has begun to hold our society's most powerful men accountable for their behavior, exemplified by the #MeToo and #TimesUp movements (Boyle, 2019). The fourth wave of feminism largely takes place online. Munroe (2013) notes the "call out" culture in which people engage in activism and discourse challenging sexism and misogyny within society. Overall, the fourth wave is responsible for facilitating a radical critique of the systems of power that allow predators to target women with impunity.

Feminist Schools of Thought

Schools of thought differ within the unique waves of feminism. Examples of feminist schools of thought include: liberal feminism, radical feminism, socialist feminism, cultural feminism, womanist theory, postmodern feminism, and Third world and postcolonial feminism. It is not uncommon for people to endorse only one school of thought or blend several of them together (Scholz, 2013). Regardless of which school of thought a person endorses, the existence of all these different ways of thinking sheds light on the harm in endorsing the idea that all women, regardless of race or class, experienced the world the same way. The success of the feminist movement was crucial for the United States to see progress for women's rights, but it ignored the realities of women with marginalized identities who did not easily fit into mainstream feminism. These waves of feminism and schools of thought show us that this thinking is harmful to the liberation of women of color, including Latinx women.

Intersectional Feminism: Womanist, Mujerista, and Womanista Approaches

As described earlier, feminism is a movement to end sexism, sexist exploitation, and oppression (hooks, 1984). Feminism has the potential to transform all our lives – men, women, and gender-expansive individuals – in significant ways. However, discussions of feminism and the history of mainstream feminism in the United States has often failed to take an intersectional approach, often centering "white, middle class, Western women" (Harrison, 2004, p. 3) and ignoring the plights of women of color and their unique lived experiences and interlocking identities.

Thus, in order to better capture how women of color understand feminism, it is critical to highlight more intersectional approaches to feminism: womanism, mujerismo, and womanista. All have their roots in feminism and share many principles, but they each speak to the unique experiences of Black, Indigenous, and women of color.

Womanism and Black Feminism

While at times used interchangeably, the terms womanism and Black feminism also have distinct differences . Alice Walker delineated between the two: "Black feminism is to womanism as lavender is to purple" (1983, n.p.). The term womanist was coined by Walker (1983): "a Black feminist or feminist of color committed to the survival and wholeness of entire people, male and female. Not a separatist, except periodically for health" (p. xi). Womanism infused Crenshaw's (1991) intersectionality, emphasizing the necessity of acknowledging race and gender in Black women's experiences and fighting for equality (Rousseau, 2013). The term is grounded in notions of possibility, hope, and change that enhance optimal living that transcends from survival to thriving (Westfield, 2007). Walker gave a psychological rationale for using the word *womanism* in her 1984 *New York Times* interview (Bradley, 1984) when she stated that a new word must be created when the old word (*feminism*) fails to capture the behavior and change that one is seeking to identify.

A womanist does not create a hierarchy between the fights against racism and sexism. Instead, a womanist sees both as necessary and central. Womanism is a sociopolitical framework that centralizes race, gender, class, and sexuality as prominent markers of women's lived experiences (Brown-Douglas, 1993). It emphasizes the "simultaneity of oppression" (p. 128) that women of color experience (Scholz, 2013). Womanists are also collectivistic and community-oriented. The focus of womanism moves beyond individual well-being to encompass the well-being of entire peoples and communities and then to humanity overall.

Similarly, Black feminism is rooted in a relational framework that understands how the histories of various marginalized groups are interconnected (Brewer, 2020; Collins, 2017). It is only through this intersectional framework that the lived experiences of multiply-marginalized communities, including Afro-Latinx women, can be fully understood. Both Black feminism and womanism developed as the result of mainstream feminism excluding Black women from the movement (Brewer, 2020). Therefore, it is crucial that we consider the intersectionality of being both Black and Latinx. It is only through a critical understanding of how systems of power intersect that we can begin to understand the unique struggles and strengths of Afro-Latinx feminists; this is especially true since as a result of racism and colonialism (Comas-Díaz, 2021), Afro-Latinx feminist plights have been ignored.

Black feminist thought birthed the concept of intersectionality. In 1977, the Combahee River Collective's manifesto stated their values: "we are actively committed to struggling against racial, sexual, heterosexual, and class oppresssion, and see as our particular task the development of integrated analysis and practice based upon the fact that the major systems of oppression are interlocking" (Combahee River Collective, 1995, p. 232). While Kimberlé Crenshaw coined the term intersectionality, other Black feminist scholars wrote about similar concepts, such as Beal's "double jeopardy," King's "multiple jeopardy," Collins' "matrix of domination," among others (Nash, 2019). These scholars laid the groundwork for expanding mainstream feminism into intersectional feminism. Because Latinx-identified persons can identify within many different racial categories, it is important to understand the history of womanism and Black feminism, especially as it relates to the experiences of Afro-Latinx women and feminists.

Mujerismo

Like womanism, mujerismo developed as a result of exclusion from White feminist movements that ignored the experiences and plights of women of color (Castañeda-Sound et al., 2016); like womanists, mujeristas embrace an interdisciplinary perspective, and mujerismo is roughly translated to mean a Latina womanism (Mejia et al., 2013). A mujerista orientation is understood as "a sensibility or approach to power, knowledge, and relationships rooted in convictions for community uplift" (Delgado-Bernal et al., 2006, p. 7). The term mujerismo was initially used during the 1970s when Peruvian women used it to dissociate themselves from feminist movements that ignored the unique needs of women of color (Vuola, 2002). Chicanx scholars have expanded upon mujerismo to better understand Latinas' lives in a complex society that often makes them feel invisible or unwelcome (Delgado-Bernal, 2006). Moreover, a Chicanx feminist perspective emphasizes both decolonization and intersectionality (Sánchez et al., 2020) which can be seen in mujerismo.

According to Comas-Díaz (2008), "mujeristas identified their marginalization from White feminism, ethnic minority patriarchy, dominant communities' oppression, neocolonization, and economic domination as impetus for their psychopolitical baptism" (p. 15). Mujerismo also has strong connections to mestiza consciousness, a concept coined by Anzaldúa (2007). According to Anzaldúa (2007), Latina women, or mujeristas, experience several different kinds of knowledge. First, there is the knowledge of feeling unwanted in the United States. Secondly, there is the knowledge born out of feeling marginalized within our own communities. Thirdly, there is the knowledge that is often made invisible by the euro-centric social practices that determine what is deemed knowledge. When these various kinds of knowledge are made known, it results in a shared emotional state of feeling seen and understood amongst Latinx women. A mestiza consciousness has been created. This consciousness motivates Latinx women to learn the strategies and tools needed to thrive in a world that was not created for them (Delgado-Bernal, 2006).

Mujerismo also has a strong spiritual foundation committed to ending oppression for all marginalized people. Comaz-Diaz & Bryant-Davis (2016) writes that the mujerista psycho-spiritual approach includes the belief in interconnectedness, holism, solidarity, communality, global liberation, and transformation. By combining mujerista psychology with mainstream psychology, mujerista psychologists become equipped with the spiritual tools to foster healing, spiritual development, and spiritual activism in the lives of their clients.

While mujerismo has resonated for many Latinx feminists, it has room for growth, and has been labeled as divisive by some. For example, mujerismo and Latinx feminism in general, excluded LatiNegras (Afro-Latinx people) and indigenous women (Comas-Díaz & Bryant-Davis, 2016). This demonstrates the influence of colonialism and racism, even when working to create a movement that is more inclusive than the original, White American feminist movement.

Womanista

In their book chapter, Comas-Díaz & Bryant-Davis (2016) noted that combining womanism and mujerismo could create a "global feminism of color" that addresses "the personal and collective plight of oppressed women around the world" (p. 284). Based upon this suggestion, Chavez-Dueñas & Adames (2021) developed the *Intersectionality Awakening Model of Womanista (I AM Womanista)* model that focuses on Latinx Women of Color, and intentionally centers the experiences of indigenous and Black (Afro-Latinx) women. While this model was created to be used as both a theory and treatment approach, it was developed to combat exclusion of women of color from other feminist movements, particularly those that promoted colorblind ideologies (Chavez-Dueñas & Adames, 2021). It is important to note that Latin America has historically demonstrated anti-Blackness, meaning that Afro-Latinx people have often been left behind and ignored which highlights the present need for intentionally centering the experiences of those who have been most harmed by colonialism (indigenous folx) and racism (Black folx; Adames et al., 2021). The *I AM Womanista* framework integrates intersectionality, womanism, and mujerismo and aims to be an inclusive answer to what other approaches and ideologies may be missing.

Centering Indigenous Ways of Knowing

The influence of Latinx and Chicanx scholars and activists highlights how Latina feminism centers indigenous ways of knowing. When discussing Latinx women navigating their multiple social identities, or group memberships, phrases such as "mestiza consciousness," "differential consciousness," and "a state of 'concientización'" are used (Hurtado, 1997, p. 313). Anzaldúa (2007) described mestiza consciousness:

The new mestiza copes by developing a tolerance for contradictions, a tolerance for ambiguity. She learns to be an Indian in Mexican culture, to be Mexican from an Anglo point of view. She learns to juggle cultures. She has a plural personality, she operates in a pluralistic mode—nothing is thrust out, the good the bad and the ugly, nothing rejected, nothing abandoned. Not only does she sustain contradictions, she turns the ambivalence into something else (p. 101).

As previously mentioned, Anzaldúa intentionally highlighted her own mestiza consciousness through her use of language in her writing. She demonstrated her experience of juggling cultures and plurality through her use of English, Spanish, and indigenous dialects.

Hernandez Castillo (2010) notes that indigenous feminism is distinct from its urban, middle-class counterpart, even if the indigenous and urban women come from the same country. In discussing intersectionality, Western approaches to considering multiple identities and oppression typically center identities such as gender and ethnicity but often fail to consider connections to indigenous culture. When discussing Latina feminism, it is important to consider all of these multiple and intersecting identities, oppressions, and privileges. One's "interlocking oppression[s]" (Collins, 1986, p. S19) must be considered as a complex spider web, not just simply as the intersectionality that is commonly discussed (Charleswell, 2014).

It is important, too, to remember how indigenous cultures viewed women pre-colonization. For example, the Aztecs had an "ambilateral system" that valued the contributions of both men and women (Chavez-Dueñas & Adames, 2021, p. 89). In fact, "women were valued, seen as powerful, and were producers and distributors of agricultural goods" (p. 89). Decolonizing feminism must emphasize indigenous practices and incorporate these key components.

Mestiza Consciousness

Anzaldúa's description of mestiza consciousness highlights the uniqueness of each individual's experience and the borders that she straddles. In my (Brooke) dissertation research, in discussing the development of their feminist identities, participants discussed their identity as it related to mestiza consciousness (Rappaport, 2019). Participants discussed their various identities as both a source of pride and struggle.

They also noted what contributed to the development of their mestiza consciousness including reading work by feminist authors, work experiences, talking with others, and attending webinars. One participant stated that though she always holds the same identities, her experience of her mestiza consciousness depends on where she is. Considering physical borders such as geographical and historical borders is important as is considering one's social location (Martinez, 2000).

Borderlands Theory

Anzaldúa (2007) defined a borderland as "a vague and undetermined place created by the emotional residue of an unnatural boundary…in a constant state of transition…[where] the prohibited and forbidden are its inhabitants" (p. 25). The inhabitants of the borderlands are labeled as the "other" or as an "alien" by the dominant White people and ultimately find themselves not belonging within the mainstream. With regard to feminism, many Latinas find themselves stuck in the borderlands; mainstream feminism does not speak to their struggles and needs but ignoring any type of women's movement is out of line with their values and desires. Patricia Arredondo noted her own mestiza consciousness development through her lived experience in the borderlands or *entre fronteras* (between borders) "as a highly ambitious Mexican American woman" (Delgado-Romero & Romero-Shih, 2016, p. 1234). Again, in my (Brooke) dissertation, one participant discussed her experiences in the borderlands: "I really love the concept of borderlands. And what it does is really authenticate life experiences…I think the borderlands applies to almost anyone when you see that there's a part of your identity that you have to manage differently…in a society that is not so accepting of differences" (Rappaport, 2019, p. 87).

Nepantla

Within Borderlands theory, Anzaldúa (2007) discusses the concept of *nepantla*, which she identifies as "a stage that women and men, and whoever is willing to change into a new person and further grow and develop, go through" (p. 237). She describes this process as uncomfortable and difficult as one navigates the in-between (Ranft, 2013). *Nepantla* allows for fluidity and ambiguity as one explores and navigates their unique space that encompasses their gender, sexuality, race, and class among other identities. This process allows for the development of a feminist identity that centers activism and liberation (De Los Santos Upton, 2019).

Tying It Together

Traditional views of Latinx cultural values would indicate that being a feminist and Latinx are incongruent, yet indigenous ways of knowing (e.g., borderlands, mestiza consciousness, mestizaje, nepantla), provide frameworks for blending all aspects of identity. For example, in one study, many participants stated that they did not experience major conflict between cultural ideals and their feminist identities; while some noted how they may not have fulfilled family expectations (e.g., motherhood, marriage), they still received support from their families. Moreover, many participants spoke specifically about the support they received from men in their cultures who promoted feminist ideals (Rappaport, 2019). Understanding their experiences of living in the borderlands formed their understanding of their own mestiza consciousnesses. This also helped them come to understand their latinidad in a variety of manners.

In conclusion, navigating the complex landscape of identity and understanding our place in this ever-changing world may feel messy, confusing, or isolating, but the journey can also feel euphoric, invigorating, inspiring, and joyful. We are not only a collection of pain and trauma; we are a collective of wisdom, resiliency, and love for our shared latinidad. It is easy to learn about the oppressive conditions and marginalization our ancestors have faced and get lost in a haze of anger and resentment. Reckoning with our history can feel deeply painful. Rather than letting anger guide us, let our anger be rooted in love so that we can continue working toward a liberated world. Let love be the motivating force behind our social justice movements – love for ourselves, for our communities, for our culture, for our ancestors. As Owens (2020) beautifully writes in *Love and Rage*, "There's no liberation without actually leaning forward and actually looking at the things we habitually run away from, in order to see things the way they really are, not as how we imagined them. This is the path of liberation through anger." Growing in our critical consciousness and learning our histories will not always be easy, but it will be revolutionary.

REFERENCES

Adames, H. Y., Chavez-Dueñas, N. Y., & Jernigan, M. M. (2021). The fallacy of a raceless Latinidad: Action guidelines for centering Blackness in Latinx psychology. *Journal of Latina/o Psychology, 9*(1), 26–44. doi:10.1037/lat0000179

Anzaldúa, G. (2002). now let us shift... the path of conocimiento... inner work, public acts. In G.E. Anzaldúa & A. L. Keating (Ed.), This bridge we call home: Radical visions for transformation (pp. 540-578). New York, NY: Routledge.

Anzaldúa, G. (2007). *Borderlands/ La Frontera: The New Mestiza*. Aunt Lute Books.

Anzaldúa, G. E. (1987). *Borderlands/La Frontera: The New Mestiza*. Aunt Lute.

Baldwin, J., & DeSouza, E. (2001). Modelo de Maria and machismo: The social construction of gender in Brazil. *Interamerican Journal of Psychology, 35*(1), 9–29.

Bernal, D. D., Elenes, C. A., & Godinez, F. E. (Eds.). (2006). *Chicana/Latina education in everyday life: Feminista perspectives on pedagogy and epistemology*. Suny Press.

Boyle, K. (2019). # MeToo, Weinstein and feminism. In # MeToo, Weinstein and Feminism (pp. 1-20). Palgrave Pivot.

Bradley, D. (1984). Novelist Alice Walker Telling the Black Woman's Story. *New York Times Magazine, 8*, 24-37.

Brewer, R. M. (2020). Black Feminism and Womanism. In N. A. Naples (Ed.), *Companion to Feminist Studies*. doi:10.1002/9781119314967.ch6

Castañeda-Sound, C. L., Martinez, S., & Durán, J. E. (2016). Mujeristas and social justice: La lucha es la vida. In T. Bryant-Davis & L. Comas-Díaz (Eds.), *Womanist and mujerista psychologies: Voices of fire, acts of courage* (pp. 237–259). American Psychological Association. doi:10.1037/14937-011

Charleswell, C. (2014, October 17). *Latina Feminism: National and Transnational Perspectives*. Retrieved July 01, 2016, from http://www.hamptoninstitute.org/latina-feminism.html#.V4klOJMrLfZ

Chavez-Dueñas, N. Y., & Adames, H. Y. (2021). Intersectionality Awakening Model of Womanista: A transnational treatment approach for Latinx women. *Women & Therapy*, *44*(1-2), 83–100. doi:10.1080/02703149.2020.1775022

Collins, P. H. (1986). Learning from the outsider within: The sociological significance of Black feminist though. *Social Problems*, *33*(6), S14–S32. doi:10.2307/800672

Collins, P. H. (2017). The Difference That Power Makes: Intersectionality and Participatory Democracy. *Investigaciones Feministas*, *8*(1), 19–39. doi:10.5209/INFE.54888

Comas-Díaz, L. (1988). Feminist therapy with Hispanic/Latina women: Myth or reality? *Women & Therapy*, *6*(4), 39–61. doi:10.1300/J015V06N04_06

Comas-Díaz, L. (2008). 2007 Carolyn Sherif Award Address: *Spirita*: Reclaiming Womanist Sacredness into Feminism. *Psychology of Women Quarterly*, *32*(1), 13–21. doi:10.1111/j.1471-6402.2007.00403.x

Comas-Díaz, L. (2021). Afro-Latinxs: Decolonization, healing, and liberation. *Journal of Latina/o Psychology*, *9*(1), 65–75. doi:10.1037/lat0000164

Comas-Díaz, L., & Bryant-Davis, T. (2016). Conclusion: Toward global womanist and mujerista psychologies. In T. Bryant-Davis & L. Comas-Díaz (Eds.), *Womanist and Mujerista Psychologies: Voices of Fire, Acts of Courage* (pp. 277–290). American Psychological Association. doi:10.1037/14937-013

Combahee River Collective. (1995). Combahee River Collective statement. In B. Guy-Sheftall (Ed.), *Words of fire: An anthology of African American feminist thought* (pp. 232–240). New Press.

Cordero, A. L.Colegio de Abogados de Puerto Rico. (1979). *Cerro Maravilla: Estudio Del Informe Del Departamento De Justicia* [Cerro Maravilla: Study of the Department of Justive Report]. Colegio de Abogados de Puerto Rico.

De Los Santos Upton, S. (2019). Nepantla activism and coalition building: Locating identity and resistance in the cracks between worlds. *Women's Studies in Communication*, *42*(2), 135–139. doi:10.1080/07491409.2019.1605232

de Sant'Anna Machado, T., & Perry, K. K. Y. (2021). Translation of "The Black Woman: A Portrait". *Feminist Anthropology*, *2*(1), 38–49. doi:10.1002/fea2.12031

Delgado-Romero, E. A., & Romero-Shih, A. (2016). Patricia Arredondo: Creating a pathway for cultural empowerment. Legacies and Traditions Forum. *The Counseling Psychologist*, *44*(8), 1212–1253. doi:10.1177/0011000016683943

Doak, R. S. (2008). *Dolores Huerta: Labor Leader and Civil Rights Activist*. Capstone.

Douglas, K. B. (1993). Womanist theology: What is its relationship to Black theology? *Black Theology*, 290–299.

Eagly, A. H., Eaton, A., Rose, S. M., Riger, S., & McHugh, M. C. (2012). Feminism and psychology: Analysis of a half-century of research on women and gender. *The American Psychologist*, *67*(3), 211–230. doi:10.1037/a0027260 PMID:22369245

Fernández, J. (2019). *The young lords: A radical history*. UNC Press Books.

Gil, R. M., & Vasquez, C. I. (1996). *The Maria paradox*. Perigee.

Ginorio, A., Guttierrez, L., Cauce, A. M., & Acosta, M. (1995). The psychology of Latinas. In C. Travis (Ed.), *Feminist perspectives on the psychology of women* (pp. 89–108). American Psychological Association.

Gonzalez, L. (1979). Primavera Para As Rosas Negras [Spring for Black Roses]. *Diáspora Africana. Editora Filhos da África, 2018*, 103–8.1.

Gonzalez, L. (1988). *Por un feminismo afro-latino-americano* [For an Afro-Latin American feminism]. Retrieved from https://edisciplinas.usp.br/pluginfile.php/271077/mod_resource/content/1/Por%20um%20feminismo%20Afro-latino-americano.pdf

Gonzalez. (2009). *Mujeres of the Young Lords*. https://www.colorlines.com/articles/mujeres-young-lords

Harrison, F. V. (2004). Global apartheid, environmental degradation, and women's activism for sustainable well-being: A conceptual and theoretical overview. *Urban Anthropology and Studies of Cultural Systems and World Economic Development, 33*(1), 1–35.

Hernández Castillo, R. A. (2010). The emergence of indigenous feminism in Latin America. *Journal of Women in Culture and Society, 35*(3), 539–545. doi:10.1086/648538

Hooks, B. (1984). *Black women shaping feminist theory*. ProQuest Information and Learning.

Hurtado, A. (1997). Understanding multiple group identities: Inserting women into cultural transformations. *The Journal of Social Issues, 53*(2), 299–328. doi:10.1111/j.1540-4560.1997.tb02445.x

Keating, A., & Anzaldúa, G. (1993). Writing, Politics, and las Lesberadas: Platicando con Gloria Anzaldúa. *Frontiers, 14*(1), 105–130. doi:10.2307/3346563

Maiorana, J. (2021). *Yolanda Guzmán (1943-1965)*. https://www.blackpast.org/global-african-history/people-global-african-history/yolanda-guzman-1943-1965/

Martinez, J. M. (2000). *Phenomenology of Chicana experience and identity: Communication and transformation in praxis*. Rowman and Littleðeld.

Mejia, A. P., Quiroz, O., Morales, Y., Ponce, R., Chavez, G. L., & Torre, E. O. Y. (2013). From madres to mujeristas: Latinas making change with Photovoice. *Action Research, 11*(4), 301–321. doi:10.1177/1476750313502553

Moraga, C. (1997). La guera. *Critical White studies: Looking behind the mirror*, 471-474.

Moraga, C. (2019). *Native country of the heart: A memoir*. Farrar, Straus and Giroux.

Moraga, C., & Anzaldúa, G. (Eds.). (1981). *This bridge called my back: Writings by radical women of color*. SUNY Press.

Moraga, C., & Anzaldúa, G. (Eds.). (1983). *This bridge called my back: Writings by radical women of color*. SUNY Press.

Munroe, E. (2013). Feminism: A fourth wave? *Political Insight*, 22-25.

Nash, J. C. (2019). *Black feminism reimagined: After intersectionality*. Duke University Press. doi:10.1215/9781478002253

Owens, L. R. (2020). *Love and rage: The path of liberation through anger*. North Atlantic Books.

Placido, S. I. (2017). *A Global Vision: Dr. Ana Livia Cordero and the Puerto Rican Liberation Struggle, 1931-1992* [Doctoral dissertation]. Harvard University, Graduate School of Arts & Sciences.

Ranft, E. (2013). Connecting intersectionality and Nepantla to resist oppressions: A feminist fiction approach. *Women, Gender, and Families of Color*, *1*(2), 207–223. doi:10.5406/womgenfamcol.1.2.0207

Rappaport, B. (2019). *Exploring the experiences of Latina feminists in psychology: navigating intersecting identities, understanding Latina feminism, and implications for allies* (Publication No. 9949333998202959) [Doctoral dissertation, University of Georgia]. https://getd.libs.uga.edu/pdfs/rappaport_brooke_s_201908_phd.pdf

Rousseau, N. (2013). Historical womanist theory: Re-visioning Black feminist thought. *Race, Gender, & Class*, 191–204.

Sánchez, B., Salazar, C., & Guerra, J. (2020). "I Feel Like I Have to Be the Whitest Version of Myself": Experiences of Early Career Latina Higher Education Administrators. *Journal of Diversity in Higher Education*. Advance online publication. doi:10.1037/dhe0000267

Scholz, S. J. (2013). *Feminism: A beginner's guide*. Retrieved from http://eds.b.ebscohost.com.proxy-remote.galib.uga.edu/eds/ebookviewer/ebook/bmxlYmtfXzkxMDczOV9fQU41?sid=2c2e0ceb-cd4b-4dae-9954-233a8e66916d@sessionmgr102&vid=14&format=EK&rid=4

Sowards, S. K. (2019). *Sí, ella puede! The rhetorical legacy of Dolores Huerta and the United Farm Workers*. University of Texas Press. doi:10.7560/317662

The Latina Feminist Group. (2001). *Telling to live: Latina feminist testimonios*. Duke University Press.

Vaughan, L. (2020). *Florinda Soriano Muñoz (Mamá Tingó) (1921-1974)*. https://www.blackpast.org/global-african-history/florinda-soriano-munoz-mama-tingo-1921-1974/

Vuola, E. (2017). Seriously Harmful For Your Health? Religion, Feminism and Sexuality in Latin America. In M. Althaus-Reid (Ed.), *Liberation Theology and Sexuality* (1st ed., pp. 137–162). Routledge. doi:10.4324/9781351153966-10

Walker, A. (1983). *In Search of Our Mothers' Gardens: Womanist Prose*. Harcourt.

Westfield, N. L. (2007). *Dear sisters: A womanist practice of hospitality*. The Pilgrim Press.

Chapter 7
Contemporary Views on Latinx Feminism:
Applying Our Collective Histories to Create a More Brilliant Future

Brooke Rappaport
Tennessee State University, USA

Lucia Quezada
https://orcid.org/0000-0002-7305-7070
University of Georgia, USA

Kiara Manosalvas
Teachers College, Columbia University, USA

Grace-Ellen Mahoney
University of Maryland, USA

ABSTRACT

This chapter discusses contemporary perspectives related to Latinx feminism. This chapter builds upon a previous chapter about the history of Latinx feminism. Ways in which feminism and gender identity intersect with other identities are discussed. The authors discuss how Latinx feminism provides avenues to resist oppression. The chapter ends with a discussion of application of feminist concepts discussed and future directions. A combination of third-person research and personal narrative is utilized.

INTRODUCTION

Mujeres, a no dejar que el peligro del viaje y la inmensidad del territorio nos asuste —a mirar hacia adelante y a abrir paso en el monte (Women, let's not let the danger of the journey and the vastness of the territory scare us—let's look forward and open paths in these woods) (Moraga & Anzaldúa, 1983, p. v)

DOI: 10.4018/978-1-6684-4901-1.ch007

The above quote was written by Gloria Anzaldúa in the forward to the second edition of her book co-edited with Cherríe Moraga entitled *This Bridge Called My Back: Writings by Radical Women of Color*. Both Anzaldúa and Moraga urged their audience to be bridges to connect their identities and experiences as important and worthy of care. This work and that of other Latinx feminist scholars, activists, writers, and artists inspired our collaborative writing of this chapter.

Making Meaning of Our Feminist and Mujerista Identities

One of the most powerful lessons feminism and mujerismo has taught me (Kiara) is that my assertiveness and boldness as a Latina woman are qualities to be celebrated rather than shamed. However, before evolving into the bold, assertive woman I am today, I was a scared, apologetic child terrified of her alcoholic father. My father was a poor immigrant from Ecuador who coveted the power, the privilege, and the respect that the White man so easily obtained. Unable to obtain the power of the White man, he chose instead to assert dominance over his family. He used his masculinity or "machismo" as a weapon to assert his authority and justify his abuse. I began to feel shame and resentment towards my culture – a culture I had associated with violence and dysfunction – and made no effort to cultivate my identity as a Latina woman.

It was not until I was forced to confront my own racial identity development and my internalized racism during my master's training in mental health counseling that I realized how hard I was working to deny my experience inside the borderlands – the discomfort of not feeling Latina "enough" to build community with others who shared my identity, yet feeling awkwardly out of place with White people. Denying this experience felt easier than sitting with the ambiguity of existing inside the borderland, of constantly living in transition. Anzaldúa (1987) writes that "borders are set up to define the places that are safe and unsafe, to distinguish us from them" (p. 3). This is certainly true, yet for me, the most painful part was recognizing how I was an accomplice in creating these divisions. In order to heal, I had to learn how to express curiosity about the contradictions within myself as I tried to belong to two different cultures. I could be both assertive and gentle. I could feel ambivalent about having kids yet also be family oriented. These things were not mutually exclusive.

Fortunately, much has changed in how I think about my racial/ethnic identity. By taking the time to understand my own mestiza consciousness and expose myself to the brilliant ancestors who came before me, I have learned how to speak from my heart, to stand up for what I believe is right, and, even if my voice trembles, to stay committed in trusting myself. I have finally arrived at a place where I see my Latinx identity as a source of strength, not as a deficit. My culture is not perfect; no culture is. I will never stop feeling irritated when my mom tells me "ahora te puedes casar!" after I've cooked a good meal. But I have come to learn that my criticism of Latinx culture no longer comes from a place of shame or anger but from a place of love. Machismo and patriarchy may have dimmed the fire I had inside of me, but it was love, community, and the inspirational writings of Latina feminists who came before me that reminded me of how easily I can strike a match to my flame once more. I no longer feel like I have to decide between cultivating my Latina identity or my American upbringing. I can be someone who sees the value in the individual and the collective.

Contemporary Views on Latinx Feminism

FEMINIST, LATINX, AND…

It is important to consider intersectionality in understanding Latinx feminism. Latinx women, like other women of color, find themselves in unique positions when navigating their various identities. Crenshaw (1991) noted:

The concept of political intersectionality highlights the fact that women of color are situated within at least two subordinated groups that frequently pursue conflicting political agendas. The need to split one's political energies between two sometimes opposing groups is a dimension of intersectional disempowerment that men of color and white women seldom confront. Indeed, their specific race and gendered experiences, although intersectional, often define as well as confine the interests of the entire group. (pp. 1251-1252)

When considering Latinx feminism, it is important to understand how identities such as class, race, sexual orientation, and spirituality intersect to create one's lived experience. While other chapters in this book address these identity variables in-depth, we want to connect our understanding of intersectionality to Latinx feminism.

Queer Perspectives

Anzaldúa (2007) wrote, "For a lesbian of color, the ultimate rebellion she can make against her native culture is through her sexual behavior. She goes against two moral prohibitions: sexuality and homosexuality" (p. 41). I (Lucia) was in eighth grade when I first questioned my sexuality. I was selling raffle tickets for my church's carnival when a girl that I knew offered to buy all of them from me. We met at a park to do the exchange and we kissed. Ironically, this all happened because of the church group I was in. Catholic guilt instantly set in. Up until that moment I identified as "straight" despite my secret attraction to women. It was during this time that I began slightly considering my bisexuality. Many of my friends described it as "bi-curiosity" or an experimenting phase. But I knew it wasn't that. I found myself in the space Anzaldúa (2002) calls *Nepantla*—caught in a cognitive tension of what it means to be queer, feeling like I don't belong in the heteronormative spaces nor queer spaces (Orozco et al., 2021). For many years I hid this side of me and kept my relationships with women on the downlow. I was always considered an ally and often frequented gay clubs with my friends; no one questioned it. I definitely had heterosexual privilege as I predominantly and openly dated men because of the compulsive heterosexuality I was socialized with. As the only daughter with two brothers, my parents often verbalized their desire for me to meet a good man to marry. It wasn't until I started college that I began embracing my bisexuality and found pride in my identity. However, I don't have a "coming out" story. I never formally "came out" to friends and family. I never felt the need to do it, but when asked I answer truthfully. In the iconic words of Mexican singer, Juan Gabriel, when questioned about his sexual orientation, "lo que se ve no se pregunta" (what is obvious isn't questioned) (Del Rincon, 2016, 6:55).

This is common in Latinx culture. Despite being a patriarchal culture that often endorses homophobia, there is an acceptance of queer identities and the existence of *jotería* that makes coming out unnecessary as it might be seen as an "exhibitionism of the self" (Hernandez, 2016). Jotería in its simplest translation is queerness (Tijerina Revilla et al., 2021). However, a distinction between queer and Jotería is that jotería centralizes racialized queer and trans Chicanx, Latinx, and indigenous experiences (Gonzalez, 2022;

Hernandez, 2016; Orozco et al., 2021). It is a way to speak from experiential knowledge. In Anzaldúa's (1987) words, "people, listen to what your jotería is saying" (p. 85). Additionally, jotería is aligned with feminist/mujerista pedagogy and praxis (Tijerina Revilla & Santillana, 2014).

Role of Spirituality

Being raised Catholic in a Mexican household means I (Lucia) was introduced to *La Virgen de Guadalupe* in early childhood. For my *quinceañera,* I was gifted a necklace with an image of her which has obtained a new meaning independently of the formal teachings on her throughout the years (e.g., Vuola, 2017). A syncretism of the Aztec goddess, Tonantzin, and the Christian Virgin Mary (Comas-Díaz, 2008; Comas-Díaz, 2016), she resembles a Latina from her dark skin color to her dark hair. Phenotypically she looks like the women in my lineage, the very same women who raised me and who epitomized a mujerista ideology for me. She is a symbol of perpetuating hope and inspiration—an icon and defender of immigrants, the poor, indigenous people, and women. Every 12th of December a *novena* is prayed to commemorate her appearance to Juan Diego (Arredondo, 2002).

Feminism and religion have often been at opposite ends throughout history (Comas-Díaz, 2008); yet central to Latinx feminism that differs from its White/traditional counterpart is the discourse around spirituality. Traditional feminist discourse typically views established religion as harmful for women, but within Latinx feminism, this can be alienating (Vuola, 2017). Thus, spiritual faith is important.

As someone who identifies as Jewish and was raised in a fairly observant home, I (Brooke) began to reject religion and identified as atheist during my college years. I remember feeling somewhat shocked when I began graduate school and was part of a team of predominantly Latinx individuals who identified more closely with their higher powers. I struggled with my own understanding of how science and religion can mix. Yet over time, I learned more about the distinction between religion and spirituality and the connection to indigenous culture and ancestral knowledge. I connected my own understanding of my identity as culturally Jewish and the meaning that held for me. For example, the Jewish concept of tikkun olam (repairing the world) has been a guiding value in both my personal and professional roles. As a White woman who identifies as a feminist, I learned that for my version of feminism to be truly intersectional, accepting spirituality as an important part of peoples' lives, even if it differed from my worldviews, was crucial; not considering this aspect of one's identity would force me to continue perpetuating harms that are prevalent in mainstream (White) feminism.

It is important to note that there is a difference between religion and spirituality. Religion involves doctrines and institutions, while spirituality promotes liberation (Comas-Díaz, 2008). Over the course of history, religion has contributed to the oppression of marginalized groups while spirituality empowers and promotes feminist consciousness. This newfound consciousness is used to liberate the self and others, a term Comas-Díaz (2008) coined as *Spirita:* the spirit of liberation among women of color. It allows women to take control of their lives, surpass their oppressed mentality, and achieve self-critical knowledge. We see this in the role that women play as healers in the Latinx community (Comas-Díaz, 2016). Additionally, the experience of multiple intersecting oppressions enables many Latinas to develop healing capacities that we see through the use of intuition, or *corazonada,* which Anzaldúa describes as *la facultad* (Comas-Díaz, 2008; Saavedra & Salazar Perez, 2017).

Racial Identity Formation for Latinx Communities

A Latinx feminist view considers the role of *nepantla* in understanding one's identity development. Oftentimes, discussions of identity amongst Latinx populations ignores the intersection of racial identity. However, with the rise of the Black Lives Matter movement in 2020, research has moved to include the unique experiences of AfroLatinx people (e.g., Adames et al., 2021; Comas-Díaz, 2021; Sanchez, 2021). Often, those who identify as AfroLatinx find themselves in the borderlands, experiencing oppression inside of the Latinx community and outside of it due to colorism which leads to the experience of "gendered-racial wounds" (Sanchez, 2021, p. 5). Lugones (2008) refers to this as "the coloniality of gender" in which AfroLatinx face oppression for the intersection of their multiple marginalized identities.

To operate from a truly intersectional feminist lens that honors decolonized perspectives (e.g., Anzaldúa, 2007), the understanding of Latinidad and oppression must be "viewed through a racialized lens" (Adames et al., p. 34). *The Intersectional Awakening Model of Womanista* (*I AM Womanista*) does just that (Chavez-Dueñas & Adames, 2021).

Because dominant views of feminism center the experiences of White and lighter skinned women, full understandings of women's experiences fail to be captured (Coles & Pasek, 2020). The component of gendered-racism from the *I AM Womanista* model highlights ways in which colonialism erased the power that Indigenous and African women had in their communities (Chavez-Dueñas & Adames, 2021). Given this understanding around the harm of gendered-racism, this model offers suggestions for healing from this gendered-racism in therapy by assessing the client's racial identity, providing counternarratives, and raising intersectionality consciousness (Chavez-Dueñas & Adames, 2021). Taking this approach empowers Latinx women to be liberated from harmful narratives and view colonization as the problem instead of themselves.

Intersection of Latinx Ethnicity, Gender, and Class

Examining how class intersects with the identities of being a cisgender Latina woman is important and lends itself to demonstrating the need to expand from mainstream (White) views of feminism. For example, equal pay has been an important concern for many people who identify as feminists. In 2021, for both part- and full-time work, women earned 77.3 cents for every dollar a manmade (Hegewisch & Mefferd, 2022). While this pay gap is infuriating, this aggregate number ignores the pay gap for women of color. In fact, for every dollar a full-time White man earned in 2021, Black women's full-time earnings were 63.1% and Hispanic/Latinx women's full-time earnings were 58.4%. Moreover, there remains segregation in areas in which women work, with one in four Hispanic women working in service positions, compared to just one in ten White women. This type of occupation has the lowest earnings and those in these jobs were considered "essential workers" during the COVID-19 pandemic. This means that not only were many Hispanic/Latinx women being underpaid compared to their White counterparts, but they were also being placed at high-risk during a global pandemic (Hegewisch & Mefferd, 2022). Each spring in the United States, Equal Pay Day is recognized. This day marks the point within the current year that it would take a woman to make what a man earned in the previous year (Zillman, 2018). However, this day fails to consider the amount of time it would take a woman of color to reach the same amount of pay as her White, male counterpart. Clearly, the predominant feminist argument for equal pay in the United States has failed to consider intersectional identities and the multiple oppressions within the broad category of being a woman.

Adding to this discrepancy among pay are the differences in college degree attainment. As of 2021, approximately 25% of Latinas obtain a college degree, whereas approximately 50% of White women do (Anthony et al., 2021). The COVID-19 pandemic contributed to fewer Latinx people obtaining college degrees as compared to previous years. Among those Latinx women that receive college degrees, less than 7 percent receive graduate degrees (Anthony et al., 2021). This does not reflect ability, but instead demonstrates barriers that Latinx women face, such as access to positive influences and mentors (Delgado-Romero et al., 2017). For example, within the field of psychology, one of the most popular undergraduate majors in the United States, Latinas are represented more than any other racial/ethnic group, yet are underrepresented in doctoral programs (Delgado-Romero & Werther, 2012). Moreover, those who do graduate from doctoral programs find themselves holding less esteemed positions within the workforce, such as lecturer and adjunct positions (Delgado-Romero & Werther, 2012). This then leads to the continued lack of Latina role models in the field to recruit, retain, and graduate Latinx students (Gloria & Robinson Kurpius, 1996). All of this contributes to the class discrepancy among Latinas and highlights the need for an intersectional and intentional approach to feminism that highlights the unique experiences of Latinx-identified people.

When I (Lucia) was in undergraduate I had a White male professor ask me what my plans were after college. I expressed to him my desire to pursue a doctoral degree in psychology and his response was that I "would not get accepted into a doctoral program, but that for a Latina like [myself], a master's in counseling was good enough." When my research mentor, who is a woman of color, found out about this transgression she advocated for me with the department chair in reporting it. Receiving the support of a woman of color at a predominately white institution granted me the assurance that I could pursue my goal. With her continued support, even beyond my undergraduate studies, I am now successfully enrolled in a doctoral program in counseling psychology. Through multicultural mentorship I was able to navigate the hidden curriculum that many first-generation Latina students like myself are unaware of.

NI UNA MENOS

On June 3, 2015, thousands of women in Buenos Aires, Argentina took to the streets in protest in front of the Argentine National Congress. The goal was to make visible the dire need to address femicide. This was following the femicide of Chiara Páez who was 14 years old and three months pregnant when her boyfriend killed her and buried her in his grandparents' backyard. In the autopsy, the doctors found that she had tried to have an abortion (Daby & Moseley, 2021). Her murder and several other high-profile murders of women in Argentina was a decisive moment for feminists there. This started the *Ni Una Menos* movement, which translates to not one (woman) less (Biglieri, 2020). This movement relies on the politics of *escraches* and memorialization as the main activist methods to document femicide and to denounce the state's institutions for being ineffective and sexist (Popescu, 2021). Escrache means to bring into light something hidden or to reveal what power hides (Grupo de Arte Callejero, 2019, p. 39, as cited in Popescu, 2021). An example of this is performative public shaming of the state and its elected officials as seen in the Chilean feminist theater collective, *Las Tesis*, with their powerful street performance, *Un Violador en tu Camino* which is a sarcastic rewording of the 1990s Chilean police slogan, *Un amigo en tu camino* (Martin & Shaw, 2021). During the performance, protestors use blindfolds, alluding to "Venda Sexy" which is an infamous estate in Chile that was used by the police as a site where they would rape and torture women detainees (Kravetz, 2018, as cited in Martin & Shaw, 2021).

This performance has been re-staged and performed in many other Spanish-speaking countries across Latin America and Europe. Memorialization focuses on creating a living, public archive for the victims that are both temporary and long-lasting. Examples of a temporary archive are protestors wearing and carrying images of the victims in marches and protests (Biglieri 2020). Examples of more permanent archives are seen within social media platforms.

In the twenty-first century we see the development of decolonial feminism, a feminist theory that considers the multiple levels of oppression at the intersections of race, gender, sexuality, and class and the impact of colonialism on these categories. Within this movement exists La Colectiva Feminista en Construcción (La Colectiva/La Cole), an Afro-feminist political collective active in Puerto Rico since 2013. The collective recognizes the influence of decolonial feminist thought and of Black feminism in their political actions and theoretical understanding of feminism and resistance; the collective defines itself as an anti-capitalist, anti-racist, anti-xenophobic, anti-colonialist, anti-patriarchal, anti-heteronormativite, eco-feminist and pro-choice organization (Crisóstomo Tejada, 2021). In 2020, La Cole released two manifestos, *La Manifesta* (Colectiva Feminista en Construcción, 2020a) and *Manifiesto antirracista de la Colectiva Feminista en Construcción* (Colectiva Feminista en Construcción, 2020b). La Cole organized what is known as the *Plantón 23N*, which was a sit-in protest that gathered hundreds of protestors in front of then-governor Rosello's mansion demanding him to sign an executive order declaring a state of emergency due to gender based violence. The protest used the "Ni una menos" slogan. As a result of this political organizing and massive public pressure, the people of Puerto Rico successfully got then-governor Rosello to resign. Moreover, after years of protest, on January 25, 2021, governor Pedro Pierluisi signed the executive order. Other organizations that are grounded in decolonial feminism include Grupo Latinoamericano de Estudios, Formación y Acción Feminista (GLEFAS), a group founded in Colombia but that now has members all across Latin America, and Junta de Prietas, an Afro-feminist collective from the Dominican Republic.

The Ni Una Menos movement also allowed for legal abortion to be rewritten in terms of *ni una muerta más por aborto clandestino* (not one woman less due to illegal abortion). It then became a matter of basic human rights. Whereas abortion is usually associated with death and murder, it now became associated with life (Biglieri, 2020). This is especially important since in Latin America restrictive laws about reproductive rights coexist with high levels of illegal abortions (Daby & Moseley, 2021). Thus, allowing abortion to become a social justice issue. We see this with *#Las3Causales* in the Dominican Republic where feminist movements and organizations demand the decriminalization of abortion, allowing a person to interrupt their pregnancy on three grounds (*3 causales*): (1) when pregnancy is a product of rape or incest, (2) the pregnant person's life is at risk, or (3) when the fetus has congenital malformations incompatible with life (Balbuena, 2018). To this day abortion remains illegal in the Dominican Republic despite President Luis Abinader reaffirming his support for *las tres causales* (the three grounds) in an interview on International Women's Day in 2022 (Nosotros a las 8, 2022).

Feminism is considered the most important social movement in Latin America (Palmeiro 2018) and protests are known to have success in achieving movement goals in places such as Argentina (Daby & Moseley, 2021). During my semester abroad in Buenos Aires in 2011, I (Brooke) interned with a woman-led organization called Grupo de Mujeres de la Argentina, a feminist organization that fights for human rights for all people. Interning with this organization demonstrated the feminist notion that the personal is political. Given the human rights abuses that took place in Argentina, including the disappearance of approximately 30,000 people (los desaparecidos) during the 1970's and 1980's, advocacy and activism is salient for many throughout the country (Hall, 2018). For example, as a student at la Universidad de

Buenos Aires (UBA), I recall classes being canceled due to student protests and protest graffiti covering the walls of the building. Protests demonstrated true liberatory and intersectional practices, protecting the rights of those who are most marginalized.

In recent years, many women across Latin America have taken to the streets in protests and demonstrations on March 8, International Women's Day, against sexual violence and femicide. This has created a transnational feminism especially in a digital age where social media makes it easier to organize (Daby & Moseley, 2021; Martin & Shaw, 2021). From this transnational feminism, a sense of sisterhood and solidarity among Latinas is seen. The women's liberation movement's idea of sisterhood was based on the idea of a shared common oppression – women's bonding was based on shared victimization and to be female meant to be a victim. However, bell hooks (1986) states that we can bond on the basis of our political commitment to a feminist movement that aims to end sexist oppression. Within Latin America, especially in Central America, feminism's origins have been in armed struggles and in rural communities with women taking on both supportive and combat roles in guerilla warfare (Martin & Shaw, 2021; Reif, 1986).

Media Coverage of Latina Organizers and Activists vs. Cis-Latino Men

Latina activists have played a crucial role in the development and promotion of human rights throughout history. Latina-led social justice efforts have influenced a wide range of causes, ranging from LGBTQ+ and workers' rights to racial justice efforts (Montoya & Seminario, 2022). Yet, the groundbreaking work of Latina activists continues to be underrepresented, unacknowledged, and/or white-washed. For instance, the highly lauded major motion picture *Frida* has been criticized for commodifying and misrepresenting the story of Frida Kahlo in an effort to fit within Eurocentric-informed Hollywood standards (Molina Guzman, 2008).

Media representation of feminist activism also erases the intersecting nature of cultural, linguistic, and geographic identities on activism and organization, thus centering the narratives of White feminists (de Onís, 2015). Well-known contemporary feminist movements exclude the voices of Latina activists. For instance, the 2017 Women's March, which gained worldwide notoriety, primarily centered narratives from White, cisgender women (Bolivar, 2021).

In addition to receiving far less coverage when compared to White female-identified activists, the work and contributions of cisgender Latino activists are often more well-known among society; the notoriety of César Chávez compared to Dolores Huerta serves as a pointed example. Despite being a cofounder of The United Farm Workers, public awareness and acknowledgement of her life work and service is scarce. Mercado Jones (2019) contends, "history has a way of positioning women as accessories to activist movements, and Dolores Huerta is no exception. Her image is often part of the background of old black and white photographs that center César Chávez as the subject" (p. 1). As an instructor for an undergraduate course at The University of Georgia entitled, "U.S. Latino/a Mental Health: An Introduction," I (Grace-Ellen) reflected on how to incorporate awareness about the lives, experiences, and contributions of Latina activists. After some research, I decided to assign students in the course to view the documentary *Dolores*, produced by PBS (Benson & Bratt, 2017). Class discussions produced two important themes. First, the vast majority of students in the class (most of whom identified as Latinx) had never heard of Dolores Huerta prior to the documentary. Second, despite the documentary's focus on Dolores Huerta, students also noticed the way in which the documentary also incorporated critical commentary on Huertas' identities as a mother, wife, and partner. We wondered, would this content be included if Huerta identified as a man?

FROM PAPER TO PRACTICE

Moving Away From Essentialist Notions of Gender in Latinx Communities

Stereotypical Gender Roles

When I (Brooke; White woman) started working on my dissertation about Latinx feminism, I was familiar with traditional understandings of gender roles within the Latinx community (e.g., machismo and marianismo). As an insider (feminist)-outsider (White, European American), I wondered how Latinx women would be able to identify as both feminist and Latinx, given the seeming contradiction between Latinx cultural values and feminism apparent in social science research. For example, research on machismo suggested that it may play out in an overt manner or may be subtler within Latin American culture, having both negative and positive outcomes (Cianelli et al., 2008; Villegas et al., 2010). Traditionally, boys were socialized from a young age to act out aggressively, demonstrating their dominance and strength; as men aged, there was an expectation of maintained dominance, independence, and sexual freedom. On the other hand, the concept of marianismo emphasizes women as remaining demure, passive, and dependent within Latinx culture (Cianelli et al., 2008) with girls being socialized from a young age to be submissive, especially to their husbands, and to seek motherhood (Cianelli et al., 2008; Castillo et al., 2010). Both of these traditional views of machismo and marianismo promote the well-being of the family (familismo) and collectivism.

However, I have learned that White people in the United States actually co-opted these terms to denote stereotypical and dysfunctional Latinx qualities that promote Latinx men as hypersexual, violent, and paternalistic and dichotomize Latinx women as either la virgen (the virgin Mary) or la puta (a whore; Anzaldúa, 2007). This dichotomy occurs as the result of Western cultures embedding underlying Christian values and patriarchy through colonization of racially and ethnically diverse groups in order to limit the roles and power of folx of color, including Latinx women within patriarchal societies (Arrizón, 2008; Conrad, 2006). This essentialist view of Latinx folx existing as these stereotypical types is harmful and in fact, the experiences of capturing and conceptualizing the meaning of one's feminist identity is complex, nuanced, and deeply personal.

To further highlight this, I refer back to my dissertation project (Rappaport, 2019) about feminist identity development among Latina feminist psychologists. The participants, who all identified as Latina feminists, stated that they did not experience major conflict between cultural ideals and their feminist identities; while some noted how they may not have fulfilled family expectations (e.g., motherhood, marriage), they still received support from their families. Moreover, many participants spoke specifically about support they received from men in their cultures who promoted feminist ideals. In her dissertation, Erin Schwartz Forehand (2012) examined the relationship between womanist identity and ethnic identity in African American and Latina women. Results indicated that there was a positive correlation between ethnic identity and womanist identity such that women who identified more strongly with their ethnicity were more likely to be in the internalization stage of womanist identity development. The internalization stage occurred when a woman was able to identify her own personalized definition of womanhood without reliance on conventional gender roles or traditional feminism (Forehand, 2012). Relatedly, Patricia Arredondo (2010) noted her own feminist identity development as being deeply influenced by her feminist father and grandmother and more traditional mother.

Again, essentialist notions of gender roles within Latinx culture are too limiting and do not allow for the richness and diversity within this ethnic group. This underscores that the Latinx culture is not a monolithic one. In fact, feminist identities are varied based on one's cultural background and lived experiences. Chavez-Dueñas and Adames (2021) note how their participants internalized, through their collective histories, an understanding that they come from a "legacy of greatness" (p. 88). This challenges the harmful stereotypes described above in favor of utilizing ancestral and indigenous ways of knowing as a means to resist oppression.

Aguantar (To Endure)

Within Latinx culture, *aguantando*, or to endure, is a cultural value that tells Latina women that they should be able to endure suffering at all costs. *Aguantando* is often a source of strength for many Latina women. It is often linked to the cultural value of familismo, meaning the decision to endure pain and suffering (i.e., harmful or violent behavior from men) is done to maintain familial harmony. However, if examined critically, to *aguantar* only reinforces patriarchy and keeps women trapped in cycles of violence. For example, Herrera & Gloria (2021) share the story of Sandra, a Latina survivor of childhood sexual abuse by her stepfather. Sandra suspected that her mother was aware of the abuse, but the trauma was never discussed. Rather, the closer her mother ever came to addressing the abuse was by sharing a story about how she had to "aguantar" the sexual advances of her uncle while immigrating from Nicaguara to the US. In sharing this story, Sandra's mother offered her daughter *un consejo (advice)*: "las mujeres temenos que echarle ganas y aguantar" (women need to work hard and endure). Through this story, we see how gender role expectations to *aguantar* encourage women to keep quiet about pain or abuse in order to maintain harmony in the family.

I (Kiara) have personally been impacted by the socialized expectations to *aguantar*. When my grandma died from COVID-19, my family reacted intensely — my uncle punched a wall, and my mom sobbed into her rosary. I, on the other hand, could not bring myself to cry and instead did what I do best: I consoled and protected my family. As the eldest daughter in a Latinx family, I have often felt the need to be strong, even when inside I do not feel strong at all. I am a first-generation college student pursuing my Ph.D., so in my working-class family, I have often been perceived as "the one who has it all together."

Mamí, however, had a special kind of magic that allowed me to let all my walls down. When I told her how insecure I felt about speaking Spanish during internship interviews, she told me to call her every day to practice together. As I opened up more to her, she opened up more to me. I learned about her pride in being a God-fearing woman, her struggle and resiliency as an immigrant, and her love for Ecuador, her home country. The vulnerability and curiosity mamí and I expressed towards one another helped me let go of my need to be strong all the time and taught me it was okay to cry. Our relationship was the catalyst in both my racial-ethnic identity development, as well as the foundation of my passion for empowering women of color and other marginalized groups in therapy. My interest in mental health and my identity as a psychologist-in-training committed to social justice and liberation started with mamí. But in order for me to do that, I had to stop aguantando. I had to let myself feel.

Grief taught me an important lesson that now influences how I understand my work as a therapist: healing does not happen in isolation; healing happens in community. To grieve my grandmother, I had to let people in and soak in their love for me, a woman who was now trying to navigate life without her compass. Rather than submitting to the expectations and demands of capitalism and grind culture, I rested. I cried. I prayed. I spent time with my family. I healed both privately and out loud.

The desire to aguantar and "keep it all together" may be tempting, but it will never be the path to wellness. Isolation and avoidance are not the medicine; community is the medicine, and this is a lesson that I strive to integrate into my professional identity. I can be strong and grieving. I can rely on others and embrace solitude. These are not mutually exclusive. Women of color constantly feel the need to be self-reliant, but I now know that pain is not meant to be felt alone.

Familismo

When I (Grace-Ellen) first began conducting interviews for my dissertation, which focuses on the experiences of Latinas following miscarriage, I was unsure what results I would find. I did recognize, however, the importance of being aware of how my own worldviews and perspectives could inform how I approached my expectations for this study, particularly given my identity as a White woman. As I started interviews with participants, it became clear early on that the experience of miscarriage could not be described without also describing familial contextual factors. In fact, "family," was one of the most salient themes to emerge from the study, aligning with the Latinx cultural value of *familismo*. Familismo is broadly understood as a Latinx value that emphasizes familial needs and cohesion before individual needs (Piña-Watson et al., 2019).

Under the umbrella of family, every participant discussed their relationships with their mothers. Although the nature of the mother-daughter relationships varied between each participant, many participants described their mothers as the glue of their family systems, both financially and socially-emotionally. Several participants shared that they strive to emulate their mothers, based on the examples that their mothers set as being hardworking, educationally focused, and career driven. Similarly, a common thread among participants was that their mothers encouraged them to pursue their goals, develop their own sense of self and identity, and advance their careers prior to starting a family. The interview results challenge potential stereotypes of machismo and Latinx men as being head of the household.

As previously discussed, Latinx women have played a pivotal role in advocating for, and advancing measures to legalize abortion and increase access to reproductive healthcare for all. Yet, the healthcare system in the United States has an extensive history of committing egregious abuse against women of color. In the fall of 2020, the Irwin County Detention Center in Ocilla, Georgia made headlines for coercing women to undergo unnecessary hysterectomies (Project South, 2020).

On June 24th, 2022, the Supreme Court of the United States overturned Roe v. Wade in a 5-4 vote, officially redacting the federal constitutional right to abortion. This day occurred while we (chapter authors) were in the midst of writing and editing this chapter. Upon hearing this news, I (Grace-Ellen) thought immediately about the participants in my dissertation. For my specific study, a medically induced miscarriage was often necessary and required to save the lives of the women I interviewed. Additionally, I reflected on the impact of this decision within a medical system that is already fraught with limited resources, a lack of attention to mental health well-being, and minimal culturally and linguistically responsive health care providers.

While the overturn of Roe v. Wade has the potential to seriously impact all birthing parents, it is important to acknowledge specific implications this ruling may have on women of color, including Latinx. First, overturning Roe V. Wade poses serious concerns to the physical health and wellbeing of

Latinx women. Latinas are much less likely to receive prenatal care than White women (Latino Policy Forum, 2022). Additionally, maternal mortality continues to rise in the United States. Maternal mortality disproportionately impacts Latinas. Between 2019-2020, maternal mortality rates of Latinas increased 44.4%, compared to a rise of 6.1% among White women (Thoma & Declercq, 2022).

The criminalization of abortion will likely further exacerbate glaring concerns related to income inequality as well. For women living in states with abortion bans, traveling to other states with fewer restrictions can require childcare, travel funds, and missing work, requiring financial means; moreover, traveling out of state for abortion access can mean significant safety concerns for Latinx who are not documented (Lozada, 2022).

It is vital to be cognizant of ways in which mainstream media and politics may conflate or misrepresent Latinx opinions on abortion. According to a 2021 poll, half of Latinx voters in the United States believe in the complete legalization of abortion without restrictions (Intersections of Our Lives, 2021). As summarized by the Latino Policy Forum, "Some will attempt to rationalize the recent decision by aligning it closely with Latino values. However, Latino culture is also rooted in a defined struggle for agency and community care, self-determination, independence, and basic rights" (2022, para. 5).

Do This by Utilizing More Qualitative Research and Strengths-Based Methodologies

Moving away from essentialist, stereotypical gender stereotypes within Latinx communities requires reevaluating how these topics are researched and published. As a White woman who has attended Primary White Institutions (PWI's) for my undergraduate, masters, and doctoral degrees, I (Grace-Ellen) had limited exposure to diverse research methodologies prior to working with Dr. Delgado-Romero. My rudimentary understanding of research methods led me to equate "rigorous" or "legitimate" research with studies involving huge sample sizes and complicated statistics. Beginning at The University of Georgia and working on a primarily Latinx research team with a Latinx advisor allowed me to confront my own biases and ignorance around approaches to research. Qualitative research, defined as "the process of collecting, analyzing, and interpreting non-numerical data, such as language," (McLeod, 2019, para 1) has great potential when working with the Latinx population. Qualitative approaches may align with the cultural values found in many Latinx communities, and offer an opportunity to capture detailed, rich narratives of participants (Delgado-Romero et al., 2018). Researchers seeking to explore gender roles among Latinx populations must be intentional about utilizing approaches that will capture the holistic experiences of participants from a strengths-based and culturally responsive framework.

In Higher Education

Approximately 20% of Latinas have at least a bachelor's degree (U.S. Census Bureau, 2020). This number has increased over the last decade meaning that more Latinas are enrolling in institutions of higher education. As diversity in enrollment increases so has the diversity in courses taught. Over the years, new ethnic studies courses have been introduced such as Mexican American Studies, Latin American studies, and Latinx feminism, among others. These courses help students develop their critical consciousness. Paulo Freire (2005) defines critical consciousness as the ability of oppressed individuals to critically analyze oppressive social forces that further perpetuate their oppressive conditions and the way they take action against them. With critical consciousness comes knowledge of the self or *conocimiento*.

Many of these courses utilize feminist epistemologies and embed students' lived experiences in the curriculum. A way these courses go about teaching the content is through the utilization of *auto-historia*, or self storytelling, which is a creative reflective process of storytelling and art-making to then theorize from (Tijerina Revilla et al., 2021). Thus, writing as an act of healing connects with Anzaldúa's concept of *conocimiento* (Solís, 2020). This is what Anzaldúa & Keating (2015) refer to as geographies of the self. This involves the environments that we interact with which in turn become part of our identities leading to higher critical consciousness. In turn, higher critical consciousness leads students to hold self-beliefs that they can induce positive change in their communities which can lead them to set higher intentions to persist in college (Cadenas et al., 2018). In addition, these courses are important for the retention of first-generation Latina students as they serve as a counter-space where students can interact with one another and be one another's support system in higher education (Marrun, 2018). It is a way for students to unlearn internalized deficit ideologies and messages about their lives (Tijerina Revilla et al., 2021).

Students in these courses describe how the curriculum and pedagogy provide a space separate from home, community, and school to process and to develop together their own narratives where they are valued. Additionally, students express how these courses help develop a new perspective on the roles and expectations of women in their families and their socialization (Marrun, 2018). Many Latinas in higher education also value the benefits of peer-to-peer mentorship and the development of community support (Moschetti et al., 2018) in their higher education journey.

Clinical Practice

In order for more Latinas to experience mestiza consciousness and increase their curiosity of existing within the borderlands, it is critical that mental health professionals make an active effort to learn about the unique challenges that exist for Latinx women that may bring them to therapy. Moreover, it is essential that mental health providers not only learn about the oppression and trauma that exist in the lives of Latinx women, but that they also put equal emphasis on the strengths and resilience found in these women. Chavez-Dueñas & Adames (2021) call for mental health providers to decenter White women as the template of womanhood and instead emphasize the importance of highlighting the collective wisdom of Latinx women of color (i.e., Black and Indigenous Latinas) who have actively resisted colonialism and attacks on their well-being. Latinx women in therapy should feel empowered to reclaim their collective histories and call upon their strengths as forms of healing. The *Intersectionality Awakening Model of Womantisa (I AM Womanista)* facilitates this therapeutic process.

The *I AM Womanista psychotherapy* treatment model was created by integrating the lessons from three analytical frameworks - intersectionality (Combahee River Collective, 1995; Crenshaw, 1991), womanism (Walker, 1983), and mujerismo (Comas-Díaz, 1988). The goal of the treatment model is to assist mental health providers working with Latinas to deliver interventions rooted in a gendered-racial-culturally responsive praxis.

Understanding the Historical-Colonial Origin of Marianismo

The *I AM Womanista* model aims to "assist psychotherapists to understand the historical-colonial origin of marianismo and interrogate its normativity by helping prevent Latina women from internalizing messages that subjugate their gendered-racial experiences and realities" (Chavez-Dueñas & Adames, 2021,

p. 86). Most psychotherapists are not trained nor socialized to reflect on how gendered-racism impacts the lives of Latinx women.

Counternarratives

Counternarratives are described as personal narratives carrying identity claims which resist those identity claims that originate from dominant discourses (Bamberg, 2004). The use of counter-narratives in clinical practice has been utilized with various different marginalized groups, including women of color (Chavez-Dueñas & Adames, 2021), LGBTQ+ communities, (Helmer, 2016), individuals with disabilities (Fisher & Goodley, 2007), and several others.

Counternarratives have a powerful purpose in psychotherapy with Latinx women. Colonization has resulted in Latinx women thinking they are weak and unimportant, or has them holding onto oppressive gender roles. However, what is often ignored is that Latinx women are the descendants of incredibly powerful, brave, and resilient women who have survived some of the most atrocious human right violations in the history of Latin America. Unfortunately, the stories of these Latinx women are often missing from mainstream culture and go unnoticed by Latinas struggling with feelings of inadequacy and low self-worth. The systemic silencing of these stories results in Latinx women thinking they need to be quiet, self-sacrificial, and submissive (Chavez-Dueñas & Adames, 2021).

Providing a therapeutic space where Latinas can be exposed to counternarratives has several important purposes. First, it allows them to closely interrogate the roles that have been ascribed to them by society (e.g., heterosexual marriage, existing in the gender binary, motherhood). By learning about other Latinas who have resisted these gender roles, Latinx women can begin to explore new options and possibilities that help them feel more in control of their life. Secondly, counternarratives encourage Latinx women to learn how systems of oppression operate, how they have been personally impacted by these systems, and – perhaps most importantly – begin to explore how they can resist oppression. This intentional exposure to womansitas in Latinx history results in womanista liberation.

I (Kiara) consider my experience integrating counter-narratives in my clinical work with Black and Latina women. Much of my clinical work has focused on supporting survivors of military sexual trauma within a VA hospital. During a group therapy session for women survivors (all of whom identify as women of color), one group member reluctantly shared with the group that she had been feeling very depressed that week. However, in an attempt to reduce the embarrassment she felt after being vulnerable, she assured the group that she is fine and to not to worry about her. Instantly, another group member said to her, "Put that pride shit aside, you don't have to go through this alone, we're here." This group of women had a beautiful way of being assertive with one another, yet in the most loving way. I used this interaction as an opportunity to encourage this particular woman to create a counter-narrative of her feelings around vulnerability. Rather than focusing on the shame and embarrassment, I encouraged the group to think about how vulnerability can be seen as a sign of strength. We processed the difficulties in creating this counter-narrative, specifically due to the socialization and patriarchal culture that exists for women of color in the military. We explicitly named the systems of power – racism, sexism, patriarchy – that caused their experiences of sexual violence to be treated as less important than a white woman's. We processed our admiration for the women who were brave enough to bring Bill Cosby's violence to the public eye. We then discussed how seeing vulnerability as a weakness may have protected them while in the military, it was no longer serving them in the present. Together, we created a counter-narrative of what it means to be an emotional woman – rather than seeing it as a sign of weakness, we agreed on how much strength there is in asking for help and how vulnerability can be the catalyst for connection, intimacy, and healing.

NLPA As a Model for Centering Feminist Perspectives

The formation of the current National Latinx Psychological Association (NLPA) in 2002 reflects the values held within counseling psychology merged with Latinx cultural values. Two prominent counseling psychologists, Melba Vasquez and Patricia Arredondo, were key founders of NLPA and have made important contributions to multicultural psychology (Chavez-Korell et al., 2012). Not only does NLPA reflect multicultural psychology, but it represents one of the few psychological organizations that successfully blends multiculturalism and feminism; NLPA infuses cultural ideals of *familismo* (family connection) and *personalismo* (interpersonal relationships) with feminist ideals including gender equality and consciousness-raising (Clay, 2011). Additionally, NLPA has consciously adopted a feminist, empowering, respectful approach that promotes gender equity (Miville et al., 2017). The founders of the National Latinx Psychological Association consciously challenged the typical Latinx language and NLPA has placed women in important leadership roles within the organization. Moreover, the leaders within NLPA purposely placed Latina in front of Latino in the original name of the organization (National Latina/o Psychological Association) to challenge traditional male-centric language. The organization recently voted to update the name to include Latinx instead of Latina/o to be more gender-inclusive. Chavez-Korell and colleagues (2012) noted that "NLPA members are committed to addressing social justice issues such as immigration, ethical treatment of immigrants (regardless of documentation status), health disparities, and the reduction of prejudice/racism" (p. 680). These members were able to fuse together the values of counseling psychology, feminist psychology, and multicultural psychology in the study of Latinx psychology.

FUTURE DIRECTIONS

Traditional theories of cultural competence tend to be ahistorical, genderless, and predominately focus on the intrapsychic experiences without acknowledging the multiple forms of oppression on a person's life (Adames, 2017). Feminist therapy tends to be colorbind. In order for Latinx feminism (and feminism, in general) to be most inclusive, we suggest a continued emphasis on utilizing an intersectional lens in understanding feminism. The *I Am Womanista* model represents this direction and we hope there can be continued research and utilization of this feminist approach to working with Latinx-identified women in therapy and beyond. This approach is congruent with our previous discussion around continued use of qualitative and strengths-based approaches.

Three out of four of the authors of this chapter were/are members of the ¡BIENESTAR! Research Team at the University of Georgia, led by Dr. Edward Delgado-Romero. Delgado-Romero was mentored by Latinx feminists like Patricia Arredondo, Azara Santiago Rivera and Melba Vasquez and critically examined and expanded his identity as a Latinx feminist man. Delgado-Romero has intentionally created a pipeline that brings more Latinx psychologists to the field; he supports students with culturally-affirming mentorship and infusion of Latinx collectivist values such as familismo and comunidad. The reciprocal nature of this pipeline means that his mentees foster this continuation in their future careers to pay it forward. We suggest other doctoral mentors utilize a similar approach to foster the growth of Latinx scholars, specifically women, in higher education and beyond.

Finally, we hope that utilizing chapters like this one in the process of decolonizing syllabi will provide both Latinx-identified and non-Latinx identified people counter-narratives to those typically taught about Latinx culture. By empowering Latina feminists to take ownership of their cultural history and to express curiosity about the wisdom and strength of the Latinas who came before them, we can build a collective of women who feel supported and encouraged as they heal the wounds inflicted by colonization, patriarchy, and White supremacy. We cannot heal in isolation; we heal in community. We hope that other Latinas can read about the powerful women who have come before them to know that they come from a "legacy of greatness" (Chavez-Dueñas and Adames, 2021, p. 88).

REFERENCES

Adames, H. Y., Chavez-Dueñas, N. Y., & Jernigan, M. M. (2021). The fallacy of a raceless Latinidad: Action guidelines for centering Blackness in Latinx psychology. *Journal of Latina/o Psychology*, *9*(1), 26–44. doi:10.1037/lat0000179

Anthony, M., Nichols, A. H., & Del Pilar, W. (2021, December 21). A look at degree attainment among Hispanic women and men and how COVID-19 could deepen racial and gender divides. *The Education Trust*. Retrieved May 8, 2022, from https://edtrust.org/resource/a-look-at-degree-attainment-among-hispanic-women-and-men-and-how-covid-19-could-deepen-racial-and-gender-divides/

Anzaldúa, G. (2002). Now let us shift... the path of conocimiento... inner work, public acts. In G.E. Anzaldúa & A. L. Keating (Ed.), This bridge we call home: Radical visions for transformation (pp. 540-578). New York, NY: Routledge.

Anzaldúa, G. (2007). *Borderlands/ La Frontera: The New Mestiza*. Aunt Lute Books.

Anzaldúa, G., & Keating, A. (2015). *Light in the Dark/Luz en lo Oscuro: Rewriting Identity, Spirituality, Reality*. Duke University Press.

Anzaldúa, G. E. (1987). *Borderlands/La Frontera: The New Mestiza*. Aunt Lute.

Arredondo, P. (2002). Mujeres Latinas—Santas y Marquesas. *Cultural Diversity & Ethnic Minority Psychology*, *8*(4), 308–319. doi:10.1037/1099-9809.8.4.308 PMID:12416317

Arredondo, P. (2010). In J. G. Ponterotto, J. M. Casas, L. A. Suzuki, & C. M. Alexander (Eds.), *Handbook of Multicultural Counseling* (3rd ed., pp. 38–44). Sage.

Arrizón, A. (2008). Latina subjectivity, sexuality and sensuality. *Women & Performance*, *18*(3), 189–198. doi:10.1080/07407700802495928

Balbuena, A. (2018). El debate sobre el aborto y las tres causales: La cuestión de la autonomía de la mujer [The Debate on Abortions and the Three grounds; The Issue of Woman's Anatomy]. *Perspectivas*, *2*(18), 1–8.

Biglieri, P. (2020). Ni Una Menos—Not One Woman Less: How Feminism Could Become a Popular Struggle. *Baltic Worlds*, *13*(1), 64–66.

Bolivar, A. (2021). "This Pussy Actually Grabs Back": A Trans Latina Expansion of "Pussy." *Frontiers*, *42*(2), 1–23. doi:10.1353/fro.2021.0020

Castillo, L. G., Perez, F. V., Castillo, R., & Ghosheh, M. R. (2010). Construction and initial validation of the Marianismo Beliefs Scale. *Counselling Psychology Quarterly*, *23*(2), 163–175. doi:10.1080/09515071003776036

Chavez-Dueñas, N. Y., & Adames, H. Y. (2021). Intersectionality Awakening Model of Womanista: A transnational treatment approach for Latinx women. *Women & Therapy*, *44*(1-2), 83–100. doi:10.1080/02703149.2020.1775022

Cianelli, R., Ferrer, L., & McElmurry, B. J. (2008). HIV prevention and low-income Chilean women: Machismo, marianismo and HIV misconceptions. *Culture, Health & Sexuality*, *10*, 297–306.

Colectiva Feminista en Construcción. (2020a). *La Manifiesta*. https://www.scribd.com/document/263057948/La-Manifiesta-Colectiva-Feminista-en-Construccion

Colectiva Feminista en Construcción. (2020b, March 6). *Manifiesto antirracista de la Colectiva Feminista en Construcción* [Anti-Racist Manifesto of the Feminist Collective in Consrutction]. https://www.todaspr.com/manifiesto-antirracista-de-la-colectiva-feminista-en-construccion/

Coles, S. M., & Pasek, J. (2020). Intersectional invisibility revisited: How group prototypes lead to the erasure and exclusion of Black women. *Translational Issues in Psychological Science*, *6*(4), 1–11. doi:10.1037/tps0000256

Comas-Díaz, L. (1988). Feminist therapy with Hispanic/Latina women: Myth or reality? *Women & Therapy*, *6*(4), 39–61. doi:10.1300/J015V06N04_06

Comas-Díaz, L. (2008). 2007 Carolyn Sherif Award Address: *Spirita*: Reclaiming Womanist Sacredness into Feminism. *Psychology of Women Quarterly*, *32*(1), 13–21. doi:10.1111/j.1471-6402.2007.00403.x

Comas-Díaz, L. (2016). Mujerista psychospirituality. In T. Bryant-Davis & L. Comas-Díaz (Eds.), *Womanist and mujerista psychologies: Voices of fire, acts of courage* (pp. 149–169). American Psychological Association. doi:10.1037/14937-007

Comas-Díaz, L. (2021). Afro-Latinxs: Decolonization, healing, and liberation. *Journal of Latina/o Psychology*, *9*(1), 65–75. doi:10.1037/lat0000164

Combahee River Collective. (1995). Combahee River Collective statement. In B. Guy-Sheftall (Ed.), *Words of fire: An anthology of African American feminist thought* (pp. 232–240). New Press.

Conrad, B. K. (2006). Neo-institutionalism, social movements, and the cultural reproduction of a mentalité: Promise keepers reconstruct the Madonna/Whore complex. *The Sociological Quarterly*, *47*(2), 305–331. doi:10.1111/j.1533-8525.2006.00047.x

Crenshaw, K. (1991). Mapping the margins: Intersectionality, identity politics, and violence against women of color. *Stanford Law Review*, *43*(6), 1241–1299. doi:10.2307/1229039

Crisóstomo Tejada, V. (2021). La Colectiva Feminista en Construcción: Puerto Rico's antiracist & feminist movement [The Feminist Collective under Construction: Puerto Rico's antiracist & feminist movement]. *Review of Education, Pedagogy & Cultural Studies*, *43*(5), 398–418. doi:10.1080/1071441 3.2021.1970466

Daby, M., & Moseley, M. W. (2021). Feminist Mobilization and the Abortion Debate in Latin America: Lessons from Argentina. *Politics & Gender*, 1–35. doi:10.1017/S1743923X20000197

de Onís, K. (2015). Lost in Translation: Challenging (White, Monolingual Feminism's) <Choice> with Justicia Reproductiva. *Women's Studies in Communication*, *38*(1), 1–19. doi:10.1080/07491409.2014 .989462

Del Rincon, F. (2016, August 29). ¿*Juan Gabriel es gay? "Lo que se ve, no se pregunta", dijo* [Is Juan Gabriel Gay? "What is seen, is not asked," he said] [Video]. CNN. https://cnnespanol.cnn.com/video/cnnee-conclusiones-entrevista-juan-gabriel-fernando-del-rincon-2002-p3/

Delgado-Romero, E. A., Singh, A. A., & De Los Santos, J. (2018). Cuéntame: The promise of qualitative research with Latinx populations. *Journal of Latina/o Psychology*, *6*(4), 318–328. doi:10.1037/lat0000123

Delgado-Romero, E. A., Unkefer, E. N. S., Capielo, C., & Crowell, C. N. (2017). El que oye consejos, llega a viejo: Examining the published life narratives of U.S. Latino/a psychologists. *Journal of Latina/o Psychology*, *5*(3), 127–141. doi:10.1037/lat0000071

Delgado-Romero, E. A., & Werther, E. (2012). Hispanic Psychologists. In R. DelCampo & D. M. Blancero (Eds.), *Hispanics @ Work: A Collection of Research, Theory and Application* (pp. 177–188). Nova Science Publishers.

Fisher, P., & Goodley, D. (2007). The linear medical model of disability: Mothers of disabled babies resist with counter-narratives. *Sociology of Health & Illness*, *29*(1), 66–81. doi:10.1111/J.1467-9566.2007.00518.x PMID:17286706

Forehand, E. S. (2012). *Multiple identities: The intersection of womanism and ethnicity in a diverse sample of women* [Unpublished doctoral dissertation]. The University of Georgia, Athens, GA.

Freire, P. (2005). *Education for critical consciousness*. Continuum Publishing.

Gloria, A. M., & Robinson Kurpius, S. E. R. (1996). The validation of the Cultural Congruity Scale and the University Environment Scale with Chicano/a students. *Hispanic Journal of Behavioral Sciences*, *18*(4), 533–549. doi:10.1177/07399863960184007

Gonzalez, S. (2022). Jotería Pedagogy. In K. K. Strunk & A. S. Shelton (Eds.), *Encyclopedia of Queer Studies in Education* (pp. 316–319). BRILL. doi:10.1163/9789004506725

Hall, N. (2018, April 23). *Argentina and "Los Desparecidos."* International Federation of Social Workers. https://www.ifsw.org/argentina-and-los-desaparecidos/

Hegewisch, A., & Mefferd, E. (2022, March 9). *Gender wage gaps remain wide in year two of the pandemic*. IWPR. Retrieved May 8, 2022, from https://iwpr.org/iwpr-publications/fact-sheet/gender-wage-gaps-remain-wide-in-year-two-of-the-pandemic/

Hernandez, E. D. (2016). Cultura Joteria: The Ins and Outs of Latina/o Popular Culture. In F. L. Aldama (Ed.), *The Routledge Companion to Latina/o Popular Culture* (pp. 291–300). Routledge.

Herrera, N., & Gloria, A. M. (2021). Latina Students' Post-IPV Healing: A Bodymindspirit Approach Using the ELLA-SANA Model. *Women & Therapy*, 1–20. doi:10.1080/02703149.2021.1982537

Latinas/xs Summary. Intersections of Our Lives. (2021). Retrieved August 1, 2022, from https://intersectionsofourlives.org/wp-content/uploads/2021/07/ISOOL_Fact-Sheet-SummarLat a-final.pdf

Lozada, C. (2022, July 2). Perspective | how three major abortion rulings reveal a fractured culture. *The Washington Post.* Retrieved September 3, 2022, from https://www.washingtonpost.com/outlook/2022/07/01/roe-casey-dobbs-abortion-supreme-court/

Lugones, M. (2008). The coloniality of gender. *Worlds & Knowledge Otherwise*, 1–17.

Marrun, N. A. (2018). "My mom seems to have a *dicho* for everything!": Family engagement in the college success of Latina/o students. *Journal of Latinos and Education*, *19*(1), 164–180. doi:10.1080/15348431.2018.1489811

Martin, D., & Shaw, D. (2021). Chilean and Transnational Performances of Disobedience: LasTesis and the Phenomenon of Un violador en tu camino. *Bulletin of Latin American Research*, *40*(5), 712–729. doi:10.1111/blar.13215

McLeod, S. A. (2019, July 30). *Qualitative vs. quantitative research.* Simply Psychology. https://www.simplypsychology.org/qualitative-quantitative.html

Mercado Jones, R. (2019). Dolores: The Silenced Cofounder of the United Farm Workers. *Women & Language*, *1*, 105.

Miville, M. L., Arredondo, P., Consoli, A., Santiago-Rivera, A., Delgado-Romero, E. A., Fuentes, M., Domenech Rodriguez, M., Field, L., & Cervantes, J. (2017). Liderazgo/Leadership Through Cultural Lenses: The National Latina/o Psychological Association. *The Counseling Psychologist*, *45*, 830–856. doi:10.1177/0011000016668413

Montoya, C., & Seminario, M. G. (2022). Guerreras y Puentes: The theory and praxis of Latina(x) activism. *Politics, Groups & Identities*, *10*(2), 171–188. doi:10.1080/21565503.2020.1821233

Moraga, C., & Anzaldúa, G. (Eds.). (1983). *This bridge called my back: Writings by radical women of color.* SUNY Press.

Moschetti, R. V., Plunkett, S. W., Efrat, R., & Yomtov, D. (2018). Peer Mentoring as Social Capital for Latina/o College Students at a Hispanic-Serving Institution. *Journal of Hispanic Higher Education*, *17*(4), 375–392. doi:10.1177/1538192717702949

Nosotros a las 8. (2022, March 8). *Abinader reafirma su apoyo al aborto en las tres causales* [Abinader reaffirms his support for abortion on all three grounds] [Video]. Youtube. https://www.youtube.com/watch?v=R3uH-c_rL8g

Orozco, R. C., Gonzalez, S., & Duran, A. (2021). Centering Queer Latinx/a/o Experiences and Knowledge: Guidelines for Using Jotería Studies in Higher Education Qualitative Research. *Journal Committed to Social Change on Race and Ethnicity, 7*(1), 117–148. doi:10.15763/issn.2642-2387.2021.7.1.117-148

Palmeiro, C. (2018). The Latin American Green Tide: Desire and Feminist Transversality. *Journal of Latin American Cultural Studies, 27*(4), 561–564. doi:10.1080/13569325.2018.1561429

Piña-Watson, B., Gonzalez, I. M., & Manzo, G. (2019). Mexican-descent adolescent resilience through familismo in the context of intergeneration acculturation conflict on depressive symptoms. *Translational Issues in Psychological Science, 5*(4), 326–334. doi:10.1037/tps0000210

Popescu, I. (2021). Memorialization and Escraches: Ni Una Menos and the Documentation of Feminicidio in Argentina. *The Latin Americanist, 65*(3), 367–392. doi:10.1353/tla.2021.0024

Project South. (2020, September 14). Retrieved July 31, 2022, from https://projectsouth.org/wp-content/uploads/2020/09/OIG-ICDC-Complaint-1.pdf

Rappaport, B. (2019). *Exploring the experiences of Latina feminists in psychology: navigating intersecting identities, understanding Latina feminism, and implications for allies* (Publication No. 9949333998202959) [Doctoral dissertation, University of Georgia]. https://getd.libs.uga.edu/pdfs/rappaport_brooke_s_201908_phd.pdf

Reif, L. L. (1986). Women in Latin American Guerrilla Movements: A Comparative Perspective. *Comparative Politics, 18*(2), 147–169. doi:10.2307/421841

Reversal of Roe vs. Wade Devastating Impact on Latina Health: Joint Statement Illinois Latino Agenda 2.0 and Illinois Unidos. (2022, July 1). Latino Policy Forum. Retrieved August 1, 2022, from https://www.latinopolicyforum.org/news/press-releases/document/SCOTUS-reversal-of-Roe-v.-Wade.pdf

Saavedra, C. M., & Salazar Pérez, M. (2017). Chicana/Latina Feminist Critical Qualitative Inquiry: Meditations on Global Solidarity, Spirituality, and the Land. *International Review of Qualitative Research, 10*(4), 450–467. doi:10.1525/irqr.2017.10.4.450

Sanchez, D. (2021). Introduction to special issue on AfroLatinidad: Theory, research, and practice. *Journal of Latina/o Psychology, 9*(1), 1–7. doi:10.1037/lat0000186

Solís, V. (2020). Writing Autohistoria through Conocimiento. In M. Cantú-Sanchez, C. de León-Zepeda, & N. E. Cantú (Eds.), Teaching Gloria E. Anzaldúa: Pedagogy and Practice for Our Classrooms and Communities (pp. 91-111). University of Arizona Press. doi:10.2307/j.ctv1595m67.12

Thoma, M. E., & Declercq, E. R. (2022). All-Cause Maternal Mortality in the US Before vs During the COVID-19 Pandemic. *JAMA Network Open, 5*(6), e2219133. Advance online publication. doi:10.1001/jamanetworkopen.2022.19133 PMID:35763300

Tijerina Revilla, A., Nuñez, J., Santillana Blanco, J. M., & Gonzalez, S. (2021). Radical Jotería-Muxerista Love in the Classroom: Brown Queer Feminist Strategies for Social Transformation. In E. G. Murillo, D. Delgado Bernal, S. Morales, L. Urrieta, E. Ruiz Bybee, J. Sánchez Muñoz, V. Sáenz, D. Villanueva, M. Machado-Casas, & K. Espinoza (Eds.), *Handbook of Latinos and Education* (pp. 22–34). Routledge. doi:10.4324/9780429292026-4

Tijerina Revilla, A., & Santillana, J. M. (2014). Jotería Identity and Consciousness. *Aztlán, 39*(1), 197–179.

U.S. Census Bureau. (2020). *Educational Attainment, 2020 American Community Survey 5-year estimates.* Retrieved from https://data.census.gov/cedsci/table?q=S1501&tid=ACSST5Y2020.S1501

Villegas, J., Lemanski, J., & Valdéz, C. (2010). Marianismo and machismo: The portrayal of females in Mexican TV commercials. *Journal of International Consumer Marketing, 22*(4), 327–346. doi:10.1080/08961530.2010.505884

Vuola, E. (2017). Seriously Harmful For Your Health? Religion, Feminism and Sexuality in Latin America. In M. Althaus-Reid (Ed.), *Liberation Theology and Sexuality* (1st ed., pp. 137–162). Routledge. doi:10.4324/9781351153966-10

Walker, A. (1983). *In Search of Our Mothers' Gardens: Womanist Prose.* Harcourt.

Zillman, C. (2018). On equal pay day 2018, there's a troubling trend behind the shrinking gender pay gap. *Fortune.* Retrieved from http://fortune.com/2018/04/10/equal- pay-day-2018-closing-gender-pay-gap/

Chapter 8
Somos Fuertes Pero También Sufrimos (We Are Strong but We Also Suffer):
La Salud Mental de Hombres Latino (The Mental Health of Latino Men)

Eckart Werther
Clayton State University, USA

Bryan O. Rojas-Araúz
In Lak'ech Counseling, Education, and Consulting, USA

Ruben Atilano
Yale University, USA

ABSTRACT

The mental health of men has recently become a topic of interest to social scientists and mental health professionals. The chapter presents a strength-based and culturally informed understanding of the interrelated factors associated with the mental health of Latinx men. Concepts such as masculine ideologies, gender socialization, help-seeking behaviors, as well as relevant trends within higher education and the mental health fields. The authors engage readers in an adapted version of the Latinx oral tradition of testimonios. The authors incorporate personal and professional experiences throughout the chapter that are relevant to the topics and to facilitate a deeper connection and appreciation with the experiences of Latinx men and their mental health.

DOI: 10.4018/978-1-6684-4901-1.ch008

Somos Fuertes Pero También Sufrimos (We Are Strong but We Also Suffer)

CHOSEN STANZAS FROM *BEHIND THE MASK OF A WARRIOR SLAM POEM WRITTEN AND PERFORMED AT COCKTALES* "STORIES OF MASCULINITY PT.1" BY BRYAN O. ROJAS-ARAUZ

It is time for us as men to start fighting back

Fight back a society that has deemed us emotionless

Fight back for ourselves and our sons

We are at war, shackled and chained, trapped in a box

We are warriors that were never given the tools for survival

A generation of fatherless sons

Single mothers raising men in fatherless homes

As young men had to figure it out all on our own

No one to show us how to be men

Hiding behind the mask of a warrior

We got it all wrong

I was built on aggression

And so I became aggressive

At 13 the first time I was jumped

Also the first time I was praised because I put up "a good fight n didn't bitch about it"

Busted lip, bloody knuckled, and dirty

The medals of honor I earned in the makings of a warrior

Like another circus attraction it was all about the show

I was angry,

Angry at the fact I was not allowed to be sad

Angry

Angry at the counselors who thought they knew what I was feeling

When truth be told, I didn't know it myself

Anger

an emotion I knew wouldn't make me less of a man

But also the emotion that stopped me from truly feeling

I found myself trying to drown my emotions

Looking for role models at the bottom of bottles

Regardless of what we've seen, we've never told

Never told about the pain

Hardship

Fear

Or sadness

Death, violence, drugs, and corruption

We've seen it all

Living in a place where if you don't become fearless then you'll always be fearful

Yet we don't even know how to spell FEAR

The weight of our memories, the chains of our experience

Neatly packed in Pandora's Box

INTRODUCTION

The mental health of men has recently become a topic of interest to social scientists and mental health professionals. The present chapter aims to present a strength-based and culturally informed understanding of the interrelated factors associated with the mental health of Latinx men. Some of the concepts reviewed include masculine ideologies and gender role socialization. A host of other relevant issues are highlighted including trends within higher education and in the mental health industry which the authors feel also have some impact on the mental health of Latinx men. Moreover, the authors provide culturally informed suggestions and recommendations relevant for students, social scientists, mental health practitioners, and policymakers interested in understanding or addressing the issues associated with Latinx men's mental health.

The authors make an effort to interject Latinx ethnocultural values that are relevant in understanding the socialization, relational, and self-care practices of Latinx men. Additionally, in the spirit of the Latinx cultural value of *personalismo* and the oral tradition of *testimonios* (see Cervantes, Fernandez, & Carmona, 2019), the authors incorporate personal and professional experiences throughout the chapter. These 1st person narratives include relevant lived experiences and perspectives associated with the topics being discussed. Our *testimonios (*testimony/story*)* share our experiential knowledge; facilitate a deeper connection and appreciation with the subject matter for readers; and legitimize our lived experiences (Cervantes, Fernandez, & Carmona, 2019).

Due to the maintenance of oppressive academic practices, there has been a call for scholar-activists to undergo a process of decolonization in order address injustice and to amplify historically marginalized voices (Camacho, 2004). Decolonization of research and knowledge calls for an examination of what's considered valuable contributions to the body of knowledge. It invites us to question who is considered an expert and whose voice is often amplified in academia and academic spaces. As scholar-activists it is important for us to recognize the significance of creating knowledge from marginalized communities themselves while understanding it is created within oppressive systems that continue to perpetuate colonialism (Zavala, 2013).

¿QUIÉNES SOMOS? (WHO ARE WE?)

The growth, heterogeneity, and demographic trends associated with the Latinx population in the United States (U.S.) have been well documented. Among the estimated 62 million persons of Latinx heritage in the U.S. (Passel et al., 2022), roughly 30 million identify as Latinx men (U.S. Census, 2020). The diversity and demographic trends seen within the larger Latinx population can be generalized and reflected by Latinx men (Noe-Bustamante, 2019). For example, similar to the greater Latinx population, Latinx men can have cultural connections with more than 20 different countries located throughout the Americas (i.e., North, Central, and South) and the Caribbean (Abalos, 2002; U.S.; Uzogara, 2019). As a result, Latinx men in the U.S. can identify and incorporate a variety of cultural affiliations, languages, religious practices, sexual orientations, immigration status, and racial identities (Abalos, 2002).

The authors represent the diversity that exists within the Latinx population. All authors identify as cisgender, heterosexual, Latinx men and are bilingual and fluent in English and Spanish. Despite these similarities, each author has unique characteristics, background, and lived experiences. The following is a brief biographical introduction of each author.

Eckart

I am a 1st generation immigrant and I come from a long line of immigrants. I am of Costa Rican and Nicaraguan heritage. I also have German heritage that originates from my paternal grandfather. He immigrated with my paternal great-grandparents to Nicaragua from Germany when he was 14 years old. He would eventually move to Costa Rica after marrying my paternal grandmother. My maternal grandmother is from Nicaragua. When she was young, she moved to Costa Rica with my maternal great-grandparents. I immigrated to the United States with my family (Father, mother and two younger sisters) at the age of 5 and grew up in South Florida.

I am the first person in my family to attend college. I had no prior role models or knowledge of the processes involved navigating higher education. Neither my father nor mother were college educated. I experienced a great deal of conflict as I navigated higher ed.

However, I stayed focused and eventually earned my B.S.W from the University of North Alabama. I worked for a few years before earning my M.S.W. from Alabama A&M University. I then worked a few more years before attending the University of Georgia where I earned my Ph.D. in Counseling Psychology.

Currently I am an associate professor of psychology, a licensed psychologist, and a licensed clinical social worker. I also serve in a variety of other important roles such as husband, father, son, brother, uncle, friend, and mentor.

Ruben

I was born to Mexican parents in California. My parents immigrated to the U.S. from Mexico in the 1980's. My parents faced many challenges coming to the U.S. including adjustment, discrimination, and language barriers. In experiencing these hardships, my parents did not want my sister and me to face the same problems, so they emphasized the value of education.

As a first-generation Latinx man, my parents motivated me through dichos (Spanish sayings) such as "No quieres trabajar como un burro" (you don't want to work manual labor like a donkey). My parents' teachings helped me recognize how success in this country starts in the classroom. Their value of education was the factor that influenced my decision to pursue a college degree. Their sacrifices gave me the determination and blue print to receive a Bachelor of Arts in Cognitive Psychology from the University of California, Irvine. I then completed a Master's in Counseling Psychology from the University of Missouri and a Ph.D. in Counseling Psychology from the University of Georgia.

I am currently a post-doctoral fellow at a university mental health center where I provide individual and group psychotherapy to undergraduate and graduate students with various presenting concerns. My enjoyment in life comes from being a husband, father, son, brother, and uncle.

Bryan

I am a bilingual, bicultural, Afro-Latino immigrant of Costa Rican and Panamanian descent. My father is Costa Rican while my mother was born and raised in Panama. At 13 years old, I came to the United States to learn English in order to go back home and help my family make ends meet. I hoped to support my family by finding employment in the tourism industry. What was supposed to be a 6-month trip became a permanent move. I spent my teenage years in the Bay Area, California. Where I became a *community organizer and DREAM activist. As a previously undocumented immigrant, I learned to value the opportunities that were not always present.*

As a first-generation undocumented immigrant scholar, I struggled to find my place in academia, often being defined out, reminded of the reasons why I shouldn't have been there or ways I was different, instead of being invited in. Even though my path was not always clear I received my B.A. in Psychology from San Jose State, earned my Master's in Counseling in Marriage, Family, and Child Therapy with a dual emphasis in College Counseling from San Francisco State, and graduated with my Ph.D. in Counseling Psychology with a Spanish Language Psychological Services and Research Specialization from the University of Oregon.

I am a trauma licensed psychologist, the co-founder of In Lak'ech Counseling, Education, and Consulting, adjunct professor in International Disaster Psychology: Trauma and Global Mental Health at the University of Denver, private practitioner, author, documentary filmmaker, slam poet, and past Director of Latinx and Spanish Language Services at a trauma clinic in Denver, CO. Additionally, I provide immigration evaluations for refugees and asylum seekers, and I am co-authoring a book on social justice engagement for psychologists and other helping professionals. My research emphases include Latinx Psychological Wellbeing, Immigrant and DREAMer Experiences, Undocumented Communities' Access to Mental Health and Education, Critical Consciousness, Cultural Sensitivity, Advocacy, and Social Justice.

MENTAL HEALTH AND PROTECTIVE FACTORS

Some of the most prevalent mental health conditions in the U.S. include depression, anxiety, trauma, and substance abuse disorders. Like other populations in the U.S, Latinx men can experience many of these same conditions. There is some evidence that Latinx individuals experience mental disorders at lower rates compared to other demographic groups (Ortega et al., 2006; Hill et al., 2019) and that they display greater resiliency when faced with stressful life situations (Myers et al., 2015).

The prevalence rates for mental health disorders amongst Latinx men can vary and can be influenced by a variety of factors. Some of the factors that contribute to the mental health of Latinx persons include family, level of acculturation, time in the U.S., racial & ethnic identity, sense of belonging, social stressors, and experiences with discrimination (Ai et al., 2015; Maldonado et al., 2018; Myers et al., 2015; Ortega et al., 2000; Ortega et al., 2006; Torres et al., 2022). Under certain instances, these factors can operate in a protective role and insulate Latinx men from psychological distress. While under separate instances they can result in Latinx men being more susceptible to developing a mental health disorder. Ai and colleagues (2015) highlighted how comorbid mental health disorders play a significant role in many chronic health conditions. For Latinx men, depression and/or anxiety symptoms can exacerbate health conditions such as asthma, cardiovascular disease, and diabetes (Ortega et al., 2006; Williams, 2018).

Difficulties in the family such as ruptured relations or discord can have a damaging effect on the mental health of Latinx persons. In one study, familial discord was associated with an increased risk of Major Depressive Disorder and an increased risk of suicidality (Ai et al., 2015). Vocational status and type of employment has also been identified as a potential risk factor for Latinx men. For example, one study found that immigrant Latinx men who sought out jobs as day laborers experienced an elevated risk of having poor mental health outcomes (Hill et al., 2019). Another study highlighted that Latinx men were at an increased risk for depression and suicide when they experienced unemployment. Ai et al., 2015). The parental status of Latinx men has also been identified as a potential risk factor for developing mental health difficulties. Garfield and colleagues (2018) found that Latinx men experienced an elevated risk of developing major depressive disorder after the birth of their first child. The role that family plays in Latinx men's mental health is expected given the Latinx cultural value of *familismo*. These risk factors arise out of the roles that Latinx men play in their respective families (ie, provider, fathers, etc).

Acculturation is another risk factor associated with Latinx men's mental health. Greater acculturative stressors were associated with an elevated risk of developing alcohol or substance abuse related disorders (Torres et al., 2022). Acculturative stress has been associated with increased risk of suicide (Hofferth et al., 2016). Language proficiency and use is also another indicator of acculturation level for persons of Latinx descent. Lower English language proficiency and use is associated with lower levels of acculturation for Latinx immigrants (Hofferth et al., 2016). Interestingly, Latinx individuals who are less acculturated have better mental health outcomes compared to their more acculturated counterparts. This has been coined in research as the "immigrant paradox" a population level phenomenon in which more highly acculturated immigrants have less optimal developmental outcomes than recently arrived immigrant youth (Marks et al., 2014)

Latinx men in U.S. society are expected to adhere to certain masculinity standards and socialized gender roles. Their inability to meet these standards or to operate within the prescribed roles results in distress known as Gender Role Conflict (GRC). While the concept will be expounded on later in the chapter, it is important to emphasize the negative effect that GRC can have on the mental health of Latinx men. For Latinx men, the psychological distress associated with GRC has been linked with poor mental health outcomes such as stress and depressive disorders (O'Neil, 2008).

Protective Factors

When it comes to Latinx men's mental health, there has traditionally been a dearth of research that identifies protective factors and strengths. There is emerging evidence that for Latinx individuals, there are certain psychosocial protective factors that reduce the risk of developing a mental illness (Ai et al., 2015). Among the many factors identified (e.g., race/ethnic identity, social support, religious beliefs, etc.), family-related variables are the most significant (Ai et al., 2015). This is a tangible example of how the Latinx cultural value of familismo operates in a protective role for Latinx men. *Familsmo* is a collectivistic value that emphasizes family loyalty, unity, and honor, which contrasts with the U.S. values of individualism (Arredondo et al., 2014). For Latinx men, *familismo* as well as the cultural value of *respeto* have been associated with how supported they feel by their respective families (Walters & Valenzuela, 2019). Fortuna and colleagues (2016) found that religiosity as well as family loyalty served as mental health protective factors for Latinx men. For Latinx men who have a preference to speak in Spanish, being able to communicate in their native language with providers facilitates help seeking and serves a protective role. Having the ability to speak in Spanish with providers allows Latinx men to accurately express their concerns and be understood by providers. Cultural gender expectations can serve dual roles as a stressor or a protective factor for Latinx men seeking mental health treatment. Incorporating awareness of these protective factors; understanding the role cultural values play; and having insight into the significance of gender expectations when supporting Latinx men can help diminish the negative stigmas behind seeking treatment. This can also facilitate the building of therapeutic rapport and trust with their provider.

Somos Fuertes Pero También Sufrimos (We Are Strong but We Also Suffer)

DISCRIMINATION AND STEREOTYPES

The existence and persistence of racial and ethnic discriminatory practices directed towards members of ethnic minority groups in the U.S. has been well documented in the scientific literature (Williams, 2018). Racial discrimination has been described as a the "unequal treatment of persons or groups on the basis of their race or ethnicity" (Pager & Shepherd, 2008, p.2). While it is distinct from associated concepts such as prejudice, stereotypes, and racism, discrimination can be directly influenced by them. As members of an ethnic minority group in the U.S., Latinx men can experience myriad forms of discrimination (Torres et. al., 2022). Examples include social exclusion or distancing, stigmatization, unfair employment practices, educational inequality, challenges finding or accessing housing, and difficulties within the banking system (Arellano-Morales et.al., 2015; Pager et. al., 2008; Torres et. al., 2022).

Racial and ethnic discrimination can take a toll on the effected persons psychological wellbeing (Vargas et.al., 2020) and has been described as one of the "pathways by which racism affects health" (Williams and Mohammed 2013). Experiencing discrimination has been linked to increased risks of developing a variety of mental health conditions. This is vital as it pertains to Latinx men because there is some evidence that suggests they have a higher prevalence of discriminatory experiences compared to Latinx women (Arellano-Morales et. al., 2015). Latinx individuals who endure discriminatory behavior directed at them in combination with other psychosocial stressors may be at a higher risk for developing major depressive disorder (Ai, et.al., 2015) and experiencing episodes of suicidality (Fortuna et. al., 2016) and substance abuse disorders (Torres et.al., 2022).

Given the deleterious impact that discrimination can have on the mental health of Latinx men, it is important to understand what factors increase their likelihood of experiencing discrimination. Research has identified a variety of variables that may increase a Latinx persons chances of being exposed to discrimination. Some of these variables may also be linked with or contribute to stereotypes held about persons of Latinx descent. Country of origin, phenotypic characteristics, and socioeconomic status (SES) are predictive variables that can determine potential exposure to discrimination. One study discovered that Latinx persons of Mexican descent; those who are of Afro-Latinx background or that have a darker complexion; or who are from higher SES were more likely to report experiences of discrimination or racism (Uzogara, 2019). Although not significant for Latinx men in the study, SES was significant for Latinx women and their experiences of discrimination. Specifically, lighter skinned Latinx women of higher SES reported more experiences w/ discrimination (Uzogara, 2019). The findings related to skin tone was in line with prior research that also found darker skinned Latinx persons experienced discrimination more often than their lighter skinned counterparts (Noe-Bustamantes et al., 2021).

There is a significant amount of evidence that points to the connection between being of darker complexion and experiences with discrimination and racism for men of color. As noted by Uzogara and colleagues (2014), darker complected men experienced greater instances of discrimination and racism compared to men of lighter complexion, even when they were of the same racial category. Phenotypically, Latinx persons, and by extension Latinx men, can come in all shades and colors. While many Latinx men may have Mestizo or indigenous heritage, African and European influences are also well represented (Abalos, 2002; González-Burchard et al., 2005). Noe-Bustamante and colleagues (2021) report that more than half of Latinx individuals identified as White (58%), about a quarter identified into the "some other race" category (27%), 8% chose two or more races, and about 2% selected Black or African American. These phenotypic variations can influence the lived experiences of Latinx men in the U.S. Within Latinx culture, racism and colorism exist. Mestizaje has been historically used to deny experiences of oppression among Latinx communities (Adames et al., 2021; Adames & Chavez-Dueñas, 2017).

There are numerous stereotypes about Latinx persons in the U.S. Some are generally applied to all Latinx's while others may be more gender specific. Some of the stereotypes may be considered positive but most of them are not. Examples of negative stereotypes generally held about Latinx persons include that *they* are loud; that *they* are emotional; that *they* are low life's or "*chusma*;" that *they* are undocumented or "*illegal.*" (Tukachinsky et al., 2017; Villenas & Deyhle, 1999) Latinx persons are also ascribed hypersexualized stereotypes that label women as "spicy" and men as "Latin lovers" (Tukachinsky et al., 2017). According to Tukachinsky and colleagues many of these stereotypes are communicated through media and can have a negative effect on minority population's identity development. Other general stereotypes include that all Latinx persons come from large families; that all Latinx persons speak Spanish; that intelligence is associated with English fluency; that all Latinx persons have the same phenotypic features (i.e., dark hair, dark eyes, light brown skin complexion etc).

For Latinx men, in addition to these general stereotypes, they are also casted as domestic abusers; gangsters; or as troublemakers who frequently get into fights. Latinx men are also stereotyped as being *machistas* or that they ascribe to hypermasculinity practices. Occupational stereotypes of Latinx men include that they work as janitors, construction workers, day laborers, landscapers, or that they are taking jobs away from "Americans."

Walters and colleagues (2019) surveyed Latinx men about their awareness of common stereotypes about Latinx men. Respondents in the study identified only a single positive stereotype which was that Latinx men are family oriented. The vast majority of the stereotypes endorsed were negative. These included that Latinx men are unskilled, undocumented, and uneducated laborers; that Latinx men are thugs, criminals or members of a gang; the Latinx men are womanizers who have multiple baby mothers that they do not support; that Latinx men are drunkards; and that Latinx men are "suave lovers" (Walters et. al., 2020). These stereotypes can be reinforced by how Latinx individuals and Latinx men are portrayed on TV, movies and media. For example, some of the most common depictions of Latinx's on TV and movies include roles such as the gangster, crime boss or uneducated hard worker (Mastro, Behm-Morawitz & Ortiz, 2007).

All of these factors can have a significant impact not only on the mental health of Latinx men but also on their lived experiences.

Eckart

Phenotypically, I have red hair, freckles, and a name with German origins. None of which suggests to anyone that I am Latinx. Before arriving in the U.S. I was often referred to as "el macho" which was an affectionate nickname due to my complexion but nothing that felt derogatory. When my family immigrated to the U.S. is when I recall my appearance becoming a source of pain.

I was frequently labeled as the "whiteboy." While I recognize the privileges that my white complexion has afforded me, in various instances growing up I felt cursed because I did not "look more ethnic." Being the "whiteboy" made me feel like an outsider in my own community and family. Growing up in a community that was largely non-white (Latinx, African American, Afro Caribbean) I often felt that I had to legitimize myself culturally, to prove that I was Latinx.

Somos Fuertes Pero También Sufrimos (We Are Strong but We Also Suffer)

My complexion never seemed like a privilege, at least not in my neighborhood. I recall the countless times I was pulled over by police because "the only white people that come around here are buying drugs." I also recall the times that I got off the public bus and the driver would say "do you know where you are getting off?" Or walking home from school and someone at the gas station saying "that's a brave white boy right there," as if I did not belong in my own neighborhood.

During my youth, experiences such as these served as reminders that I did not fit in. They were sources of pain and shame.

Bryan

Racially, I am of Afro-Caribbean, Spanish, and indigenous descent; whereas ethnically, I identify as Latino; therefore, I today identify as a proud Afro-Latino man. After migrating to the United States I have become more sensitive to these identities. I have learned to embrace my otherness, the color of my skin, and the curls on my head. I've learned to embrace all of my identity not as fractions or pieces but instead as the whole person I am, but that was not always the case. As someone who is biracial, I've struggled with my identity. I remember growing up and not feeling like I was enough of anything. Having a Costa Rican father and Panamanian mother meant that to my Costa Rican family and peers I was their darker Panamanian cousin or classmate, while visiting my Panamanian family I was their light skin Costa Rican family member. This made it difficult to feel as if I had a place to belong. My ambiguity allowed me to play between the two worlds. I identify with the biracial development model that Poston (1990) proposes in which biracial individuals feel pressure to first choose one racial or ethnic group which is influenced by many factors including phenotype. Because of the way I looked I always felt closer to my Panamanian family; however, since I had been born in Costa Rica, I felt it was important for me to name my "ticoness." Trying to fit within both of them meant identifying as a "Panatico" culturally while denying any influence of Blackness in my family or racial background. Growing up in a bicultural family made me appreciate the cultural differences that exist even within two neighboring countries. My experiences helped me become more aware, tolerant, and accepting of cultural differences. However, race was not something we discussed in my family.

As a child I remember exploring my otherness and at times wanting to look more like my father who is a tall light skinned individual. I didn't love my features, color of my skin, or hair. Wanting answers to my questions, my mother explained to me that my grandfathers' parents, like many other Panamanians, are of Afro-Caribbean heritage but grew up in Panama in a time period in which racism erased our Caribbean heritage and culture. She explained to me that I was beautiful because I looked like her as she did her father. However, my grandfather would have told you that he was a proud Panamanian man. Identifying with his country of origin while ignoring the influence that race had in his experience as an Afro-Latino man. This is a representation of the influence colonialism and internalized racism has had on many Afro-Latino individuals. Chavez-Dueñas, Adames and Organista (2014), argue that colonization, lack of awareness, and mestizaje promote and maintain racist ideologies and colorism in Latinx communities.

Once I migrated to the United States I would be considered "Latino" a term that prior to my move had little meaning to me. At first even though I was Latino, I had a hard time adapting to the Latino community since my accent, word choices, and customs were different from the majority Mexican communities in the Bay Area. I pushed away both my racial and ethnic identities to protect myself from rejection. Once I started college and joined the Puente program, I would learn to identify with my Latinoness, and the diversity that entailed being in a classroom representative of students from Mexico, Centro, and South American, while still pushing away notions of blackness within myself. I did not "look black enough," therefore I couldn't claim my racial and ethnic background without feeling like I would be questioned or asked for a burden of proof. Colorism and lack of critical consciousness were likely partially responsible for my response. In Latin America race relations are complicated as they stand in a continuum in which blackness is reserved for a specific social representation (Wade, 2010) and like my grandfather people learn to identify with their country of origin. According to Poston (1990), biracial individuals may feel guilty for not embracing themselves fully or denying group differences to better fit their schemas, to then explore and adopt parts of identities not previously chosen. This provides an opportunity for appreciation and integration of a whole person. For me this development was no different. As an adult I began to ask questions that at times were considered taboo while understanding that for me it was important to explore the influence of race within my family. Learning to be unapologetically me has been a process, I have learned to integrate my racial and ethnic identities in my work. As an immigrant Afro-Latino man I try to name and honor the histories and ancestral influence of those I come from in all of my roles. This gives me the opportunity to reclaim my heritage and racial identities.

LATINX MALE SOCIALIZATION AND MASCULINITY

Gendered role socialization practices are influenced by various contextual and cultural standards which impact the role that men play in society (Addis & Mahalik, 2003; Levant & Richmond, 2007). These socialization practices can change over time and can also vary from one culture to the next (Courtenay, 2000; Davis & Liang, 2014). Addis and Mahalik (2003) noted that masculine ideologies and masculine gender-role conflict are two prominent factors associated with the gender role socialization of men in U.S. society.

Masculinity Ideologies

The predominant masculine ideology in the U.S. is based on Eurocentric, heteronormative, and hegemonic standards (Addis et al., 2003; Griffith et al., 2016; Hall, 2016; Torres-Pagán & Toro-Alfonso, 2017). Hegemonic masculinity provides a framework for understanding how hypermasculine practices generally shape the status and norms of men (Abbott & Geraths, 2021). These hegemonic norms influence the traits considered to represent what is "masculine" or what it means to be "a man." Examples of these hegemonic traits include: being physically tough, rugged, and strong; being stoic and assertive/ a decision maker; sexual conquest/dominance of others; being self-reliant and not needing /depending on others; and restricted display of emotions, particularly those considered "not masculine" such as sadness, pain, or fear (Evans et al. 2011; Griffith et al., 2016; Kennedy & Moorhead, 2021; Levant et al. 2016; Lindinger-Sternart, 2015). Hegemonic ideologies also influence how members of society accept and often expect men to operate (Connell & Messerschmidt, 2005).

Eckart

Somos Fuertes Pero También Sufrimos (We Are Strong but We Also Suffer)

I played on the football team in high school and college. Throughout my athletic experiences, it was clearly reinforced to me that I had to be "tough". I learned early on that there was a difference between being injured and being hurt. Coaches would ask "are you injured or are you hurt?" The implication was that if I was injured, I could not play, but I could play hurt. The expectation oftentimes was that I had to "man up" and fight or play through the pain.

Gender Role Conflict

The value ascribed to Latinx men in U.S. society is closely linked to how they adhere to these masculine standards (Abalos, 2002). The psychological stressors and negative consequences of not meeting these standards result in what is known as Gender Role Conflict (GRC: O'Neil, Helms, Gable, David, & Wrightsman, 1986; O'Neil, 2008). GRC is a detrimental psychological state wherein socialized gender roles have unhealthy consequences for the person or others (O'Neil, 2008). GRC is a multidimensional framework of psychological factors, situational contexts, and personal experiences. According to O'Neal and colleagues (1986), GRC operates at four intersecting levels: Cognitive, Affective, Behavioral, and Unconscious. These levels capture how persons in U.S. society generally think and are influenced by masculinity standards and gender role expectations (O'Neil et al., 1986). The GRC framework can help understand the distress that men can experience if or when they fail to meet hegemonic masculinity standards (O'Neil et al., 1986; O'neal, 1990, 2008; Davis et al., 2015).

Eckart

Depending on the circumstances, not being able to "man up" had its consequences. While this concept came up in many aspects of my lived experience it was very evident in sports. Being tough and rugged was a desired quality. I recall one time injuring my hand in practice and the pain was so excruciating that I shed tears as the trainer was tending to my injury. This was noticed by teammates which resulted in jokes and insinuations during practice. Not showing toughness or displaying an emotional vulnerability was seen as a weakness and may run the risk of being called a variety of derogatory labels. In some instances, a situation where others are calling you names might result in a physical confrontation which would then create additional stressors to respond in a tough manner. The last thing you wanted to be labeled was a push over which would just result in more problems. The best thing to do to avoid these potential circumstances was to simply "man up."

Bryan

For the first 8 years of my life I had both of my parents present. Both were good role models and in many ways my dad was my hero. I was growing up in a loving home where I had the ability to be as gentle and sentimental as I wanted to be. After my parents' divorce, I was being raised by a single mother who played both roles at times. This lack of gendered role performance made it where, at a young age, I viewed traditionally gendered behaviors (cleaning, cooking, fixing things) as things that need to get done. At 8 years old I had become the right-hand man to my mom and caregiver to my younger brother. I learned to clean, cook, and iron uniforms before school. My experience and family make up made me challenge traditional gender roles and influence my feminist identity. However, growing up in a single parent household did not protect me from displays of toxic masculinity. I witnessed domestic violence, and lived in fear for my mother, my brother, and myself, at the hands of a stranger. A man who my mother dated, who eventually moved in with us and introduced me to living in a home marked by substance use and domestic violence. These experiences help me understand the impact violence against women can have on their children, families, and community. It also made me want to do better for my future wife and daughters. Even through the experiences of DV I was not a violent person.

Once I arrived in the Bay Area at 13 years old, I had to learn quickly what gang politics entailed and had to learn to fight and defend myself. I learned to perform masculinity in the ways needed. I became a jock that was praised for my toughness and ability to endure in sports such as football, wrestling, and rugby. I also made a name for myself in a neighborhood in which it was necessary to be fearless and willing to fight at the drop of a dime. I learned that any look, word, or action that threatened my manhood needed to be confronted with violence. I was not an aggressive person but had learned to become someone else. The influence of my upbringing faded away and I became hyperaware of anything that would make me feel or look like less of a man. Something I would continue to struggle with for many years later.

Latinx Masculinities

Westernized masculinity standards and GRC (Torres-Pagán & Toro-Alfonso, 2017) transcend race and ethnicity as they are applied to and expected of all men regardless of background (see Walters & Valenzuela, 2020). Torress and colleagues (2002) highlight the current understanding of masculinity in the U.S. tends to be too generalized and overlooks the role that ethnicity and race play. Because these standards are generally imposed on men, a narrow understanding has developed about the masculinity of men of color that has traditionally undervalued the role of culturally relevant practices (Torres et al., 2002; Torress, 1998). It also has created a definition of Latinx masculinity that does not allow for deviance outside of the accepted norm. However, it is our understanding through our education, clinical, practice, and lived experience that Latinx masculinities need to include the diversity of ways in which Latinx men express their identity.

Latinx cultural standards generally expect men to serve in a mixture of roles, including provider, protector, and/or impregnator (Abolos, 2002). The concept of *machismo* is commonly associated with Latinx male socialization and masculinity (Perez et al., 2020). Some scholars argue that the concept of *machismo* is misunderstood, has not been comprehensively studied, and that it lacks a proper definition (Arciniega, Anderson, Tovar-Blank, & Tracey, 2008; Perez et al., 2020). The term *machismo* has often been used to describe stereotyped hypermasculine norms, behaviors, attitudes, and gender roles of Latinx men (Torres et al., 2002). The concept of *machismo* has social and cultural origins (Wong, 2013) and illustrates the set of values, attitudes, and beliefs within Latinx culture about masculinity (Nuñez et al., 2016). Often leaving little room for other masculinities to be represented.

Colonialism and Masculinity

The influences of colonialism may provide some understanding about the origins of Latinx masculinity standards. Some argue that the remnants of colonialism are typified in the hyperrmasculine behaviors of Latinx men. Historically Aztec, Mayan and pre-colonial societies did not prescribe to the current notions of masculinity. Worldwide there has been a push back against colonial masculinity including in Hawaii (Tengan, 2002), India (Sinha, 1999; 2017), South Africa (Morell, 1998), Latinx (Mirandé, 1997), and

Chicano Culture (Martinez, 2019). Colonialism is a violent endeavor that shaped the historical, cultural, and social hierarchies of those who were colonized, it "undermined the position of women. It brought a system which carried rigid gender ideologies which aided and supported the exclusion of women from the power hierarchy" (Amadiume, 1987, p.185). According to Morell ``Colonialism created new and transformed existing masculinities" (1998).

It is also important for us to recognize, masculinity was not socially conceptualized in vacuum and it invites the analysis of the intersection of race, sexuality, and gender and the ways they have and continue to be used to create a power hierarchy in society and among men e.g. "white men" vs black "boys", emasculation of colonized societies or non white body types, emasculation of non-heteronormative relationships, and the demonization of LGBTQ communities. Pre-colonial societies had a more fluid understanding of gender e.g. inclusion, recognition, and celebration of two spirited individuals, and third or more genders (Robinson, 2019). Colonialism stripped cultural ways of being and understanding from those being colonized, additionally it created a representation of masculinity for survival. The introduction of catholicism and patriarchal perspectives further shaped the hierarchy that is accepted as normal within many Latinx communities. However, "much of the Latinx culture revolves around religion that stemmed from colonization" (Martinez, 2019). Mirandé (1997) presents in his book "Hombres y Machos: Masculinity in Latino Culture" that machismo was not a response to Spanish conquest but instead a form of assimilation to hypermasculine conquistadores who shared many of the characteristics associated with toxic Latinx masculinity.

Machismo and Caballerismo

Much of the research on *machismo* has overwhelmingly focused on its negative/ hypermasculine aspects; and overlooked the positives (Arciniega et al., 2008; Perez et al., 2020; Torres et al., 2002; Wong, 2013). For example, Latinx men are often characterized as *machistas* (Galanti, 2003). Torres and colleagues (2002) identified 5 distinct categories of *machismo*: 1) *Contemporary Masculinity* (egalitarian; family-oriented; collaborative gender role; not demanding, controlling, nor domineering); 2) *Machismo* (respect for family, caring, emotionally expressive; is not demanding, controlling, or domineering); 3) *Traditional Machismo* (Authoritarian personality, demanding, conflicts within their life roles; not emotionally expressive; aligns with the negative aspects of machismo); 4) *Conflicted/Compassionate Machismo* (authoritarian, demanding, traditional views about gender roles, kind, thoughtful, competitive, and conflicted with life roles); and 5) *Contemporary Machismo* (moderate level of authoritarianism; demands obedience and respect; has traditional views on gender roles; emotionally expressive; balanced life roles and competitiveness). While the Latinx men in this study endorsed a variety of beliefs, only a small percentage endorsed the hypermasculine and hegemonic behaviors associated with the *traditional machismo* category. The majority of the Latinx men in the study endorsed masculinity standards that embraced being emotionally expressive; being collaborative with family members; being moral, honorable and reliable; and being a protective and provider (Torres et al., 2002).

Arciniega and colleagues (2008) also explored the concept of *machismo* and offered a bidimensional perspective. They proposed that machismo has two dimensions: *traditional machismo* and *caballerismo*. *Traditional machismo* is associated with the negative masculine qualities that have been previously highlighted (i.e., aggression, chauvinism, hypermasculinity, etc.) (Arciniega et al., 2008). *Caballerismo* represents the positive qualities associated with Latinx masculinity, such as being emotionally connected with others, being chivalrous, being a provider & protector of the family, and being spiritual (Arciniega et al., 2008). *Traditional machismo* and *caballerismo* are both considered independent constructs. Therefore, a Latinx man can endorse one, neither and/ or both in varying degrees (Arciniega et al., 2008; Ojeda & Piña-Watson, 2014). The reality is that researchers rarely focus on the positive qualities of Latinx masculinity, such as *caballerismo* (Arciniega et al., 2008).

The concept of *caballerismo* has been related to a host of positive behaviors and outcomes for Latinx men. These include improved problem-solving & coping strategies, being emotionally connected & responsive, exhibiting nurturing qualities, and having a strong family orientation (Perez et al., 2020). Ojeda and Piña-Watson (2014) note that despite the limited literature, the available evidence on *caballerismo* has revealed that it is a strength for Latinx men and related to positive psychological well-being. *Caballerismo* operates as the underlying prosocial aspect of *machismo* and serves as a protective factor for Latinx men (Ojeda et al., 2014; Paredes & Parchment, 2021).

Ruben

I grew up in a very traditional Mexican household in terms of gender roles in the sense that my father was the provider of the family and my mother took on the caretaker role. From a young age, I learned to be Latinx man through interacting and observing my father. My father demonstrated his love to me in a very tough and macho way. My father never told me that he loved me, but he would constantly call me a pendejo. I knew my father loved me by the way he would put his needs second, but he did not know how to properly communicate his feelings.

As I began to solidify my academic identity and aspirations, my father passed away. I was acutely aware of my cultural gender role as the only male in the family. Mexican cultural values dictated that I carried the responsibility to take care of my family when my dad passed away. I was the bearer of the family name and also immediately responsible to take care of my family. I struggled to know how best to take care of my family. Should I return home? Or should I pursue a master's degree? It was a difficult decision to make, and I was only 22 years old.

After my father passed away, moving to a small college town for my masters and PhD was personally the worst and best thing that could have happened to me. It was difficult because, like my father, I coped with hardships through humor. Being around others helped distract me from all the emotions I was dealing with after my father's death. I was finding any excuse to socialize to avoid the feelings of loneliness and having to deal with negative emotions. I did not realize that my first year leaving California would force me to deal with these things by disconnecting from the community I left behind. It was best because I started making small changes to grieve, such as working out, processing what life would be like without my father, and allowing myself to be alone. I saw a major difference when I went back home, and I was able to be mentally present with family and friends.

As a husband and father, there are things that I am still learning and unlearning as a Latinx man to become the best version of myself for my family. One of those things is being more communicative with my emotions. For example, communicating throughout the day to my wife and son how much I love them. Mentally, I knew I loved them, but it was still uncomfortable for me because I did not see it in my household growing up. My wife has played a major role in normalizing this behavior from the beginning of our relationship, constantly verbalizing her love and appreciation for me, which I have loved.

Somos Fuertes Pero También Sufrimos (We Are Strong but We Also Suffer)

Additionally, my father worked long hours growing up, so I saw it as the man's responsibility to work hard to provide for their family. As a result, I am still working on being comfortable with saying no to research projects, it brings me more joy to be out with my son and wife. Moreover, it has helped me to recognize that my mother and father were fortunate enough to put me in a position where I did not need to work long hours to provide for my family. Being able to grow through my relationship with my wife and son has been the best thing for me than all the things I accomplished academically.

Bryan

Growing up in a single parent household meant I didn't always have a male role model around. My father had always been a gentle, kind, and loving father. However, after he left my family, I learned that toxic masculinity did not always show up as demands, traditional gender roles, or control. Sometimes, toxic masculinity looked like unmet responsibilities as a father and husband. Machismo and patriarchy are in some ways part of Latinx culture and socially accepted in ways that harm us at times without our own consciousness. As I grew up, I maintained a relationship with my father but saw him sporadically. At a young age, as the oldest son in my family, I had taken on the role of "man of the house." I believed it was my responsibility as a man to help and protect my family. In many ways, migrating to the United States was connected to the sense of responsibility I felt and understanding that I needed to "man up" and do what I had to do to help. I had asked my mother to leave her abuser and to choose her children over him. Without a second thought, she had left him but struggled to make ends meet. At 12 years old, I internalized the idea that I needed to help provide for my family, and planned to do so by migrating to the United States on my own, learning English, and returning to Costa Rica to work in tourism. Once I arrived in the United States, I was a guest in relatives' homes; I learned to be self-reliant and to make do by needing nothing from anyone. I learned to suppress my emotions and quiet my needs.

When I was 14, my father moved to the United States and we rekindle our relationship. Having to learn to live with one another after not having the opportunity to do so for many years was a challenge at times. The young boy that he had left with my mother was no longer there, but I was not a fully grown man yet. He figured out ways to provide for us and tried to make up for lost time. My father taught me then the importance of hard-work, dedication, and grinding determination. He was as gentle, kind, and loving as I remembered him to be. However, his love language was not always expressed through words or emotional expression but instead as opportunities to spend the day working with each other. I was his assistant plumber, painter, roofer, handyman, and odd job facilitator. I was often reminded that as a man, I needed to know how to do all the things these jobs would teach me so I could take care of my home and my family. I remember for my 15th birthday, he planned a demolition day; we rebuilt a roof and he paid me at the end of the day. Even though this was the first birthday we had spent together in a long time, there were no parties, gifts, or surprises but instead a welcome to manhood that included working hard for your own money. I remember feeling sad and heartbroken but not knowing how to communicate it; instead, I convinced myself those were the emotions of a child, something for which I no longer had time or space.

Now, as he has gotten older, I have witnessed my father soften even further. I see him interact with children in gentle ways telling them stories from the bible, playing, and supporting their communities through missionary work and pastoral duties. In many ways, he is now helping children who are less fortunate or who come from single parent homes. He has also become more affectionate and often sends texts and videos reminding my brother and I that he loves us. I love our relationship now more than ever. This is a reminder that masculinity is not a fixed identity but instead an ever changing and evolving way of being. I am excited to see the way he will once again change as he becomes a grandfather. I look forward to having kids of my own and to try my best to teach them to be strong feminist, loving, caring, and socially just people. Regardless of their gender, I want to make sure that they are able to embrace equity, inclusion, support, and kindness. If I have sons, I hope to have them learn healthier expressions of masculinity, to support them in exploring their softness, interests, and ways of being that may or may not fit in traditional views of masculinity. As men, we live a great tragedy in which we are taught as boys that we need to be hard, reserved, and emotionless, yet the qualities that make us great fathers and husbands are quite the opposite. The mask we wear to fit in as men is one we then need to learn to deconstruct and remove to be authentically ourselves in all the loving, caring, and wonderfully human ways we were always meant to be.

Eckart

My father modeled a mixture of traditional machismo and caballerismo. My father viewed his primary role as being "the provider." He was an incredibly hard-working individual who operated his own business for more than 40 years. My dad worked long hours. It was common for him to leave before my sisters, and I awakened and not return until night. While I learned a great deal of work ethic, integrity and resiliency from my father, I learned less about being nurturing, loving, or how to manage my emotions. My father was not very skilled with the intimate aspects of parenting such as saying "I love you" or displaying physical affection (i.e. kissing or hugging). My father did not clean dishes, vacuum, change diapers, nor help with homework. Those duties were my mother's responsibility.

Unlike my father, I am very family oriented, and I openly model affection to my children, wife, and other family members. I am very vocal in letting my children know that I love them and value them. I try to teach them and prepare them for life as much as possible. My children and I connect on activities that my father and I never had the chance to explore because he was always working. He rarely was able to attend any events or activities. I on the other hand carve out time to coach them up and play a variety of sports with them; I consistently volunteer at or attend their respective events; and enjoy having shared interests with them like fishing, martial arts and hiking trails. I enjoy helping around the house with duties such as cooking, laundry and cleaning. I try to openly model and practice egalitarian gender roles. I do not see any of this as "special" but rather feel that it is my role as husband, father, and member of my family. In these respects, I am very different from my father.

HELP SEEKING BEHAVIORS

Men in the U.S. have a higher mortality rate for many of the top causes of death (e.g., heart disease, cancer), are more likely to die from suicide, and have higher rates of substance abuse disorders (Jarrett et al. 2007; Murphy et.al., 2021; Vogel et. al., 2011). Despite these morbid health outcomes, men do not disproportionately seek out health-related services. When men experience a health-related condition (i.e., physical or medical), they generally do not seek health-related services at similar rates as women

(Addis & Cohane, 2005; Jarrett et al., 2007: Kennedy & Moorhead, 2021). Service utilization rates are even lower when men experience mental health issues (Call & Shafer, 2018). Male socialization has been highlighted as a factor that deters men from seeking mental health services (Sager-Ouriaghli et al., 2019).

Masculinity standards that expect men to be strong and to fight through challenges are generally not congruent with help-seeking behaviors (Mahalik et al., 2003; Rochlen, 2005; Vogel et al., 2011). For Latinx men, their conformity to these negative masculinity standards (traditional machismo) is linked with reduced help-seeking behaviors (Gast et. al., 2020; Martinez, 2020; Vogel et al., 2011). The results in these studies also note that the opposite is true. When Latinx men align themselves less with hyper-masculine *machismo* ideology, they tend to be more receptive to seeking help.

Regardless of the label used to describe mental health services (i.e., therapy, counseling, psychotherapy, mental health counseling, treatment, etc.), Latinx individual seek "it" out at much lower rates (Ishikawa, Cardemil, Falmagne, 2010). Similar to other men of color in the U.S., Latinx men are less likely than their White male counterparts to seek out and utilize mental health services (Chandra et al., 2009; Cho et al., 2014; Vogel et al., 2011). Attempts to explain these low help seeking rates have often focused on a variety of structural barriers. Examples of structural barriers that inhibit the help-seeking behaviors of Latinx men include lack of insurance; lack of cultural and linguistic competent providers; and immigration concerns (Schwatken, 2011, Cabassa, 2007). Attitudes held by Latinx men about mental health and mental health services have also been associated with their help seeking behaviors. Viewing services as a sign of weakness; believing that services are only for those with severe mental illnesses; preferences for talking with a friend or family member vs. a professional; and/or believing that they would experience something that goes against their masculine identity (i.e., that counseling would cause them to be vulnerable or emotional like a woman) are examples of such attitudes (Velasquez, et.al., 2004). In addition to structural barriers and attitudes, the stressors associated with GRC have also been found to negatively influence mental health help seeking behaviors (Levant, Wimer, & Williams, 2011; Nguyen, Liu, Hernandez, & Stinson, 2012).

Cultural factors that are influential to the help-seeking behaviors of Latinx men include: religious beliefs, country of origin &/or affiliation, preferences regarding resources, acculturation status, educational level, age, and gender (Schwatken, 2011). As highlighted earlier in this chapter, the Latinx cultural value of *familismo* is significant as Latinx men prefer leaning on family when mental health or emotional support is needed instead of utilizing professional services (Cho et al., 2014; Chang & Biegel, 2018). Chiang and colleagues (2004) found that Latinx individuals rated family and social support as more favorable options than professional mental health services. We contend that these "barriers" should be reclassified as manifestations of the protective qualities of culture. Latinx men are culturally socialized to lean on family and close social networks in addressing distress and mental health concerns. The supportive nature of the Latinx family when men experience mental health concerns is also highlighted as a possible reason for underutilization of services by Latinx men (Chang and Biegel, 2018).

Bryan

As an undocumented immigrant, you learn to be invisble; you learn to move in silence and to never be "a molestia" (a bother). As a man, you learn to be tough and to not need anything from anyone. Therefore, it is not surprising that as an immigrant man, I learned to never go to any kind of medical service unless I felt my life depended on it, and sometimes, even that would not be enough to get me to a hospital or doctor. I had learned to ignore emergencies, thinking that my suffering was not as important as the suffering of others. From dislocated shoulders, to a broken clavicle, to a concussion, I always figured out an alternative to getting medical care.

Similarly, I also found it difficult to ask for psychological and emotional help. I had been providing mental health services for five years before ever receiving my own. I was selling a product that I believed everyone was deserving of but me. I also told myself that the issues I was facing were not as difficult as what others faced. I kept telling myself that the cost or the stigma were enough of a reason to not ever attend. It was not until my second year in my doctoral program after 45 was elected as president and I considered dropping out, that I decided to go into counseling services. I had gone in with a list of issues to discuss at a surface level: 1) ADHD – I had always felt I was diagnosable but a lack of insurance and understanding of the help I deserved stopped me from exploring further or asking for help; 2) Racial Trauma – Living in a majority white state and city under a 45 presidency made me feel the color of my skin in ways I never had before; 3) Dropping out – I felt like a sellout and that the work I was doing in academia was not real activism because it lacked impact and purpose; it was performative at best, unhelpful and meaningless at worst. These were the three things that brought me to counseling services. They were important and impactful in my life; however, they were not attached to any kind of emotion or feeling. They were all means to an end: learn to deal with ADHD to improve academically, learn to deal with a majority white state and decide how you can best support "the movement," and then decide what to do next. They were all problems that if addressed would improve my life but did not resolve the deeper needs or the core of the real issues. Through exploring these areas, we got to the heart of what was really going on in my life, at times without knowing it myself. These were the things that actually needed to be addressed: 1) I was emotionally disconnected and unhappy in my relationships; 2) I had trauma I had never discussed or processed; and, 3) I needed or rather, I wanted to learn how to cry. I realized that at 30 years old, I had cried a handful of times since my 16th birthday and felt as if I was broken, unable to reach my emotions unless it was under the most extreme circumstances. I remember sharing with my first therapist, at times feeling like crying but not knowing how to. She asked me to share my story with her and as she cried with empathy, in some ways, it gave me permission to cry in session. She explained CPTSD, ADHD, masculinity, and the ways in which my experiences had created a recipe for emotional suppression and disconnection. It made me realize the support I had needed and deserved for so long. It rekindled my motivation and commitment, and helped me find reasons, along with the tools and support I needed, to finish my doctoral education.

RELEVANT TRENDS

Trends in the Mental Health Industry

There are certain trends within the mental health professions that have direct and indirect impacts on the mental health of Latinx men. The mental health professionals generally include the fields of psychology, psychiatry, social work, counseling, and marriage & family therapy. In order to meet the needs of the Latinx community and of Latinx men, it is imperative that the U.S. mental health industries develop a workforce that is diverse; that has adequate representation of Latinx professionals; and that is culturally and linguistically competent (Delgado-Romero et al., 2012). This workforce must also be multidisciplinary. No one mental health profession has demonstrated the capacity to meet the mental health needs of the Latinx community on their own. Unfortunately, this workforce does not currently exist. Although some progress has been made, much more needs to be accomplished.

In professional psychology for example, despite decades long efforts to diversify, it is still a white dominated profession. According to an American Psychological Association (APA) study, 84% of active psychologists identified as white, 16% as a racial minority, and only 5% identified as Latinx (Lin et al., 2018). Psychologists are considerably less diverse (84% white) than the U.S. workforce (61% white, 5% Asian, 12% Blatck, 18% Latinx). Although there may be subtle demographical improvements in other mental health professions, the trends remain consistent. A recent survey within social work revealed that despite having better representation of ethnic minorities (28%) and of Latinx (14%), the field also remains heavily white dominated (66%) (Salsberg, et. al., 2020). These same trends are witnessed within the fields of counseling as well as in marriage and family therapy.

These trends result in a psychological workforce that does not mirror many of the communities that they intend to serve and is not properly equipped to address the needs of those communities. Not having stronger representation of Latinx professionals, not having a culturally and linguistically competent workforce increases the potential for cultural malpractice (Hall, 1997). The lack of representation also results in an underrepresentation of intellectual and theoretical contributions that influence practice, research and training.

Bryan

I remember my first interaction with a counselor being less than ideal. She was at our school providing services after another gun violence incident had taken the life of a student at the high school I was attending. The school had invited students to speak with counselors and some of us were required to do so. I remember walking into a room and meeting a young white woman, she was likely a young clinician still learning to navigate clinical interactions. Her opening "I know that what you are going through is difficult" served as nothing more than an invitation for my anger to spill out. I responded harshly reminding her, she had no idea what I was going through or what it was like to grow up in the neighborhood I was living in. I questioned how she spent her 16th birthday and if she even knew how the other half of the world lived. I demanded for her to tell me if she had any idea what it was like to lose a friend to gun violence. I wanted her to tell me she knew what it was like to leave your family behind as a child or what it was like to be on her own by 16 years old. She froze and said nothing. I walked out of that room furious. I didn't think of that interaction until many years later when I was navigating my own education and identity development as a healer.

I had never envisioned what life would look like after high school beyond working and helping my family. Luckily, during my senior year of high school I had a 15 minute conversation that changed my life. A student who was two years older was on campus getting his transcripts and asked what I was doing out of class and what my plans were after college. I said "not much." He invited me to attend community college, I jokingly laughed and pointed out barely graduating high school didn't make much of a college student. At the time I didn't even know if I was going to be able to graduate. He said "if nothing else it would at least give you the opportunity to party and meet some people... and as I remember you into that." I now tell my students that I went to college to party and stayed for a PhD.

When I first started college I wanted to be a firefighter. I didn't really know everything that was available to me or what a career or degree were. I had believed the narrative that college was not for everyone, specially not for an Afro-Latino undocumented immigrant. That first semester I started dropping classes, and nearly dropped out. I decided to focus and gave myself a semester to figure it out or drop out. During that semester I took a random child & adolescent development & psychology class that was supposed to be nothing more than a credit filler to maintain my financial aid. In that class I learned about myself like never before. I also remembered that first interaction with a counselor and decided that I wanted to give kids like me something I had not been given. A therapist that came from where they came from, who understood their stories, and who looked like them.

The higher up I went into education the more isolated I felt. Often becoming one of the few or only males of color in my psychology classes. While in graduate school it came to my attention that I had gone most of my undergraduate years without ever meeting a Latinx psychologist. As I provided services I noticed often being the only BIPOC male provider even in a state like California, while serving a majority of clients (80%) that were Black and Latinx kids in juvie and probation. I was the exception and not the norm. During my masters I had my first BIPOC Immigrant male professor, Dr. Alvarez, who changed what I believed possible. He and Dr. Toporek became my first academic mentors, took me to my first conference, gave me my first authorship, and pushed me to go beyond a masters.

During my first conference I met Dr. Joseph White, after he had just given a talk and gotten a standing ovation in an auditorium full of people, he pointed to me and invited me to sit with him and to ask him questions. I really had no idea why someone of his importance would want to talk to someone like me. I also didn't know Dr. Alvarez and Dr. Toporek had made it a point to let him know I was coming and wanted me to connect with him. During that first conversation I asked if I would ever feel like I belonged in academia, he smiled and kindly replied "we can not be validated by places that were not created for us but think what it would mean to your community." Dr. White sat me down and told me I would become a psychologist one day. On a napkin he wrote down the schools I would apply to and without knowing it then mapped out my life for me. He invited me to ride the Freedom Train and explained the cost to come aboard was to "pay it forward". From that moment on we began to write to each other. Soon after, Dr. Alvarez took me to my first NLPA, "Undocumenetd Immigrants, DREAMers and Social Justice," it was there that I decided a PhD was something within my grasp. A few years later at the same conference we had met, Dr. White introduced me as the "caboose" of the freedom train and let an auditorium full of people know I was going to be attending the University of Oregon in the fall. His lessons I still carry with me many years later. I'm now taking students to their first conferences and mentoring them to come aboard the freedom train like I once was asked to.

Now as a psychologist and entrepreneur I'm reminded of the importance of representation in academia and the field. I have gotten mentorship that has helped me start my own practice. I was told during a workshop for BIPOC clinicians "For BIPOC healers, private practice is an act of Liberation." Private practice was something I had never considered. Private practice was like a bad word that shouldn't be spoken in academic spaces. However, being in private practice has allowed me to work with the clients I want, to continue to be involved with students through supervision and teaching as an adjunct faculty member, to create and support immigrant communities, and to continue to work in publishing with colleagues and friends who are in academia.

Somos Fuertes Pero También Sufrimos (We Are Strong but We Also Suffer)

Trends in Higher Education

Ruben

During my doctoral program, I felt like my work mattered to the Latinx community, the majority whom are Mexican and undocumented. Researching and counseling the Latinx community was a humbling experience. Hearing them share their stories helped me stay motivated and grounded in my work. Like the supportive relationship I was able to form with Dr. Jeanett Castellanos, known as Dr. C, I was able to work closely with Dr. Ed Delgado-Romero, known as DR. Like me, he was a first-generation Latinx student, and he explicitly talked about his journey and his struggle balancing both family and school. Unlike most faculty where you get to only see the work life of the person, DR shared his family life as well. I've met his wife, kids, siblings and even his mother. I saw first-hand that it is possible to have both a career and family which is important to me.

There is no denying that my advisors, friends, and mentors have played a central role in my academic success. I do not feel comfortable talking about the things that I have been able to accomplish academically without first recognizing the fact that I did not do it alone. My collectivist values, desire to learn and create my own academic family, led me to surround myself with individuals that have shaped me in many different ways. The person that I am today is shaped by the characteristics that I most admire of these individuals.

Eckart

I pursued a higher education for no other reason than to pursue my athletic ambitions of playing football in college. I had no idea what being a college student entailed given that I was the first person in my family to attend college.

I first enrolled at a small college in rural Nebraska. The college had a population about the size of my high school and the town had one intersection. We would drive 35 minutes to get fast food or get groceries and the closest major city was 2 hours away. This was a major culture shock for me coming from South Florida. The football team was the only source of diversity on that campus. I elected to transfer to a larger school in Texas. There, I became ensnared in the social life and ended up earning all F's. Although I was not dismissed after earning a 0.0 GPA, I was encouraged not to return. I ended up moving back home and worked odd end jobs for the next year and a half.

One of the most jarring moments after returning home involved an incident where I and a group of friends had an encounter with police. Suffice to say that getting thrown to the ground, having a gun pointed at you by a cop and being handcuffed face down on the ground made me have a moment of clarity. I recall thinking something to the effect of "I gotta get my shit together." Thankfully, unlike many others who find themselves in those types of situations, my friends and I were able to walk away from that incident alive and free. I started to get myself together and save money to return to school.

After spending that year and a half at home, I transferred a 3rd time to a school in Alabama. This time I was much more focused and knowledgeable about navigating the college environment. I would eventu-

ally graduate with my bachelor's degree and a very respectable GPA. The excitement of becoming the first person in my family to graduate with a college degree blinded me to what I was going to do next. It was not until the last week of my senior seminar course that I realized college was ending and I had to get a job. It was also at that time where I first considered graduate school.

When I attempted to pursue my master's degree I had to send transcripts not only from the school I graduated from but from all institutions I had attended. The 0.0 GPA was factored into the calculations which lowered my overall GPA making me ineligible for admissions. As I researched options I learned that I could still improve my overall GPA by taking additional undergraduate courses as a post baccalaureate student. To achieve my goal of raising my GPA enough to be eligible for admissions into a master's program, I had to take courses that I had not previously completed, and I had to earn an "A" in every one. Earning "B's" or anything less would not help me. While working full time at a social service agency, I enrolled at a community college and completed 2-3 courses each semester for 2 years. I was able to raise my overall GPA enough to apply to an M.S.W. program.

The only M.S.W program that would consider me for admissions was over 100 miles away from where I lived and worked. Nevertheless, I applied and got accepted. For the next 2 years, I continued to work full-time at the social service agency and drove more than 200 miles round trip each time for class. In those days there were no online or hybrid options so all classes were in-person. I would go on to earn my MSW. Subsequently I was promoted to a therapist position and began my work as a mental health professional.

The trends that are occurring in the higher educational landscape have a direct effect on the number of Latinx professionals found in the mental health industry. One relevant trend is the underrepresentation of men within higher education. Generally, fewer men are attending college and fewer men are obtaining college degrees (Postsecondary National Policy Institute, 2021). Men of color are further underrepresented across the higher educational landscape. Latinx men attend college and obtain degrees at disproportionately lower rates when compared to Latinx women (Saenz & Ponjuan, 2009; Postsecondary National Policy Institute, 2022). The lack of Latinx men within the academic pipeline (Delgado-Romero & Werther, 2012) results in fewer men that can elect to pursue careers in the helping professions.

Another issue is that among the men that do attend college, few elect to pursue careers in the mental health professions. This contributes to the growing gender gap that has emerged within the mental health professions. Delgado-Romero and colleagues (2015) pointed out that the helping professions are becoming female dominated. For example, in the field of psychology, the majority of psychologists (65%) identify as women and amongst psychologists that identify as Latinx the gender ratio is 5:1 (Lin et al., 2018). These trends within the mental health professions should not be ignored and the underrepresentation of Latinx men should be cause for alarm. These trends inhibit efforts within the mental health professions to develop a diverse and culturally competent workforce that reflects and is able to meet the needs of diverse populations (Goforth et al., 2016; Luan et al., 2018; Pedrotti & Burnes, 2016).

These trends are salient because all of the mental health professions are graduate level disciplines (ie., the lowest educational requirement is a master's degree). A master's degree is the general educational requirements for clinical social workers, professional counselors, and marriage & family therapists. In the case of psychology and psychiatry, doctoral level training is the minimum educational requirement to enter into each profession. Psychiatrists are medical doctors and they attend medical school, psychologists attend graduate doctoral programs in psychology. Latinx men are underrepresented across each of these disciplines and academic trajectories.

Ruben

At UCI, I attended a talk by Dr. C, where she shared her experience as a first-generation Latinx college student and faculty member. I didn't know anything about academia, but what got my attention was when she said she was from South Gate in her speech. Here she was, a Latinx professor from my hood.

It is an unwritten rule that if you ever need help, someone from your hood is bound to help you. With this rule in mind, I placed the responsibility on Dr. C to help me before we even knew each other. As part of Dr. C.'s lab, I learned about research and the way that research could be used to give voice to those communities that were often marginalized in education. Dr. C created a space where students were able to explore their passions and learn from one another. Through empowering students of color about college and career options, she taught me about the research that already exists within the Latinx community, and how I personally could contribute to the field of psychology.

Bryan

Education is often a measure of success and attainment in the United States. It has been linked to higher financial stability and achievement of the American Dream (Bernstein, 2003). For me, being a highly educated person is a key aspect of my identity. It permeates all aspects of my life and dictates many of the roles within it. Thanks to my educational experiences I have been able to better understand my identity, my experience, and the tools needed to become an effective clinician and scholar-activist. My experiences in academia have also been a measure of things beyond academic learning. It is at times a measure of resilience, determination, and strength. In some ways, academia is a well-oiled machine that perpetuates and maintains systems of oppression (Corntassel, 2003; Hursh & Martina, 2003). At times, academia is no more than a gatekeeping, antiquated, self-serving "hazing" practice keeping the "unworthy' outside of the ivory tower (Corntassel, 2003).

I often felt as if I was "the unworthy." I came to the United States alone when I was 13 years old. I was not lucky enough to arrive in a neighborhood that fostered or encouraged academic development. Instead, I arrived in a place where violence, poverty, and misguided lessons were the compass that guided me. Through navigating these challenges with the support of others, I was able to achieve more than I ever believed possible. I graduated college, earned a Master's degree in Counseling, and I am now a licensed psychologist and entrepreneur. In my academic experience I have been able to teach, research, author, publish, and provide mental health counseling to family and individuals, things I could not have imagined growing up. I can leverage my past to help diverse clients reach their potential, change academia by becoming a part of it, and also contribute to research that addresses immigrant experiences in the United States (Cardenas et al., 2021; McWhirter et al., 2019; 2020, Rojas-Araúz, 2021). The confidence I now feel was not always present.

When I was 18 years old, I set foot on a college campus for the first time. I knew nothing about higher education and had no guiding resources. As a first-generation undocumented college student, there are specific challenges that I have encountered including lack of cultural capital, lack of financial support, feelings of isolation, anxiety, and depression. Through the eventual support of faculty and the connections I forged with my professors, I received something that I had not been able to get on my own - hope. This hope guided me on my academic path. While this path was filled with questions and unknowns, the commitment of the people with whom I had the opportunity to come in contact with helped me find my own answers. I have witnessed the important role that being connected, represented and understood can play in ensuring student success. On the other hand, academia has been historically normed on individualistic and Eurocentric ideals. Because of this I often feel like my cultural and personal values did not fit in it. It serves as a reminder that my identities, values, and histories are often not represented in academic spaces and that I can easily be "defined out" (Turner, 2002). At times my lack of academic capital has helped maintain feelings of doubt and a lack of belonging, often feeling like an impostor in a place with familiar faces. Turner (2002) captures this experience as being newcomers to a world defined and controlled by ideals and practices that do not address our realities, that do not affirm our intellectual contributions, and that do not understand our experience.

Being a college student has always had its challenges for me. I felt caught between spaces, not from here and no longer from there either, streets and academia, immigrant yet American, split in opposite directions. At every step of the way I have had doubts and felt like an impostor. Being in a doctoral program only increases those insecurities. I found myself questioning my purpose, because at times being in academia did not feel like enough. For example, it was seeing my community attacked by a presidential candidate with xenophobic and racists promises. To then witness him become president. I was worried for my community, my family, and friends. I was an activist before I was a college student. I wanted to be in the streets organizing and helping my community. I wanted to demonstrate, resist, and support a movement. I felt like I needed to go home. I felt like I could do more there than in academia. A mentor, Dr. Joe White, reminded me to trust my community would have someone to take my place in the streets, because my persistence in academia was a form of resistance. My ability to stay and ride "the freedom train" to its destination became a form of activism within itself. I have had to learn to resist in different ways, and learn what it means to be a scholar-activist. The hardest part was learning to trust the process and believing we belonged all along.

At times I still worry I may be perceived as less prepared, less "academic," and undeserving of the opportunities I've been given. I have learned to find mentors and role models in the field that support and guide me in this process. Dr. White would often remind me to find validation within myself and my community after all academia was not created for men of color in mind. He would often say "Bryan, do not look for validation from your oppressors... find it in the places that matter."

Eckart

The therapist position I was promoted into after getting my M.S.W. gave me the opportunity to work and be supervised for the first time by a Spanish speaking therapist (Consuelo). Another person I worked closely with during those years was the director of a violence prevention program (Wes) who was not of Latinx background but who had deep connections to the Latinx community. Wes was also fluent in Spanish. Both Consuelo and Wes had vested interests in serving the Latinx community and both (whether they knew it or not) played a significant role in my early professional development.

Somos Fuertes Pero También Sufrimos (We Are Strong but We Also Suffer)

After a few years in this position my interests were piqued into pursuing a doctoral degree in psychology. I began to research programs but encountered a great deal of internal doubts. I wavered about going back to school for many months. One defining moment in my decision making process came during lunch with my wife's graduate professor (Karen). I shared with her my concern about the years it would take; and if it was worth it to spend that much more time in school. Karen told me "Eckart, do you hope to be alive in 5-6 years?" I answered "yes." Karen said, "well you're either going to be 5 or 6 years older with a Ph.D. or 5-6 years older without a Ph.D."

After I submitted my doctoral applications, I was invited to interview at a few programs and would eventually be extended multiple offers of admission. I elected to accept the offer at UGA and work under DR. Starting the doctoral program was thrilling and at the same time extremely intimidating. Here I was a first generation immigrant; first generation college student; and former college flunk out starting a doctoral program. I experienced a great deal of imposter syndrome and stereotype threat. During the first few years in training, I was the only Latinx male and native Spanish speaker in the program. I was also the only student with an M.S.W. background. Microaggressive statements by peers and by others made me feel tokenized and unwelcomed, I felt "out of place" in academia, a foreigner in the ivory tower. I strongly considered quitting multiple times.

DR played a significant role in dispelling many of these feelings and doubts. As I interacted with him there was always this sense of familiarity in how he spoke to me, how he phrased things, and how he responded to my experiences. He welcomed me not only into his professional space but also into his home and into his family. I got a chance to get to know DR on a professional and personal level. I was able to connect culturally with him as another Latinx man. I learned to recognize and appreciate my value; to feel like I belonged in the space I was navigating; felt understood; and I was reminded repeatedly that I was not alone on this journey. I saw a lot of myself in DR which humanized the process for me allowing me to persevere.

I never envisioned when I left South Florida that my journey would be capped off by earning a Ph.D. Coming from where I grew up and the origins of my family, I definitely never envisioned myself being a tenured professor nor doing many of the things I have accomplished in my career. My journey may have been unconventional but I would not have done it any other way. I appreciate the decision my parents made to come to this country. I appreciate the sacrifices and resiliency they had. I value the community that has mentored, advised, supervised, and supported me throughout my journey, despite my failures and imperfections. This network helped this kid from Homestead go from a 0.0 GPA to Ph.D.

CONCLUDING THOUGHTS AND RECOMMENDATIONS

Chosen Stanzas From *Behind The Mask Of A Warrior Slam Poem Written and Performed at CockTales* "Stories of Masculinity Pt.2" by Bryan O. Rojas-Arauz

The lessons we were given were wrong

Like a scratched disk we keep repeating the song

Somos Fuertes Pero También Sufrimos (We Are Strong but We Also Suffer)

The message my father, his father, and my father's father, received was the same

It's time for us to relearn what it is to be a man

Time for us to forgive and love our fathers

Time for us to break the cycle of this coil

Provide for our seeds, for we are their soil

The present our gift, our sons got tomorrow

Real men are able to cry, feel, change

It is time to start practicing self-compassion

Real men address their problems,

They don't self-destruct.

Talk it out, express yourself, ask for help

Be your brother's keeper

Real men have Courage

They have the ability to take risks,

Strength to be compassionate

Wisdom to be humble

Real men can be themselves and define who they are

They don't act or react with violence

Real men trust their hearts

love others, and themselves

Be quick to smile, slow to anger, and treat all people with the respect they deserve

It is time to redefine what it is to be a man.

Somos Fuertes Pero También Sufrimos (We Are Strong but We Also Suffer)

Let's stop hiding behind the armor

Stop hiding behind

the mask of a warrior

Eckart

As I reflect on the process of writing this chapter with my colleagues, the concepts of resiliency; degrees of separation; and mentorship stand out to me.

Each of us has overcome and endured odds that could have easily derailed our respective trajectories. In each of our lived experiences, we found a way to remain resilient and to persevere in our educational and professional pursuits.

We share a number of overlapping professional and personal relationships despite the different points in time that we navigated higher ed. and the differences in institutions attended. Ruben and I knew each other prior to collaborating on this project. He and I met at the National Latinx Psychological Association (NLPA) conference when he was first starting his doctoral training. Ruben also attended the same program I graduated from and we both studied under the same advisor. Bryan and Ruben had met previously and collaborated on a presentation. They also met at an NLPA conference. I met Bryan as a result of collaborating on this chapter. He is the only other Tico (Costa Rican) psychologist that I have met here in the U.S. Although he attended graduate training on the west coast, he and I connected quickly as a result of our shared cultural background and similarities in interests. Additionally, Bryan was close with one of my former undergraduate students who is a doctoral candidate in the same program Ruben and I graduated from. These connections created a sense of familiarity for me that I really valued in this writing process and at this point in my career.

We met virtually throughout the writing process to discuss the direction and progress of the chapter. During these meetings, in addition to our work related to the chapter, we connected on our shared cultural experiences and perspectives as Latinx men. We would often get off track and share resources or professional advice; discussed developments in our respective families; shared accomplishments; or processed challenges associated with our professional roles. It was nice not only to collaborate with each of them on this chapter but also to learn about them on a personal level.

Bryan

As I reflect on the process of writing this chapter I think of both the honor and responsibility we have in creating knowledge that comes from the community that is for the community. Collaborating allowed me to have a healing experience by joining with my Latinx brothers in telling a story we wished had been given to us in our education and creating a chapter that hopefully captures the complexities of Latinx masculinities.

Ruben and I had met at NLPA a few years back and have collaborated in different projects along the way. We have shared parallel experiences and gone through milestones at similar times. We share a network of Latinx psychologists and NLPA familia that have supported us every step of the way. I have been connected to UGA counseling psychology doctoral students and professors through mentors, mentees, friends and colleagues. As well as similar interests and areas of study. From the beginning we have clicked in ways that would later make sense including being part of the same academic family tree. Prior to this book I had not known Eckart but I can say that without a doubt meeting him was probably a gift I was not expecting when I accepted to collaborate in the chapter. Knowing another immigrant Tico psychologist was special and something I had never had before. In a field where men of color are rare, finding someone with my same ethnic background is nearly impossible. As we wrote this chapter he became a colleague, friend, and mentor. Getting together as Latinx men allowed for a different experience in writing. It challenged me to be more vulnerable and to lean into the discomfort of sharing our narratives with one another and eventual readers. It also served as a way of validating and normalizing the struggles of being Latino male students, practitioners, and scholar-activists.

I hope this chapter gives the reader an introduction to the many factors we need to take into account when talking about Latinx men. I hope it invites them to challenge what they have learned in their graduate programs while expanding the way they think of Latino men. I hope it can be a resource for clinicians to better serve Latinx communities and especially men who need their services. Lastly, I hope academic spaces can challenge their leadership to better support Latinx men's academic success and that the field of psychology can commit to increasing the representation of Latinx men in the field.

Based on the authors collective experience navigating the higher educational pipeline as Latinx men, and in conjunction with the available scientific literature on the matter, we present the following recommendations.

Higher Education- Institutional

- Systemic introduction of support services targeted at BIPOC students during freshman or transfer student orientation prior to attending the institution. Name the services and how they might help students, and make overt statements about the support and commitment at the institution.
- Systematic outreach to parents that helps them understand the challenges of college, how family cultural assets can support college students, and the resources available to Latinx students. This will allow families to better understand systems and their son's experiences.
- Institutions and programs often support the notion of inclusiveness and diversity but rarely address the underlying structures that make these efforts unproductive. External new hires for leadership positions, in-service workshops for faculty, offering affordable CEU's for faculty, and hiring outside trainers are methods to begin addressing some of the structural issues (Smith & Werther, 2017).
- We charge academic departments to develop and provide opportunities for faculty and staff to collaborate and develop interdisciplinary collaboration skills. Too often academic departments and disciplines operate in silos, never interacting with other related disciplines on campus. Students must not be indoctrinated to operate in this fashion.

- An infusion of diverse perspectives, theories, modalities, and skills is needed within the helping professions to better develop culturally responsive research and treatment strategies. The lack of demographic and curricular diversity may be making graduate training for many students of color (and Latinx men) unattractive.
- Creation of target services that center the Latinx men experience including:
  - The creation of Latinx Men Resource Centers or related physical spaces that can serve as safe spaces for Latinx men and locations for connecting with community leaders, families, and sharing cultural wisdom.
- Create opportunities for collective healing and celebration of cultural traditions, histories, and strengths of the community through programing and outreach events (e.g., Dia de los Muertos, Posadas Navideñas, Cultural celebration months).
- Provide cultural competence training and empathy building programs for staff, faculty, and other students so they can better understand Latinx men experiences.
- Increase diversity of faculty and staff to represent the identities, histories, and lived experience of Latinx men.
- Create structures for formal and informal peer and faculty mentoring for Latinx men.
- Promote collaboration among different departments, services, and resources designed to improve responsiveness of staff and faculty to Latinx men.
- Secure funding and invest in programs and organizations that work with the Latinx men (e.g., Counseling services, MCC, MSAS, student organizations, etc.). Research exploring Latinx students experience in higher education has noted the significance that student organizations play in helping them navigate academia and build a support network (Luedke, 2019)
- Institutions should create streamlined processes for funding and reimbursement for faculty and student travel. Procedural barriers can discourage faculty students from engaging in such efforts. These are some of the most rewarding experiences for students and institutions should recognize the value of supporting student development.
- The field of psychology (and other helping professions) must make a concerted effort in outreaching, recruiting, and supporting Latinx men into their respective disciplines.

Higher Education- Faculty and Staff

- We charge members of the academy to:
  - Be productive as scholars, mentors, and educators committed to diversity, equity, and inclusion efforts.
  - Actively recruit, train and retain Latinx men into the academia. Benefiting programs with an infusion of new blood, energy, and ideas. We must move away from labeling the work of emerging scholars of color as controversial or unconventional simply because it makes white faculty uncomfortable.
  - ¡ Stay up to date with information about career and educational trajectories so that you are able to provide accurate information and advice for students and not just "the way you did it."
  - Lectures and reading material should include research, authors, and knowledge about diverse figures within the helping professions.

- Support and work towards increasing the number of Latinx men who pursue careers in one of the mental health fields. This can be accomplished through admissions, funding opportunities, targeted recruitment, mentorship programs, outreach, and faculty representation.
- Provide opportunities for relationship building through office hours or visual meetings
- Implement cultural values such as *personalismo, platica*, and *familismo* into your interaction with students.
- Use expertise and academic skills to write policy briefs or op-eds, and engage in and present research that educates and raises consciousness of the community and Latinx men.
- Incorporate flexible and adaptive teaching methods that offer a balance of rigor, empathy, and support the development of skills to navigate life stressors and circumstances.
- Continue to develop cultural competence by actively engaging in trainings, empathy exercises, and continuing to learn beyond individual trainings (e.g., readings, documentaries, etc.).
- Stay up to date with information pertaining to challenges, services, and political climate of Latinx students.
- Add to syllabi a standard message informing students of course policies and sensitivity to student challenges including a list of resources and services available at the University. This allows for students to receive support without having to disclose their barriers.
- In the creation of class accommodations center those most marginalized.

For Mental Health Practitioners and Counseling Centers

- Current mental health practitioners should:
    - Assure that the services being provided are ethically and legally sound as well as culturally and linguistically competent. The authors believe that you cannot be clinically competent if you are not culturally competent.
    - Process their views associated with gender, ethnicity and assumptions of Latinx men. The goal is for mental health providers to explore their own biases and reflect on their privileges to explore values and beliefs that may impact how they interact with Latinx men.
    - Support the development and introduction of culturally and linguistically appropriate services for Latinx men.
    - Provide or support outreach and educational workshops for Latinx men that aim to counter mental health stigmas; that promotes and normalizes Latinx men experiences; that builds community and collective healing; and that promotes the benefits of mental health.
    - Become proficient in different modalities of care inclusive of individual, group, and family services. Given the significant role that family dynamics have, mental health practitioners working with Latinx men should aim to understand the familial relationships and the dynamics of those relationships.
    - Work towards increasing as well as supporting the diversity and representation of Latinx men within the mental health professions.
    - Support the conscientization and empowerment of Latinx men by disseminating research findings on the protective factors and psychological strengths of Latinx communities (Chavez-Dueñas, et al., 2019 ; Rojas-Araúz, 2021).

- Support and attend training that helps mental health providers to integrate traditional healing practices (e.g., curanderismo, energy work, ancestral knowledge) with more traditional western practices (e.g., CBT, ACT, IPT).
  - Take on the responsibility of increasing cultural competence and understanding by attending training, reading, and viewing documentaries on Latinx experiences and challenges. Also for those who are able, work towards developing linguistic competency.
  - Challenge stereotypical views of Latinx masculinity that are deficit based or that promote unhealthy hypermasculinity standards for Latinx men. .
  - Aim to have a physical presence and visibility in the community you serve; participate in spaces outside of counseling centers or offices to build awareness and relationships with clients and increase a sense of safety in seeking services.
  - Use multiple avenues to reach Latinx men and increase visibility including social media, email, and word of mouth.
  - Use images, art, and symbols in the décor of your office or treatment facility that can help Latinx men feel more welcomed and safer in the space.
- The final charge we leave for mental health professionals is to stop engaging in the inter and intra disciplinary conflicts that plague the mental health professions. Members of one profession should not be ostracizing other professionals simply because they are in a separate discipline (Psychiatry vs Psychology) or earned a different degree in the field (Counseling Psychology vs Clinical Psychology), or based on level of education (doctoral level professional vs masters level professional). These inter and intra disciplinary conflicts are unproductive in addressing disparities amongst various groups, including Latinx men.·

Research

- Given that research informs practice, it is imperative that more emphasis be placed on conducting research on Latinx men and also having research samples with greater representation of Latinx men.
- Instead of focusing on the experience of Latinx males from a deficit model, research should instead utilize a strength-based framework and approach. The author's shared narratives demonstrate a change in the typical experience of Latinx men. However, most studies continue to exclude the lived experience of this community from a strength based perspective. Research with Latinx communities needs to focus on creating counter narratives that highlight the strength and resilience as much as the challenges represented (Rojas-Araúz, 2021). The authors suggest research can break down miss conceptions of Latinx men through qualitative studies that assess and define characteristics of their lived experiences (Delgado-Romero, Singh, & De Los Santos, 2018).
- Faculty at undergraduate programs must create opportunities for Latinx men to have opportunities to connect and develop working relationships with faculty; to work with faculty conducting research; and to attending professional conferences.
  - Latinx students identified having unequal access to professional development opportunities and faculty mentorship as one of the most significant barriers in their doctoral experiences. At the same time, supportive peers and faculty mentors serve as key protective factors (Ramirez, 2017). Being a Latinx man in psychology often becomes a double negative in which academic and clinical experiences can be isolating and alienating. Building communi-

ties that promote mentorship and create cultural capital that can be shared and passed down may be a way to combat these barriers.

Policy Makers

- Support policy and legislature that expands access to tuition equity and financial support.
- Support policy and legislation that support loan forgiveness options for professionals within the mental health fields.
- Support policy and legislature that expands access to education, health and mental health services.
- Reject efforts that attack or vilify intellectualism; That criminalize the teaching of diversity and inclusion concepts; or that promote a whitewashed history.
- Secure funding to support programs and organizations that work with Latinx men.
- Take the time to build genuine relationships with Latinx communities.
- Continue to develop cultural competence by actively engaging in trainings, empathy exercises, and continuing to learn beyond those spaces (e.g., readings, documentaries, etc.).

REFERENCES

Abalos, D. T. (2002). *The Latino Male: A Radical Redefinition*. Lynne Rienner Publishers.

Abbott, J. Y., & Geraths, C. (2021). Modern Masculinities: Resistance to Hegemonic Masculinity in Modern Family. *Journal of Contemporary Rhetoric, 11*(1/2), 36–56.

Adames, H. Y., & Chavez-Dueñas, N. Y. (2017). *Cultural foundations and interventions in Latino/a mental health: History, theory, and within group differences*. Routledge.

Adames, H. Y., Chavez-Dueñas, N. Y., & Jernigan, M. M. (2021). The fallacy of a raceless Latinidad: Action guidelines for centering Blackness in Latinx psychology. *Journal of Latina/o Psychology, 9*(1), 26–44. doi:10.1037/lat0000179

Addis, M. E., & Cohane, G. H. (2005). Social scientific paradigms of masculinity and their implications for research and practice in men's mental health. *Journal of Clinical Psychology, 61*(6), 633–647. doi:10.1002/jclp.20099 PMID:15732091

Addis, M. E., & Mahalik, J. R. (2003). Men, masculinity, and the contexts of help seeking. *The American Psychologist, 58*(1), 5–14. doi:10.1037/0003-066X.58.1.5 PMID:12674814

Ai, A. L., Pappas, C., & Simonsen, E. (2015). Risk and protective factors for three major mental health problems among Latino American men nationwide. *American Journal of Men's Health, 9*(1), 64–75. doi:10.1177/1557988314528533 PMID:24707037

Amadiume, I. (1987). *Male daughters, female husbands: Gender and sex in an African society*. Zed Books Ltd.

Arciniega, G. M., Anderson, T. C., Tovar-Blank, Z. G., & Tracey, T. J. G. (2008). Toward a Fuller Conception of Machismo: Development of a Traditional Machismo and Caballerismo Scale. *Journal of Counseling Psychology*, *55*(1), 19–33. doi:10.1037/0022-0167.55.1.19

Arellano-Morales, L., Roesch, S. C., Gallo, L. C., Emory, K. T., Molina, K. M., Gonzalez, P., Penedo, F. J., Navas-Nacher, E. L., Teng, Y., Deng, Y., Isasi, C. R., Schneiderman, N., & Brondolo, E. (2015). Prevalence and Correlates of Perceived Ethnic Discrimination in the Hispanic Community Health Study/Study of Latinos Sociocultural Ancillary Study. *Journal of Latina/o Psychology*, *3*(3), 160–176. doi:10.1037/lat0000040 PMID:26491624

Arredondo, P., & Tovar-Blank, Z. G. (2014). Multicultural competencies: A dynamic paradigm for the 21st century. In F. T. L. Leong, L. Comas-Díaz, G. C. Nagayama Hall, V. C. McLoyd, & J. E. Trimble (Eds.), APA handbook of multicultural psychology: Vol. 2. *Applications and training* (pp. 19–34). American Psychological Association. doi:10.1037/14187-002

Bernstein, A. (2003). Waking up from the American dream. *Business Week*, *1*, 54-58.

Cabassa, L. J. (2007). Latino Immigrant Men's Perceptions of Depression and Attitudes Toward Help Seeking. *Hispanic Journal of Behavioral Sciences*, *29*(4), 492–509. doi:10.1177/0739986307307157

Call, J. B., & Shafer, K. (2018). Gendered Manifestations of Depression and Help Seeking Among Men. *American Journal of Men's Health*, *12*(1), 41–51. doi:10.1177/1557988315623993 PMID:26721265

Cervantes, A., Fernandez, I. T., & Carmona, J. F. (2019). Nosotros importamos (we matter): The use of testimonios with Latino male adolescents in group counseling. *Journal of Creativity in Mental Health*, *14*(2), 181–192. doi:10.1080/15401383.2019.1568941

Chandra, A., Scott, M. M., Jaycox, L. H., Meredith, L. S., Tanielian, T., & Burnam, A. (2009). Racial/ethnic differences in teen and parent perspectives toward depression treatment. *The Journal of Adolescent Health*, *44*(6), 546–553. doi:10.1016/j.jadohealth.2008.10.137

Chang, C. W., & Biegel, D. E. (2018). Factors affecting mental health service utilization among Latino Americans with mental health issues. *Journal of Mental Health (Abingdon, England)*, *27*(6), 552–559. doi:10.1080/09638237.2017.1385742 PMID:28980838

Chavez-Dueñas, N. Y., Adames, H. Y., & Organista, K. C. (2014). Skin-color prejudice and within-group racial discrimination: Historical and current impact on Latino/a populations. *Hispanic Journal of Behavioral Sciences*, *36*(1), 3–26. doi:10.1177/0739986313511306

Chavez-Dueñas, N. Y., Adames, H. Y., Perez-Chavez, J. G., & Salas, S. P. (2019). Healing ethno-racial trauma in Latinx immigrant communities: Cultivating hope, resistance, and action. *The American Psychologist*, *74*(1), 49–62. doi:10.1037/amp0000289 PMID:30652899

Chiang, L., Hunter, C. D., & Yeh, C. J. (2004). Coping attitudes, sources, and practices among Black and Latino college students. *Adolescence*, *39*, 793–815. PMID:15727415

Cho, H., Kim, I., & Velez Ortiz, D. (2014). Factors Associated with Mental Health Service Use Among Latino and Asian Americans. *Community Mental Health Journal*, *50*(8), 960–967. Advance online publication. doi:10.100710597-014-9719-6 PMID:24659219

Cokley, K., Hall-Clark, B. N., & Hicks, D. (2011). Ethnic Minority-Majority Status and Mental Health: The Mediating Role of Perceived Discrimination. *Journal of Mental Health Counseling*, *33*(3), 243–263. doi:10.17744/mehc.33.3.u1n011t020783086

Connell, R. W., & Messerschmidt, J. W. (2005). Hegemonic Masculinity: Rethinking the Concept. *Gender & Society*, *19*(6), 829–859. doi:10.1177/0891243205278639

Corntassel, J. J. (2003). An activist posing as an academic? *American Indian Quarterly*, *27*(1/2), 160–171. doi:10.1353/aiq.2004.0029

Courtenay, W. (2000). Constructions of masculinity and their influence on men's wellbeing: A theory of gender and health. *Social Science & Medicine*, *50*(10), 1385–1401. doi:10.1016/S0277-9536(99)00390-1 PMID:10741575

Davis, J. M., & Liang, C. T. H. (2015). A test of the mediating role of gender role conflict: Latino masculinities and help-seeking attitudes. *Psychology of Men & Masculinity*, *16*(1), 23–32. doi:10.1037/a0035320

Delgado-Romero, E. A., Espino, M., Werther, E., & Gonzalez, M. J. (2012). Building infrastructure through training of bilingual mental health providers. In L. P. Buki & L. M. Piedra (Eds.), *Building Infrastructures for Latino Mental Health*. Springer.

Delgado-Romero, E. A., Merrifield, J., & Werther, E. (2015, Fall). Latina/o Psychologists: Who decides who we are? *Latina/o. Psychology Today*, *2*, 22–25.

Delgado-Romero, E. A., Singh, A. A., & De Los Santos, J. (2018). Cuéntame: The promise of qualitative research with Latinx populations. *Journal of Latina/o Psychology*, *6*(4), 318–328. doi:10.1037/lat0000123

Delgado-Romero, E. A., & Werther, E. (2012). Hispanic Psychologists. In R. DelCampo & D. M. Blancero (Eds.), *Hispanics at Work: A Collection of Research, Theory, and Application* (pp. 177–188). Nova Science Publishers.

Evans, J., Blye, F., Oliffe, J., & Gregory, D. (2011). Health, illness, men and masculinities (HIMM): A theoretical framework for understanding men and their health. *The Journal of Men's Health*, *8*(1), 7–15. doi:10.1016/j.jomh.2010.09.227

Fortuna, L., Álvarez, K., Ramos Ortiz, Z., Wang, Y., Mozo Alegría, X., Cook, B., & Alegría, M. (2016). Mental health, migration stressors and suicidal ideation among Latino immigrants in Spain and the United States. *European Psychiatry*, *36*, 15–22. doi:10.1016/j.eurpsy.2016.03.001 PMID:27311103

Garfield, C. F., Abbott, C., Rutsohn, J., & Penedo, F. (2018). Hispanic Young Males' Mental Health From Adolescence Through the Transition to Fatherhood. *American Journal of Men's Health*, *12*(5), 1226–1234. doi:10.1177/1557988318765890 PMID:29577835

Gast, J., Peak, T., & Hunt, A. (2020). Latino health behavior: An exploratory analysis of health risk and health protective factors in a community sample. *American Journal of Lifestyle Medicine*, *14*(1), 97–106. doi:10.1177/1559827617716613 PMID:31903089

Goforth, A. N., Pham, A. V., Chun, H., Castro-Olivo, S. M., & Yosai, E. R. (2016). Association of acculturative stress, Islamic practices, and internalizing symptoms among Arab American adolescents. *School Psychology Quarterly*, *31*(2), 198–212. doi:10.1037pq0000135 PMID:27243243

González-Burchard, E., Borrell, L. N., Choudhry, S., Naqvi, M., Tsai, H. J., Rodriguez-Santana, J. R., Chapela, R., Rogers, S. D., Mei, R., Rodriguez-Cintron, W., Arena, J. F., Kittles, R., Perez-Stable, E. J., Ziv, E., & Risch, N. (2005). Latino populations: A unique opportunity for the study of race, genetics, and social environment in epidemiological research. *American Journal of Public Health*, *95*(12), 2161–2168. doi:10.2105/AJPH.2005.068668 PMID:16257940

Griffith, D. M., Gilbert, K. L., Bruce, M. A., & Thorpe, R. J. Jr. (2016). Masculinity in men's health: Barrier or portal to healthcare? In J. J. Heidelbaugh (Ed.), *Men's health in primary care* (pp. 19–31). Springer. doi:10.1007/978-3-319-26091-4_2

Hall, C. C. I. (1997). Cultural malpractice: The growing obsolescence of psychology with the changing U.S. population. *The American Psychologist*, *52*(6), 642–651. doi:10.1037/0003-066X.52.6.642 PMID:9229997

Hall, W. D. (2016). *Masculine ideology in adolescent male relationships: a quantitative study* [Master's Thesis]. Smith College, Northampton, MA. https://scholarworks.smith.edu/theses/1691

Hill, C. M., Williams, E. C., & Ornelas, I. J. (2019). Help Wanted: Mental Health and Social Stressors Among Latino Day Laborers. *American Journal of Men's Health*, *13*(2). Advance online publication. doi:10.1177/1557988319838424 PMID:30880547

Hofferth, S. L., & Moon, U. J. (2016). How do they do it? The immigrant paradox in the transition to adulthood. *Social Science Research*, *57*, 177–194. doi:10.1016/j.ssresearch.2015.12.013 PMID:26973039

Hursh, D., & Martina, C. A. (2003). Neoliberalism and Schooling in the US: How state and federal government education policies perpetuate inequality. *The Journal for Critical Education Policy Studies*, *1*(2). http://www.jceps.com

Ishikawa, R. Z., Cardemil, E. V., & Falmagne, R. J. (2010). Help seeking and help receiving for emotional distress among Latino men and women. *Qualitative Health Research*, *20*(11), 1558–1572. doi:10.1177/1049732310369140 PMID:20448272

Jarrett, N. C., Bellamy, C. D., & Adeyemi, S. A. (2007). Men's Health Help-Seeking and Implications for Practice. *American Journal of Health Studies*, *22*(2), 88–95.

Kennedy, A., & Moorhead, A. (2022). Help-seeking and masculinity in opposition: A quantitative study investigating the potential of coaching to increase men's engagement in help-seeking. *The Coaching Psychologist*, *17*(2).

Levant, R. F., Hall, R. J., Weigold, I. K., & McCurdy, E. R. (2016). Construct validity evidence for the Male Role Norms Inventory-Short Form: A structural equation modeling approach using the bifactor model. *Journal of Counseling Psychology*, *63*(5), 534–542. doi:10.1037/cou0000171 PMID:27598043

Levant, R. F., & Richmond, K. (2007). A review of research on masculinity ideologies using the Male Role Norms Inventory. *Journal of Men's Studies*, *15*(2), 130–146. doi:10.3149/jms.1502.130

Levant, R. F., Wimer, D. J., & Williams, C. M. (2011). An evaluation of the psychometric properties of the Health Behavior Inventory-20 (HBI- 20) and its relationships to masculinity and attitudes towards seeking psychological help among college men. *Psychology of Men & Masculinity, 12*, 26–41. doi:10.1037/a0021014

Liang, C. T. H., Salcedo, J., & Miller, H. A. (2011). Perceived racism, masculinity ideologies, and gender role conflict among Latino men. *Psychology of Men & Masculinity, 12*(3), 201–215. doi:10.1037/a0020479

Lin, L., Stamm, K., & Christidis, P. (2018). How diverse is the psychology workforce? *Monitor on Psychology, 49*(2). https://www.apa.org/monitor/2018/02/datapoint

Lindinger-Sternart, S. (2015). Help-seeking behaviors of men for mental health and the impact of diverse cultural backgrounds. *International Journal of Social Science Studies, 3*(1), 1–6. doi:10.11114/ijsss.v3i1.519

Liu, W. M. (2005). The study of men and masculinity as an important multicultural competency consideration. *Journal of Clinical Psychology, 61*(6), 685–697. doi:10.1002/jclp.20103 PMID:15732087

Luedke, C. L. (2019). "Es como una familia": Bridging emotional support with academic and professional development through the acquisition of capital in Latinx student organizations. *Journal of Hispanic Higher Education, 18*(4), 372–388. doi:10.1177/1538192717751205

Mahalik, J. R., Locke, B. D., Ludlow, L. H., Deimer, M. A., Scott, R. P. J., Gottfried, M., & Freitas, G. (2003). Development of the Conformity to Masculine Norms Inventory. *Psychology of Men & Masculinity, 4*(1), 3–25. doi:10.1037/1524-9220.4.1.3

Maldonado, A., Preciado, A., Buchanan, M., Pulvers, K., Romero, D., & D'Anna-Hernandez, K. (2018). Acculturative stress, mental health symptoms, and the role of salivary inflammatory markers among a Latino sample. *Cultural Diversity & Ethnic Minority Psychology, 24*(2), 277–283. doi:10.1037/cdp0000177 PMID:29154561

Marks, A. K., Ejesi, K., & García Coll, C. (2014). Understanding the US immigrant paradox in childhood and adolescence. *Child Development Perspectives, 8*(2), 59–64. doi:10.1111/cdep.12071

Martinez, M. (2019). Toxic masculinity: An outcome of colonialism and its effects on the Latinx/Chicanx LGBTQ+ community. *McNair Research Journal SJSU, 15*(1), 6. doi:10.31979/mrj.2019.1506

Martinez, R. (2020). Hispanic Men's Perceptions About Depression and Attitudes Toward Mental Health Treatment. *UC Merced Undergraduate Research Journal, 12*(1). Retrieved from https://escholarship.org/uc/item/93x0104f doi:10.5070/M4121046071

Mastro, D., Behm-Morawitz, E., & Ortiz, M. (2007). The Cultivation of Social Perceptions of Latinos: A Mental Models Approach. *Media Psychology, 9*(2), 347–365. doi:10.1080/15213260701286106

Mirandé, A. (2018). Hombres y machos: Masculinity and Latino culture [Men and Males: Masculinity and Latino Culture]. Routledge. doi:10.4324/9780429500008

Morrell, R. (1998). Of boys and men: Masculinity and gender in Southern African studies. *Journal of Southern African Studies, 24*(4), 605–630. doi:10.1080/03057079808708593

Murphy, S. L., Kochanek, K. D., Xu, J. Q., & Arias, E. (2021). Mortality in the United States, NCHS Data Brief, no 427. Hyattsville, MD: National Center for Health Statistics. icon. doi:10.15620/cdc:112079external

Myers, H. F., Wyatt, G. E., Ullman, J. B., Loeb, T. B., Chin, D., Prause, N., Zhang, M., Williams, J. K., Slavich, G. M., & Liu, H. (2015). Cumulative burden of lifetime adversities: Trauma and mental health in low-SES African Americans and Latino/as. *Psychological Trauma: Theory, Research, Practice, and Policy*, *7*(3), 243–251. doi:10.1037/a0039077 PMID:25961869

National Latinx Psychological Association. (2020). Ethical guidelines of the National Latinx Psychological Association. *Journal of Latina/o Psychology*, *8*(2), 101–111. doi:10.1037/lat0000151

Nguyen, C. M., Liu, W. M., Hernandez, J. O., & Stinson, R. (2012). Problem-solving appraisal, gender role conflict, help-seeking behavior, and psychological distress among men who are homeless. *Psychology of Men & Masculinity*, *13*(3), 270–282. doi:10.1037/a0025523

Noe-Bustamante, L. (2019). *Key Facts About U.S. Hispanics and Their Diverse Heritage*. Pew Research Center. https://www.pewresearch.org/fact-tank/2019/09/16/key-facts-about-u-s-hispanics/

Noe-Bustamante, L., Gonzalez-Barrera, A., Edwards, K., Mora, L., & Lopez, M. H. (2021). *Majority of Latinos Say Skin Color Impacts Opportunity in America and Shapes Daily Life*. Pew Research Center. https://www.pewresearch.org/hispanic/2021/11/04/majority-of-latinos-say-skin-color-impacts-opportunity-in-america-and-shapes-daily-life/

Nuñez, A., González, P., Talavera, G. A., Sanchez-Johnsen, L., Roesch, S. C., Davis, S. M., Arguelles, W., Womack, V. Y., Ostrovsky, N. W., Ojeda, L., Penedo, F. J., & Gallo, L. C. (2016). Machismo, Marianismo, and Negative Cognitive-Emotional Factors: Findings From the Hispanic Community Health Study/Study of Latinos Sociocultural Ancillary Study. *Journal of Latina/o Psychology*, *4*(4), 202–217. doi:10.1037/lat0000050 PMID:27840779

O'Neil, J. M. (1990). Assessing men's gender role conflict. In D. Moore & F. Leafgren (Eds.), *Problem-solving strategies and interventions for men in conflict* (pp. 23–38). American Association for Counseling and Development.

O'Neil, J. M. (2008). Summarizing 25 years of research on men's gender role conflict using the gender role conflict scale: New research paradigms and clinical implications. *The Counseling Psychologist*, *36*(3), 358–445. doi:10.1177/0011000008317057

O'Neil, J. M., Helms, B. J., Gable, R. K., David, L., & Wrightsman, L. S. (1986). Gender-Role Conflict Scale: College men's fear of femininity. *Sex Roles*, *14*(5-6), 335–350. doi:10.1007/BF00287583

Ojeda, L., & Piña-Watson, B. (2014). Caballerismo may protect against the role of machismo on Mexican day laborers' self-esteem. *Psychology of Men & Masculinity*, *15*(3), 288–295. doi:10.1037/a0033450

Ortega, A. N., Feldman, J. M., Canino, G., Steinman, K., & Alegría, M. (2006). Co-occurrence of mental and physical illness in US Latinos. *Social Psychiatry and Psychiatric Epidemiology*, *41*(12), 927–934. doi:10.100700127-006-0121-8 PMID:17013767

Ortega, A. N., Rosenheck, R., Alegría, M., & Desai, R. A. (2000). Acculturation and the lifetime risk of psychiatric and substance use disorders among Hispanics. *The Journal of Nervous and Mental Disease*, *188*(11), 728–735. doi:10.1097/00005053-200011000-00002 PMID:11093374

Pager, D., & Shepherd, H. (2008). The Sociology of Discrimination: Racial Discrimination in Employment, Housing, Credit, and Consumer Markets. *Annual Review of Sociology*, *34*(1), 181–209. doi:10.1146/annurev.soc.33.040406.131740 PMID:20689680

Paredes, T. M., & Parchment, T. M. (2021). The Latino father in the postnatal period: The role of egalitarian masculine gender role attitudes and coping skills in depressive symptoms. *Psychology of Men & Masculinity*, *22*(1), 113–123. doi:10.1037/men0000315

Passel, J. S., Lopez, M. H., & Cohn, D. (2022). *U.S. Hispanic population continued its geographic spread in the 2010's*. Pew Research Center. https://www.pewresearch.org/fact-tank/2022/02/03/u-s-hispanic-population-continued-its-geographic-spread-in-the-2010s/

Pedrotti, J. T., & Burnes, T. R. (2016). The new face of the field: Dilemmas for diverse early-career psychologists. *Training and Education in Professional Psychology*, *10*(3), 141–148. doi:10.1037/tep0000120

Pérez, O. F. R., & Morales, A. (2020). Machismo. In B. J. Carducci, C. S. Nave, J. S. Mio, & R. E. Riggio (Eds.), *The Wiley Encyclopedia of Personality and Individual Differences*. doi:10.1002/9781118970843.ch305

Poston, W. C. (1990). The biracial identity development model: A needed addition. *Journal of Counseling and Development*, *69*(2), 152–155. doi:10.1002/j.1556-6676.1990.tb01477.x

Poston, W. C. (1990). The Biracial Identity Development Model: A needed addition. *Journal of Counseling and Development*, *69*(2), 152–155. doi:10.1002/j.1556-6676.1990.tb01477.x

Postsecondary National Policy Institute. (2021). *Factsheets: Women in Higher Education*. https://pnpi.org/women-in-higher-education/

Postsecondary National Policy Institute. (2022). *Factsheets: Men of Color*. https://pnpi.org/men-of-color/

Ramirez, E. (2017). Unequal socialization: Interrogating the Chicano/Latino (a) doctoral education experience. *Journal of Diversity in Higher Education*, *10*(1), 25–38. doi:10.1037/dhe0000028

Robinson, M. (2019). Two-spirit identity in a time of gender fluidity. *Journal of Homosexuality*. PMID:31125297

Rochlen, A. B. (2005). Men in (and out of) therapy: Central concepts, emerging directions, and remaining challenges. *Journal of Clinical Psychology*, *61*(6), 627–631. doi:10.1002/jclp.20098 PMID:15732139

Rochlen, A. B., Land, L. N., & Wong, Y. J. (2004). Male restrictive emotionality and evaluations of online versus face-to-face counseling. *Psychology of Men & Masculinity*, *5*(2), 190–200. doi:10.1037/1524-9220.5.2.190

Rojas-Araúz, B. O. (2021). *Undocumented Healing: Strengths and Resilience from the Shadows* [Doctoral dissertation]. University of Oregon.

Saenz, V. B., & Ponjuan, L. (2009). The Vanishing Latino Male in Higher Education. *Journal of Hispanic Higher Education*, *8*(1), 54–89. doi:10.1177/1538192708326995

Sagar-Ouriaghli, I., Godfrey, E., Bridge, L., Meade, L., & Brown, J. (2019). Improving Mental Health Service Utilization Among Men: A Systematic Review and Synthesis of Behavior Change Techniques Within Interventions Targeting Help-Seeking. *American Journal of Men's Health*, *13*(3). doi:10.1177/1557988319857009 PMID:31184251

Salsberg, E., Quigley, L., Richwine, C., Sliwa, S., Acquaviva, K., & Wyche, K. (2020). The Social Work Profession; Findings from three years of surveys of new social workers. Fitzhugh Mullan Institute for Health Workforce Equity, The George Washington University.

Schwatken, S. (2011). *Latino/a help-seeking behavior and endorsement of common factors* [Master's Thesis]. Iowa State University, Ames, IA. doi:10.31274/etd-180810-3000

Sinha, M. (2017). Colonial masculinity: The 'manly Englishman' and the 'effeminate Bengali' in the late nineteenth century. In *Colonial masculinity*. Manchester University Press. doi:10.7765/9781526123640

Smith, D., & Werther, E. (2017). *Invisible Color: The Continued Lack of Diversity in Professional Psychology*. Poster presented at the Southeastern Psychological Association Annual Conference, Atlanta, GA.

Tengan, T. K. (2002). (En) gendering colonialism: Masculinities in Hawai'i and Aotearoa. *Cultural Values*, *6*(3), 239–256. doi:10.1080/1362517022000007194

Torres, J. B. (1998). Masculinity and gender roles among Puerto Rican men: A dilemma for Puerto Rican men's personal identity. *The American Journal of Orthopsychiatry*, *68*, 16–26. doi:10.1037/h0080266 PMID:9494638

Torres, J. B., Solberg, V. S. H., & Carlstrom, A. H. (2002). The myth of sameness among Latino men and their machismo. *The American Journal of Orthopsychiatry*, *72*(2), 163–181. doi:10.1037/0002-9432.72.2.163 PMID:15792057

Torres, V., Hernández, E., & Martinez, S. (2019). *Understanding the Latinx Experience: Developmental and Contextual Influences* (1st ed.). Stylus Publishing.

Torres, V. N., Williams, E. C., Ceballos, R. M., Donovan, D. M., & Ornelas, I. J. (2022). Discrimination, acculturative stress, alcohol use and their associations with alcohol-related consequences among Latino immigrant men. *Journal of Ethnicity in Substance Abuse*, 1–16. Advance online publication. doi:10.1080/15332640.2022.2077273 PMID:35634786

Torres-Pagán, L., & Toro-Alfonso, J. (2017). Hegemonic Masculinity as a Key Factor on Health Beliefs and Seeking Help in Puerto Rican Men with Hypertension: A Qualitative Study. *Puerto Rican Journal of Psychology. Revista Puertorriqueña de Psicología*, *28*(1), 134–147.

Tukachinsky, R., Mastro, D., & Yarchi, M. (2017). The effect of prime time television ethnic/racial stereotypes on Latino and Black Americans: A longitudinal national level study. *Journal of Broadcasting & Electronic Media*, *61*(3), 538–556. doi:10.1080/08838151.2017.1344669

Turner, C. (2002). Women of Color in Academe: Living with Multiple Marginality. *The Journal of Higher Education*, *73*(1), 74–93. doi:10.1080/00221546.2002.11777131

U.S. Census Bureau. (2020). *Sex by Age (Hispanic or Latino), 2020 American Community Survey 5-Year Estimates.* Retrieved from https://data.census.gov/cedsci/table?q=Hispanic%20by%20sex,%20 2020&tid=ACSDT5Y2020.B01001I

Uzogara, E. E. (2019). Gendered Racism Biases: Associations of Phenotypes with Discrimination and Internalized Oppression Among Latinx American Women and Men. *Race and Social Problems*, *11*(1), 80–92. doi:10.100712552-018-9255-z

Uzogara, E. E., Lee, H., Abdou, C. M., & Jackson, J. S. (2014). A comparison of skin tone discrimination among African American men: 1995 and 2003. *Psychology of Men & Masculinity*, *15*(2), 201–212. doi:10.1037/a0033479 PMID:25798076

Vargas, S. M., Huey, S. J., & Miranda, J. (2020). A critical review of current evidence on multiple types of discrimination and mental health. *The American Journal of Orthopsychiatry*, *90*(3), 374–390. doi:10.1037/ort0000441 PMID:31999138

Velasquez, R. J., & Burton, M. P. (2004). Psychotherapy of Chicano men. In R. J. Velasquez, L. M. Arrellano, & B. W. McNeill (Eds.), *The handbook of Chicana/o psychology and mental health* (pp. 177–192). Lawrence Erlbaum Associates, Inc.

Villenas, S., & Deyhle, D. (1999). Critical race theory and ethnographies challenging the stereotypes: Latino families, schooling, resilience and resistance. *Curriculum Inquiry*, *29*(4), 413–445.

Vogel, D. L., Heimerdinger-Edwards, S. R., Hammer, J. H., & Hubbard, A. (2011). "Boys Don't Cry": Examination of the Links between Endorsement of Masculine Norms, Self-Stigma, and Help-Seeking Attitudes for Men from Diverse Backgrounds. *Journal of Counseling Psychology*, *58*(3), 368–382. doi:10.1037/a0023688 PMID:21639615

Wade, P. (2010). *Race and Ethnicity in Latin America.* Pluto Press. doi:10.26530/OAPEN_625258

Walters, A. S., & Valenzuela, I. (2019). "To me what's important is to give respect. There is no respect in cheating": Masculinity and Monogamy in Latino Men. *Sexuality & Culture*, *23*(4), 1025–1053. doi:10.100712119-019-09615-5

Walters, A. S., & Valenzuela, I. (2020). More Than Muscles, Money, or Machismo: Latino Men and the Stewardship of Masculinity. *Sexuality and Culture, 24*(3), 967. https://link.gale.com/apps/doc/A621914271/HRCA?u=anon~a27a5c2d&sid=googleScholar&xid=a6f3e8ca

Williams, D. R. (2018). Stress and the Mental Health of Populations of Color: Advancing Our Understanding of Race-related Stressors. *Journal of Health and Social Behavior*, *59*(4), 466–485. doi:10.1177/0022146518814251 PMID:30484715

Williams, D. R., & Mohammed, S. A. (2013). Racism and Health I: Pathways and Scientific Evidence. *The American Behavioral Scientist*, *57*(8), 1152–1173. PMID:24347666

Wong, S. J. (2013). Machismo. In K. D. Keith (Ed.), *The Encyclopedia of Cross-Cultural Psychology.* doi:10.1002/9781118339893.wbeccp339

Chapter 9
Higher Education:
Latinx Individuals *Luchando* for Higher Education

Leslie Espinoza
University of Georgia, USA

Monica Sanchez
University of Georgia, USA

Alexina Pilo
University of Georgia, USA

Nancy Muro-Rodriguez
University of Georgia, USA

ABSTRACT

This chapter focuses on the history and educational experiences of current and past Latinx students. It helps understand governmental policies and systemic barriers that Latinx students and faculty face in the education system. This chapter provides information regarding higher education by highlighting the different experiences of first-generation college students. Authors help identify multicultural considerations when working with Latinx students both in higher education and in the counseling space. Lastly, the authors focus on future directions and resources to support and better help Latinx students create a pipeline towards higher education.

INTRODUCTION

This chapter is about the history and educational experiences of current and past Latinx students. It examines the educational pipeline of Latinx Persons from undergraduate education to the professoriate. It helps understand systemic barriers that Latinx students and faculty face in the education system in the U.S. This chapter also identifies multicultural considerations when working with Latinx students

DOI: 10.4018/978-1-6684-4901-1.ch009

in higher education. Lastly, it acknowledges supporting factors that better help Latinx students cope in higher education.

Positionality

Latinx people with graduate degrees have helped guide and pave the way for many Latinx persons through mentorship, community, support, and the mere fact of being a Latinx individual succeeding through the advancement of their higher education. Through our positionality, we would like to give the reader insight into the experiences of Latinx mentorship, peer support, and the positive impact Latinx culture and identity have had on the author's educational journey.

I, Leslie Espinoza, have roots from Zacatecas, Mexico, born in Riverside, California and raised in Houston County, Georgia. I am a counseling psychology student working on my doctoral degree under the mentorship of Dr. Delgado-Romero at the University of Georgia (UGA). My academic journey has always been a lonely one due to the *Mexicana* minority status I hold and the *Español* that is my first language. My lonely journey changed when I met my colleague Dr. Ruben Atilano and my future mentor Dr. Delgado-Romero who both looked and spoke like me. I was amazed by their work and how both individuals gave back to the Latinx community within their profession. I always believed that it was challenging to work in an ethnocentric monocultural space when catering to clients that are multicultural, bilingual, and hold different world views from what students are taught in textbooks and research. Dr. Delgado-Romero has helped me feel safe in my views, research, and therapy work as a psychologist-in-training. He has provided unique spaces for his mentees that have been composed of support, familiarity, value, security, and an amazing academic family. In the Latinx culture the concept of closeness is very important, and Dr. Delgado-Romero has fostered and shown that value to all of his students both in academic and personal settings. Having a Latino as a mentor has been inspiring, but most importantly, has made me feel heard.

I, Monica Sanchez, was born and raised in Georgia, but my family is from Tarimoro, Guanajuato, México. I am a first-generation PhD student at UGA in the Counseling Psychology program where I also completed my master's degree. Within my academic journey, building a community has always been very important to me. I rarely met Latinas who were on the same academic journey as I was, so it was so refreshing coming to UGA and seeing so many Latinas working towards the same goal. As I began connecting with these women, I felt so seen and understood. Their reassurance, support, stories, guidance, and authentically showing up as themselves within academic spaces has helped me to refine my academic goals and pursue a doctoral degree. Mentorship for Latinx students is so important in fostering academic growth and wellness. Latinx individuals in higher education uplift our communities by being an example of *"Si se Puede!"* because sometimes it may feel as if these spaces are not for us. As I continue my education, I hope to also be a support for other Latinx students. The authors of this chapter (and many more throughout the book) have been a great support system and I am so grateful to have so many Latinx individuals with me for my academic journey!

I, Alexina Pilo, am a doctoral student in Counseling Psychology at UGA, under the mentorship of Dr. Edward Delgado-Romero. Prior to attending UGA, I obtained my master's degree from Boston College (BC) and my bachelor's degree from the University of California, Irvine (UCI). At UCI, I began to learn the power of mentorship. Being mentored by Dr. Jessica Ortega and Dr. Jeanett Castellanos, I was challenged and embraced with love and passion while pursuing my degree and furthering my journey of self-love and self-discovery. While at UGA, I continue to be mentored by Dr. Delgado-Romero who continues to provide support and guidance throughout one of my most challenging pursuits. With time, I have begun to formulate what I see as my academic family and am thankful for the love and guidance my mentors continue to provide. I aspire to one day follow in the footsteps of my mentors and engage in the mentorship of other Latinx students while continuing to expand my academic family.

I, Nancy Muro-Rodriguez, am a doctoral candidate at UGA, under the mentorship of Dr. Delgado-Romero. Prior to attending UGA, I attended the University of Wisconsin-Milwaukee (UWM) and was mentored by Dr. Shannon Chavez-Korell. As a first-generation Latina college student, navigating a Predominantly White Institution (PWI) came with many challenges such as code switching, family responsibilities, and navigating the higher education system. Finding peers or professors who had similar cultural backgrounds as I was often difficult. During a panel, I met Dr. Chavez-Korell, as she discussed her education experience from living in a rural town in Texas to obtaining her doctoral degree. Dr. Chavez-Korell took the time to mentor me and encourage me to continue to pursue a doctoral degree. She supported me every step of the way, by helping me apply to my master's program and always being there to advocate for me. We often talked about the difficulties of leaving family, but it was often needed to help them down the road. She was the first professor that I felt understood how complex cultural values can interfere with career decisions. Throughout my master's and doctoral education, mentorship has been a pillar of my education. Oftentimes, I have found myself with other students who are first generation and often are scared of continuing a master's or doctoral degree. I truly believe that if my path did not cross with Dr. Chavez-Korell, my life would be so different from now and I would have not pursued a doctoral degree.

GOVERNMENTAL POLICIES

The undocumented Latinx student population has been drastically affected by frequent policy and administration changes. During the Clinton administration, a large proportion of immigrants filled the United States (U.S.) and grew the economy (Suárez-Orozco & Suárez-Orozco, 2009). Due to the influx of Latinx children, important educational policies needed to be put in place to help both their skills and language development to achieve academically. Unfortunately, different policies and administrations continue to make it difficult for Latinx students to overcome educational and legal barriers.

Bush Administration

The 2001 Bush administration was concerned about English Language Learners (ELLs) spending 6 years or more in English Speakers of Other Languages (ESOL) classes. This administration proposed restrictions on ELL services and sanctions for states who failed to get language minorities to perform at school standards and speak fluent English within a 3-year time frame. This was not only a threat to equal educational opportunities for the Latinx community, but it also restrained Spanish speaking students from overcoming language barriers (Mora, 2002). Despite the new proposed No Child Left Behind policy, it still hindered many ELLs in their process of learning. This new policy also contradicts the case of Castaneda V. Pickard in 1980, which affirmed that schools must address barriers and provide services to ELLs without time restrictions to protect the civil rights of full equal educational opportunities (Mora, 2002).

DREAM Act

Millions of children continue to identify as mixed-status or undocumented, which is why it is important to be aware of the historical context impacting today's educational climate. Policies have evolved with each president and their administration, impacting students and their families who may be part of the mixed-status or undocumented status households. Millions who were planning to graduate high school encountered barriers that would prevent them from higher education due to their status (Suárez-Orozco & Suárez-Orozco, 2009). The Development, Relief, and Education for Alien Minors (DREAM) Act is a law that would have provide undocumented high school graduates a path to residency and eventually citizenship through college, work, or armed services (Herrera & Obregón, 2018). As of 2022, the DREAM Act continues to be discussed with no action taken due to the failure of government officials to support this legislation. There are two versions of the DREAM Act currently before Congress: The DREAM Act of 2021 (S. 264) and a version of the DREAM Act that is incorporated into a larger bill known as the Dream and Promise Act of 2021 (H.R. 6) in hopes of being passed (American Immigration Council, 2022). The DREAM Act bill involves a three-step process: 1.) the ability to obtain conditional permanent residence, 2.) a lawful permanent residence (LPR) which can be obtained by receiving a degree, working for three years, or military service for 2 years, and 3.) naturalization which one can obtain by having LPR status for at least five years (American Immigration Council, 2022).

DACA

On June 15, 2012, then-president Obama's administration enacted the Deferred Action Childhood Arrivals (DACA) Act when it was clear the DREAM Act would not pass. DACA is a relief program that protects immigrants who come to the U.S., which gives them protection from deportation and a work permit for two years (Herrera & Obregón, 2018). DACA has been a way for the individuals within the undocumented community to be protected in the U.S. Unfortunately, due to former President Trump's administration, the possibility of DACA being taken away has created fear throughout the undocumented population. As future administrations will continue to change policies regarding both education and citizenship, advocacy and social justice work will be important to ensure that the U.S. preserves or expands DACA. Both the DREAM Act and DACA program are important for the Latinx community. These two laws can create a pipeline of educators and employers that are needed to support the U.S. ever-growing Latinx community.

LATINX HIGHER EDUCATION

According to Martinez (2018), Latinx students are receiving doctoral degrees higher than ever before. Between the years of 2019 and 2020, a total of 14,868 of doctoral degrees were conferred to Latinx students (National Center of Educational Statistics, 2019). Latinx individuals are rapidly becoming the new majority in the U.S. which is why it is important to support our Latinx community in creating an educational pipeline to higher education. The total Hispanic college enrollment in 2020 by students 18-24 years old in degree-granting postsecondary institutions, was 36% (NCES, 2019). In the U.S., college enrollment differs by ethnic backgrounds and is broken down from 33 different Latinx countries including: Cuban 45%, Dominican 38%, Nicaraguan 39%, Mexican 35%, Chilean 64%, and Venezuelan

Higher Education

59%. Between 2000 and 2016, Hispanics who applied to post-baccalaureate education doubled from 111,000 to 260,000 and degrees awarded increased from 77,700 to 235,000. Master's degrees awarded almost tripled between 2000 and 2016 from 21,700 to 62,900, and Doctoral degrees doubled from 5,200 to 11,800 (National Center of Educational Statistics, 2019). Unfortunately, Latinx undergraduate students are often discouraged from applying to graduate school for numerous reasons, including a lack of social capital, mentorship, financial, academic, and emotional support (Martinez, 2018). Therefore, it is important to provide academic support and put in place programs that will help and encourage underrepresented groups to attend college and graduate. For example, the Penn Center for Minority Serving Institutions (PCSI) developed a program specifically for Hispanic Serving Institutions (HSIs) to provide support to a scholar with aspirations of becoming a professor in the humanities area of study (Martinez, 2018). The McNair Scholars Program, also a federally funded program, is a pipeline for underrepresented students who come from disadvantaged backgrounds: first-generation, low socioeconomic status (SES), and marginalized racial identity (Martinez, 2018). This federal program provides universities with funds to support college students and connect them with mentors for research opportunities throughout their doctoral journey (Martinez, 2018). Support programs as discussed above are important for Latinx undergraduate students to help them be more competitive when they leave college, as well as to open the possibility of applying for a graduate degree.

First-Generation College Students

First-generation college students are defined as students who are the first in their family to attend college and receive their bachelor's degree, but this does not encompass the experiences of Latinx students (Vega, 2016). Carrying the label of "first-generation college student" as a Latinx individual means navigating two worlds with different responsibilities simultaneously. Many Latinx first-generation college students navigate cultural factors such as family responsibility, English as a second language, acculturation, guilt, documentation status, and gender expectations (Vega, 2016). Other crucial tasks to consider are entrance exams, applications, student aid, housing, and school demands without help from others. This lonely educational road is due to the lack of role models or elders that have not had the eligibility to experience college education.

A report from Excelencia in Education reported 44% of first-generation students are Hispanic or Latino compared to other racial groups (2019). Thus, a majority of Latinx students are learning how to navigate higher education for the first time. The literature has captured data that highlights the challenges of first-generation college students, including how these students are less academically prepared for college, less knowledgeable about how to apply to college, and the difficulties of acclimating to the environment once enrolled in a higher education (Tym et al., 2004). Fortunately, their *orgullo* of being the first in their family to *seguir adelante* with their education can be a significant motivator for students, so highlighting their accomplishments and achievements throughout their education can serve as a way to combat imposter syndrome within their academic journey.

LATINX CULTURAL CONSIDERATIONS

In providing support for Latinx students there are cultural considerations one should be aware of while helping them navigate academic environments. Studies (e.g., Von Robertson et al., 2016; Cuellar, 2019) have indicated that having mentorship, professors of color, Latinx organizations, counter spaces, and mental health support in college and universities has benefited Latinx students in their academic journey. Latinx counter spaces can include school organizations, academic clubs, research teams, volunteer work, and Greek life.

Familismo

Martinez (2013) defines *familismo* "as the tendency to hold the wants and needs of family in higher regard than one's own and has been considered a common trait of Latina/o families" (p. 23). Often, we see students continue to hold the value in familismo while pursuing their education, which is true of all the authors of this chapter. *Familismo* and collectivism have many similar parallels in the sense that individuals' thoughts, actions, and behaviors are often thought about as how one person's actions impact the family or those around the individual (Greenfield & Quiroz, 2013; Raeff et al., 2000). This is quite different compared to White Western counterparts, who have been raised in individualistic cultures, reinforced by mainstream culture. Individuals from individualistic cultures uphold behaviors and cognitive decision making that tends to impact oneself without thinking of others (Arevalo et al., 2016).

One example where *familismo* shows up for students is when they select where to apply for college. Often that may look like applying to nearby in-state colleges because they may have responsibilities at home that they cannot disregard (Vasquez-Salgado et al., 2015; Covarrubias et al., 2019). One avenue of support is talking to the students and having the family involved during the application process. Oftentimes, Latinx students can be the first in their families to graduate high school and apply to higher education, thus the process of applying to a college can be very daunting. In having the family involved, it allows the student to have less pressure relaying information to their parents regarding navigating systems they have little information on (Engle, 2007). It is common for parents to find themselves not knowing or understanding how to best support their child through applying for higher education. In comparison, children whose parents have obtained some level of college education are able to assist their child during the early start of applying to college. Parents who have only completed middle school education or less, may not have the tools or be equipped to help their child, not because they don't want to but because they do not have the knowledge, experience, or comprehension of the application process. Although Latinx parents may not always understand the process and pressures of being in college, parents can support students with verbal affirmations, social support, financial support, and little reminders of home.

Mentorship

Another way to support Latinx students in higher education is having a faculty mentor. Research has shown a positive impact on Latinx students when they interact with a faculty mentor at all levels of education: undergraduate, master, and doctoral level. Research has shown that having a faculty mentor provides students with a higher college self-efficacy and an increased ability to meet academic goals (Holloway-Friesen, 2021). Santos and Reigadas (2002) found that students with same-ethnic mentors had significant satisfaction in their education and furthered their personal and career development. They also highlighted the importance of the frequency of contact between students and mentors and how it positively correlated to students' adjustment to college, perceived mentor supportiveness, and program satisfaction (Santos & Reigadas, 2002; Santa-Ramirez, 2022). As mentioned by the authors of this chapter, both faculty and peer mentorship have provided a positive experience, allowing the authors to continue to pursue their next level of higher education (Delgado-Romero & Hernández, 2002; Liou et al., 2021).

The four authors in this chapter have had a positive outcome in obtaining mentorship during their educational journey. Oftentimes, faculty or university staff underestimate the support they provide to students. Faculty may not be aware of the trust and comfort a student may experience under their supervision; however, it is important to mention that faculty support is very much appreciated by students. Without faculty giving students like us, the authors, a chance, we would have missed out on many opportunities for growth. If it wasn't for the trust and confidence that Dr. Delgado Romero has in his students, we would not have had such an incredible opportunity to write alongside him in this textbook.

INSTITUTIONAL EXPERIENCES

Navigating PWIs and HSIs

The majority of Latinx students attend predominantly white institutions (PWIs) which may be due to Hispanic Serving Institutions (HSIs) only being in locations where the majority of the population is Latinx and the limited amount of HSIs across the nation (Von Robertson et al., 2016). PWIs are institutions in which White individuals account for 50% of the student population (Solorzano, 2000). Research indicates that Latinx students frequently report racism, discrimination, and isolation while attending PWIs (Von Robertson et al., 2016). The unfair treatment of Latinx students has impacted students to the point where they feel they need to assimilate or separate themselves from the dominant culture or their cultural heritage. The belief that one can integrate both cultures and prevail in a PWI can be contradicted when institutions have systems that are put in place that hinder marginalized communities. It is also impossible to attempt to integrate when individuals in these institutions create toxic environments that include microaggressions, racism, and invalidating spaces. According to Solorzano and colleagues (2000), Latinx students do well in PWIs when there are faculty of color, Latinx historical content in curriculum, programs that support Latinx recruitment, and institutional commitment to diversity. The first author reflected:

As a Mexicana, going to a PWI was difficult because there was no sense of community and space of security. I will forever remember the fear of speaking up in class due to my differential views and ways of thinking. I was always scared of being scrutinized or misinterpreted when speaking my truth because people made me feel like I was a false college student, setting up my future imposter syndrome. Fortunately, as a Latina, I have an amazing culture that values family and friendship; with this beautiful aspect of my life, it has motivated me to keep moving forward in my education.

PWIs can be difficult for Latinx students for a multitude of reasons, and even so, Latinx students pull strength from their cultural values and history to persevere within higher education spaces.

HSIs are defined as institutions with at least 25% percent of the student body made up of Latinx students. This federal designation comes with additional federal funding to help support institutions in increasing the degree attainment of Latinx students (Cuellar, 2019). In 2015 there were a total of 239 HSIs across the nation (Cuellar, 2019). It is important to invest in these institutions to best serve the growing population of Latinx college students because these institutions cultivate environments that are inclusive of their culture, language, and demographic characteristics (Martinez, 2018). As the Latinx population is diverse in terms of ethnic and racial backgrounds, it is important to note that Central American populations from countries like El Salvador, Puerto Rico, and Guatemala are more likely to attend HSIs than Mexican Americans and Multiracial Latinx individuals (Cuellar, 2019). This may be due to immigrational history and financial stability (Cuellar, 2019).

Latinx communities with fewer economic resources, such as family income and financial aid, are also more likely to enroll at HSIs compared to those with more financial resources because HSIs have lower tuition rates and more scholarships for Latinx students than PWIs. Latinx individuals who choose and are more likely to enroll in HSIs tend to express family encouragement as being an important factor in attending college. Family engagement is salient at HSIs because family support positively impacts Latinx college students' academic self-perceptions (Cuellar, 2019). HSIs embody factors that include economic, human, social, familial, and resistant capital that are important to Latinx students. These factors inform how HSIs put together environments in ways that authentically serve Latinx students (Cuellar, 2019). As the Latinx college population increases overall, some PWI's have crossed the threshold to also be considered HSIs. This practice is considered controversial for many reasons including the fact that enrolling Latinx students is not the same as serving them and the fear that PWIs may begin to siphon off grant funding from smaller HSI.

Graduate School Experiences

Within graduate school, Latinx students see little Latinx representation within most academic spaces, with fewer students of color and fewer faculty of color within the classrooms in many majors other than Romance Languages (Dominguez-Rebollar & Acevedo-Polakovich, 2021). Peer and faculty mentors can be a supportive factor in the success of Latinx students by sharing resources, experiences, and similar cultural values that provide students with an example of how their Latinx identity impacts their academic journey (Dominguez-Rebollar & Acevedo-Polakovich, 2021; Gomez, 2020; Holloway-Friesen, 2021; Moschetti et al., 2018). Even just having someone to discuss how hard it is to navigate family drama or whose *cafecito* is better, Latinx students need that time to express themselves authentically and unapologetically with peers, mentors, or faculty members who understand what it's like to be in graduate school. It is important for colleges and universities to hire and admit people of color within their institution. Representation between student diversity, faculty, the recognition of the accomplishments of faculty, and students who hold marginalized identities can help inspire other students to continue within higher education (Gomez, 2020). It is critical for Latinx students to feel validated in their work and that they have access to representations of what the future could look like for them after completing their graduate programs.

Across many universities, Latinx graduate students in various programs are unable to get adequate training or education in working with Latinx people or having bilingual experiences (Rosales et.al., 2018). The second author of this chapter shares:

Within my academic experience, I was unable to find a class for my major that addressed Latinx issues, nor did I have a supervisor who spoke Spanish until my graduate program at a larger university.

Although this may not be the case for students within all universities, smaller universities may not have the same resources, which creates a concern for Latinx students that may attend rural or smaller universities closer to home. Having this unequal access to training and professional development that is culturally relevant and unequal access to faculty members with culturally relevant expertise could bring undue hardships for Latinx students (Santa-Ramirez 2022).

Latinx Research Experiences

Universities have prided themselves in being inclusive and diverse, and yet these institutions continue to endorse dominant ideologies and policies that erase the history, stories, knowledge, and emotions of the lived experiences of communities of color (Salinas, 2017). Working on research projects with faculty within PWIs leaves students feeling disparate or disconnected to the people, the curriculum, or research they are conducting. The second author reflected:

I remember being in two research labs at my undergraduate university and I felt very disconnected from the research we would do in the lab, almost as if my interests and my experiences were not worthy of exploring. Similarly, in class, I was never taught about Latinx scholars, researchers, or theories until my graduate program in a Latinx-specific class.

Within the classroom, Latinx students can feel unwelcome; they have a lack of Latinx faculty and staff to connect with, little to no representation in curriculum, and a curriculum that does not discuss historical oppression or the accomplishments of people of color (Salinas, 2017). Promoting Latinx curriculum, students, faculty, and experiences can provide incoming and existing students with examples of what is possible, what they are capable of, and help students *pa'lante* with their education!

Within research, there is not enough data about the Latinx community, with most data being generalized or non-proportional to the actual demographic information of the area in which the research is being conducted. As an act of resistance to this phenomenon, Latinx students, faculty, and staff should uplift *voces perdidas*, in which Latinx scholars produce and publish non-English research projects, create accessibility to scholarship and academic resources for the Latinx community, and translate existing theoretical frameworks (Salinas, 2017). There is also a lack of access to theories, treatment, or frameworks that examine Latinx identities specifically within the methodology (Salinas, 2017). Latinx students could greatly benefit from learning frameworks that center on Latinx experiences, such as Chicana Feminist Epistemology or Latino/a Critical Race Theory (López et al., 2020; Gutierrez, 2022). Acknowledgement of Latinx theories, frameworks, and methodologies within classrooms can encourage researchers to reexamine past research or nurture future research to bridge the gap in Latinx information across multiple fields of study.

By encouraging liberatory consciousness for Latinx individuals in academia, Latinx academics and researchers can build linguistic capital and validate the experiences of Spanish and Portuguese speakers who can then challenge the dominant ideologies present within academic research (Salinas, 2017). Approximately 70 percent of academic writing across the world is written in English, forcing Latinx bilingual students to choose academic success or working to help their cultural community by using *sus voces* (Salinas, 2017). Although bilingual students navigate these challenges of creating academic work in English, this is a strength that not many students possess and should be rewarded for having the capacity to engage in different languages. Schools and universities should foster Latinx students' work in multiple languages and help their academic development. Bilingual Latinx students and faculty can feel more comfortable producing research in both languages to minimize losing meaning or interpretation from the translation process when conducting research in a non-English language.

LATINX COUNSELING: HURDLES AND PERSEVERANCE

Described as a "rare commodity" (Smith, 2018), the number of Latinx psychologists is slim in comparison to the continuously growing Latinx population. Despite the substantial population of Latinx individuals who reside in the U.S., only 7 percent (8,203 people) of available psychologists across the nation identify as Latinx (American Psychological Association, 2020). Additionally, survey data released by the APA highlights that only 10.8 percent of psychologists can offer bilingual services, and only 5.5 percent are able to provide services in Spanish (Hamp et al., 2016). Prior to the COVID-19 pandemic, the need for Latinx counselors was evident. A study completed in 2019 highlighted that approximately 49 percent of Latinx individuals residing in the U.S. experienced at least one poor mental health day within the past 30 days (Basurto, 2020). Barriers including lack of access to bilingual and bicultural counseling resulted in many individuals being left without services.

With the rise of the global pandemic, the need for Latinx counselors is more apparent than ever. The Latinx community has been affected by the pandemic at disproportionate rates, affecting the population's mental health, heightened barriers pertaining to the ability to seek services, and access to care (Garcini et al., 2022). Stressors including separation from loved ones, health concerns, job insecurity, financial stressors, and unequal access to technology affecting access to health services, school, and social interaction were all linked to increased struggles with mental health for the Latinx community due to the COVID-19 pandemic (Paulsen, n.d.). With the rise of the pandemic, barriers have continued to flourish, including a lack of access to stable internet and privacy to engage in services.

Barriers

In higher education, Latinx students, especially undocumented Latinx students, continue to face disparities in relation to overall well-being and mental health (Cha et al., 2019) . When seeking mental health services, university-specific structural barriers including uncertainty regarding policies and procedures, fear of documentation on academic records, hours of clinic operation, language proficiency among providers, fear surrounding documentation status, and lack of multicultural sensitive providers are some additional barriers that may affect one's ability to seek treatment (Samlan et al., 2021). Underrepresented students are historically susceptible to marginalization and a decreased sense of belonging across college campuses (Dueñas & Gloria, 2017). Social isolation due to the pandemic has significantly increased symptoms of stress, anxiety, and depression among college students, specifically racial-ethnic students (Molock & Parchem, 2022). Limited access and barriers to counseling resources continue to impede Latinx college students' mental health. Many colleges continue to lack bilingual and bicultural services and often if services are available, extraordinary waitlists persist. Across college campuses, mental health resources are also often correlated with session limits, further exacerbating barriers. The need for services continues to outweigh the number of bilingual and bicultural clinicians available, adding to the barriers that the Latinx community faces.

Theoretical Orientation

Training clinicians who are working to obtain their degrees are often fielded with questions pertaining to their theoretical orientation. Specifically, for clinicians working with the Latinx population, questions about applicability and appropriateness of specific theoretical orientation comes into question. The third author of this chapter states:

As a graduate student, if not for my Latinx mentors, I believe I would continue to significantly struggle with the question "what is your theoretical orientation?".

Throughout the course of obtaining a graduate degree in counseling, students are often required to engage in courses pertaining to both theory and multicultural psychology. Depending on the program, the multicultural degree requirements can often be fulfilled within one semester and briefly, if at all, touch on theoretical approaches best suited for use with Latinx communities.

In a 2010 interview in which she discussed theoretical orientation, Dr. Arredondo noted the importance of understanding the role that our biases and beliefs have within our perception of the social learning theory (Cardona & Softas-Nall, 2010). The interview also highlights the use of the Racial Minority Identity Model to help understand the experiences of marginalized individuals (Cardona & Softas-Nall, 2010). Latino/a Critical Theory (LatCrit), an extension of Critical Race Theory (CRT), specifically considers Latinx intersectionality and the way gender, classism, sexism, and racism affect the individual (Bernal, 2002). LatCrit acknowledges the lived experiences of the individual specifically considering cultural values, immigration, and language (Bernal, 2002).

Multicultural theoretical perspectives such as Racial Identity Model and LatCrit, can be helpful while working with Latinx student clients and remaining aware of intersecting social aspects, cultural components, barriers, conceptualizing client presenting concerns, and formulating treatment plans and goals to adequately treat these clients. Engaging in individual research pertaining to these frameworks while working with Latinx clients can aid clinicians in further understanding the client's lived experiences, connecting culturally with clients, and helping clients recognize forms of resilience and cultural assets.

CONCLUSION

Latinx individuals have historically been underrepresented in academic spaces. The number of Latinx individuals in this country is not equal to the success of Latinx individuals within higher education. By examining the history, cultural values, importance of mentorship, educational experiences, and systemic barriers for students and faculty, this chapter has explored the Latinx student identity and highlights different supports and barriers to the success of these students within higher education. *¡El futuro de los latinos está aquí!* Latinx's are here and they are not leaving! As the number of Latinx students continues to rise, they will make an everlasting and significant impact on future Latinx individuals in higher education.

Although many educational systems do not fully accept the Latinx identity and the complexities that come with it, we must work to decolonize academic spaces to include Latinx experiences. The Latinx identity becomes embedded within being a student, creating this unique and rare way that shapes their experiences in higher education because their identities are not binary (Gutierrez et al., 2022). Therefore, it is crucial for Latinx students to have images of what higher education can look like through role models and mentors. Faculty and peers should work with Latinx students in navigating educational systems that historically oppress their voices and implement supports. Teachers and professionals have the ability to uplift and promote Latinx students and research, which could in turn help guide others into higher education. From the first author's educational experience:

I was fortunate enough to learn and study under a white faculty member in my doctoral program that was willing to teach and guide me without hesitation.

Uplifting Latinx voices and creating equitable opportunities for Latinx students is everyone's responsibility, not just Latinx faculty or faculty of color.

Latinx people belong in these academic spaces as authentically as they want to be, and it is up to us to create space from within for the future Latinx scholars in higher education. Existing and promoting Latinx voices is a form of resistance that can empower and support Latinx students and faculty in higher education to promote more history, stories, and knowledge about Latinx experiences. In the words of the second author:

When I am my authentic self in class and bring in stories about my culture and experiences, I show that I am here, I have a history, and I have an identity that demands recognition.

Others may describe Latinx's as resilient, cultural, and family oriented but they are more than just values. *Los Latinos tienen historia, perspectiva, conocimiento, y lenguaje,* which makes them valuable and capable of being successful in academic settings. Latinx history will not be erased, silenced, or dismissed by those who marginalize this beautiful ever-growing community. Overall, being a Latinx individual in higher education is a form of resistance.

Future Directions

Our country needs to focus on educating and accommodating students to bridge the gap from elementary school to higher education. Past U.S. administrations have separated Latinx students into categories from the day they step foot in school. They create barriers by separating ELLs and implementing policies to hinder their growth. As Latinx individuals, our language is not a barrier, and our history is not false. Instead of making us feel unwelcome because of our differences, we should be praised for our intellectual abilities, of understanding more than one language, more than one culture, and having an ability to succeed despite laws created for our downfall. As future administrations will continue to change policies regarding both education and citizenship, advocacy and social justice work will be important to ensure that the U.S. preserves the DACA act.

University systems should challenge the ways in which its system impacts Latinx students by funding and promoting bicultural mental health resources and more opportunities for bilingual training within different programs. Although it is not always possible for universities to have access or resources to a variety of training opportunities, faculty and graduate programs should make more efforts to seek opportunities for students that allow them to explore training or professional development opportunities that are for Latinx or bilingual students. The classroom curriculum should integrate more culturally relevant material and promote the work of multiple marginalized identities, not just by presenting one or two cultural examples and then never discussing those identities again for the rest of the semester. By bringing in more awareness of Latinx identities within the curriculum, faculty can help stop the perpetuation of an educational system that historically has hidden or erased Latinx scholars from academic spaces.

Within academic departments, programs, and organizations, Latinx students should be provided with networking and mentorship opportunities with other Latinx faculty and peers. Universities should promote and urge more culturally relevant curriculum, practices, research, and training opportunities that include ways for bilingual students to gain that knowledge and experience within these programs. University employers should challenge how they recruit faculty, staff, and students. It's about time for PhD student and professoriate populations to reflect the Latinx demographics of this diverse country. Overall, the authors hope that you take this chapter and listen to the voices of Latinx students as they work to create a pipeline towards higher education and use their strengths to find solutions for their growth. As a final message for our readers, we leave you with some affirmations to remember:

You are capable. You are strong. You are enough.

Eres capaz. Eres fuerte. Eres suficiente.

Você é capaz. É forte. Você é o suficiente.

RESOURCES

Undocumented Students

- Please go to https://www.uscis.gov/DACA if you are interested in applying to DACA. The website will provide you with in-depth information on what DACA is, the process for first-time applicants, the filing process for renewals, travel information, fee exemptions, and much more (Consideration of DACA, 2022). Please be sure to renew or apply 6 months or more prior to your DACA expiration date. DACA requirements include:
    - Arrived to the U.S before the age of 16
    - Being under 31 years old as of June 15th, 2012
    - Lived continuously in the U.S. since June 15th, 2007
    - Has been physically present in the U.S on June 15, 2012, and at the time one applies
    - Came to the U.S without valid documents before June 15th, 2012
    - Currently studying, has graduated from high school or has been honorably discharged from the military
    - Has not been convicted of a felony or misdemeanor (Consideration of Deferred Action for Childhood Arrivals, 2022).
- Grants and Internships https://latino.cornell.edu/scholarship-internship-resources
- American Immigration Council https://www.americanimmigrationcouncil.org/topics/immigration-benefits-and-relief

Student Scholarships

- Penn Center for Minority Serving Institutions (PCSI)
- AAHHE Undergraduate Fellowship Program (UFP)
- AAHHE Graduate Student Fellowship Program (GSFP)
- LULAC National Scholarship Fund (LNSF)
- Hispanic Scholarship Fund (HSF)
- The McNair Scholars Program

College Resources

- American Association of Hispanics in Higher Education (AAHHE) https://www.aahhe.org/
- Federal Student Aid FAFSA https://studentaid.gov/h/apply-for-aid/fafsa
- Hispanic Association of Colleges and Universities (HACU) https://www.hacu.net/hacu/default.asp

Latinx Research Resources

- *Multicultural Care: A Clinician's Guide to Cultural Competence* (Comas-Díaz, L. 2012)
- *Culturally responsive counseling with Latinas/os* (Arredondo, Gallardo-Cooper, Delgado-Romero, & Zapata, 2014)
- Chicana Feminist Epistemology (López et. al., 2020)
- Latina/o Critical Race Theory (LatCrit) (Solorzano, & Yosso, 2001)
- Cuéntame: The promise of qualitative research with Latinx populations (Delgado Romero, Singh, & De Los Santos, 2018)

REFERENCES

American Psychological Association. (2020). *Demographics of U.S. Psychology Workforce* [Interactive data tool]. http://www.apa.org/workforce/data-tools/demographics.aspx

Arevalo, I., So, D., & McNaughton-Cassill, M. (2016). The role of collectivism among Latino American college students. *Journal of Latinos and Education, 15*(1), 3–11. doi:10.1080/15348431.2015.1045143

Arredondo, P., Gallardo-Cooper, M., Delgado-Romero, E. A., & Zapata, A. L. (2014). *Culturally responsive counseling with Latinas/os*. American Counseling Association.

Basurto, L. E. (2020, October 22). *Why we should be talking about mental health among Latinx communities*. Urban Institute. Retrieved May 1, 2022, from https://www.urban.org/urban-wire/why-we-should-be-talking-about-mental-health-among-latinx-communities

Bernal, D. D. (2002). Critical race theory, Latino critical theory, and critical raced-gendered epistemologies: Recognizing students of color as holders and creators of knowledge. *Qualitative Inquiry, 8*(1), 105–126. doi:10.1177/107780040200800107

Cardona, B., & Softas-Nall, L. (2010). Family therapy with Latino families: An interview with Patricia Arredondo. *The Family Journal, 18*(1), 73–77. doi:10.1177/1066480709356543

Cha, B. S., Enriquez, L. E., & Ro, A. (2019). Beyond access: Psychosocial barriers to undocumented students' use of mental health services. *Social Science & Medicine, 233*, 193–200. doi:10.1016/j.socscimed.2019.06.003 PMID:31212126

Comas-Díaz, L. (2012). *Multicultural care: A clinician's guide to cultural competence*. American Psychological Association. doi:10.1037/13491-000

Consideration of deferred action for childhood arrivals (DACA). (2022, April 12). USCIS. Retrieved May 1, 2022, from https://www.uscis.gov/DACA

Covarrubias, R., Valle, I., Laiduc, G., & Azmitia, M. (2019). "You never become fully independent": Family roles and independence in first-generation college students. *Journal of Adolescent Research, 34*(4), 381–410. doi:10.1177/0743558418788402

Cuellar, M. G. (2019). Creating Hispanic-Serving Institutions (HSIs) and emerging HSIs: Latina/o college choice at 4-year institutions. *American Journal of Education, 125*(2), 231–258. doi:10.1086/701250

Delgado-Romero, E. A., & Hernandez, C. A. (2002). Empowering Hispanic students through student organizations: Competencies for faculty advisors. *Journal of Hispanic Higher Education, 1*(2), 144–157. doi:10.1177/1538192702001002004

Domínguez-Rebollar, R., & Acevedo-Polakovich, I. D. (2021). Factors and interventions that foster success of Latinx students in public community colleges: A theory-driven systematic review and content analysis of psychological research. *Journal of Hispanic Higher Education*.

Dueñas, M., & Gloria, A. M. (2017). ¿Pertenezco a esa universidad?: The mediating role of belonging for collective self-esteem and mattering for Latin@ undergraduates. *Journal of College Student Development, 58*(6), 891–906. doi:10.1353/csd.2017.0070

Engle, J. (2007). Postsecondary access and success for first-generation college students. *American Academic, 3*(1), 25-48.

Garcini, L. M., Rosenfeld, J., Kneese, G., Bondurant, R. G., & Kanzler, K. E. (2022). Dealing with distress from the COVID-19 pandemic: Mental health stressors and coping strategies in vulnerable Latinx communities. *Health & Social Care in the Community, 30*(1), 284–294. doi:10.1111/hsc.13402 PMID:33894080

Gomez, R. (2020). Success is being an example: Trajectories and notions of success among Latinx faculty, staff, and students in academia. *Journal of Latinos and Education, 19*(3), 258–276. doi:10.1080/15348431.2018.1507909

Greenfield, P. M., & Quiroz, B. (2013). Context and culture in the socialization and development of personal achievement values: Comparing Latino immigrant families, European American families, and elementary school teachers. *Journal of Applied Developmental Psychology, 34*(2), 108–118. doi:10.1016/j.appdev.2012.11.002

Gutierrez, D., Gonzalez, C., & Seshadri, G. (2022). We are the unicorns: Exploring experiences of Latina graduate women utilizing an intersectional Latino/a critical theory framework. *Peace and Conflict*, *28*(1), 130–139. doi:10.1037/pac0000595

Hamp, A., Stamm, K., Lin, L., & Christidis, P. (2016). *2015 APA survey of psychology health service providers*. American Psychological Association. https://www.apa.org/workforce/publications/15-health-service-providers/

Herrera, L. J. P., & Obregón, N. (2018). Challenges facing Latinx ESOL students in the Trump era: Stories told through testimonios. *Journal of Latinos and Education*, *19*(4), 383–391. doi:10.1080/15348431.2018.1523793

Holloway-Friesen, H. (2021). The role of mentoring on Hispanic graduate students' sense of belonging and academic self-efficacy. *Journal of Hispanic Higher Education*, *20*(1), 46–58. doi:10.1177/1538192718823716

Liou, D. D., Martinez, J. A. L., & Rotheram-Fuller, E. (2021). Latinas at a Hispanic-serving institution: Resilient resistance affirming race–gender expectancies for college attainment. *Journal of Diversity in Higher Education*. Advance online publication. doi:10.1037/dhe0000340

López, R. M., Valdez, E. C., Pacheco, H. S., Honey, M. L., & Jones, R. (2020). Bridging silos in higher education: Using Chicana feminist participatory action research to foster Latina resilience. *International Journal of Qualitative Studies in Education: QSE*, *33*(8), 872–886. doi:10.1080/09518398.2020.1735566

Martinez, A. (2018). Pathways to the professoriate: The experiences of first-generation Latino undergraduate students at Hispanic serving institutions applying to doctoral programs. *Education Sciences*, *8*(1), 32. doi:10.3390/educsci8010032

Martinez, M. A. (2013). (Re)considering the role familismo plays in Latina/o high school students' college choices. *High School Journal*, *97*(1), 21–40. doi:10.1353/hsj.2013.0019

Molock, S. D., & Parchem, B. (2020). The impact of COVID-19 on college students from communities of color. *Journal of American College Health*, 1–7. PMID:33502970

Mora, J. K. (2002). Caught in a policy web: The impact of education reform on Latino education. *Journal of Latinos and Education*, *1*(1), 29–44. doi:10.1207/S1532771XJLE0101_3

Moschetti, R. V., Plunkett, S. W., Efrat, R., & Yomtov, D. (2018). Peer mentoring as social capital for Latina/o college students at a Hispanic-serving institution. *Journal of Hispanic Higher Education*, *17*(4), 375–392. doi:10.1177/1538192717702949

National Center for Education Statistics. (2016). *The condition of education 2016, characteristics of postsecondary faculty*. https://nces.ed.gov/fastfacts/display.asp?id=61

Paulsen, E. (n.d.). *Covid-19 mental health facts - american psychiatric association*. Retrieved May 1, 2022, from https://www.psychiatry.org/File%20Library/Psychiatrists/APA-COVID-19-Mental-Health-Facts-Hispanics.pdf

Raeff, C., Greenfield, P. M., & Quiroz, B. (2000). Conceptualizing interpersonal relationships in the cultural contexts of individualism and collectivism. *New Directions for Child and Adolescent Development*, *2000*(87), 59–74. doi:10.1002/cd.23220008706 PMID:10763567

Rosales, R., Figuereo, V., Woo, B., Perez-Aponte, J., & Cano, M. (2018). Preparing to work with Latinos: Latino-focused content in social work master's degree programs. *Journal of Teaching in Social Work*, *38*(3), 251–262. doi:10.1080/08841233.2018.1472175

Salinas, C. Jr. (2017). Transforming academia and theorizing spaces for Latinx in higher education: Voces perdidas and voces de poder. *International Journal of Qualitative Studies in Education: QSE*, *30*(8), 746–758. doi:10.1080/09518398.2017.1350295

Samlan, H., Shetty, A., & McWhirter, E. H. (2021). Gender and racial-ethnic differences in treatment barriers among college students with suicidal ideation. *Journal of College Student Psychotherapy*, *35*(3), 272–289. doi:10.1080/87568225.2020.1734133

Santa-Ramirez, S. (2022). Sink or swim: The mentoring experiences of Latinx PhD students with faculty of color. *Journal of Diversity in Higher Education*, *15*(1), 124–134. doi:10.1037/dhe0000335

Santos, S. J., & Reigadas, E. T. (2002). Latinos in Higher Education: An Evaluation of a University Faculty Mentoring Program. *Journal of Hispanic Higher Education*, *1*(1), 40–50. doi:10.1177/1538192702001001004

Smith, B. L. (2018, June). *Spanish-speaking psychologists in demand*. Monitor on Psychology. Retrieved April 14, 2022, from https://www.apa.org/monitor/2018/06/spanish-speaking#:~:text=Yet%20there%20are%20only%20about,ago%2C%20according%20to%20Census%20data

Solorzano, D. G., Ceja, M., & Yosso, T. J. (2000). Critical race theory, racial microaggressions, and campus racial climate: The experience of African American college students. *The Journal of Negro Education*, *69*(1), 60–73.

Suárez-Orozco, C., & Suárez-Orozco, M. (2009). Educating Latino immigrant students in the twenty-first century: Principles for the Obama administration. *Harvard Educational Review*, *79*(2), 327–340. doi:10.17763/haer.79.2.231151762p82213u

The DREAM act: An overview. (2022, March 7). American Immigration Council. Retrieved May 1, 2022, from https://www.americanimmigrationcouncil.org/research/dream-act-overview

Tym, C., McMillion, R., Barone, S., & Webster, J. (2004). *First-generation college students: A literature review. TG*. Texas Guaranteed Student Loan Corporation.

Vasquez-Salgado, Y., Greenfield, P. M., & Burgos-Cienfuegos, R. (2015). Exploring home-school value conflicts: Implications for academic achievement and well-being among Latino first-generation college students. *Journal of Adolescent Research*, *30*(3), 271–305. doi:10.1177/0743558414561297

Vega, D. (2016). "Why not me?": College enrollment and persistence of high achieving, first-generation Latino college students. *School Psychology Forum*, *10*, 307–320.

Von Robertson, R., Bravo, A., & Chaney, C. (2016). Racism and the experiences of Latina/o college students at a PWI (predominantly White institution). *Critical Sociology*, *42*(4-5), 715–735. doi:10.1177/0896920514532664

Chapter 10
Yo Nací Aquí:
Maintaining a Connection With One's Country of Origin

Alejandra Martínez Villalba
University of Georgia, USA

Marta J. González
Latinx Mental Health, USA

Julia Roncoroni
https://orcid.org/0000-0003-2931-9202
University of Denver, USA

ABSTRACT

This chapter will focus on cross-border ties that Latinx immigrants maintain with their countries of origin. The authors discussed factors related to ethnic identity, language, and biculturalism/multiculturalism and explored issues associated with navigating changes faced when returning to their native countries, such as shifts in roles and social identities. The authors also engaged in reflecting about the significance of support and finding symbolic ways for individuals to uphold a connection with their roots. Finally, the chapter ends with a discussion on the importance of representation and advocacy for the Latinx immigrants.

Developing a transnational identity when migrating to another country entails multiple aspects that bring challenges and growing opportunities for Latinx immigrants. Although each individual's experience is different, some of the nuances can be shared with others, as evidenced by the authors' stories presented below.

DOI: 10.4018/978-1-6684-4901-1.ch010

Yo Nací Aquí

ALEJANDRA

Quito, Ecuador is my home. My first time living outside the country was when I moved to the United States (U.S.) in 2018 to pursue a master's degree at the University of Miami. I did not have expectations for my time in the U.S., but I was certainly surprised by the experiences I encountered. Some of the statements I heard about me were: "*The White American*", "*Oh... you have an accent*", and "*Are you really from Ecuador?*". It was shocking how many people questioned my ethnicity and where I was from. *Ecuatoriana* and *mestiza* were the ways I used to identify myself, but I was suddenly expected to adopt a generic "Latinx/Hispanic" identity, and to be okay with others describing me merely as "White", since I was "not *mestiza* enough" due to my light-tone skin color. Having my identity questioned and altered brought the words of singer Facundo Cabral to my mind, "*no soy de aquí, ni soy de allá*[1]", as I found myself struggling to stay connected to my roots while at the same time feeling *ajena*[2] to life in the U.S. However, I have been fortunate to be able to visit my home country frequently over the years and retain a connection with my culture, while continuing to settle in the U.S. Whenever I go to Ecuador, I get to meet family and friends, see my dogs, hike on volcanoes, eat *ceviche* and *locro* (and other delicious traditional foods), be surrounded by the Ecuadorian culture... be home. I also face the reality of how much everything changes whenever I travel, including me. Being an immigrant is not easy, and leaving my home country was (and continues to be) challenging, as I have always felt strongly attached to it. I left Ecuador to go in search of opportunities that I could not find in the country, but I sometimes wish I could have stayed. The days prior to my return to the U.S. are always hard and I continuously ask myself, "is it worth it to keep coming back home?" I believe and hope so. The unconditional support I have received from my family and friends has kept me motivated, even when I have felt like giving up (videocalls and messages have become vital to me). I have found ways to stay connected with the Ecuadorian culture and be able to bond with the essence of who I am, have a richer understanding of myself both in the U.S. and in Ecuador, and continue to integrate these two realities. In fact, this chapter was written while I was in three different cities: Quito, Miami, and Athens (GA).

MARTA

"*Alcanza las estrellas aunque solo llegues a la luna*[3]" was one of my grandmother's *dichos*[4]. While swinging in a hammock watching the nearby active volcano, I received exciting news. "I was going to the U. S. for three years with the purpose of learning the English language." The idea of visiting and discovering another country was exhilarating. I had not gone further than the neighboring borders of Mexico and El Salvador where my native language was spoken. As an exploratory trip, I came to the U.S. with my mother and sister when I was a teenager. Little did I know that this experience would have a profound impact on my personal and professional life. Being a newcomer and an English language learner was difficult. I was fearful of the unseen, but I was eager to explore the host culture and the educational system. Two years later, the excitement was short lived when my mother became ill and went back to my country of origin with my younger sister. I made the decision to stay in the U.S. Being alone in a foreign country was frightening as I faced the reality of not having my nuclear and extended family to provide emotional support. I missed the traditions that accompanied folk cuisine and music, which brought family and friends together. Through phone conversations, I received emotional support from my mother and maternal grandmother. I was encouraged by my mother's words, "*No te des por vencida, sigue adelante⁵*" which gave me strength. I learned to cope with the separation of my loved ones by emerging in cultural traditions that represented my nationality. Through this journey, I explored the acculturation and ethnic identity phases. *Ladina* or *mestiza* was my original ethnic identity of a mixed ancestry of Spanish and indigenous descent. Guatemalan and Hispanic were the terms I used when I came to Los Angeles. Although many people looked like me, everyone identified ethnically with their country of origin. When I reached higher education, I began to identify as "*Latina*" and currently as "Latinx." I learned to adapt to the host culture. In the corporate workforce, there was an implicit expectation to be assimilated in order to succeed. Nevertheless, motherhood helped connect myself to my own cultural beliefs. I felt a responsibility as a parent to share with my child about our ancestors, our culture, and the connection with my country of origin. Subsequently, education helped me understand the acculturation process. After all, my mother brought me to the U.S. [for better educational opportunities]. The support of friends and the guidance of mentors enabled me to navigate the higher education system, which eventually led me to obtain a doctorate in Counseling Psychology. Over the years, I have learned to become bicultural, immersing to both cultures equally. Hence, I continue having a deep and strong connection with my country of origin where is also my home.

JULIA

I was born and raised in Buenos Aires, Argentina, during the Dirty War, a period when a military junta naturalized the recourse of violence as legitimate means of resolving conflict. In this climate, the message was clear: success equated to working hard and minding your own business. At a privileged middle-upper class school, my interests and efforts to understand how people's identities placed them at intersections that determined their life experiences were met with confusion and disapproval. I was a preschool and elementary school English teacher for several years prior to moving to the United States, at age 25, on a student visa. Then, I studied psychology at San Diego State University. My first approximation to psychology was not based on an interest to understand human emotion but was, instead, fueled by my passion for social justice. I aimed to emulate lessons learned from my father, a renowned physician who much preferred working in the slums around Buenos Aires for free than making public appearances. When I moved to the United States, my interest in diversity grew exponentially. Initially, I felt lucky: for the dominant majority, I can pass for White – I speak fluent English and my skin is their shade of white. Soon, however, I realized: "[as a minority], you may wear the jersey, but you are not on [their] team" (Torres, 2013). The work I did to redefine myself in the face of discrimination, added to the curiosity I had always felt towards learning about others, and led me to get a PhD in Counseling Psychology from the University of Florida in 2016. I was an Assistant Professor at the University of Denver from 2016-2022, when I got tenure and became Associate Professor. My immigration experiences have sensitized me to the experiences of other immigrants, in particular from Latin America, who are my community. My research, teaching, and clinical practice are primarily oriented to serve Latinx. I maintain an active connection with Argentina. I visit with my children and Puerto Rican partner at least once a year, often for months at a time, and call and text multiple times a day. Existing in The Borderlands, as labeled by Gloria Anzaldúa, between Argentina and the U.S. ongoingly challenges me to critically reflect on my intersecting identities and how they may impact my access to resources and relationship with others.

Yo Nací Aquí

BRIEF HISTORY OF LATINX IMMIGRATION TO THE U.S.

The story of the Latinx community in the U. S. starts with a reflection on migration patterns. While the coronavirus pandemic has deeply impacted the ability of foreign nationals to travel to the U.S. on any status (Budiman, 2020), the U.S. still has the largest percentage of immigrants of any country in the world. Immigrants to the U.S. represent almost 14% of the total population and, in 2018, Mexico was the top birthplace for Latinx immigrants in the country (25%; Budiman, 2020). Immigrants from other countries in Latin America account for 25% of all immigrants to the U.S., with 10% from the Caribbean, 8% from Central America, and 7% from South America. The Latinx population has become the fastest growing ethnic minority group in the U. S. This unprecedented growth is four times higher than the total U.S. population growth (10%) and varies by Latinx groups: Mexicans (54%), Cubans (44%), Puerto Ricans (36%), and other (22%) such as Central and South Americans (Lopez et al., 2019). With this rapid growth trend, it is estimated that one in three U.S. residents will be of Latinx/Hispanic descent by the year 2050 (Passel & D'Vera Cohn, 2008).

The complicated economic and political realities of different countries in Latin America have contributed to a shift in Latin American migration patterns to the U. S. Between 2010 and 2017, Venezuelans, Dominicans, and Guatemalans have seen the fastest population growth (Noe-Bustamante, 2020). As an example, in the case of Venezuela (the fifth-largest immigrant group from South America), the economic and political destabilization linked to the mismanagement of the country's oil wealth by President Hugo Chávez and his follower, Nicolás Maduro, has led to a mass exodus of Venezuelans to the Americas, including the U.S. (Gallardo & Batalova, 2021). Immigrants from the Dominican Republic, the fourth-largest Hispanic immigrant group in the U.S., have grown since the political and economic turmoil that followed the assassination of longtime dictator Rafael Trujillo in the early 1960s (Babich & Batalova, 2021). The increase in Guatemalan family migration to the U.S. has been primarily linked to rural poverty and agricultural stress produced by climate change (Bermeo et al., 2022).

While immigrants to the U. S. are often clustered for research purposes as "foreign-born Latinx," great diversity exists amongst them. Latin America has a history and culture involving indigenous cultures, European colonization, African slavery, and global migration that make its communities hard to describe by a single label (Turner-Trujillo et al., 2017). Instead, Latin America is characterized by being multiethnic and multicultural. For instance, Ecuador is a pluricultural country with a population of at least 14 Indigenous groups (7.03%), Afro-Ecuatorians (5.35%), montubios (7.39%;), mestizos (mixed-race; 71.93%), Whites (6.09%), and other ethnicities (0.37%; Instituto Nacional de Estadísticas y Censos, 2015). Additionally, Guatemala is a multiethnic country with a population of 17.4 million [i.e., Ladina o mestizo (56%), Mayan (41.7%), Xinca (1.8%; non-mayan indigenous group) and Garífuna (0.1%; Afro-Latinx community)]. There are 25 languages spoken (i.e., 22 of those are Mayan languages, Spanish, Garifuna, and Xinca), although Spanish is the official and most spoken language (Instituto Nacional de Estadística, 2022).

Immigration and Connection

Now, beyond the migration patterns and the reasons for it, relocating means leaving behind family, traditions, and specific characteristics that each country has. For instance, Latin America is well known for its natural habitat, much of which cannot be found in the U.S. (e.g., cities that are surrounded by both active and inactive volcanoes, or towns that are over 15,000 feet above sea level). The losses immigrants face when leaving their country of origin can cause cultural bereavement and grief (Beauregard, 2020), as they may lose touch with their culture and encounter differences even in daily life activities. For example, listening to the radio or watching TV shows (those that are in English are usually translated to Spanish in Latin America) become a different experience when one lives in the U.S.

Moreover, despite having a large number of immigrants from Latin America, the U.S. culture and media have failed to represent the diversity of Latinx origins. Since the majority of the Latinx population in the U.S. is of Mexican descent (Budiman, 2020), the media relies mainly on Mexican traditions and pan-ethnic stereotypes to represent the Latinx community. Thus, making it difficult to find representation of a diversity of cultures in the country in any form, including traditional music, food, and/or festivities. The separation from one's native country and a lack of representation in the host country can create distance with one's ethnic and cultural identity. This can be evidenced by the lack of participation of U.S. born Latinx individuals in cultural activities, which minimizes their self-identification as Hispanic or Latinx (Lopez et al., 2017).

Despite the threats to one's ethnic identity by being disconnected from one's culture and country of origin, not everyone who has migrated can continue to have a relationship with their native country for reasons related to sociopolitical factors, migratory experiences, and trauma, to name a few. In some of these cases, Latinx immigrants can even develop a fear of associating with their culture, creating a disconnection and lack of desire to return to their countries of origin (Chávez-Dueñas et al., 2019). Nevertheless, regaining ties with one's home country can provide a space for Latinx immigrants to grow and heal through cultural strength, and increase connection with their own cultural values (Chávez-Dueñas et al., 2019; Lopez et al., 2017). Similarly, resilience in Latinx immigrants is associated with a connection to cultural values (Morgan et al., 2021), and immigrant resiliency can be associated with strong ethnic identities, community and social support, and biculturalism (Consoli et al., 2018). Thus, the following chapter will delve deeper into Latinx immigrants' cross-border ties, and will present a critique on the existing barriers to maintain a connection with their culture and countries of origin.

Culture and Identity

Immigration has an effect on every aspect of an individual's life, starting from their essence. The interplay found within the layers of identity has an impact on an individual's objective and subjective experiences, and translocation can greatly influence it (Comas-Díaz, 2012). Latinx immigrants' identities and worldviews should be observed through a contextual lens, keeping in mind their history of immigration, and considering all the places that have guided their interpretation of the world and themselves. One important aspect to consider is that Latinx immigrants can potentially become a minority for the first time when entering the U.S. and this can pose as a challenge to maintain their ethnic identity, creating a separation from what is familiar and what constitutes as their identities. This can result "in disorientation, cultural fatigue, adjustment, dislocation, and even trauma" (Comas-Díaz, 2012, p. 78). Keeping ties with one's country of origin can strengthen one's ethnic identity and become a protective factor for Latinx immigrants' mental health (Torres et al., 2016).

Acculturation

Berry (1997) defined acculturation as the adjustment that takes place when individuals from different cultural backgrounds come into continuous and direct contact with each other. Acculturation is also defined as a process of perceptions and affect, which is mostly measured by language development and friendships (Santiago-Rivera et al., 2002). Many ethnic minorities may retain their native culture versus fully adapting to the dominant culture. Thus, one may or may not have to adhere to acculturation standards. Specifically, those who immigrate and do not plan to stay in the host culture may not perceive a need to acculturate. On the other hand, high-acculturated individuals who immigrate and remain in the host country tend to have higher resiliency than those who return to their country of origin (Comas-Diaz, 2006). As the Latinx population in the U.S. acculturate or adapt to their new environments, their identity continues to evolve in different contexts.

Ethnic Identity

Ethnic identity encompasses the process of defining oneself within a larger social context which, in turn, provides individuals with a clear sense of self. For Latinx in the U.S., ethnic identity is known to be fluid (Suro, 2006) as it continues to evolve across cultural contexts over the lifetime. Latinx born in Central or South America may identify as *Ladino/a* or *mestizo/a,* which describes a race of a mixed ancestry of Spanish and indigenous descent (Funk and Lopez, 2022). Thus, there may be a loss of identity when adapting to new ethnic terms. Over the last decades, there has been an evolution on the ethnic identification terms for Latinx and/or Hispanics in the U.S. Although both terms (i.e., Hispanics and Latinx) have been used interchangeable in the literature, the term Latinx has been adopted as a term that is representative of the inclusivity and intersectionality of this ethnic group in the U.S. (Lozano et al., 2020).

Moreover, race differs from ethnicity as the former is a social construct that is associated with phenotypical characteristics, such as skin color or hair texture. Skin color in Latin America has been historically associated with privilege, class, discrimination, oppression, and marginalization. For instance, Latinx with darker skin have reported experiencing more discrimination than Latinx with light skin color. A recent study by Pew Research Center (Noe-Bustamante et al., 2021) found that 64% of Latinx with darker skin color reported experiencing some type of discrimination versus 54% of Latinx with light skin color experiencing the same in the U.S. To this day, skin color remains a major determinant of personal and professional outcomes. Historical and current oppression can create intergenerational racial trauma, but resiliency can also potentially be passed through generation (Comas-Díaz et al., 2019), which can be sustained through cross-border ties with families and friends.

Biculturalism and Multiculturalism

Due to the great variability within the Latinx community, having more than one cultural identity is very common. However, individuals seem to identify more with one of their multiple identities than with the rest, potentially due to external forces that had led individuals to choose between them (Morgan et al., 2021). Maintaining contact with one's roots could possibly increase a connection between an individual and their multiple identities, and preserve traditional practices that are key to enhance their sense of ethnic pride. The latter can keep traditions alive, such as eating 12 grapes during New Year's celebrations (at 12 am on the dot) while making 12 wishes, or celebrating the day of the dead, which is represented in different ways according to the country, although the Mexican festivity is more known across the globe. Combining old and new practices, and finding a balance in the context of the new place can create a stronger sense of identity. This means reconciling aspects of one's identity while navigating through changes and being able to incorporate new practices.

Language

Language is a cultural expression that can strengthen one's ethnic identity (Machado-Casas, 2012), and Latin America has a myriad of Native languages: Spanish, English, Portuguese, Quechua, Waorani, among others. Due to *el mestizaje* (the mix of races), it is common for individuals who speak Spanish as a first language to have words from native indigenous languages in their vocabulary (Rendón, 2008). For instance, in the highlands of Ecuador, it is very common to hear *mestizos* use words in Quichua such as "*achachay*[6]" "*ayayay*[7]", "*ñaña*[8]", "*guagua*[9]". Moreover, there are also words that cannot be directly translated to English, such as "*te quiero*[10]" (Spanish), "*apapacho*[11]" (In Náhuatl), "*ndumui*[12]" (in Otomí) (Pineda Santiago, 2021). Some of these words cannot even be translated to Spanish, despite it being the most spoken language in Latin America (Lopez et al., 2017). Being able to express using these particular words could connect individuals to their roots.

Many people decide to preserve the language of their ancestors in their households, and even language brokering can promote the maintenance of the family's native language (López et al., 2019). However, many lose touch with it, which can create a disconnection with one's ethnic identity. For instance, some Latinx families seem to lose their native language throughout generations, as there might be a stronger connection with the host country's language; in this case, English. This tends to happen more in generations where English becomes the first language and, throughout this process, Latinx immigrants may even stop self-identifying as Hispanic/Latinx (Lopez et al., 2017). Thus, individuals may choose to promote the use of their native language in the household and pass verbal wisdom throughout generations to remain connected with their roots. Language is rich in culture and its preservation can bring strong ties with one's identity and a deep sense of belonging (Pineda Santiago, 2021).

Moreover, language can also carry deep cultural knowledge through *dichos/refranes*. These are short sentences that tend to be subjective in nature and encapsule native wisdom, address any life-circumstances, and represent collectivistic values and a high-context communication style (Comas-Díaz, 2006). Some examples are, "*al que madruga Dios le ayuda*[13]", "*no hay mal que por bien no venga*[14]", "*la pereza es la madre de todos los vicios*[15]". Retaining a connection with this verbal expression can work as a form of cultural resiliency. *Dichos* can act as protective factors as they help with cognitive reframing, emphasize the ability to overcome adversity, and highlight positive aspects of life (Comas-Díaz, 2006).

CROSS-BORDER TIES: NAVIGATING CHANGES

Differences in Roles and Family Structures

Migration can create a disconnection with social roles, as the way these are enacted (in both social and intrafamilial ways) changes. Thus, readjusting to roles and novel family structures in the new context is imperative. For example, if a Spanish-speaking family migrated to the U.S. and had a child in school that was learning English, the roles that the child played at home will most likely expand as they become their family's translator (e.g., language brokering; López et al., 2019). However, if returning to their country of origin, this will no longer be necessary, changing -once again- the role of the child. Similarly, many Latinx immigrants have siblings and extended family in their country of origin, and one can gain the role of a sibling, nephew/niece, aunt/uncle, among others. An individual can go from being the only child in the household to being an older or younger sibling (Chung et al., 2022). Thus, it is important to keep an understanding of how these changes in roles can become challenging, but at the same time can demonstrate the capacity of people to shift from role to role, while gaining different skills in the process.

Social Identities

Maintaining a connection with one's native country entails balancing alterations in social identities, as one exists differently according to the context. Immigrants face changes in social norms when leaving their home country (Beauregard, 2020) and suddenly being a friend, a partner, a worker, a citizen, or an individual becomes a completely new experience. When returning to their country of origin, the person who left may start noticing changes in themselves and their surroundings; some old places have closed and new have opened, the park that used to be visited weekly is now an apartment complex, the close friend with shared common interests seems like a stranger now, and other people also start noticing how the person who left has changed as well. Going through the process of understanding these transformations can be perplexing, and it takes time, especially since all of this change can increase feelings of alienation (Chung et al., 2022). Additionally, social identities that have the potential to be scrutinized in the home country, such as being in a same-sex relationship, can create feelings of discomfort or fear of returning home (Anzaldúa, 1987). Thus, there is a need to understand and manage personal (real and perceived) identities in the new and old space, as well as expectations of social norms.

Breaking Patterns

Living in a new country can expose an individual to different environments and experiences that will provide them with new information that can add to their worldviews. Thus, breaking old thought patterns within oneself. It is likely that when returning to their native countries, immigrants will encounter situations that were normalized in the past but are now being challenged (e.g., heteronormative expectations), which in turn can create conflict within Latinx families due to acculturative stress (Chung et al., 2022; Miville et al., 2018). This process can present a challenge to family cohesion (Dillon et al., 2013) but the amplified worldviews could also act as change agents and be a positive attribute as it can disrupt maladaptive patterns (whether in social or familial groups) that had not been questioned in the past. Thus, keeping a connection with one's country of origin can influence not only the way the individual operates, but also their environments.

Being a Chameleon

It is crucial for individuals to adapt to the host country's culture, and this process could be facilitated through the multiethnic and multiracial nature of the Latinx community. For instance, multiracial individuals appear to be able to connect more easily with people from different backgrounds due to their capacity to act like a chameleon (Morgan et al., 2021; Miville et al., 2005). Leaving one's country of origin provides an opportunity to expand inner circles and meet people from diverse contexts, providing an opportunity to learn about new realities and different points of view. It can sometimes be challenging to undertake new perspectives, so being willing to include new information onto old thought patterns can allow individuals to expand their worldviews. The ability to merge with different cultures can potentially strengthen the more connected a person is to their country of origin, as they would constantly be exposed to the need of adapting to the contrasting social norms and experiences of both the host and home country.

Support

Comas-Díaz (2006) stated that Latinx individuals have a relational worldview, which entangles one's identities with collectivities that include culture, family, and ethnicity. Additionally, Latinx immigrants have reported that ties with families are stronger in their native countries than in the U.S. (Lopez and Moslimani, 2022), and Comas-Díaz (2012) emphasizes that separation can lead to disconnection. Thus, being connected with family is vital for Latinx immigrants, which is congruent with the Latinx value of *Familismo*. For instance, it can allow for individuals to stay connected with family when illness comes around and caring for family members could strengthen the family bond. However, this connection can pose as a challenge due to acculturative stress (Dillon et al., 2013) and an increased fear of family or friends being deported or criminalized (Chavez-Dueñas et al., 2019; Arredondo, 2018). Additionally, feelings of betrayal from those in the country of origin are common when the individual starts making connections with people in the host country (Comas-Díaz, 2012; Chung et al., 2022), and symptoms of guilt can easily appear in those who left.

Despite the challenges, being able to maintain a connection means opening ways to receiving support in various forms, from emotional care to facilitating economic stability. By addressing the rising tension within family or friends, individuals could potentially improve their communication and strengthen relationship with both groups and start making peace with change. Similarly, connection with one's roots can allow the preservation of cultural values and cultural strength, which can be attained through familial support from members who continue to be in their country of origin (Machado-Casas, 2012).

Support provided in one's native country can mean getting support from a culture that only exists within one's ethnic group. This is particularly true in cases of indigenous communities, as groups share a specific cosmovision that may not be found anywhere else (e.g., Mantilla Falcón & Solís Ruiz, 2016). Along with this, as Latinx individuals migrate, they may encounter new forms of discrimination, particularly in a country so racialized as the U.S; and cross-border ties can act as buffers to the effects of discrimination (Torres et al., 2016). Similarly, due to collective formative events (Comas-Díaz, 2012), maintaining a connection with one's native country could potentially increase resiliency through intergenerational wisdom. Support is a vital resource when moving to a new country as resilience can potentially be passed through generations (Comas-Díaz et al., 2019).

Finding Ways to Stay Connected

Latinx immigrants seem to maintain a direct line of contact with their countries of origin. For instance, a large percentage of Latinx immigrants have stayed connected by making phone calls to family/friends, visiting their native country, and sending remittances (Torres et al., 2016). However, as discussed previously, being able to stay connected to one's country of origin is not always possible. Visiting family and friends, or just travelling for tourism is a privilege. Even making phone calls can sometimes be close to impossible. Economic factors can prevent someone from getting round-trip tickets as they can be expensive, and make it impossible to take days off from work. Migratory and health status can prevent someone from leaving the country, and sociopolitical factors could make the return to the native country unsafe (Torres et al., 2016; Consoli et al., 2018).

In cases in which being physically present in one's native country is not possible; individuals could find ways to symbolically connect with it. This could mean listening to folk music, engaging in dances that represent their culture (salsa, merengue, bachata), making or having traditional foods, speaking in their native languages or dialects (including colloquialisms), attending cultural events, or visiting areas that represent of one's roots (such as Little Havana in Miami). Other ways to increase this connection could be by having an emblematic representation of the individual's roots in one's current home, such as having a decorative national flag, a national soccer jersey, or a painting that represents the country. Being able to find connections with one's origins can stimulate a sense of belonging (Torres et al., 2016), even if it is through a symbolic way.

Building a bridge between host and home countries can be a powerful experience. For instance, having one's social group from the U.S. visit one's native country can unite the person to their roots and deepen their connection with both places by opening a route for their two realities to coexist. Even if a physical journey is not possible, narratives could be used as an alternative, as storytelling is a way Latinx individuals connect with their roots (Comas-Díaz, 2012). Being able to bring one's country of origin to the host country by telling stories can bring back memories and parts of someone's life that were left behind. It can also reconnect an individual with parts of themselves that got lost somewhere along the line and allow for the start of a journey of connection with their personal identities.

IMPLICATIONS

Latinx immigrants have endured hardship in both their home countries and in the U.S., yet they have demonstrated to be a resilient group. Cross-border ties may have a positive effect on the resiliency and ethnic pride of Latinx immigrants but, despite the growing numbers of Latinx in the U.S., the literature on this subject is scarce. More research should address the effects and impact that cross-border ties can have on ethnic identity, cultural identity, and resiliency of Latinx immigrants in the U.S. Additionally, expectations of acculturation has led to an oversimplified impression of what a person needs in order to endure life in their host country. The development of measurements that capture the holistic view of an individual (e.g., traditional attitudes and behaviors, language, connection with country of origin, length of time in the U.S., etc.) could provide a better understanding of acculturation and adaptability of Latinx immigrants.

Moreover, maintaining a connection with one's country of origin appears to strengthen one's ethnic identity, which can have both beneficial and detrimental effects on the mental health of Latinx immigrants. A strong ethnic identity can act as a protective factor, but aggravated effects of discrimination resulting from having one's core identity antagonized can threaten one's mental health (Lopez et al., 2016). For this, social justice initiatives should aim to undertake discrimination against Latinx immigrants, starting by acknowledging the uniqueness of this community and increasing representation of the many different ethnicities that exist within Latin America. Simplistic efforts of representation such as having a "Latin American" section in supermarkets or commercializing festivities such as *5 de Mayo* can be very damaging, as it sends an erroneous message of what it means to be Latin American. There is an urgent need for political advocacy to increase the representation of Latinx immigrants and facilitate cross-border ties.

Oppression and marginalization towards Latinx immigrants in the U.S. are fairly common, and some groups are vulnerable to different types of discrimination. Intersectionality research should focus on the variability within the Latinx community and the particular experiences of Afro Latinx and members of indigenous communities, as these groups encounter added structural discrimination due to racism, colorism, and classism. By continuing to promote a generalization of Latinx communities, these experiences become invisible. It is imperative to give a space to celebrate diversity and to recognize the unique struggles that Latinx immigrants face. This could promote more liberatory practices in the field of psychology when working with the Latinx community. Similarly, it is important to consider the cosmovision of indigenous groups both in research and in the clinical aspect of the field, as cross-border ties may be particularly important to cultivate for members of these groups.

The oversimplifications of Latinx cultures and traditions in the U.S. could, at first, bring feelings of belonging to Latinx immigrants, as they appear to provide recognition of Latin America in the host country. However, this could lead to "cultural Stockholm syndrome, a condition in which members of an oppressed group accept the dominant cultural values, including the stereotypes of their own group" (Comas-Díaz, 2020, p. 1320). The generalization of Latin Americans creates an amalgamation of different cultures, ethnicities, and experiences that makes the existence of most Latinx immigrants invisible. Adopting a generic "Latinx" identity can be detrimental to the self as the variabilities amongst Latin Americans can make a person not feel represented by the stereotypes of who they are supposed to be. Thus, living in the borderlines of the host and home country can arise feelings of not belonging due to not having a U.S. nationality and not being "Latinx" enough (Anzaldúa, 1987). Building a bridge between these two seems imperative to alleviate the mental health effects that this ambivalence can cause.

Lastly, psychologists in the U.S. must engage in a collaborative relationship with colleagues from Latin American countries. The limited amount of involvement with foreign psychologists prevents the exchange of knowledge, skills, and experience between professionals. Perhaps a collaboration between mental health professionals in the U.S. and Latin American countries could allow a deeper understanding of mental health in Latinx communities that maintain cross-border ties. One alternative can be initiatives like "*Psicólogos sin Fronteras*" or "*Salud Mental sin Fronteras*" in which mental health professionals collaborate and share knowledge and skills for the benefit of the Latinx communities. Organizations such as the National Latinx Psychological Association or the Interamerican Society of Psychology can initiate exploratory groups to develop ideas on fomenting cross-border ties with other mental health professionals.

We (Alejandra, Marta, and Julia) have realized the importance of cross-border ties in our lives through academic, professional, and personal experiences. I (Alejandra) have been at La Clínica in La'Kech under the supervision of Dr. Edward Delgado-Romero for the past year. La Clínica is, as expressed by my advisor, a rare find, as it is uncommon to have so many Latinx counselors-in-training in the same space in the U.S. As a Latinx international student, I have struggled with continuous feelings of not belonging and homesickness. While I have continued to stay in contact with my family and friends from back home, being surrounded by colleagues and supervisors who understand and represent my own culture, as well as being able to provide services to the Latinx community have shortened the distance with my Latinx ties.

For me (Marta), having a strong connection with my country of origin has provided me with a strong sense of ethnic identity and it has allowed me to acculturate to the host culture while retaining my own. This process has impacted my personal, academic, and professional realms. I am able to travel quite often to Guatemala and learn from other professionals in the field of psychology. More importantly, I continue to learn about the current ethnic groups as well as staying connected with my family and my country of origin.

The experiences I (Julia) have had as an immigrant have challenged me to recognize, master, and defy the space "in-between" temporal and geographic locales. From a pragmatic stance, modern technology has made it easier to stay tuned to life in these different locales; the entire world is one WhatsApp (or a similar app) call away. Logging into social media (Facebook, Instagram) feeds the fantasy that the "in-between" can be eradicated, that it is simply possible to exist in various spaces at the same time.

The challenge resides in defining my first-generation Latina immigrant identity in the "in between" and relaying this identity with all its vicissitudes to my children and students.

REFERENCES

Anzaldúa, G. (1987). *Borderlands/La Frontera: The new mestiza.* Aunt Lute Books.

Arredondo, P. (2018). Latinx immigrants set the stage for 2050. In *Latinx Immigrants* (pp. 1–13). Springer. doi:10.1007/978-3-319-95738-8_1

Babich, E., & Batalova, J. (2021). *Immigrants from the Dominican Republic in the United States.* Migration Policy Institute. Retrieved from https://www.migrationpolicy.org/article/dominican-immigrants-united-states-2019

Beauregard, C. (2020). Being in between: Exploring cultural bereavement and identity expression through drawing. *Journal of Creativity in Mental Health, 15*(3), 292–310. doi:10.1080/15401383.2019.1702131

Berry, J. W. (1997). Immigration, acculturation, and adaptation. *Applied Psychology, 46*(1), 5–33.

Budiman, A. (2020). *Key findings about U.S. immigrants.* Pew Research Center. Retrieved from https://www.pewresearch.org/fact-tank/2020/08/20/key-findings-about-u-s-immigrants/

Chavez-Dueñas, N. Y., Adames, H. Y., Perez-Chavez, J. G., & Salas, S. P. (2019). Healing ethno-racial trauma in Latinx immigrant communities: Cultivating hope, resistance, and action. *The American Psychologist, 74*(1), 49–62. doi:10.1037/amp0000289 PMID:30652899

Chung, R. C. Y., Bemak, F., & Sánchez, R. O. (2022). Latinx adolescent migrant challenges in reuniting with family members. *International Review of Psychiatry (Abingdon, England)*, 1–10. doi:10.1080/09540261.2022.2072192

Comas-Díaz, L. (2000). An ethnopolitical approach to working with people of color. *The American Psychologist, 55*(11), 1319–1325. doi:10.1037/0003-066X.55.11.1319 PMID:11280941

Comas-Díaz, L. (2006). Latino healing: The integration of ethnic psychology into psychotherapy. *Psychotherapy (Chicago, Ill.), 43*(4), 436–453. doi:10.1037/0033-3204.43.4.436 PMID:22122135

Comas-Díaz, L. (2012). *Multicultural care: A clinician's guide to cultural competence.* American Psychological Association. doi:10.1037/13491-000

Comas-Díaz, L., Hall, G. N., & Neville, H. A. (2019). Racial trauma: Theory, research, and healing: Introduction to the special issue. *The American Psychologist, 74*(1), 1–5. doi:10.1037/amp0000442 PMID:30652895

Consoli, A. J., Bunge, E., Oromendia, M. F., & Bertone, A. (2018). Argentines in the United States: Migration and Continuity. In *Latinx Immigrants* (pp. 15–32). Springer. doi:10.1007/978-3-319-95738-8_2

Dillon, F. R., De La Rosa, M., & Ibañez, G. E. (2013). Acculturative stress and diminishing family cohesion among recent Latino immigrants. *Journal of Immigrant and Minority Health, 15*(3), 484–491. doi:10.100710903-012-9678-3 PMID:22790880

Funk, C., & Lopez, M. H. (2022). *A brief statistical portrait of U.S. Hispanics*. PEW Research Center. Retrieved from https://www.pewresearch.org/science/2022/06/14/a-brief-statistical-portrait-of-u-s-hispanics/

Gallardo, L. H., & Batalova, J. (2021). *Venezuelan immigrants in the United States*. Migration Policy Institute. Retrieved from https://www.migrationpolicy.org/article/venezuelan-immigrants-united-states-2018

Instituto Nacional de Estadística Guatemala. (2022). *Censo de Población* [Publication Census]. Retrieved from https://www.ine.gob.gt/ine/

Instituto Nacional de Estadísticas y Censos (INEC). (2015). *Estadística de Etnicidad en Censos, Encuestas de Hogares, y Registros Adminitrativos* [Ethnicity Statistics in Censuses, Household Surveys and Administrative Records]. Retrieved from https://www.inei.gob.pe/media/dme/17.MarleneHaro.pdf

López, B. G., Lezama, E., & Heredia, D. Jr. (2019). Language brokering experience affects feelings toward bilingualism, language knowledge, use, and practices: A qualitative approach. *Hispanic Journal of Behavioral Sciences, 41*(4), 481–503. doi:10.1177/0739986319879641

Lopez, M. H., Gonzalez-Barrera, A., & López, G. (2017). *Hispanic identity fades across generations as immigrant connections fall away*. Pew Research Center. Retrieved from https://www.pewresearch.org/hispanic/2017/12/20/hispanic-identity-fades-across-generations-as-immigrant-connections-fall-away/

Lopez, M. H., Krogstad, J. M., & Passel, J. S. (2021). *Who is Hispanic?* Pew Research Center. Retrieved from https://www.pewresearch.org/fact-tank/2021/09/23/who-is-hispanic/

Lopez, M. H., & Moslimani, M. (2022). *Latinos See US as Better Than Place of Family's Ancestry for Opportunity, Raising Kids, Health Care Access*. Pew Research Center. Retrieved from https://www.pewresearch.org/race-ethnicity/2022/01/20/latinos-see-u-s-as-better-than-place-of-familys-ancestry-for-opportunity-raising-kids-health-care-access/

Lozano, A., Salinar, C. Jr, & Orozco, R. C. (2021). Constructing meaning of the termLatinx: A trio-ethnography through Pláticas. *International Journal of Qualitative Studies in Education: QSE*, 1–18. Advance online publication. doi:10.1080/09518398.2021.1930251

Machado-Casas, M. (2012). Pedagogías del camaleón/Pedagogies of the chameleon: Identity and strategies of survival for transnational indigenous Latino immigrants in the US South. *The Urban Review, 44*(5), 534–550. doi:10.100711256-012-0206-5

Miville, M. L., Calle, C. Z., Mendez, N., & Borenstein, J. (2018). Colombians in the United States: History, values, and challenges. In *Latinx Immigrants* (pp. 53–73). Springer. doi:10.1007/978-3-319-95738-8_4

Miville, M. L., Constantine, M. G., Baysden, M. F., & So-Lloyd, G. (2005). Chameleon Changes: An Exploration of Racial Identity Themes of Multiracial People. *Journal of Counseling Psychology, 52*(4), 507–516. doi:10.1037/0022-0167.52.4.507

Morgan, M., Pigg, E. N., Consoli, A., Pavone, D., & Meza, D. (2021). Like a chameleon: Resilience among self-identified latinx mixed adults. *Revista Interamericana de Psicología. Interamerican Journal of Psychology, 55*(1), e988–e988. doi:10.30849/ripijp.v55i1.988

Noe-Bustamante, L. (2020). *Key facts about U.S. hispanics and their diverse heritage*. Pew Research Center. Retrieved from https://www.pewresearch.org/fact-tank/2019/09/16/key-facts-about-u-s-hispanics/

Noe-Bustamante, L., González-Barrera, A., Edwards, K., Mora, L., & López, M. H. (2021). *Majority of Latinos Say Skin Color Impacts Opportunity in America and Shapes Daily Life.* Pew Research Center. Retrieved from https://www.pewresearch.org/hispanic/2021/11/04/majority-of-latinos-say-skin-color-impacts-opportunity-in-america-and-shapes-daily-life/

Passel, J. S., & D'Vera Cohn, D. (2008). *US population projections, 2005-2050.* Pew Research Center.

Pineda Santiago, I. (2021). *Intraducibles.* Libro Intraducibles. Retrieved from https://intraducibles.org/libro/

Rendón, J. A. G. (2008). *Mestizaje lingüístico en los Andes: génesis y estructura de una lengua mixta* [Linguistic Miscegenation in the Andes: Genesis and Structure of a Mixed Language]. Editorial Abya Yala.

Santiago-Rivera, A., Arredondo, P., & Gallardo-Cooper, M. (2002). *Counseling Latinos and La Famila.* Sage.

Suro, R. (2006). A developing identity: Hispanics in the United States. *Carnegie Reporter, 3*(4), 1–5.

Torres, J. M., Alcántara, C., Rudolph, K. E., & Viruell-Fuentes, E. A. (2016). Cross-border ties as sources of risk and resilience: Do cross-border ties moderate the relationship between migration-related stress and psychological distress for latino migrants in the United States? *Journal of Health and Social Behavior, 57*(4), 436–452. doi:10.1177/0022146516667534 PMID:27803264

Torres, M. (2013, March 29). College feminisms: Elementary feminisms: Majoring in English. *The Feministe Wire.* https://thefeministwire.com/2013/03/majoring-in-english/

Turner-Trujillo, E., Del Toro, M., & Ramos, A. (2017). *An overview of Latino and Latin American identity.* Getty. Retrieved from https://www.getty.edu/news/an-overview-of-latino-and-latin-american-identity/

ENDNOTES

1. *I am not from here, nor I am from there*
2. *Like an outsider*
3. *Reach for the stars, even if you land on the moon*
4. *Sayings*
5. *Do not give up, keep going*
6. *Expression used when something is/someone feels cold*
7. Expression used when something is/someone feels hot
8. *Sister*
9. *Child*
10. *Closest translation: I love you*
11. Hugging from the soul
12. *Deep sadness that can be felt from the stomach to the heart*
13. *The early bird gets the worm*
14. *Every cloud has a silver lighting*
15. *Laziness is the mother of all vices*

Chapter 11
Rompiendo Cadenas:
Breaking Down Intergenerational Trauma in the Latinx Community

Charmaine Mora-Ozuna
University of Georgia, USA

Inés Rodriguez
Georgia State University, USA

Marjory Vazquez
Kaiser Permanente, USA

Jacqueline Fuentes
University of Georgia, USA

ABSTRACT

Four first-generation Latinxs use their personal lived experiences and the experiences that they bear witness to as mental health practitioners to provide a critical lens on the decolonization of intergenerational trauma (IGT) in the Latinx community. The authors acknowledge that IGT is rooted in systemic oppression and colonization. They explore the systemic, cultural, interpersonal, and intrapersonal bidirectional impact that these areas have on the well-being of Latinxs. They highlight the inherent resistance and resilience skills that Latinxs have to survive and thrive from trauma. The authors share culturally responsive interventions that reclaim the cultural values of Latinxs to promote holistic healing and end the transmission of trauma.

BREAKING DOWN INTERGENERATIONAL TRAUMA IN THE LATINX COMMUNITY

Like other chapters, this chapter speaks not only from an academic perspective but includes the professional and lived experiences that have impacted the authors of this book. Although these four practitioners come from different paths of life, one thing that the authors have in common is their passion to eradicate the intergenerational trauma that is present in their beloved Latinx community. None of the authors are immune to the impact that intergenerational trauma has had on their families, communities, and clients that they serve in their respective roles.

The first author, Charmaine Mora-Ozuna is a cisgender woman, a *Mexicana* from California, and currently a doctoral candidate in the Counseling Psychology program at the University of Georgia. Charmaine provides therapy to marginalized communities across the lifespan, and her niche is supporting the healing journey of survivors of intimate partner violence. The second author, Inés Rodriguez, is a gender non-conforming *afro-latine* with their Master's of Social Work, who was born in New York and has roots in the Dominican Republic. They work with Black, queer, and migrant community leaders and social service organizations as an equity trainer, dialogue facilitator, and program manager. The third author, Marjory Vazquez, is a Mexican and Salvadorian cisgender woman from Southern California who is currently working as a psychologist at Kaiser Permanente Hospital in Northern California. Marjory also has a private practice, The Sana House, in which she serves Latinas and women of color in healing past traumas. The fourth author, Jacqueline Fuentes, is a cisgender *Xicana* from Southern California and is currently a doctoral candidate in the Counseling Psychology program at the University of Georgia. Jacqueline provides bilingual Spanish and English counseling to Latinx individuals across the lifespan, college students, and African American women who have experienced trauma.

We four have searched for ways to resist the difficulties of being first-generation Latinx college students while also uplifting other women of color. Charmaine and Ines are co-founders of the Alpha Pi Chapter of Sigma Lambda Upsilon/ Señoritas Latinas Unidas Sorority Inc., at Georgia State University and Marjory and Jacqueline are co-founders of the Zeta Chapter of Phi Lambda Rho at The University of California at Irvine. Although these individuals attended their undergraduate institutions on two different coasts, their intentions were similar; to create counter spaces that honored and nurtured their whole selves, while also making space for others coming after them.

Much like the authors of this chapter, who thrived in institutions not created for them, Latinx folks hustle to make a way out of nothing in the U.S. Their very presence is an act of resistance and resilience. We believe this is how the Latinx community deals with trauma and hardships. However, just because we push through as individuals or as a collective, does not mean that the oppressive systems do not need to change. Because along the way to thriving, surviving entails struggling, breaking down, and doubting our capabilities, all of which can be re-traumatizing. Dismantling intergenerational trauma is an act of liberation, and we hope that this chapter highlights how we can collectively work together towards ending this cycle of trauma and retraumatization.

INTRODUCTION

Intergenerational trauma (IGT) is the transmission of trauma or the effects of trauma from one generation to the next. Symptoms can include things such as depression, anxiety, shame, guilt, and physical health problems (Dass-Brailsford, 2007; Sangalang & Vang, 2017). While the concept of IGT is not new, the term was originally utilized to speak about survivors of the Holocaust. Researchers noticed that children of Holocaust survivors, even if they were not in the Holocaust, were overrepresented with mental and physical health disorders (Cerdena, Rivera, & Spak, 2021). Thus, there was some pathway for trauma to be transmitted across generations.

The conversation about IGT within the Latinx community is relatively new but has come to the forefront for healers, clinicians, clients, and the Latinx community at large. With the recent release of the Disney movie *Encanto*, which focuses on the transmission of trauma, IGT within the Latinx community is something that people are not only actively talking about, but also something that people are actively trying to heal (Conroy, 2022). Before the conversation of IGT came into the mainstream, trauma within the Latinx community was historically seen through isolated events such as being diagnosed with Post-Traumatic Stress Disorder (PTSD) from war, violence, or abuse. Given the conspiracy of silence, in which families do not discuss past traumas to protect future generations (Danieli, 2007), IGT encountered within the Latinx community is not commonly discussed. This lack of conversation creates a breeding ground for trauma to be passed down.

Although there is still a great deal of research and work that can be done around IGT within the Latinx community, the research that has been done up to date has primarily been viewed through the mother-child dyad (Cerdena et al., 2021). In the context of therapy, the topic of IGT commonly comes up when doing postpartum work with mothers with depression and/or anxiety who are fearful of passing down unhealed aspects of their past or themselves, to their children. Research focusing on Latina teenagers has revealed that they are one of the highest groups who have attempted suicide rates amongst adolescents due to conflict with their mothers and bicultural stress (Zayas, 2011). The problem with existing narratives of women being the gatekeepers of intergenerational trauma is that it also places the burden of healing on women. This bypasses the role of men as it does not consider that they also play an active role in the transmission of trauma from one generation to the next. Perhaps even more importantly, the existing narratives do not consider how men also need to play an active role in healing IGT.

Another reason that trauma is not discussed is due to the resiliency and strength within the Latinx community. It is not common for Latinxs to label their hardships as "trauma" because these hardships are just experiences that they must overcome. For example, the idea that Latinx folx must work twice as hard to be in the same spot as white individuals is commonly known and accepted amongst nearly all Black, Indigenous, and People of Color (BIPOC) folx. Although having a strong work ethic and being resilient are indeed strengths, not speaking about struggles can create paradigms such as imposter syndrome and perfectionism. Imposter syndrome and perfectionism are ways in which IGT can present itself and be passed down to future generations. Latinxs are under constant pressure because they must work harder than their white counterparts and, given the realities of systemic inequality, it can make people feel like they are always falling short or behind - a cycle that feeds itself. This cycle is often manifested in how Latinx immigrants never have the time and space to make mistakes, as their lives and their families' depend on their ability to keep moving their work along, and make their sacrifices "worth it". The inherent pressure that Latinx children experience has always been a reality, but it is finally being labeled intergenerational trauma. When speaking about the relationship of IGT in the Latinx community, it is imperative to acknowledge the systemic, cultural, interpersonal, and intrapersonal bidirectional impact that these areas have on the well-being of the Latinx community.

Systemic

Systems theory reminds us that many factors work together to influence behavior. Specifically, family, friends, social settings, economic class, the environment, among other factors, all work as a system to influence how people think and act. (Friedman & Allen, 2011). This definition grounds us in the reality that systems are essential to understanding Latinx mental health, and that within this framework we must understand the convergence of place and time. When we reclaim the impact of place and time, we can recontextualize the impact of the political and socio-economic decisions made by nations within history, and how these systems are both the cause and effect of collective, cultural, and intergenerational traumas shared by many of the of people in Latin-America.

Our goal within this section is to reorient you, the reader, to 1) the impact that systems have had on our collective wellbeing, 2) name ways Latinxs have resisted, and 3) begin decolonizing *Latinidad* in favor of reclaiming racial, cultural and Indigenous visibility, knowledge, and power to begin healing from IGT. We would like to say upfront that no one story is the same, and that identity, politics, and mental health are nuanced, evolving, and complex. Rather than try to tell one story, we will be sharing a broad analysis of histories and connection points in hopes of further pushing the conversation on Latinx mental health and the role that histories, politics, and systems play within them.

Now before we start, we have an ask of you. We would like you to hold this quote by Resmaa Menakeem (2021), Somatic Abolitionist, in the foreground of your mind:

Trauma decontextualized in a person looks like personality. Trauma decontextualized in a family looks like family traits. Trauma in a people looks like culture (ch.3).

If certain thoughts or feelings come up for you as you read along, jot them down in your journal, or in the margins. Consider everything that comes to mind as an invitation to explore how you relate to the text or as a prompt towards what you would like to learn more about. You do not have to do anything else - now let us get started.

We have all been colonized. The authors of this chapter, this book, our communities, and all peoples of Latin America have been colonized. For most of us in our lineage, we have also been the colonizer. Part of healing from IGT is naming the truths of our mixed race, mixed status, and pluralistic cultural lineages. The other part is reclaiming our responsibility to decolonize our internalized colonized-colonizer psyches which is something we have the privilege to restore and make right.

Latin America is composed of people of European, African, Asian, Southeast Asian, and Indigenous descent; all with varying cultural identities, journeys, and ancestral contributions to the shaping of present-day Americas. Latin America was colonized by Spain, France, the Netherlands, the United States, and Portugal starting with Columbus' first voyage to Hispaniola in 1492 and ending with revolutions and wars for independence across the Caribbean, South, and Central Americas by 1825. In addition to colonization, the United States (U.S.) Imperialism ran rampant in Latin America starting with the Monroe Doctrine in 1823 until the handing over of the Panama Canal in 1999. Economically dominating a nation, as the U.S. Imperialist projects did, was a way of "indirectly controlling the internal affairs of other sovereign nations without resorting to colonial administration" (Imperialism in Latin America, n.d., 2). The U.S. strategically destabilized Latin American nations, which is equally as important given its' promise of democratization under the veil of further racial stratification (Gobat, 2013) and corporate colonial devastation.

Why are the transnational economics of colonization and U.S. imperialism important to understand? Because these transnational histories and political forces are inextricably linked to how we experience ourselves. The reality is that Latin America has been in ongoing conflict with many *conquistadores* and *guerrilleros* which we believe primed our interpersonal, economic, and sociopolitical landscape for gender-based violence and present-day drug wars and gang violence. It is the economic and social collapse of a nation that forces people to flee their homes for safety while facing equally as terrorizing odds during their migration journey.

In the words of poet and writer, Warsan Shire (2011):

no one leaves home unless

home is the mouth of a shark

you only run for the border

when you see the whole city running as well

...

you have to understand,

that no one puts their children in a boat

unless the water is safer than the land

...

i want to go home,

but home is the mouth of a shark

home is the barrel of the gun

and no one would leave home

unless home chased you to the shore

unless home told you

to quicken your legs

leave your clothes behind

crawl through the desert

wade through the oceans

drown

Rompiendo Cadenas

save

be hunger

beg

forget pride

your survival is more important

...

no one leaves home until home is a sweaty voice in your ear

saying leave,

run away from me now

i don't know what i've become

but i know that anywhere

is safer than here

excerpt from "Home"

In a conversation about IGT, we must name the ways our lineages have been militarized, exploited, enslaved, displaced, violated, and erased. These are the systemic causes of structural and strategic decisions made by peoples and nations. Some we have participated in and perpetuated, and others we have revolted against and rebuilt from.

Cultural

Understanding intergenerational trauma by accounting for the impacts of colonialism is relevant to situating our present-day cultural values. Doing so will push us forward in ameliorating and discarding historical and colonial trauma's embodied nature while also understanding Latinx cultural values and scripts utilizing a more nuanced, decolonial, and critical analysis.

We seek to acknowledge the role colonial legacies of Spanish colonization and the Spanish Catholic Church have had in creating the cultural values and scripts we hold today. We begin by noting how our cultural values encompass remnants of our Indigenous ways of being that have allowed for our resistance as a people. Cultural values like *personalismo, respeto, familismo,* and *compadrazgo* have allowed us to foster connections and create strong bonds at the individual, familial, and community levels. Similarly, the benefits of faith and spirituality are also essential to highlight, as sources of spirituality assist in our ability to cope with the various forms of oppression. Nevertheless, through our work, we have been privy to the difficulties our communities face when seeking to assert their needs, especially when adhering to strict aspects of these cultural values. Challenging such values can be difficult because many values and scripts are intertwined within aspects of our gendered socialization. For example, the cultural values of *familismo* are supported by the gender socialization of *machismo* and *marianismo*, prescribing how men and women enact varying gender norms and behaviors within the Latinx culture.

Through repression and punishment, the Spanish Church established strict gender and social roles (Hardin, 2002) and the gender socialization of *machismo* and *marianismo*. Focusing on the Aztec people of Mexico, we highlight how this gender socialization occurred. The identity of Mexican men was created through the conflicting relationship between the *conquistador* and *Indio*, resulting in our present-day concept of *machismo* (Hardin, 2002). The Conquistadores and the Spanish Catholic Church attacked the beliefs held by Indigenous Aztecs regarding gender expansiveness, as records indicate that Aztecs venerated deities that "shifted their sex" (as cited in Hardin (2002); Brundage (1979), p. 54) and "were androgynous" (as cited in Hardin (2002); Clendinnen (1991). pp. 167, 168). Our knowledge of such remains limited due to one-sided historical accounts primarily written by "the Spanish scribes and missionaries who were so eagerly prosecuting" (Hardin, 2002, p. 9). Mexican women's gender socialization of *marianismo* occurred through the Spanish Catholic Church utilizing *Tonantzin*, the Aztec deity of motherhood to convert Indigenous folxs to venerate La Virgen de Guadalupe, a Catholic representation of motherhood. Today, La Virgen is a symbolic representation of *marianismo*, as she embodies "sacred duty, self-sacrifice, and chastity [along with] dispensing care and pleasure, not receiving them." (Gil & Vazquez, 1996, p. 7).

In noting this specific historical account, our respective work also provides us with examples of cultural scripts when working with folxs from the Latin diaspora and the Caribbean, especially through their interpersonal dynamics. As professionals accompanying people in navigating through the impacts of IGT, we emphasize that naming gendered-racial colonialism (Chavez Ducñas et al., 2022) also requires noting the multiple oppressions people across the gender spectrum are subjugated to, which complicate these interpersonal dynamics. Without doing so, we fall into limited and harmful ways of perpetuating Eurocentric and deficit-based understanding of behaviors espoused by individuals and thus limits the utilization of culturally relevant understandings.

For instance, a lack of understanding of gender fluidity may be due to feelings of constraint, and limited notions of gender expression or exploration, that inherently exist in our Indigenous cultures due to colonization. Thus, challenging binary thinking of being "this or that" requires assisting Latinxs to (re)member and become privy to such historical accounts while also noting how forced conversion to Catholicism forced heteronormative-patriarchal gender norms. The Muxes from Oaxaca, Mexico, who do not ascribe to gender labels but instead note that "labels should be their self-identification" (Olita, 2018) can be one way in which gender binary trauma can be challenged. In popular culture, Puerto Rican Reggaetón Artist Bad Bunny also challenges gender norms through his music and personal aesthetics, which has increased conversations around gender norms within the Latinx community.

Alternatively, challenging aspects of *marianismo* and *machismo* are growing. This includes deviating away from the "ride or die" culture, that emphasizes *aguantando* toxic relationships (Avila, 2022) and engaging in sacrificial acts Latinx women experience when navigating both motherhood and their professions (Torres, 2021). In challenging machismo, we emphasize that utilizing an intersectional analysis of Latinx masculinities is necessary to challenge the "complicated sense of self" (Hurtado 2003c, p. 56) men experience because of social injustices due to "their class, their race, their ethnicity, their sexuality" (Hurtado 2003c, p. 56).

As we collectively continue to access new language and understanding of IGT, we hold the responsibility to share such knowledge and hold systems of oppression responsible for the harm, while also moving towards reclaiming aspects of cultural values that do not perpetuate heteronormative-patriarchy. By not critically challenging colonial legacies and this "imposed European-brand patriarchy" (Muñoz, 2017), we will continue to enact biased and colonial ways of healing.

INTERPERSONAL ASPECTS IMPACTING TRAUMA

Familia carries the culture forward and sets the stage for relationships. For better or worse, the cultural value of *familismo* impacts how Latinxs relate to others. This section will highlight the strengths and risk factors of Latinx familial relationships, and how many of these interpersonal styles are re-enacted in relationships and impact Latinxs mental health journey.

The family dynamics in Latinxs vary greatly from the Eurocentric family makeup, as Latinx families face unique immigration and economic conditions that impact interpersonal relationships. Since trauma impacts the entire family system, it is also important to consider how Latinx families make sense of traumatic experiences. As healers, we witness the inevitable transmission of trauma to Latinx children from their ancestors starting with grandparents, to parents, and extended family members. We also witness differences in their healing journey. Many factors impact these generational differences in healing including cultural beliefs and access to resources. A reoccurring trend that the authors have witnessed is the reality that the first time immigrant parents interact with the mental health system is to access services for their children. This demonstrates the transmission of intergenerational trauma as a result of unresolved trauma and is exacerbated by a lack of access to mental health services (Delgado-Romero et al., 2021). When immigrant parents finally do receive mental health services, it is common for them to have held their unprocessed trauma for so long that it impacts the way they can show up for their children because they are dealing with their own triggers.

The sacrifices that Latinx immigrant parents make to improve their children's quality of life can become the children's pressure to succeed and repay their parents for their sacrifices. An example of this was expressed on an Instagram page (So Mexican, 2022) that shared a reel of a first-generation Latino reporting his realization of being his parents' 401-k retirement fund and how his parents' security was dependent upon his success. Such realities may predispose children of immigrants to experience exacerbated mental health symptoms. It is important to note that this is a direct result of systemic oppression relegating many immigrants from access to retirement funds and other benefits due to a lack of legal documentation status. This oppressive system leaves employers profiting from cheap labor, while children of immigrant parents struggle to balance education, work, and familial obligations.

Additionally, "*La ropa sucia se lava en la casa*[1]," is a *dicho*[2] that upholds the silence culture and cycle of IGT. Adherence to this *dicho*, often preached by parents and elders to protect their family, also has the consequence of silencing Latinxs as they are explicitly being taught to not speak about their problems outside of the home. Unfortunately, *la ropa sucia* can go unaddressed preventing the ability to cope, manage, or solve the issue at hand. These issues more often than not, are symptoms or root causes of IGT that become normalized through generations. Silence is then reinforced through beliefs that those who speak up or seek psychological or therapeutic services *estan locos*[3].

Despite the stigma of mental health services being perpetuated by the idea of not seeking outside support, Latinx families also proclaim their strength and resilience. A Latinx motto, *¡Si Se Puede!* is used to motivate people to believe in themselves, despite hardships. Likewise, "*no hay mal que por bien no venga*" serves to reclaim someone's challenging experiences and reorient and motivate them to continue to push through.

Crediting the Latinx community's survival strategies allows healers to uncover and build on their inherent resiliency. Healers can lean in on the collectivistic value of Latinxs by making them and their families a part of their own treatment plans especially when working within interdisciplinary teams. In doing so, we not only learn from the experts but also empower Latinxs with the choices that they have. It is equally important for healers to validate people's pain and to disrupt the personalization and self-blame that survivors of trauma often experience. To dismantle such burdensome experiences, people in positions and systems in power must engage in the same difficult work that individuals and families engage in within healing spaces.

Intrapersonal Factors

To survive, Latinxs have continuously found coping strategies. Although the literature has historically focused on at-risk behaviors that Latinxs engage in, we invite you to reframe your thinking and create space to acknowledge that these behaviors have served Latinxs. Latinxs' choice of self-soothing activities, even when they do put them at-risk, should not negate their resiliency or their luchas.[4] With this disclaimer, we share relevant findings to highlight some consequences when trauma goes unhealed. There is an indirect impact that emotional dysregulation has on the relationship between posttraumatic symptoms and drinking alcohol in Latinxs (Paulus et al., 2019). Similarly, there is a positive correlation between acculturative stress in Latinas and depressive symptoms and binge eating (Higgins et al., 2017). These examples emphasize the power in the relationship between emotions, behaviors, and cognitions, all occurring within the individual and impacting how the individual functions.

Van der Kolk (2014) also underlines the impact that trauma has on one's body, such that the body keeps a score and remembers what people experience, even when the brain may not be able to recall those events. He notes that survivors of trauma may also experience physical reactions that can mimic autoinflammatory diseases (van der Kolk, 2014), suggesting that an exhausted nervous system can lead to more harm. What is more, somatic symptoms are the chief presenting concern that Latinxs identify (Escovar et al., 2018), making it imperative for healers to approach the treatment of trauma holistically. The process of regulating and healing should start introspectively, and we must teach our community how to do so from childhood and continue this psychoeducation throughout adulthood.

Innovative approaches such as the use of media to provide psychoeducation have been on the rise. The movie *Inside Out*, for instance, portrays the various emotions one can experience, highlighting that even difficult emotions are not bad and can be regulated. Although a simple concept, it often contradicts what Latinxs are taught regarding expressing their feelings and overall experiences, as it can come off as complaining and being ungrateful. By using Martín-Baró's (1994) liberation psychology framework, we can balance honoring unhealthy learned reactions, but also help people change the narrative by teaching them how to 1) question where their feelings are coming from and make sense of oppressive factors (*Problematización*) and 2) help create new awareness, knowledge, and skills that consider all historical experiences and individual strengths (*Concientización*). In the same vein, this framework should be used when teaching Latinxs about cognitive distortions and ways to manage and heal. By giving Latinxs these strategies to manage various emotions, cognitions, behaviors, and somatic symptoms, we are empowering them to center their inner strength.

Rompiendo Cadenas

From Surviving to Thriving

Latinxs have the ability and strength to heal, but we must entrust them with the power to do so. Figure 1 illustrates examples of the various factors discussed in this chapter (systemic, cultural, interpersonal, and intrapersonal). Before you continue reading, reflect on the following prompt: *What power and privilege do I hold, and how can I leverage it to support the healing of Latinxs' intergenerational trauma?* By acting on this reflection, you would honor what Crenshaw (1989) describes as intersectionality and the value of naming and using one's power and privilege to support those who are most marginalized.

When working with Latinxs with trauma in a therapeutic setting, various evidence-based practices can be used. Although this section will describe a few helpful practices, it is vital to be flexible and to trust your client. What may work with one person, may need to be tailored with another, regardless of if they both identify with similar identities, presenting concerns, and/or experiences. Using genograms and trauma treatments such as Eye Movement and Desensitization and Reprocessing (EMDR) Therapy can help address intergenerational trauma. Genograms are a tool used in counseling that outlines a person's family history, and intergenerational patterns of behavior, and can map developmental trauma. Genograms can help assist both patients and clinicians in processing a client's family dynamics and in creating a treatment plan. There are genograms specifically tailored to acquire trauma histories such as the *Color-Coded Timeline Trauma Genogram* (Jordan, 2004) and the *transgenerational trauma and resilience genogram* (Goodman, 2013). Genograms can also be used as an assessment tool in the first phases of EMDR. EMDR is a widely researched therapy that utilizes bilateral stimulation to access and change the way that memories are stored in the brain. EMDR adheres to the Adaptive Information Processing (AIP) model, which sees symptoms of trauma including PTSD because of previous memories that were not adequately processed (Shapiro, 2017). Unlike other popular evidence-based trauma treatments, EMDR allows for and invites attention to body sensations that come up for patients because of trauma. Given that Latinx populations experience things very somatically, EMDR can be a good fit as a trauma treatment.

Cognitive Processing Therapy (CPT) is also a recommended evidence-based treatment for trauma and posttraumatic stress disorder (APA, 2017). Although originally developed for survivors of rape (Resick & Schnicke, 1992) it can be tailored to fit the cultural needs of Latinxs with other traumatic experiences. Not surprisingly, Marques and her colleagues (2016) noted that although traumas in Latinxs can be similar to non-Latinxs, Latinxs are more likely to report trauma about immigration experiences. In their study, Latinx participants tended to self-blame more when the violent act was perpetrated by a family member. When working with Latinx families, we recommend using *familismo* as support for treatment. In prior clinical practice, the authors have included multiple family members (i.e. parents and siblings) in an adolescent's treatment of sexual abuse. Having support from family members validated this teenager and mitigated the self-blame that she originally expressed for "messing up her family." Including family members also allowed them to support her on her healing journey and be included in her safety plan for suicidal ideations

Herrera and Gloria (2021) provide the ELLA-SANA Model to support survivors of interpersonal violence reclaim the disconnection to their mindbodyspirit as a result of not only intimate partner violence but also oppression. Healing, thus, includes restoring the ruptured "whole" by assisting survivors in becoming *poderosas*[5] by claiming their ability of self-healing (Gloria & Castellanos, 2012). The ELLA-SANA model emphasizes the healing and unearthing of one's inner *ponderosa* through self, family, community, and attention to ancestors through the following four tenants: Envision transformation, Live through, Live-out patron and cultural values, and Act with Intent (Herrera & Gloria, 2021). More recently, the seven psychological strengths of Latinxs, identified and described by Adames and Chavez-Dueñas (2017, p. 29) note overall survival strategies consisting of "determination, esperanza, adaptability, strong work ethic, connectedness to others, collective emotional expression, and resistance." Together, these culturally-rooted interventions illuminate the continued necessity to include and center our cultural strengths to heal.

Chaves Dueñas and her colleagues (2019) developed the Healing Ethno and Racial Trauma (HEART) Model to specifically support Latinx immigrant communities. Like other trauma-informed treatments, the first step identified is to create safety. Due to the complexity that immigration status raises, creating sanctuary spaces is invaluable, but may need flexibility and creativity from providers because it may not always be as easily attainable. Phase two encourages the *concientización*[6] of individuals to understand experiences from a historical lens, considering the oppression that existed to perpetrate such traumas and experiences. The authors highlight creating connections for Latinxs, not just individually, but within their families and communities, to embed their culture and survival skills into their healing journey. The last phase raises the importance of embedding social justice throughout the work of healing. The HEART model offers many aspects needed to liberate individuals from their traumatic experiences, which often keeps individuals, and in the case of intergenerational trauma, families, and communities, imprisoned. Among youth, programs like Xinachtli (Haskie-Mendoza et al., 2021) and Joven Noble (Tello, 2010) foster youth to develop kinship networks that facilitate mental health promotion, advocacy, and healing against oppression. Growing *conocimiento*[7] has also emphasized that when we solely borrow from "external, oppressive, and nonnative systems" (Comas-Diaz, 2006, p.176, as cited in Gloria & Castellanos, 2016) we deviate away from utilizing our respective cultural strengths. Efforts to include interventions centering on culturally responsive aspects honor the necessity to ensure that healing is derived through the reclamation of cultural values that promote wholeness.

ROMPIENDO CADENAS, UN PASO A LA VEZ [BREAKING CHAINS, ONE STEP AT A TIME]: CHAPTER TAKEAWAYS

Ultimately, using creative and cultural approaches to empower Latinxs will increase their ability to resist the transmission of intergenerational trauma, and eventually *romper las cadenas*[8] of such ill fate and rejoice in the power to create their liberated life journey.

Although one may think about intergenerational trauma on the individual level, IGT begins at a systemic level. Going as far back as colonization, we have all been colonized and have colonized others. Our ancestors have been put through things such as wars, imperialism, and collective traumas that may not be spoken about daily, but the effects continue to be passed down. The effects of systemic trauma might in turn be passed down as what we call culture. Concepts such as gender socialization, cultural scripts, and gendered-racial socialization were all influenced by colonization. For instance, take the role of the Catholic Church and the Spanish language. Indigenous people were colonized and forced to speak Spanish and follow the teachings of the Catholic church. Both the Spanish language and the Catholic church are now seen as pillars of Latinx culture and influence topics such as gender, race, and sex.

The family system constitutes interpersonal aspects of intergenerational trauma. The concept of *familismo* is deeply ingrained within the Latinx Culture and comes with its own sets of rules and guides. The culture of silence is the idea that trauma should not be spoken about so that future generations are not impacted by the trauma. The well-intended belief that trauma should not be spoken about can sometimes do the opposite and stifle healing. Thus, it is important to build upon the culture's strengths and intentionally disrupt negative cognitions that may impact the family system. On an intrapersonal level, trauma may be passed down through coping strategies such as perfectionism and anxiety that lives in the body. To combat intergenerational trauma, Martín-Baró's (1994) liberation psychology framework can be a foundation for making sense of oppressive factors and how to navigate those factors from a strengths-based perspective. Therapy can be another alternative to a healing modality for intergenerational trauma. Cognitive Processing Therapy (CPT) and Eye Movement Desensitization Reprocessing (EMDR) therapy are well-known therapies for trauma. Lastly, the ELLA SANA model can be used for survivors of intimate partner violence and the HEART MODEL can be used to support Latinx immigrant communities in healing (Haskie-Mendoza, et al., 2021; Tello, 2010).

CLOSING EXERCISE

Dear Amigxs,

We know that after such a lengthy analysis it can feel overwhelming to know how to move forward. The prompts below will support your embodied processing of the material via metacognition, reflective thinking, and somatic integration. Take a moment to allow the mind to release all it has learned and listen to what is left in the body.

Reflection. Take the space below to answer the prompts and free write your answers.

No judgment- just dump out all that rises to the surface.

Some Questions I have:

Thoughts, Images and/or Feelings that came up for me:

Somatic Integration. Choose as many of the following exercises as you would like. Set aside at least 5-15 minutes to enter each practice slowly and consciously. Allow your body to move freely.

1. Choose a song that feels good or comes to mind at this moment. Notice how your body wants to move and allow it to. Repeat until you feel settled or complete.
2. Find a brief Guided Body Scan video on youtube. Get comfortable in your space and gently stretch if/as needed before starting. Repeat until you feel settled or complete.
3. Grab a blank sheet of paper or coloring book. Set up your space and art supplies in a way that feels good to you. Allow yourself to free draw, color, or sketch what comes to you.

Word Association Collage. Grab a blank sheet of paper and write down the words HEALING on one side, and STRENGTHS on the other side. Set a timer for 2 minutes and write down (or sketch out) all that comes to mind for you when you think about yourself, your family, your culture, and/or your community. Flip to the other side, reset the timer, and repeat.

Thank you for journeying with us, hasta que *rompamos las cadenas*.

REFERENCES

Avila, L. (2022, June 29). It's time to retire toxic ride-or-die culture. In *Hot Girl Somos*. Refinery29. https://www.refinery29.com/en-us/2022/06/11027589/marianismo-ride-or-die-culture-toxic

Cerdeña, J. P., Rivera, L. M., & Spak, J. M. (2021). Intergenerational trauma in Latinxs: A scoping review. *Social Science & Medicine, 270*, 113662. doi:10.1016/j.socscimed.2020.113662

Chavez-Dueñas, N. Y., Adames, H. Y., & Perez-Chavez, J. G. (2022). Anti-colonial futures: Indigenous Latinx women healing from the wounds of racial-gendered colonialism. *Women & Therapy, 45*(2-3), 1–16. doi:10.1080/02703149.2022.2097593

Chavez-Dueñas, N. Y., Adames, H. Y., Perez-Chavez, J. G., & Salas, S. P. (2019). Healing ethno-racial trauma in Latinx immigrant communities: Cultivating hope, resistance, and action. *The American Psychologist, 74*(1), 49–62. doi:10.1037/amp0000289 PMID:30652899

Conroy, S. (2022). Narrative Matters: Encanto and intergenerational trauma. *Child and Adolescent Mental Health, 27*(3), 309–311. Advance online publication. doi:10.1111/camh.12563 PMID:35394693

Danieli, Y. (2007). Assessing trauma across cultures from a multigenerational perspective. In J. P. Wilson & C. S.-K. Tang (Eds.), *Cross-cultural assessment of psychological trauma and PTSD* (pp. 65–89). Springer. doi:10.1007/978-0-387-70990-1_4

Dass-Brailsford, P. (2007). A practical approach to trauma: Empowering interventions. *Sage (Atlanta, Ga.)*.

del Valle, L. E., & Alvelo, J. (1996). Perception of post traumatic stress disorder symptoms by children of Puerto Rican Vietnam veterans. *Puerto Rico Health Sciences Journal, 15*(2), 101–106. doi:10.4135/9781452204123

Delgado-Romero, E.A., Mahoney, G.E., Muro-Rodriguez, N., & Atilano, R., Cardenas-Bautista, E., De Los Santos, J., Duran, M., Espinoza, L., Fuentes, J., Gomez, S., Ingram, R., Jiminez-Ruiz, J., Monroig, M., Mora-Ozuna, C., Ordaz, A.C., Rappaport, B., Suazo-Padilla, K. & Vazquez, M.S. (2021). Clinica In Lak'ech: The establishment of a practicum site to integrate practice, advocacy, and research with Latinx clients [The Counseling Psychologist – Special Issue, the Integration of Practice, Advocacy, and Research in Counseling Psychology]. *The Counseling Psychologist, 49*(7), 987–1012. doi:10.1177/00110000211025270

Escovar, E. L., Craske, M., Roy-Byrne, P., Stein, M. B., Sullivan, G., Sherbourne, C. D., Bystritsky, A., & Chavira, D. A. (2018). Cultural influences on mental health symptoms in a primary care sample of Latinx patients. *Journal of Anxiety Disorders, 55*, 39–47. doi:10.1016/j.janxdis.2018.03.005 PMID:29576380

Friedman, B. D., & Allen, K. N. (2011). Systems theory. *Theory & Practice in Clinical Social Work, 2*(3), 3-20.

Gil, R. M., & Vazquez, C. I. (2014). *The Maria paradox: How Latinas can merge old world traditions with new world self-esteem*. Open Road Media.

Gobat, M. (2013). The Invention of Latin America: A Transnational History of Anti-Imperialism, Democracy, and Race. *The American Historical Review, 118*(5), 1345–1375. doi:10.1093/ahr/118.5.1345

Goodman, R. D. (2013). The transgenerational trauma and resilience genogram. *Counselling Psychology Quarterly*, *26*(3-4), 386–405. doi:10.1080/09515070.2013.820172

Haskie-Mendoza, S., Serrata, J. V., Escamilla, H., & Jaimes, C. (2021). Xinachtli: A Healing-Informed, Gendered, and Culturally Responsive Approach with System-Involved Latinas. *Latinas in the Criminal Justice System: Victims, Targets, and Offenders*, *18*, 315–332. doi:10.18574/nyu/9781479804634.003.0015

Herrera, N., & Gloria, A. M. (2021). Latina Students' Post-IPV Healing: A Bodymindspirit Approach Using the ELLA-SANA Model. *Women & Therapy*, 1–20. doi:10.1080/02703149.2021.1982537

Higgins Neyland, M. K., & Bardone-Cone, A. M. (2017). Tests of escape theory of binge eating among Latinas. *Cultural Diversity & Ethnic Minority Psychology*, *23*(3), 373–381. doi:10.1037/cdp0000130 PMID:27831694

Hurtado, A., & Sinha, M. (2008). More than men: Latino feminist masculinities and intersectionality. *Sex Roles*, *59*(5), 337–349. doi:10.100711199-008-9405-7

Imperialism in Latin America. (n.d.). Retrieved May 11, 2022, from https://web-clear.unt.edu/course_projects/HIST2610/content/06_Unit_Six/19_lesson_nineteen/06_imp_lat_am.htm

Jordan, K. (2004). The Color-Coded Timeline Trauma Genogram. *Brief Treatment and Crisis Intervention*, *4*(1), 57–70. Advance online publication. doi:10.1093/brief-treatment/mhh005

Marques, L., Eustis, E. H., Dixon, L., Valentine, S. E., Borba, C. P. C., Simon, N., Kaysen, D., & Wiltsey-Stirman, S. (2016). Delivering cognitive processing therapy in a community health setting: The influence of Latino culture and community violence on posttraumatic cognitions. *Psychological Trauma: Theory, Research, Practice, and Policy*, *8*(1), 98–106. doi:10.1037/tra0000044 PMID:25961865

Martín-Baró, I. (1994). *Writings for a liberation psychology*. Harvard University Press.

Martinez, M. (2021). Toxic Masculinity: An Outcome of Colonialism and its Effects on the Latinx/Chicanx LGBTQ+ Community. *McNair Research Journal SJSU*, *17*(11). Advance online publication. doi:10.31979/mrj.2021.1711

McLaughlin, K. A., & Lambert, H. K. (2017). Child Trauma Exposure and Psychopathology: Mechanisms of Risk and Resilience. *Current Opinion in Psychology*, *14*, 29–34. doi:10.1016/j.copsyc.2016.10.004 PMID:27868085

Menakem, R. (2021). *My grandmother's hands: Racialized trauma and the pathway to mending our hearts and Bodies*. Penguin Books.

Mendoza, S., Serrata, J., Escamilla, H., & Jaimes, C. (2021). 14. Xinachtli: A Healing- Informed, Gendered, and Culturally Responsive Approach with System- Involved Latinas. In V. Lopez & L. Pasko (Eds.), *Latinas in the Criminal Justice System: Victims, Targets, and Offenders* (pp. 315–332). New York University Press. doi:10.18574/nyu/9781479804634.003.0015

Muñoz, M. (2017). *10 Reasons Why Colonialism Strengthened Rape Culture In Latinx Communities*. Everyday Feminism. Retrieved May 6, 2022, from https://everydayfeminism.com/2017/07/colonialism-latinx-rape-culture/

Olita, I. (2018, January 29). *The Third Gender* [Video]. The Atlantic. https://www.theatlantic.com/video/index/551738/muxes-mexico-third-gender/

Paulus, D. J., Tran, N., Gallagher, M. W., Viana, A. G., Bakhshaie, J., Garza, M., Ochoa-Perez, M., Lemaire, C., & Zvolensky, M. J. (2019). Examining the indirect effect of posttraumatic stress symptoms via emotion dysregulation on alcohol misuse among trauma-exposed Latinx in primary care. *Cultural Diversity & Ethnic Minority Psychology, 25*(1), 55–64. doi:10.1037/cdp0000226 PMID:30714767

Resick, P. A., & Schnicke, M. K. (1992). Cognitive processing therapy for sexual assault victims. *Journal of Consulting and Clinical Psychology, 60*(5), 748–756. https://doi.org/10.1037//0022-006x.60.5.748

Sacks, V., & Murphey, S. (n.d). *The prevalence of adverse childhood experiences, nationally, by state, and by race or ethnicity*. https://www.childtrends.org/publications/prevalence-adverse-childhood-experiences-nationally-state-race-ethnicity

Sangalang, C. C., Jager, J., & Harachi, T. W. (2017). Effects of maternal traumatic distress on family functioning and child mental health: An examination of Southeast Asian refugee Journal Pre-proof 48 families in the U.S. *Social Science & Medicine, 184*, 178–186. doi:10.1016/j.socscimed.2017.04.032

Shapiro, F. (2017). *Eye movement desensitization and reprocessing (EMDR) therapy: Basic principles, protocols, and procedures*. Guilford Publications.

Shire, W. (2011). *Home*. Teaching My Mother How to Give Birth.

So Mexican [@somexican]. (2022, July). *Have u thought about this? #somexican via:tiktok/thenosabokidhtx"* [Video]. Instagram. https://www.instagram.com/reel/CgpIvKcj0Cw/?igshid=YmMyMTA2M2Y

Tello, J., Cervantes, R. C., Cordova, D., & Santos, S. M. (2010). Joven Noble: Evaluation of a culturally focused youth development program. *Journal of Community Psychology, 38*(6), 799–811. https://doi.org/10.1002/jcop.20396

van der Kolk, B. A. (2014). *The body keeps the score: Brain, mind, and body in the healing of trauma*. Viking.

Zayas, L. H. (2011). *Latinas attempting suicide: When cultures, families, and daughters collide*. Oxford University Press.

ENDNOTES

[1] Don't air your dirty laundry
[2] Saying
[3] Are crazy
[4] Struggles
[5] Powerful
[6] Consciousness raising
[7] Consciousness
[8] Break the chains

Chapter 12
Juntos Resistimos y Sanamos:
The Strength of Latinx Families

Jacqueline Fuentes
University of Georgia, USA

Violeta J. Rodriguez
University of Georgia, USA & Department of Psychiatry and Behavioral Sciences, University of Miami Miller School of Medicine, USA

Madison L. Rodriguez
University of Georgia, USA

Ana Carina Ordaz
University of Georgia, USA

ABSTRACT

The authors seek to provide a more holistic, compassionate, and liberatory understanding of Latinx families. This chapter will highlight the importance of understanding families from a historical, culturally centered manner that honors their layered experiences of contextual factors, intergenerational trauma, and strengths-based approach. This chapter seeks to honor ethnic heterogeneity and cultural strengths and expand the notion of what consists of the family constellation. In doing so, the chapter will focus on central aspects of la familia, including child development, parenting, and recommendations focused on engaging Latinx families and improving the assessment and family interventions.

JUNTOS RESISTIMOS Y SANAMOS [TOGETHER WE RESIST AND HEAL]: THE STRENGTH OF LATINX FAMILIES

The experiences of Latinx families living in the United States are vast, ever-changing, and uniquely experienced within all ethnic or national groups. Although our colonial legacies, language, and some of our customs connect us, the impacts of intergenerational trauma, discrimination, and sociopolitical context are all uniquely felt. We thus seek to situate familial dynamics and experiences as not solely occurring

DOI: 10.4018/978-1-6684-4901-1.ch012

within interpersonal relationships but rather actively occurring through citizenship, immigration, and racialization, influenced by institutional discrimination (i.e., U.S. policies). We challenge oppressive, apolitical, and ahistorical accounts missing from our therapeutic practices and seek to emphasize the role of the U.S. in creating familial conditions, such as family separation, to not only note the legacies of intergenerational trauma but oppressive ecologies (Carlo et al., 2022) that affect parenting, family processes, adjustment, and development.

Our understanding of the complex Latinx familial experiences remains limited due to the hegemonic analysis of families and our overreliance on the pan-ethnic term Latinx. The lack of ethnic representation in psychological research samples continues to perpetuate a lack of understanding of cross-cultural variations impacting behavior (Arnett, 2016; Nielsen et al., 2017). The existing research holds Whites as the comparative standard of psychological functioning, resulting in cultural (mis)attribution bias (Causadias et al., 2018; Sue, 1999). Consequently, we are unlikely to note Latinx families' survival and resistance strategies by strictly adhering to deficit approaches (Rodriguez & Morrobel, 2004).

We also note that the overreliance on the pan-ethnic term Latinx, in addition to the broader concept of Latinidad, has resulted in limited ethnic group and geographic diversity in research (Delgado-Romero et al., 2017). Due to the overwhelming focus on Mexican families in research, there is an increased risk of negating and erasing the experiences of other ethnic minority groups (Mendez & Cortina, 2021). Within Latinidad, the all-encompassing term fails to name the legacies of "anti-Blackness, femicide, anti-Indigeneity, and inarticulation of violence" (Pelaez Lopez, 2018, Color Bloq's X Collection). Efforts to understand Latinx families within their specific ethnic and cultural histories are necessary to capture essential family factors, including Indigenous ancestry, Black ancestry, proximity to Whiteness, bilingualism, acculturation, and multilingualism. These factors have a significant function and impact on familial well-being and distress and broaden the often-narrow scope by which Latinx culture is examined and understood. Thus, this chapter will address the impact of Latinx adolescent development, parenting, and interventions focused on expanding assessment tools and seek to illuminate essential considerations when working with Latinx families.

LATINX ADOLESCENCE

We begin by bringing attention to the unique and layered development stage of adolescence Latinx youth undergo. Until the past decade, research has focused on deficits, primarily comparative between-ethnic/ racial group differences (Azmitia, 2021) and psychopathology (Rodriguez & Morrobel, 2004) among Latinx youth. The shift to more asset-based research (Azmitia, 2021) acknowledges unique facets within this stage, including ethnic and racial-ethnic socialization, biculturalism, language brokering, and connection to cultural values. The recent inclusion of ethnic and racial identity (ERI) development indicates that stronger ethnic and racial identity protects youth from discrimination, thus fostering positive self-esteem (Umaña-Taylor & Updegraff, 2007) and offsetting mental health challenges beginning in early childhood (Meca et al., 2020; Serrano-Villar & Calzada, 2016; Torres et al., 2011). Additionally, ERI development includes caregivers and family members as agents of socialization, highlighting their pivotal role in building youth's view of the world and developing themselves (Meca et al., 2021). Efforts to contextualize Latinx youth's ERI development, specifically within their contexts and within the backdrop of oppression, are growing and offer adaptive strategies enacted by youth to navigate oppressive forces (Sladek et al., 2022; Torres et al., 2020). Nevertheless, gaps in our understanding are especially lacking for AfroLatinx and Indigenous youth (Azmitia, 2021), necessitating that we challenge our denial of anti-Blackness and anti-Indigeneity within Latinx culture to support Latinx youth who are very much affected by racialization in the U.S.

Biculturalism is another crucial factor to consider in Latinx adolescent development. Defined as the co-existence of diverse cultures, where one integrates traditions, customs, and languages from both cultures into their daily life (Schwartz & Unger, 2010), biculturalism is often understood through speaking Spanglish and/or retention of one's Indigenous languages. This choice of language is an act of resistance that often gets dismissed, especially as youth navigate the pressures to acculturate are most challenged within school systems. Oppressive policies, such as English-only laws implemented in schools, have long-lasting impacts on youth and older generations. Thus, ensuring schools strive to support students through ethnic studies and noting their funds of knowledge (Moll et al., 1992) can promote ethnic-racial socialization.

In discussing language, specifically bilingualism and language brokering, we seek to highlight these competing realities experienced by Latinx youth. Bilingualism promotes connection to their community, thus creating an asset for the individual and their family (Cardoso & Thompson, 2010). Similarly, language brokering is a developmental niche in Latinx families (Dorner et al., 2008; Fuller & Coll, 2010), where youth may take on the translator role in varying capacities to assist caregivers. Research findings on language brokering are mixed, such that on the one hand, language brokering may allow college students to maintain their first language and enhance their problem-solving abilities (López et al., 2019), whereas those who self-classified as high language brokers displayed more negative mental health outcomes and intergenerational conflict (Martinez et al., 2009; Morales & Wang 2018; Shen & Dennis, 2019). Such findings are worrisome because they fail to recognize how Latinx youth, within their families, utilize the cultural value of interdependence to assist their caregivers when navigating the systematic racism evident through language inequity. Enacting such interdependence comes at a cost, where youths are exposed to discrimination early on. Given these findings, it is vital to ensure that language brokering is understood strengths-based while attending to the emotional toll this may have on adolescents.

COMPONENTS OF THE FAMILY

Familismo is an essential aspect of Latinx adolescent development. The connection among family members buffers against negative mental health symptoms over time and in multiple situations for Latinx adolescents (Ramos et al., 2021; Reyes & Elias, 2011; Taylor et al., 2020) while also protecting against the negative effects of associating with deviant peers and externalizing behaviors (Germán et al., 2009; Piña-Watson et al., 2019). Perceived family resilience also buffers the adverse effects of perceived discrimination on self-reported depressive and somatic symptoms (Ramos et al., 2021). Therefore, *familismo* is crucial for mental health providers to consider as it contributes to positive youth development in Latinx youth.

In recognizing that the family contributes to the ethnic identity of Latinx youth, we must also identify how differences in ethnic identity arise through family dynamics. The perceptions of youth regarding their family ethnic socialization led to greater ethnic identity exploration and resolution during adulthood. The segmented assimilation theory explains how children of immigrants assimilate into different sections of society, in which there may be individual-level and contextual factors (Zhou, 1997). Individual-level factors include English-language ability, place of birth, and education. Contextual factors include socio-economic and racial statuses. This theory stresses the importance of multiple factors that contribute to the various pathways for children of immigrants. For example, this theory allows us to understand why some individuals take the upward mobility pattern to integrate into middle-class America while others take the downward mobility pattern.

While families can buffer against adverse mental health outcomes for Latinx youth, acculturative pressures and lack of citizenship also impact Latinx families. Latinx youth and their families are subject to larger pressures to acculturate thus resulting in acculturative conflict due to cultural discrepancies (Lawton & Gerdes, 2014). The acculturation gap-distress model also illustrates how Latinx youth, with varying levels of acculturation compared to their parents, may challenge traditional views of their parents (Telzer, 2010). This can include Latina youth challenging cultural gender socialization and seeking to diverge from such expectations. Given the detrimental outcomes associated with acculturative conflict, mental health professionals need to consider the role of cultural discrepancy when working with Latinx youth and their parents/ caregivers as this conflict predicts more significant depressive symptoms in Latinx youth (Huq et al., 2016). Providing parents psychoeducation on acculturative stress could mitigate conflict and facilitate generative communication (Galvan & Gudino, 2019). This includes providing families with bicultural effectiveness training to develop the capacity to manage their cultural differences within their household (Szapocznik & Kurtines, 1993).

Immigration-related stressors, such as lack of citizenship and anti-immigrant policies, also impact families. Undocumented parents endure substantial stress as they aim to provide the best environment for their children while managing the stress of deportation threats, placing them at greater risk for anxiety and depressive symptoms (Potochnick & Perreira, 2010). Consequently, these impacts also affect their children's well-being and development (Torres et al., 2018) and may lead to their confusion about their own legal status. For undocumented Latinx youth, this includes a greater risk for negative mental health challenges, such as perceiving their future as hopeless, as well as experiencing anxiety and depressive symptoms (Gonzalez et al., 2015).However, in the face of immigration related stressors, the family can be a source of encouragement (Rios Casas et al., 2020) in addition civic and political participation, which can promote help learned hopefulness (Zimmerman, 1990) and critical consciousness-raising (Diemer, 2021) as being part of organizations, extracurricular activities, or in spaces where individuals feels they can contribute.

Parenting

To understand Latinx parenting, mental health professionals shall seek to not to overlook how Latinx parents incorporate intergenerational healing practices while also seeking to balance competing cultural values as they raise their children. Our work must consider non-traditional parenting, such as transnational mothering (Falicov, 2008), a common reality among immigrant communities. To so do, we utilize the *Seven Psychological Strengths of Latinxs* proposed by Adames and Chavez-Dueñas (2017), to understand Latinx parenting. The seven strengths include: (1) Determination, (2) *Esperanza*, (3) Adaptability, (4) Strong Work Ethic, (5) Connectedness to Others, (6) Collective Emotional Expression, and (7) Resistance (Adames & Chavez-Dueñas, 2017, p. 29). Let us consider the case of Elisa and her children and how these strengths provide a holistic and culturally oriented understanding of how Latinx parents resist systems of oppression while parenting (Parra, 2019).

Elisa is a 31-year-old cisgender woman from Escuintla, Guatemala. She currently lives in Georgia with her two teenage sons, who are 13 and 15 years old. Elisa has sought mental health services for her 15-year-old, Antonio, who is "*portandose mal (misbehaving)*" at home and school. Antonio has been living with her for five months since being reunified after immigrating from Guatemala. Before immigrating, Antonio lived with his paternal grandmother in Guatemala and the last time he saw his mother in person was when he was one year old. They have communicated through phone calls, video calls, and Facebook. Elisa expressed her frustrations with parenting as she compared Antonio to her 13-year-old Manuel, *"el [Manuel] siempre me respeta y no se porta mal (Manuel is always respectful and never misbehaves)."*

Elisa shared that she is a single mother, and her reason for immigrating to the U.S. without Antonio was that she only had enough money to pay for her *coyote*. She explained that making ends meet as a single mother in Guatemala was difficult. When she came to the U.S., his paternal grandmother was the only person willing to care for Antonio. She agreed that she would support them financially until Elisa had enough money to bring him. She expressed, *"siempre trabaje duro y nunca perdi la fe de traermelo pero no fue facil juntar el dinero (I always worked hard and never lost faith in reuniting with him, but it was not easy to work to obtain the money to do so.)*

While Elisa shares her story as an undocumented immigrant from Guatemala, this is only a portion of her story. Beyond this intake, she embodies determination, as she dared to leave her home not fully knowing what to expect on her journey to the U.S. to provide a better life for her newborn in Guatemala *"nunca pedi las esperanze de volver a estar con mi hijo (I never lost faith in reuniting with my child)."* She maintained a strong work ethic that today allows her to be physically connected to her son, Antonio Elisa's resilience and strength also made her adapt, allowing her to exist and resist in spaces that have not been safe or welcoming.

Culturally responsive parent training interventions remain limited. More so, they fail to shed light on how inequities and heightened levels of oppression hinder parents' abilities to endorse positive parenting (Parra, 2019). To address the realities parents face, culturally adapted interventions must address socio-cultural contexts and cultural values, such as *familismo* and *respeto*, to foster acceptance and engagement of parenting interventions (Parra, 2019). These interventions must also move away from parent blaming and seek to honor cultural strengths that parents exhibit in their parenting. In the same vein, interventions acknowledge and promote biculturalism among Latinx immigrant families by addressing parents' ability to communicate their emotions with their children (Parra, 2019) and the *resentimiento* (resentment) that may arise due to compromised attachment amongst reunified transnational families (Menjivar, 2006).

As healers, psychologists, social workers, counselors, and other helping professionals, we play a significant role in introducing Elisa to these strengths while also being critical that we not pathologize Elisa for engaging in "creative family practices for survival" (Abrego & Hernández, 2021, p. 174). Utilizing the *Seven Psychological Strengths of Latinxs* (Adames & Chavez-Dueñas, 2017) within our therapeutic approaches can provide parents with tools to resist oppressive realities.

Transnational Families and Reunification

We expand on the focus of reunification of unaccompanied immigrant children with parents residing in the U.S. and emphasize the need to consider the challenges and strengths found within transnational families prior to reunification. This includes noting the cultural beliefs and values that sustain them during the lengthy periods of separation while gaining insight into their coping (Boss, 1999; Falicov, 2008). Additional challenges parents face include the interactions with various systems (i.e. child welfare, educational and health care systems) that can either support or hinder reunification efforts. Children separated from their parents are commonly toddlers who reunite with their parents at later ages (i.e., preteens, adolescence) after being cared for by extended family members. Thus recognizing parents' decision to prioritize protecting them from immigration journeys (Becker Herbst et al., 2018) while also utilizing Boss' (1999) theory of ambiguous loss, can provide understanding in how transnational families experience living in a state of uncertainty that includes being physically absent but psychologically present. Transnational mothering (Falicov, 2008) can also clarify how Elisa's mothering differs from transnational fathering. The gendered differences in transnational parenting posit that mothers may experience a more significant toll as they not only navigate the expectations to be caregivers, nurturers, and breadwinners, while transnational fathers adopt a more honorary role of solely being a breadwinner (Dreby, 2006).

Attending to the separation and reunification of immigrant children with their parents is necessary, given its adverse effects on children's well-being. Adverse effects of separation include literacy difficulties and increased risk for emotional and behavioral problems (Lu et al., 2020). Play therapy is a modality we propose can assist in processing the traumatic encounters children experience in their immigration journey and promote the reunification process to move towards resiliency (Pizarro, 2021). This child-centered counseling modality includes parents in the therapeutic process and promotes family healing, learning, and unlearning while also moving away from child-blaming. The utilization of culturally relevant toys allows children to engage in play therapy in a culturally attuned manner, thus allowing them to vocalize and make sense of their experiences through play, thus decreasing internalized and externalized behaviors (Garza & Bratton, 2005). We highlight the need to avoid blaming children for their externalized behaviors once reunified with their parents while also focusing on cultural and family-specific dynamics that move away from a one size fits all model.

Emotion Socialization in the Latinx Family

Attention to the expression and socialization of emotions needs to be explored in familial therapeutic processes. Specifically, language considerations, such as being bilingual and trilingual, are of focus. Attending to bilingualism and trilingualism allows us to understand the expression or suppression of emotions (Chen et al., 2012; Kassem et al., 2022). Certain immigrant families retain Indigenous languages, which is especially relevant as unaccompanied minors may meet their US-born siblings who speak English and reconnect with caregivers who predominantly speak Spanish. In the case of Antonio and Elisa, they both speak *Poqoman*, a Mayan language spoken in Escuintla. For Antonio, primarily raised by his grandmother, Poqoman is his primary language, while Spanish is his second. Antonio may face language barriers that hinder the ability of his family to understand and express his emotions congruently. Attending to this reality should be a therapeutic priority.

We also note how gender roles impact emotional socialization. For instance, exploring who gets to express their feelings through cultural scripts of *marianismo* and *machismo* and how such emotions are expressed in the household provides vast information on therapeutic interventions at increasing and promoting emotional expression. This is especially relevant as girls are more likely to express submissive emotions while boys are more likely to express disharmonious emotions (Chaplin et al., 2005).

Immigrant Families and Grief

In discussing grief in the Latinx community, it is essential to consider cultural heritage, belief systems, norms, values, generational status, and family systems to capture how grief is expressed and understood.

We note that grief does not always involve death but extends when families face divorce or separation from family due to immigration or deportation. Centering the cultural values of *familismo, respeto, and personalismo* can aid in capturing how grief is expressed more broadly. Movies like *Coco* further provide conversations about grief that attends to belonging, ancestors, *cuentos*, and life after death. Equally important is considering the barriers mixed-status families face when navigating the death of a loved one. Immigrant familial grief also includes noting forced absence from ceremonies (e.g., burial, dispersing ashes) due to the inability to travel across borders due to the lack of documentation or legal status and financial burdens.

The Covid-19 pandemic has forced families to have conversations about death beyond *ofrendas* and *altares* (Bermúdez & Bermúdez, 2002) due to the health inequalities that have ravaged our communities and led to disproportional deaths. These realities have led Latinx families to experience death in the family and grief for the first time or experience navigating end-of-life care and international burial services (i.e., international shipment) while considering financial factors. Depending on family members' language proficiency, navigating burial services may fall on the oldest child or grandchild of the deceased family member. Amid all the pain and loss, the *Seven Psychological Strengths* of Latinx families are displayed fiercely (Adames & Chavez-Dueñas, 2017, p. 29). This includes extended family convening, sharing meals, *cuentos*, and laughter while crying as they collectively remember their loved ones. Yet, we also note that closure and goodbyes with parted loved ones, especially within mixed-status families, can create unique circumstances where only specific individuals can travel. This includes children partaking in international burial services while their parents and other family members stay behind due to lack of documentation. In such instances, we must recognize how families adapt and utilize social media, such as Facebook and Facetime, to be virtually present while attending virtual burial services internationally. Together, Latinxs continue to find ways to connect with their *esperanza* to overcome all the unknowns.

Recommendations and Implications

Thus far, we have reviewed distal and proximal factors influencing Latinx parenting and child development, and how psychological researchers and practitioners can capitalize on unique factors and the strengths of Latinx families to generate opportunities to support Latinx families and the development of Latinx children. These complex, multifaceted, distal, and proximal factors, limitations, and strengths underscore the importance of using multifaceted and multilevel approaches in working with Latinx families to maximize the benefit of psychological assessment and interventions. It is hopefully now evident that interventions and assessments that consider distal (e.g., systematic) and proximal (e.g., parenting, Latinx adolescent development) factors influencing Latinx families and the development of Latinx children are more likely to yield the greatest benefit for them. Based on the review of these factors, we make the following recommendations for assessment of, and interventions in, Latinx families:

Validate Parenting and Family Assessments Among Latinx Families

Though the adaptation of psychological interventions for use among specific groups has generally received attention in the literature, the adaptation of quantitative measures for use with specific groups (i.e., Latinx non English speaking populations) is less frequently discussed and in the case of parenting and family measures, neglected (Rodriguez et al., 2021). However, quantitative assessments are important for screening parents and families into interventions, 2) identifying additional needs requiring support during interventions, and 3) monitoring progress once families have been engaged in interventions. Therefore, researchers and clinicians that view Latinx families as homogeneous may continue to try to quantify Latinx parenting using assessments traditionally validated in middle-class European American families, which may in turn fail to identify and accommodate their unique needs in interventions (Rodriguez et al., 2021). For this reason, we argue that adapting quantitative assessments used with Latinx parents, families, and children's merits as much attention as adapting interventions.

Specifically, the exploration of important psychometric properties for assessing racial and ethnic minorities has received little attention in the literature, including the psychometric property of measurement equivalence, which is of even greater relevance to homogenous groups such as Latinx families and parents. Measurement equivalence refers to whether constructs, such as psychological terms, have a similar meaning across the diverse groups assessed in a sample. For example, assessing positive and negative parenting may carry different meanings across racial and ethnic groups, particularly because of systemic, historical, structural, and contemporary challenges that Latinx families face. An illustrative example is assessing neglect via resources that may not be available to historically marginalized groups. For example, a previous study showed that racial and ethnic minorities were less likely to report having someone take them to the doctor, which is in the physical neglect subscale of the Childhood Trauma Questionnaire (Rodriguez et al., 2019). However, such an item may measure healthcare access, as opposed to parental neglect. In such cases, establishing measurement equivalence is vital for making conclusions about the types of parenting that may be promoted in parenting interventions for Latinx families, and how we conceptualize different psychological constructs.

For Latinx families, who hold various levels of Spanish and English proficiency (in addition to, potentially, other languages, including Indigenous dialects), the understanding of assessments may be further complicated by linguistic equivalence. Linguistic equivalence refers to whether certain words in a language have the same meaning for multiple groups in a population. For example, it has been shown that different words for physical maltreatment may be used by different racial and ethnic groups (Rodriguez et al., 2019). Further, a systematic review of the literature examining measurement equivalence of parenting constructs across racial and ethnic groups showed that measurement equivalence across racial and ethnic groups, including Latinx parents, was only assessed for 6 parenting scales out of only 10 studies examining 8 parenting assessments' psychometric properties. Considering that an earlier review in 2014 identified 164 parenting measures, this shows the tremendous amount of work needed to further the study of Latinx parenting using quantitative measures (Hurley et al., 2014).

Quantitative measures are used for monitoring the efficacy of interventions adapted for Latinx families, and the results of quantitative assessments are used to evaluate the performance of Latinx children for educational and psychological purposes. As such, the availability of Spanish assessments that are not simply literally translated into Spanish is needed. Existing guidelines for the rigorous and judicious translation adaption of measures in counseling research exist, and these should be disseminated and implemented widely (Lenz et al., 2017).

Providing a clinical and experiential perspective, the second author has worked with Indigenous families for the purposes of IQ testing. Although the second author is Spanish-English bilingual, in her work with Indigenous families she has encountered barriers in accessing materials to accurately assess trilingual children, particularly considering the families' hesitance in recognizing that they speak an Indigenous language at home due to stigma. Without adapting these assessments and developing methods to evaluate multilingual children, middle-class European American families will continue to be the standard, and multilingual children will continue to be disadvantaged by standardized testing.

Challenge the Deficit-Based Discourse on Latinx Families

Related to the use of unvalidated quantitative measures of parenting and family factors among Latinx families with middle-class the tendency to use European American families as the standard has yielded a deficit-based perspective of racial and ethnic minorities in the U.S. Specifically, when using middle-class European American families as the norm, Latinx parents and their children are often viewed as deficient, regardless of whether that deficiency is to their benefit or detriment. Challenging such deficit-based perspectives of Latinx children and their families can impact the low degree attainment rates among Latinx children, highlighting the importance of using innovative strategies to study Latinx families to inform programs and policies affecting Latinx families (Grosso Richins et al., 2021).

Emerging research points to ways exemplary teachers have begun to do this in school environments, starting with learning more about Latinx students and families' backgrounds. Not being aware of the unique living situations of families can prevent assumptions about why certain circumstances may occur in this historically misunderstood group. For example, Latinx parents may not have the same transportation or time resources to attend appointments, and as a health or social service employees, one should not assume this refers to unwillingness to participate in services. That is, some navigational and social factors to promote awareness of unique living circumstances among Latinx families have included recognizing that some Latinx families may have fewer transportation and economic resources (e.g., no license or car), and greater time constraints to meet with teachers (Grosso Richins et al., 2021). Greater awareness of these circumstances has helped accommodate their unique needs to better promote home literacy practices. To this end, exemplary teachers often incorporate or develop creative (and at times unconventional) ways of generating awareness for themselves about Latinx families and their living situations. This includes expanding their availability to the weekends, and/or other times, coming to areas where a substantial proportion of their students live (i.e., mobile home areas) to get to know their students and families. Other ways of capitalizing on the cultural wealth of Latinx families may include recognizing their challenges and communicating high expectations despite the challenges families may face. Exemplary teachers have used their awareness of challenges to help family's problem-solve around the barriers/ challenges they face by asking Latinx families and parents what may work for *their particular* family. That is, lowering expectations in the face of adversity should not be the first solution. Similarly, simply setting expectations based on traditional middle-class European American parents without recognizing challenges is another blind approach that will continue negatively impacting Latinx children's academic achievement.

Recognizing Latinx families' communication preferences can also facilitate engagement (Grosso Richins et al., 2021). For example, teachers reported that using social media to communicate with families, rather than expecting them to learn to use email, improved their communication with families. Though social media usage for clinical interventions may be an unrealistic solution in these times of constant privacy threats, this highlights the need to develop easier and more accessible methods of communicating with Latinx families, likely using innovative mobile health interventions, e.g., videos, text messaging (Gonzalez et al., 2021). Communication with parents is important: Communicating with families about fathers' tight schedules made it possible for teachers to modify their schedules to facilitate fathers' engagement in parent-teacher meetings, and resulted in higher attendance rates by parents (Grosso Richins et al., 2021). Furthermore, facilitating a culturally and linguistically responsive environment may include involving extended family and having bilingual staff, given that extended family are more frequently involved in the care of Latinx children than in other groups. It is therefore important to recognize the role that *familismo* plays in Latinx families and how integrating this value may make an unfamiliar environment more welcoming for Latinx families.

Though these accommodations are emerging out of the field of education, these practical solutions emerging from innovative research with Latinx families may be reasonably extrapolated to psychological assessment and interventions until further research specific to psychological assessments and interventions emerges. This may include further research on whether mobile health interventions (i.e., app-based interventions) facilitate or hinder participation among Latinx families. Parenting and family researchers and practitioners are encouraged to think about the multiple ways by which Latinx children development can be promoted beyond traditional parenting practices generated from research with European American families.

WORKING WITH LATINX FAMILIES USING CULTURALLY RESPONSIVE STRATEGIES AND VALIDATING LATINX STRENGTHS

Considering the factors reviewed in this chapter, culturally responsive strategies for working with Latinx families may include:

Advocacy. Integrating advocacy into practice is essential for working with Latinx families. Working with Latinx families may involve multiple roles as advocates, including advocacy as mental health professionals and as civically engaged community members (Delgado-Romero et al., 2021). It has previously been acknowledged that these multiple roles may often conflict with professional ethical guidelines. However, such ethical codes need to acknowledge their role in burdening and limiting access for Latinx families, for example, by increasing paperwork requirements by Latinx families. The National Latinx Psychological Association has published their own ethical guidelines that address ethical issues in the psychological treatment and training of Latinx people (see National Latinx Psychological Association, 2020).

Carefully tailor interventions - beyond literal translations. Tailoring and adapting interventions for Latinx families should involve more than literal translations of intervention content (Cabrera et al., 2021). Instead, tailoring interventions for Latinx families should involve systematically adapting interventions to ensure the fit of the interventions with Latinx values and culture. This is an area where the use of implementation science frameworks, such as the Exploration, Preparation, Implementation, and Sustainment framework, to systematically adapt interventions for specific groups may make substantial contributions to our work with Latinx families (Moullin et al., 2020). Similarly, just because an intervention is shown to promote the desired behavior among middle-class European American families, this does not indicate that increase in such behavior is compatible with Latinx values and cultures. By the same token, when incorporating extended family and fathers in interventions, these should be smooth and specific integrations for how extended family and fathers are involved in Latinx families, rather than simple "add-ons" to interventions (Cabrera et al., 2021).

Using interventions for Latinx families. When possible, using interventions that were specifically developed for Latinx families is preferred. For example, Brief Strategic Family Therapy (BSFT) is an evidence-based intervention for families of adolescents who engage in problematic behaviors (i.e., substance use). BSFT was developed for Latinx youth and their families by practitioners who work with Latinx youth (Szapocznik & Hervis, 2020). Specifically, BSFT was developed with and for Latinx immigrant families experiencing intergenerational family conflict related to cultural issues, with the goal of reducing conflicts that influenced youth problem behaviors (i.e., drug use, delinquency). Superficially adapted interventions that omit or dismiss acculturative stress or intergenerational conflict may result in decreased engagement.

Minimizing bureaucracy. Because of the high proportion of undocumented immigrants among the growing Latinx population in the United States, asking Latinx families to provide proof of documentation may influence whether Latinx families access services. Asking families to navigate these complex bureaucratic systems not only creates more barriers for undocumented families, but also those from low socioeconomic or immigrant backgrounds who do not know how to navigate these systems. These bureaucratic procedures are further complicated by limited English proficiency in Latinx immigrant families. More so, they can put an undue burden on children to provide language brokering while navigating such bureaucracies.

CONCLUDING THOUGHTS

Accompanying Latinx families in their healing is a social justice endeavor requiring constant learning and unlearning on our part.. As noted in this chapter, expanding our concepts of Latinx adolescence and parenting highlights the necessity to move beyond comparative analysis and understand how adolescence and parenting are situated within contextual realities perpetuated by citizenship, immigration, and racialization. Families are affected in myriad ways, and by dismissing such realities and the ethnic heterogeneity of families, our work will fall short in addressing the oppressive ecologies families succumbed to (Carlo et al., 2022). Our work must also extend to the literal translation of assessments to ensure diligent adapted assessments are available to families to challenge thus deficit-based discourses that dismiss the knowledge, creativity, and strengths Latinx families possess. More so, assessment tools utilized within systems, such as education and child welfare, may utilize assessments that are not culturally appropriate and further perpetuate oppression based on these findings. Challenging and creating assessment tools by us and for us is of high importance. Finally, this work is a political act that simultaneously challenges our unreasonable expectations and beliefs about Latinx families, challenging systems of oppression and assisting families in their consiensazation. Thus, practicing patience, grace, accountability, and compassion with our clients and ourselves is necessary to ensure that we allocate the difficulties of this work to our broader socio-political realities and legacies of intergenerational trauma.

REFERENCES

Abrego, L. J., & Hernández, E. (2021). 13.# FamiliesBelongTogether: Central American Family Separations from the 1980s to 2019. In Critical Dialogues in Latinx Studies (pp. 173-185). New York University Press.

Adames, H. Y., & Chavez-Dueñas, N. Y. (2017). *Cultural foundations and interventions in Latino/a mental health: History, theory, and within group differences*. Routledge.

Arnett, J. J. (2016). Life stage concepts across history and cultures: Proposal for a new field on indigenous life stages. *Human Development, 59*(5), 290–316. doi:10.1159/000453627

Azmitia, M. (2021). Latinx Adolescents' Assets, Risks, and Developmental Pathways: A Decade in Review and Looking Ahead. *Journal of Research on Adolescence, 31*(4), 989–1005. doi:10.1111/jora.12686 PMID:34820953

Becker Herbst, R., Sabet, R. F., Swanson, A., Suarez, L. G., Marques, D. S., Ameen, E. J., & Aldarondo, E. (2018). "They were going to kill me": Resilience in unaccompanied immigrant minors. *The Counseling Psychologist, 46*(2), 241–268. doi:10.1177/0011000018759769

Bermúdez, J. M., & Bermúdez, S. (2002). Altar-making with Latino families: A narrative therapy perspective. *Journal of Family Psychotherapy, 13*(3/4), 329–347. doi:10.1300/J085v13n03_06

Boss, P. (1999). *Ambiguous loss: learning to live with unresolved grief.* Harvard University Press.

Cabrera, N. J., Alonso, A., & Chen, Y. (2021). Parenting contributions to Latinx children's development in the early years. *The Annals of the American Academy of Political and Social Science, 696*(1), 158–178. doi:10.1177/00027162211049997

Cardoso, J. B., & Thompson, S. J. (2010). Common Themes of Resilience among Latino Immigrant Families: A Systematic Review of the Literature. *Families in Society, 91*(3), 257–265. doi:10.1606/1044-3894.4003

Carlo, G., Murry, V. M., Davis, A. N., Gonzalez, C. M., & Debreaux, M. L. (2022). Culture-Related Adaptive Mechanisms to Race-Related Trauma Among African American and US Latinx Youth. *Adversity and Resilience Science*, 1-13.

Causadias, J. M., Vitriol, J. A., & Atkin, A. L. (2018). Do we overemphasize the role of culture in the behavior of racial/ethnic minorities? Evidence of a cultural (mis) attribution bias in American psychology. *The American Psychologist, 73*(3), 243–255. doi:10.1037/amp0000099 PMID:29355353

Chaplin, T. M., Cole, P. M., & Zahn-Waxler, C. (2005). Parental socialization of emotion expression: Gender differences and relations to child adjustment. *Emotion (Washington, D.C.), 5*(1), 80–88. doi:10.1037/1528-3542.5.1.80 PMID:15755221

Chen, S. H., Kennedy, M., & Zhou, Q. (2012). Parents' expression and discussion of emotion in the multilingual family: Does language matter? *Perspectives on Psychological Science, 7*(4), 365–383. doi:10.1177/1745691612447307 PMID:26168473

Delgado-Romero, E. A., Mahoney, G., Muro-Rodriguez, N. J., Atilano, R., Cárdenas Bautista, E., De Los Santos, J., Durán, M. Y., Espinoza, L., Fuentes, J., Gomez, S. N., Ingram Estevez, R. E., Jimenez-Ruiz, J., Monroig Garcia, M. M., Mora-Ozuna, C. J., Ordaz, A. C., Rappaport, B., Suazo-Padilla, K., & Vazquez, M. (2021). La Clinica In LaK'ech: Establishing a practicum site integrating practice, advocacy, and research with Latinx clients. *The Counseling Psychologist, 49*(7), 987–1012. doi:10.1177/00110000211025270

Dorner, L. M., Orellana, M. F., & Jiménez, R. (2008). "It's one of those things that you do to help the family" language brokering and the development of immigrant adolescents. *Journal of Adolescent Research, 23*(5), 515–543. doi:10.1177/0743558408317563

Dreby, J. (2006). Honor and virtue: Mexican parenting in the transnational context. *Gender & Society, 20*(1), 32–59. doi:10.1177/0891243205282660

Falicov, C. J. (2019). Transnational journeys. In M. McGoldrick & K. Hardy (Eds.), *Revisioning culture, race and class in family therapy* (3rd ed., pp. 108–122). Guilford Press.

Fuller, B., & García Coll, C. (2010). Learning from Latinos: Contexts, families, and child development in motion. *Developmental Psychology*, *46*(3), 559–565. doi:10.1037/a0019412 PMID:20438170

Galvan, T., & Gudino, O. (2019). Understanding Latinx youth mental health disparities by problem type: The role of caregiver culture. *Psychological Services*, *18*(1), 116–123. Advance online publication. doi:10.1037er0000365 PMID:31192675

Garza, Y., & Bratton, S. (2005). School-based child centered play therapy with Hispanic children: Outcomes and cultural consideration. *International Journal of Play Therapy*, *14*(1), 51–80. doi:10.1037/h0088896

Germán, M., Gonzales, N. A., & Dumka, L. (2009). Familism Values as a Protective Factor for Mexican-origin Adolescents Exposed to Deviant Peers. *The Journal of Early Adolescence*, *29*(1), 16–42. doi:10.1177/0272431608324475 PMID:21776180

Gonzales, R. G., Suárez-Orozco, C., & Dedios-Sanguineti, M. C. (2013). No Place to Belong: Contextualizing Concepts of Mental Health Among Undocumented Immigrant Youth in the United States. *The American Behavioral Scientist*, *57*(8), 1174–1199. doi:10.1177/0002764213487349

Gonzalez, C., Early, J., Gordon-Dseagu, V., Mata, T., & Nieto, C. (2021). Promoting Culturally Tailored mHealth: A Scoping Review of Mobile Health Interventions in Latinx Communities. *Journal of Immigrant and Minority Health*, *23*(5), 1065–1077. doi:10.100710903-021-01209-4 PMID:33988789

Gonzalez, L. M., Stein, G. L., Prandoni, J. I., Eades, M. P., & Magalhaes, R. (2015). *Perceptions of Undocumented Status and Possible Selves Among Latino/a Youth*. The Counseling. doi:10.1177/0011000015608951

Grosso Richins, L., Hansen-Thomas, H., Lozada, V., South, S., & Stewart, M. A. (2021). Understanding the power of Latinx families to support the academic and personal development of their children. *Bilingual Research Journal*, *44*(3), 1–20. doi:10.1080/15235882.2021.1998806

Huq, N., Stein, G. L., & Gonzalez, L. M. (2016). Acculturation Conflict Among Latino Youth: Discrimination, Ethnic Identity, and Depressive Symptoms. *Cultural Diversity & Ethnic Minority Psychology*, *22*(3), 377–385. doi:10.1037/cdp0000070 PMID:26460666

Hurley, K. D., Huscroft-D'Angelo, J., Trout, A., Griffith, A., & Epstein, M. (2014). Assessing parenting skills and attitudes: A review of the psychometrics of parenting measures. *Journal of Child and Family Studies*, *23*(5), 812–823. doi:10.100710826-013-9733-2

Kassem, N., Rum, Y., & Perry, A. (2022). To feel and talk in a language of conflict: Distinct emotional experience and expression of bilinguals among disadvantaged minority members. *Journal of Multilingual and Multicultural Development*.

Lawton, K. E., & Gerdes, A. C. (2014). Acculturation and Latino adolescent mental health: Integration of individual, environmental, and family influences. *Clinical Child and Family Psychology Review*, *17*(4), 385–398. doi:10.100710567-014-0168-0 PMID:24794635

Lenz, A. S., Gómez Soler, I., Dell'Aquilla, J., & Uribe, P. M. (2017). Translation and cross-cultural adaptation of assessments for use in counseling research. *Measurement & Evaluation in Counseling & Development*, *50*(4), 224–231. doi:10.1080/07481756.2017.1320947

López, B. G., Lezama, E., & Heredia, D. Jr. (2019). Language brokering experience affects feelings toward bilingualism, language knowledge, use, and practices: A qualitative approach. *Hispanic Journal of Behavioral Sciences*, *41*(4), 481–503. doi:10.1177/0739986319879641

Lu, Y., He, Q., & Brooks-Gunn, J. (2020). Diverse experience of immigrant children: How do separation and reunification shape their development? *Child Development*, *91*(1), e146–e163. doi:10.1111/cdev.13171

Martinez, C. R. Jr, McClure, H. H., & Eddy, J. M. (2009). Language brokering contexts and behavioral and emotional adjustment among Latino parents and adolescents. *The Journal of Early Adolescence*, *29*(1), 71–98. doi:10.1177/0272431608324477 PMID:19898605

Meca, A., Gonzales-Backen, M., Davis, R., Rodil, J., Soto, D., & Unger, J. B. (2020). Discrimination and Ethnic Identity: Establishing Directionality among Latino/a Youth. *Developmental Psychology*, *56*(5), 982–992. doi:10.1037/dev0000908 PMID:32105119

Meca, A., Moreno, O., Cobb, C., Lorenzo-Blanco, E. I., Schwartz, S. J., Cano, M. Á., Zamboanga, B. L., Gonzales-Backen, M., Szapocznik, J., Unger, J. B., Baezconde-Garbanati, L., & Soto, D. W. (2021). Directional effects in cultural identity: A family systems approach for immigrant Latinx families. *Journal of Youth and Adolescence*, *50*(5), 965–977. doi:10.100710964-021-01406-2 PMID:33599938

Mendez, L. O., & Cortina, K. S. (2021). Within Group Ethnic Diversity in Latinx Psychological Research: A Publication Analysis. *Hispanic Journal of Behavioral Sciences*, *43*(1-2), 114–130. doi:10.1177/0739986321996478

Menjívar, C. (2006). Liminal legality: Salvadoran and Guatemalan immigrants' lives in the United States 1. *American Journal of Sociology*, *111*(4), 999–1037. doi:10.1086/499509

Moll, L. C., Amanti, C., Neff, D., & Gonzalez, N. (1992). Funds of knowledge for teaching: Using a qualitative approach to connect homes and classrooms. *Theory into Practice*, *31*(2), 132–141. doi:10.1080/00405849209543534

Morales, A., & Wang, K. T. (2018). The relationship among language brokering, parent–child bonding, and mental health correlates among Latinx college students. *Journal of Mental Health Counseling*, *40*(4), 316–327. doi:10.17744/mehc.40.4.04

Moullin, J. C., Dickson, K. S., Stadnick, N. A., Albers, B., Nilsen, P., Broder-Fingert, S., Mukasa, B., & Aarons, G. A. (2020). Ten recommendations for using implementation frameworks in research and practice. *Implementation Science Communications*, *1*(1), 1-12.

National Hispanic and Latino MHTTC. (2019, October 28). *Complicated grief: Cultural considerations when working with loss in Hispanic and Latino Students and their families*. https://mhttcnetwork.org/centers/national-hispanic-and-latino-mhttc/product/complicated-grief-cultural-considerations-when

National Latinx Psychological Association. (2020). Ethical guidelines of the National Latinx Psychological Association. *Journal of Latina/o Psychology*, *8*(2), 101–111. doi:10.1037/lat0000151

Nielsen, M., Haun, D., Kärtner, J., & Legare, C. H. (2017). The persistent sampling bias in developmental psychology: A call to action. *Journal of Experimental Child Psychology*, *162*, 31–38. doi:10.1016/j.jecp.2017.04.017 PMID:28575664

Parra, C. J. R. (2019). Healing through parenting: An intervention delivery and process of change model developed with low-income Latina/o immigrant families. *Family Process*, *58*(1), 34–52. doi:10.1111/famp.12429 PMID:30786004

Pelaez Lopez, A. (2018). *The X in Latinx is a wound, not a trend.* Color Bloq's X Collection. Retrieved May 11, 2022, from https://www.colorbloq.org/article/the-x-in-latinx-is-a-wound-not-a-trend

Piña-Watson, B., Gonzalez, I. M., & Manzo, G. (2019). Mexican-descent adolescent resilience through familismo in the context of intergeneration acculturation conflict on depressive symptoms. *Translational Issues in Psychological Science*, *5*(4), 326–334. doi:10.1037/tps0000210

Pizarro, C. (2021). Children with unspeakable trauma: Unaccompanied minors and family separations. *Play Therapy*, *16*(3), 20–23.

Potochnick, S. R., & Perreira, K. M. (2010). Depression and Anxiety among First-Generation Immigrant Latino Youth: Key Correlates and Implications for Future Research. *The Journal of Nervous and Mental Disease*, *198*(7), 470–477. doi:10.1097/NMD.0b013e3181e4ce24 PMID:20611049

Ramos, G., Ponting, C., Bocanegra, E., Chodzen, G., Delgadillo, D., Rapp, A., Escovar, E., & Chavira, D. (2021). Discrimination and Internalizing Symptoms in Rural Latinx Adolescents: The Protective Role of Family Resilience. *Journal of Clinical Child and Adolescent Psychology*, 1–14. doi:10.1080/15374416.2021.1923018 PMID:34038290

Ramos-Zayas, A. Y., & Rúa, M. M. (Eds.). (2021). *Critical Dialogues in Latinx Studies: A Reader.* NYU Press. doi:10.18574/nyu/9781479805198.001.0001

Reyes, J. A., & Elias, M. J. (2011). Fostering social–emotional resilience among Latino youth. *Psychology in the Schools*, *48*(7), 723–737. doi:10.1002/pits.20580

Rios Casas, F., Ryan, D., Perez, G., Maurer, S., Tran, A. N., Rao, D., & Ornelas, I. J. (2020). "Se vale llorar y se vale reír": Latina immigrants' coping strategies for maintaining mental health in the face of immigration-related stressors. *Journal of Racial and Ethnic Health Disparities*, *7*(5), 937–948. doi:10.100740615-020-00717-7 PMID:32040841

Rodriguez, M. C., & Morrobel, D. (2004). A review of Latino youth development research and a call for an asset orientation. *Hispanic Journal of Behavioral Sciences*, *26*(2), 107–127. doi:10.1177/0739986304264268

Rodriguez, V. J., La Barrie, D. L., Zegarac, M., & Shaffer, A. (2021). A systematic review of parenting scales the literature on measurement invariance/equivalence of parenting scales by race and ethnicity: Recommendations for inclusive parenting research. *Assessment*. Advance online publication. doi:10.1177/10731911211038630

Rodriguez, V. J., Shaffer, A., Are, F., Madden, A., Jones, D. L., & Kumar, M. (2019). Identification of differential item functioning by race and ethnicity in the Childhood Trauma Questionnaire. *Child Abuse & Neglect*, *94*, 104030. doi:10.1016/j.chiabu.2019.104030 PMID:31181398

Schwartz, S. J., & Unger, J. B. (2010). Biculturalism and context: What is biculturalism, and when is it adaptive?: Commentary on Mistry and Wu. *Human Development, 53*(1), 26–32. doi:10.1159/000268137 PMID:22475719

Serrano-Villar, M., & Calzada, E. J. (2016). Ethnic identity: Evidence of protective effects for young, Latino children. *Journal of Applied Developmental Psychology, 42*, 21–30. doi:10.1016/j.appdev.2015.11.002 PMID:26778873

Shen, J. J., & Dennis, J. M. (2019). The family context of language brokering among Latino/a young adults. *Journal of Social and Personal Relationships, 36*(1), 131–152. doi:10.1177/0265407517721379

Sladek, M. R., Umaña-Taylor, A. J., Hardesty, J. L., Aguilar, G., Bates, D., Bayless, S. D., Gomez, E., Hur, C. K., Ison, A., Jones, S., Luo, H., Satterthwaite-Freiman, M., & Vázquez, M. A. (2022). "So, like, it's all a mix of one": Intersecting contexts of adolescents' ethnic-racial socialization. *Child Development, 93*(5), 1284–1303. doi:10.1111/cdev.13756 PMID:35366330

Sue, S. (1999). Science, ethnicity, and bias: Where have we gone wrong? *The American Psychologist, 54*(12), 1070–1077. doi:10.1037/0003-066X.54.12.1070 PMID:15332528

Szapocznik, J., & Hervis, O. E. (2020). *Brief strategic family therapy*. American Psychological Association. doi:10.1037/0000169-000

Szapocznik, J., & Kurtines, W. M. (1993). Family psychology and cultural diversity: Opportunities for theory, research, and application. *The American Psychologist, 48*(4), 400–407. doi:10.1037/0003-066X.48.4.400

Taylor, Z. E., Ruiz, Y., Nair, N., & Mishra, A. A. (2020). Family support and mental health of Latinx children in migrant farmworker families. *Applied Developmental Science*, 1–18. doi:10.1080/10888691.2020.1800466

Telzer, E. H. (2010). Expanding the acculturation gap-distress model: An integrative review of research. *Human Development, 53*(6), 313–340. doi:10.1159/000322476

Torres, L., Yznaga, S. D., & Moore, K. M. (2011). Discrimination and Latino Psychological Distress: The Moderating Role of Ethnic Identity Exploration and Commitment. *The American Journal of Orthopsychiatry, 81*(4), 526–534. doi:10.1111/j.1939-0025.2011.01117.x PMID:21977938

Torres, S. A., Santiago, C. D., Walts, K. K., & Richards, M. H. (2018). Immigration policy, practices, and procedures: The impact on the mental health of Mexican and Central American youth and families. *The American Psychologist, 73*(7), 843–854. doi:10.1037/amp0000184 PMID:29504782

Torres, S. A., Sosa, S. S., Flores Toussaint, R. J., Jolie, S., & Bustos, Y. (2022). Systems of Oppression: The Impact of Discrimination on Latinx Immigrant Adolescents' Well-Being and Development. *Journal of Research on Adolescence, 32*(2), 501–517. doi:10.1111/jora.12751 PMID:35365889

Umaña-Taylor, A. J., & Updegraff, K. A. (2007). Latino adolescents' mental health: Exploring the interrelations among discrimination, ethnic identity, cultural orientation, self-esteem, and depressive symptoms. *Journal of Adolescence, 30*(4), 549–567. doi:10.1016/j.adolescence.2006.08.002 PMID:17056105

Zhou, M. (1997). Segmented assimilation: Issues, controversies, and recent research on the new second generation. *The International Migration Review*, *31*(4), 975–1008. doi:10.1177/019791839703100408 PMID:12293212

Zimmerman, M. A. (1990). Toward a theory of learned hopefulness: A structural model analysis of participation and empowerment. *Journal of Research in Personality*, *24*(1), 71–86. doi:10.1016/0092-6566(90)90007-S

Chapter 13
Un Paso Adelante (A Step Forward):
A Family's Migration Testimonino and Recommendations for Mental Health Providers

Elizabeth Cárdenas Bautista
Cambridge Health Alliance, Harvard Medical School, USA

Gabriela Cárdenas
Independent Researcher, USA

Manuela Silvia Bautista Gil
Independent Researcher, USA

Mario Cárdenas Villanueva
Independent Researcher, USA

ABSTRACT

This chapter includes powerful testimoninos in Spanish and English of the history and impact of immigration on individual and familial levels. Framed from the perspective of different family members, the authors share their migration experience to the U.S. South between 1980 and 1990. Topics of pre-migration, acculturation, trauma, the impact of post-migration experiences, and psychological growth are addressed from the perspective of first-generation Mexican immigrants and children of immigrants. The chapter also provides recommendations for mental health providers as they assess and conceptualize Latinx immigrant communities in the U.S. South.

DOI: 10.4018/978-1-6684-4901-1.ch013

Un Paso Adelante (A Step Forward)

INTRODUCTION

All the authors of this chapter are members of the Cardenas-Bautista family. In it we share the migration experiences of our family to the United States between (U.S.) 1980 and 1990. The *testimoninos* that we share describe the pre- and post-migration experiences from the perspective of a father, mother, and two siblings. In particular, we talk about how our family experiences in the U.S. South. Our migration stories, shared from four different perspectives, provide an insightful description of the history and impact of immigration on an individual and familial level. Our *testimoninos* seek to connect with readers who may share similar experiences and provide mental health providers with recommendations to consider while working with Latinx immigrant populations in the southern regions of the U.S. We conclude our chapter by providing recommendations that go beyond considerations of language acquisition and acculturation. Through our stories and recommendations our objective is to move away from the generalization of complex personal history of a community and encourage the introspective dive of rich *historias* that we carry beyond borders and time. It is also our intention to keep the *testimonios* of our father and mother in the language they chose to write their stories. Readers can find the English versions of their stories in the X. We note that not including the English version of their testimonios represents our intention to relocate our gaze of the reader.

LA DESCENDENCIA DE UN SOBREVIVIENTE ANTIGUO

Un Testimonio de Padre

Mario Cárdenas Villanueva

Yo nunca pensé que pudiera compartí mi historia, pero mi familia tiene una historia de inmigración que vino más antes de mi propio viaje al Norte. Siendo yo nacido de una población de San Miguel Enyege, Municipio de Ixtlahuaca, Pueblo Masagua, podría decir que yo estaba creciendo sin presencia de mi padre pues nos frecuentaba seguido, en mi hogar esta mi mama y mis hermanos. Soy el penúltimo de siete hermanos y nuestra responsabilidad era estudiar hasta que pudiéramos y trabajar. En una ocasión, salí de clases y le pedir un *ride* a una camioneta. Al bajar se me quedó un pie atorado y la camioneta me arrastró. Ese día, yo perdí parte del cuero cabelludo de mi cabeza. Por este accidente yo estuve hospitalizado un año y al salir mis padres emigraron al Estado de México con nuestra vacas y puercos. Comenzando a sobrevivir en colonia era fuerte. Empezaba trabajando duro con más necesidades de agua, luz, drenaje, nueva escuela. Para ayudarnos económicamente mis padres pusieron una tienda, y yo cuida a mis vacas y asistir a clases. Con el resto de mi tiempo surtir la tienda de mercancía, con transporte público. Yo recuerdo que llevaba costales de papá, cajas de plátano, cajas de jitomate, un costal de naranja, y todo era en bultos. Pasaron los años y los hermanos se casaron y se acabó la tienda. Se vendieron las vacas, y mi vida era muy presionada por la zona urbana que era grande. Mis medios me permitieron estudia hasta el sexto año y empecé a trabajar en una fábrica de piezas de carro.

 No había nada de superación. La policía presionaba al joven. Todo el tiempo lo arrestaba, golpeaba, y en el año 1980 era fuerte, como hasta hoy. Mis amigos estaban en toda la colonia, y de tantos amigos había un jovencito, que en paz descanse, había venido a Houston, Texas. Y me invitó a que viniéramos para la oportunidad de supéranos. Yo era muy aventado al trabajo, pues mi niñez siempre era de trabajo.

Un Paso Adelante (A Step Forward)

Trate de venirme sin permiso de mamá, ya que yo era el brazo derecho de mamá para todo y sabía que ella no quería que me fuera. Pero me fui de todos modos, al salir a la terminal de camiones de la Ciudad de México a Matamoros, mi mamá, sin yo saber, me alcanzó atravesando una avenida, y con un fuerte grito me dijo:

Dijo mi mamá: "¿Y a dónde vas Mario!?"

Yo contesté: "¡A Estado Unidos, con plan de trabajar!"

Dijo mi mamá: "Por favor regresa!"

Yo contesté: "No, yo me voy."

Dijo mi mamá (con voz anhelante): "Que Dios te acompañe mi hijo."

En mi primer viaje llegamos a Matamoros con frontera a Brownsville, Texas. Hicimos travesía de dos días con una noche, caminamos, nos subimos en tren, y en camión. A fin llegar a Houston, me gane mi vida de jornalero. Tres meses después, con mucho esfuerzo, mande $300 USD a mi mamá. En ese tiempo el dólar lo pagaban a 12 Pesos. Y mi mamá me manda a decir que lo iba a guardar en mi cuenta de banco.

A reflexionar mi experiencia en este País (Estados Unidos) era no estar en casa con una comida recién hecha por mamá. Aquí no había comodidad, había uno que otro hombre con fisonomía Hispana, pero no querían hablar español. Los negocios que frecuentábamos eran de Negros, Asiático y Blancos. Trabaje en un restaurante limpiando mesas de 9:00 am a 12:00 pm y mi transporte era una bicicleta. No me molestaba nadie. Era muy diferente a mi país. Vivíamos solo hombres y era solitario en parte. Regresé a los Estado Unidos con una visión más clara, había mejor oportunidad para tener una vida mejor y poder ayudar a mis hermanos. Pero como había posibilidad también había tragedia. Durante mi camino de regreso, pase una experiencia muy desagradable. Perdí a un amigo en el Río Grande de Matamoros, que en paz descansé.

Regresé a México y continué mi noviazgo y me casé con mi amada Silvia, *Mi Chivís*. Construimos nuestra casa con dos cuartos y un baño, se me acabó el dinero en casamiento y poca construcción. Y otra vez me fui a Houston, Texas y trabajé por temporadas de un año y medio. Y hacía mis viajes de regreso a México. Tuvimos tres hermosas niñas, Eva, Gaby, y Eli. Las cuales siempre han formado mucha fortaleza en mi vida. Fortaleza de no ver obstáculos. Aunque cada que me despedía lloraban y yo también lloraba en el camión, solo por horas. Esta parte de mi vida son mucho recuerdo, muchos vacíos, soledad, tristeza, pero al final uno se hace fuerte y vive la aceptación que emigrar de un país a otro es muy devástate y peligroso. Pero uno lo hacía por la familia y la familia es lo que te da la fortaleza de necesitamos.

En estos tiempos, a llegar a Georgia me di cuenta como acceso a clases básicas de inglés me podían ayudar a apoyarme e integrar. Me hubiera ayudado tener acceso a un psicólogo o consejero, una terapia en español, pero en este tiempo no había nadie. Normalmente tomamos un ritmo, que la vida es solitaria, caminar adelante, trabajar y luchar. Pero la realidad es que lo más importante es tener familia con uno. La vida si es de luchar y sobrevivir, pero no te puedes olvidar, que la vida puede ser más que sobrevivir. Antes que mi familia llego a Georgia, yo pensaba que tenía todo, pero no estaba completo. A llegar mi esposa, fue a renacer, era mi refuerzo. Después de un gran esfuerzo y gracias a Dios llegaron mis hijas, era una cosa tan profunda, mi vida era completa. Estar la familia separada era difícil, pero tratas de no darte cuenta. Se me olvidaba que había sufrido. Pero a estar juntos en familia te encuentras con una profunda alegra, energía y a través del apoyo de sientes fortalecido. Te das cuenta de que te faltaba. A llegar mi familia, casi fue como otra vez ser un niño, ahí compartiendo con todos.

UN PASO ADELANTE

Un Testimonio de una Madre

Manuela Silvia Bautista Gil

"En la vida se toman decisiones que no entendemos en ese momento, porqué las hacemos: pero con el paso del tiempo descubrimos para que lo hicimos."

Manuela Silvia Cardenas es el nombre de casada, mi nombre es Manuela Silvia Bautista Gil, tengo 56 años, mi esposo Mario Cardenas y nuestras 3 hijas: Eva María Cardenas, Gabriela E. Cardenas y Elizabeth Cardenas Bautista. Tengo 28 años en Estados Unidos, llegue en Mayo 22 de 1995, entre por San Isidro California, venia en una peregrinación religiosa de la iglesia de mi lugar de origen en México, y para mayo 24, me encontraba ya en Atlanta, Georgia, lugar al que llegue y continuo aquí.

Cual fue la razón que me hizo emigrar a este país; saben la mayoría de la gente lo hace por buscar un futuro mejor, por la necesidad económica, por la guerra, por razones políticas, pero mi historia es diferente, nunca lo pensé como un plan a futuro, solo sabía que mi esposo ya estaba en Estados Unidos, que trabajaba, con lo que ganaba envía remesas para mantenernos y después de un periodo determinado regresaba, estaba con nosotros un tiempo breve y volvía a regresar, ese era el sistema de vida que llevábamos, al cual me había acostumbrado, pero no me daba cuenta que eso no era correcto, que eso no era un matrimonio, que no era una familia y sobre todo no era sano para nuestras hijas y para nosotros como pareja, pero había necesidades en la familia y el esposo buscaba la oportunidad y esa oportunidad estaba en Estados Unidos.

En febrero de 1995, estando mi esposo en Atlanta, trabajando en la construcción sufre un accidente del cual queda en mala condición, el accidente es la caída de una altura aproximada de 2 pisos y al caer cae de espalda sobre unos botes, eso le hiso tener una lesión en su espalda, en su columna vertebral, me entere de lo sucedido y a partir de ahí empieza la razón por la cual tuve que emigrar a Estados unidos. Esa noticia me lleva a pensar lo más extremoso de la realidad, las ideas vinieron a mi mente; Que hacer?, Como podría yo ir a verle?, Como dejar a nuestras hijas?, Eran tan pequeñas Eva 7 años, Gaby 5 años, Eli 2 años, como dejarlas?, Si las cosas no estaban bien con papa, que les diría yo a ellas?, Que explicación les daría para irme, eran pequeñas, ellas no entenderían?, Y si algo me sucede y mi regreso se demora?; muchas preguntas sin respuesta pasaron por mi mente. Hable con mis padres y me apoyaron, ese era un buen comienzo, gracias a Dios el Párroco de mi Parroquia, me permitió ingresar en el grupo de peregrinos que venían para California, en peregrinación de nuestra Señora de Rosario de Talpa y pude venir sin enfrentar esos riesgos tan grandes que sufren todos nuestros hermanos migrantes.

Mi razón, mi motivo, mi necesidad fue buscar y ayudar en la salud y rehabilitación de mi esposo y padre de mis hijas, poder decirles a ellas, su papi está bien y pronto regresaremos con ustedes. En mi vida la decisión más difícil fue esa, dejar a mis hijas, buena madre no fui, pero las amaba, a mi manera, con lo que tenía para darles y tuve que tomar una decisión, la tome porque debía de hacerlo, pero no la tome porque quisiera hacerlo.

Los primeros 3 años fueron los más difíciles y desgastantes de mi vida, en un país lejano, sin familia, solo mi esposo y yo, sin amigos, un idioma que no hablaba, una cultura diferente, no documentos para trabajar, estar siempre en la angustia de no poder estar en libertad, trabajos fuertes y mal pagados a causa de no saber manejar para buscar otros trabajos mejores, angustia de saber que las hijas están lejos, que necesitan su ayuda económica, no poder comunicarse con ellas con la frecuencia que debería, por el salario tan poco, pagar renta, agua, luz, gas, comida y tener que enviar para ellas, mes con mes tratar de economizar lo más posible. En muchas ocasiones una sola comida para mi esposo y para mí en todo el día; la frustración de ir al médico con mi esposo y no poder expresar sus condiciones de salud, no poder tener un tiempo para descansar, esperando la pronta mejora de salud de mi esposo, su recuperación para poder empezar a trabajar, fue difícil, pero gracias a Dios vivido y trascendido.

Cuales eran mis expectativas. Recuerdo que cuando salí de mi país no esperaba nada, solo quería llegar para saber el estado real de salud de mi esposo y ver qué es lo que podía hacer por él, sabiendo que no sería algo bueno, que iba a pasar un momento fuerte pero me preparaba para ello.

La realidad de lo que pasaba era fuerte ya que cuando yo llegue, Mario estaba en malas condiciones, vivía con algunos amigos, pero vivía mal, en un pequeño cuarto con un sillón por cama todo en malas condiciones y el con su daño de espalda, lo primero que pensé fue: esta situación le está empeorando su condición, debemos de cambiar todo esto. Agradecí que no fueran tan grandes como lo había pensado, gracias a Dios podía moverse con dolor y dificultad pero lo podía hacer.

Al llegar a este país, tuve que trabajar de inmediato no había tiempo para esperar, la conexión fue mediante la mano de obra que podía yo proporcionar, integrarme a la cultura de ellos por medio del trabajo, no tuve la oportunidad de hacerlo de otro manera. Lo que me admiro fue el orden, la capacitación, el desempeño que se tiene en los trabajos, en aquel tiempo siempre fui mano de obra no calificada, trabaje de limpiadora de cuartos housekeeper, trabajo demasiado pesado, mis respetos para estos trabajadores ya que están en trabajos duros, pesados y mal remunerados y se mantienen ahí, trabaje limpiando cocinas de hoteles, trabajo de limpieza en restaurantes-bufet, limpieza de oficinas, mesera. En estos trabajos siempre había juntas de seguridad, de poder exponer las necesidades del trabajador, tenía uno un horario y se respetaba, tiempo que se pasara o tuvieran uno que trabajar más, tiempo que era pagado como extra, eso nunca lo vi en mi país, en los lugares que trabaje, y trabaje en oficinas como secretaria, ahí se veía la preferencia, la barbería, quedar mejor con el jefe para que tuviera preferencia, sueldos mal pagados, no respetaban el horario, eran abusivos. En el tiempo que trabaje aquí como trabajador no calificado pensaba que si esta situación estaba bien como debería estar la situación en los trabajos calificados; en las ocasiones que me toco ir al doctor, o alguna oficina de servicio me daba cuenta de cómo era el ambiente ahí y como se portaba el personal y entendí que este país tiene buenos puntos en su cultura y para mí se debe a su nivel de educación que tiene sus habitantes, se cómo en todos los países hay personas que tal vez no tienen educación pero entre más el país ponga empeño en la educación de sus habitantes, ese país será más de progreso. Una cultura muy independiente, pero con oportunidades para los que tiene el deseo y la oportunidad de aprovechar. En México, mi país es muy penoso lo que voy a mencionar, pero esa es mi experiencia la gente con educación es la menos accesible, es la más déspota, la que cree que todo se lo merece y desprecia a la gente sin educación y se aprovecha de ella. Aquí lo que me ha tocado experimentar, la gente te da respeto y atención sin importar tu apariencia o tu grado de escuela y eso lo hace la persona que trabaja contigo como trabajador general y también aquel profesional que

Un Paso Adelante (A Step Forward)

te atiende te da ese mismo respeto sin importarle tu apariencia o escuela, puedes ir de tu trabajo con tu uniforme y sucio y te respetan y te atienden. La autoridad que tiene la usan adecuadamente con todos, puede tener sus casos diferentes, pero en mi experiencia cuando yo llegue a este país fue de la manera que les comento. Cada quien tiene sus valores y principios que nos ensenar en casa, esos nunca los cambiare, esos seguirán conmigo y espero que mis hijas y mas generaciones los conserven. La familia es algo muy importante que siempre tiene que permanecer y perseverar con sus principios y valores y eso no se debe perder.

La educación de este país también forma parte de su cultura, y eso a mí me impacto al darme cuenta de la importancia que se le da que cada niño asista a la escuela, saber que la educación básica en este país es hasta el nivel de preparatoria (high school), como base de educación, vaya eso si me sorprendió, ya que cuando yo crecí, el educarte era demasiado difícil, primero por la situación económica, la escuela desde el kínder tiene un costo, supuestamente la educación es por ley gratuita, laica y obligatoria, mentira, desde kínder pagas colegiatura, uniforme, libros, conserje, y si no pagas no estudias. Si alguien termina la primaria ósea la elementary school es un logro ya que para estudiar la secundaria (middle school) pagas colegiatura, libros, uniforme, uso de biblioteca, uso de computado. Es difícil lograr a terminar preparatoria (high school).

Cuando supe todo esto, mi sueño ya era otro, era que mis hijas llegaran a este país y se educaran y lograran lo que se propusieran. Este pensamiento me mantuvo firme en cada momento de tristeza, de desánimo, de soledad, de angustia, siempre me decía un día vamos a reunirnos y empezar una vida juntos, en un lugar con oportunidades. Cuando me pregunto si perdí o gane algo al dejar mi país, me digo: Si perdí el valioso tiempo de niñez con mis hijas, la convivencia con mis familiares, mis niñas no tuvieron esa convivencia con sus primos, tíos, se perdieron ese gran amor de los abuelos; también perdí mi apellido Paterno "Bautista", al momento de pedir mi naturalización a inmigración, eso no fue fácil para mí, pues mi apellido es mi persona. Tuve que hacerlo para poder emigrar a mis padres como ciudadana de este país. Eso perdí, pero le doy gracias a Dios porque dio la oportunidad que nuestras hijas estuvieran en este país, se educaran y alcanzaran sus metas que se propusieron y lo están logrando, permitió que podamos estar juntos como familia y que nuestras generaciones nazcan en este país. Que el esfuerzo de nuestro trabajo se vea en los frutos y a la vez podamos aportar algo a nuestra familias, a nuestra comunidad y tratar de mejorar e ir avanzando en nuestros propósitos.

El espacio en el que me he mantenido ha sido pequeño; pero le he tratado de enseñar y compartir mis experiencias, haciéndoles saber que cada persona vale y tiene que ser respetada sin importar la situación que tenga o como viva, que tenemos los mismos derechos, pero que también tenemos que respetar los derechos de los demás y adaptarnos a lo que se presenta pero sin perder la esencia de lo que soy, mi ser, mi yo. Y sentirme orgulloso de mis raíces, de donde vengo, de mi familia, de mi origen y todo esto transmitirlo a mis generaciones, los valores y principios nacen en casa, se transmiten en el hogar, se viven en la familia y deben de mantenerse siempre en cada uno de nosotros. Mi cultura soy yo, yo la represento.

Cada vez que volteo a ver a mi esposo y nuestras hijas, me siento tan orgullosa de cada uno de ellos y de lo que han logrado y doy gracias a Dios por todo lo que he vivido y por lo que pasare.

"La familia siempre estará unida,

sin importar la distancia que exista,

ya que en cada uno de nuestros corazónes

cada una de nuestras almas permanecen unida."

Para una mama es muy difícil iniciar el proceso familiar en un nuevo país, con un diferente idioma, cultura, y sobre todo poder educar y dirigir a los hijos. Tenemos las costumbres de nuestras madres y queremos aplicar lo mismo que ellas nos dieron para poder educar a nuestros hijos y eso es lo que nos lleva a no hacer en ocasiones lo correcto.

Es importante que consideren que nos educaron a respetar, proveer, aceptar, y conformarse con lo que nos tocó en la vida y con lo que fue nuestra elección, rara vez nos decían que era nuestra decisión, que podíamos cambiar el rumbo de nuestra vida, que podríamos mejorar nuestra situación, aunque eso significara terminar con lo que teníamos y poder tener otra opción e iniciar de nuevo. Mi generación es lo que nos enseñaron, las nuevas generaciones han cambiado un poco, pero nuestra idiosincrasia sigue siendo la misma.

Necesitamos sentirnos apoyadas, entendidas y sobre todo a confiar en nosotras mismas y tener seguridad propia. Cuando inicie el nuevo proceso con mis hijas en este país me hubiera gustado tener un apoyo en la información en español, saber de consejería sobre la educación de los hijos, las opciones de escuelas, tanto de gobierno, como privadas, saber que también mis hijos pueden asistir a ese tipo de escuelas, mediante becas, saber de los medios de ayuda de gobierno con la cual uno puede contar, saber que si mi hijo tiene alguna situación emocional existe un apoyo para ellos y para los padres de familia, sentirnos incluidas como miembros de las escuelas para poder apoyar a nuestros hijos, somos trabajadoras de 8 horas al día, pero aun así, buscaríamos el tiempo para participar más con nuestros hijos en relación a su educación. Que se nos permita expresar nuestras necesidades por medio de grupos de apoyo para los padres de familia, porque hago tanto hincapié en relación de la educación de nuestros hijos? Bueno porque para mí es muy importante la educación de ellos ya en un futuro serán la base de la sociedad en que nos movemos, tanto joven que se pierde por no ser orientados como se debe, una parte importante es en el hogar, pero la segunda y de igual importancia en la escuela, de donde nuestros hijos toman también la decisión importante de su vida, para continuar y llevar acabo sus sueños, que tantas veces son realidades y la gran mayoría son las decisiones que los llevan a no continuar, por no ser entendidos, por los profesores por sus amistades y por los mismo padres de familia. Esto fue, es y será siempre una situación que debe de mejorar para nuestras generaciones, si los padres de familia se sienten aceptados e incluidos nuestras generaciones podrán tener un buen futuro. Saben en nuestros países la educación no es importante, al gobierno de nuestros países no les interesa, tal vez por esa razón nosotros nos conformamos, si mi hijo estudia o no, pero aquí, gracias a Dios, la educación básica es High School, y para nosotros como padres de familia, es un gran logro el que nuestros hijos terminen la High School, Y sin darnos cuenta esto es solamente el inicio de la educación de nuestros hijos, ellos pueden alcanzar más y eso es lo que como madres y padres de familia debemos de tratar de inculcar a nuestros hijos, su superación educativa, porque lo pueden lograr, ya sea a nivel técnico o nivel superior.

Ayudemos a tener las herramientas necesaria para poder cambiar y mejorar nuestra percepción de ver el futuro de nuestros hijos y sentir que podemos hacer algo más por ellos y no sentirnos frustradas por no haber hecho un buen trabajo para el futuro de ellos.

Un paso adelante por pequeño que sea, hace gran diferencia.

Un Paso Adelante (A Step Forward)

CHANGES/CAMBIO

The Testimonio of a Middle Child and Daughter

Gabriela Cárdenas

The decision to immigrate was out of my control. My parents had finally settled in Atlanta, Georgia and it was time for our family to reunite. Prior to our arrival my father, Mario Cardenas, had immigrated back and forth for most of my primary years. He suffered a work-related accident and my mother, M. Silvia Cardenas, had to leave us to care for him. While most of my early childhood has been repressed as a means of self-preservation. I do remember parts and bits of our actual journey to the States.

My parents were born into a working poor class. They lacked everyday essentials. However, these circumstances created a strong desire to attain upward mobility. My parents shared a similar goal of giving my sisters and me a better starting point. That desire drove them to leave everyone they knew behind in a search of a better life.

My expectations of American culture came from mainstream media and stories told by others who had been in the US. Whiteness was glorified. Whiteness was a standard of beauty. Endless possibilities were depicted as easily available to all. Acceptance and tolerance of others seemed to be the standard. However, that was far from reality. We arrived in South Atlanta. We lived in a predominantly African American neighborhood. At that time there were a handful of others that looked like me or spoke Spanish. Division amongst African Americans and Mexicans was clearly defined yet there was never a real platform to address differences and similarities between these two communities. Socializing with anyone different was unwelcomed. Rather, it was discouraged and made me feel like an outcast among Mexican peers. Most of this prejudice came from experiences of violence against those parents who arrived prior to 1996. The most important skill that helped the transcend and navigate my new world was dominating my new language, English. I understood that being able to speak, read and write would open doors that had been closed off to my parents. Being able to dominate English allowed me to exit ESOL and blend with other classmates outside my race. I quickly learned all things Southern heavily influenced by African American culture and most important music. I believe that socializing with peers from different backgrounds helped me grasp a sense of my new home. I began to realize that my family shared more things in common with other than we realized. Fitting into one specific box was no longer the goal, rather being able to navigate different spheres.

My life benefited from going to school. It was there where I realized my disadvantages and lack of privilege. However, I also realized that all my trauma and hurdles had prepared me to take on everything that came my way. College was difficult to navigate given that I lacked lifelines or guidance. But I could not allow myself to give up. With each class that I took, professors that I encountered and experiences with peers I became more assertive that I did belong in that sphere. Classes were challenging, professors were not always welcoming, and I was not academically prepared, but I tried my best. During the entirety of my undergraduate degree, I worked full time. I was able to gain real life experiences through my work. I was able to gain a better understanding of school material because I used it every day while working.

I am now a parent who is guiding two beings in this world. My goal as a parent is to provide them with support and guidance. I want my children to experience a life where they are open to other cultures and can navigate in any sphere they are placed. More important, I want them to hold on to their culture while embracing any new one they decide to take on.

Reflecting on my migration experience, I would have benefited from having someone to teach me to identify and address my childhood trauma, setting boundaries and teaching me to heal rather than repress. Mental health was overlooked by my caregivers and not even a part of school requirements. Government agencies in particular the educational system would better service students by making basic cognitive behavioral therapy classes part of curriculum.

EL DESEO DE DAR FRUTO AL ESFUERZO DE MIS PADRES: MY DESIRE FOR MY PARENT'S LABOR TO BEAR FRUIT

The Testimonio of a Younger Daughter

Elizabeth Cárdenas Bautista

Many of my childhood memories of my life in Mexico before immigrating to the United States are hazy, but one memory often replays in my mind and impacted my career to train as a psychologist working with immigrant populations.

The morning of my mother's departure, I rolled over to seek comfort in the warmth of her arms as the chilly air creeped in, only to be woken in a frigid daze, my mother was no longer by my side. Due to chronic poverty, restricted social mobility, and the deep necessity to provide for her children with the opportunity of a better future, my mother made the unimaginable decision to leave the sanctuary of her home and family in Mexico to immigrate to the United States to reunite with my father. Never knowing when she would return, she left, solely focused on paving a better future for her children. Behind she left her 7, 4, and 2-year-old daughters in the care of her parents and extended family as she embarked on this uncertain journey. I was the confused 2-year-old toddler, who at such a young age, faced the emptiness of separation, a palpable sensation of constant longing that has transported borders and life stages, a longing that would be my companion for years to come.

The departure of my mother, although it left me with an unresolved pain, provided me with the opportunity to be raised with my maternal grandparents, who did their best to show me the love I couldn't physically receive from my mother and father and kept my sister and I together while we were separated from our parents. My grandparents also help me understand transnational parenting that happened over phone calls, and weekly reports of our accomplishments or behavioral concerns. Most importantly my grandparents reminded me that my parents were attentive of my needs, present in my life and demonstrated it by sending what little money they had, even if this often symbolized overlooking their own needs. What unfortunately no one prepared me for was the tension I would feel when I were to be reunited with my biological parents, because this meant losing my normality again, right at a moment when I started to feel more grounded.

After years of tireless and harsh working conditions, my parents were able to bring our family back together. Although there was joy in reuniting, as an immigrant child, I once again at a young age faced the loss of connection with my caregivers and land, detaching from my second parents, not knowing *cuando te volveré a ver/* when I would see them again. From this reunion, I experienced grief and distress of living between borders, feeling a sense of incompleteness while attempting to recreate a new beginning, longing for what I lost, while attempting to flourish in new surroundings, and recreate the bond with my parents. As a child and adolescent, I struggled internally but outwardly I learned to camouflage and presented overall positively. My adjustment and grief concerns went unnoticed by teachers and counselors because I learned to blend in and contain.

As children we learned to create connections with others, particularly children who had recently arrived. Although rarely verbally addressed within us, there was an understanding we shared experiences of migration and learned from each other to make sense of our shared circumstances. Some things we often struggled with was feeling the purpose of our journeys, dealing with grief of what we lost, stumbling to feel the togetherness of our family, making sense of prejudice we witness to our community.

As a child and adolescent, I struggled internally with determining to what degree I will lay my roots in the United States. I struggled to remain connected and feel connected to family in Mexico. Our calls became shorter and more distant throughout the years, visiting as often as we could, while living apart. Due to these early experiences retaining connections has been imperative for me and at times has been the median to self-love. Along with retaining connections I experienced grief around feeling that I was surrounded by the loss of mother figures and connection to Mexico. As a child I had many questions including: When will I go home? How long will we stay here? What if I never go back? Questions that never got asked out of fear of not liking the answer I would receive.

Although I deeply loved my mother, my adolescent mind often grappled with how and why my mom had to leave us in Mexico. I interpreted this as being unwanted or easily forgotten. Now as an adult and after years of compassionate self-reflection for both my mother and father, I understand the complexities of their decision and the pain this caused. The professional and inner child in me, would advocate for age-appropriate transparency and communication. I would have benefited from being provided space to grief my mother leaving and the space to prepared me for the upcoming move without my grandmother. My parents, loving so, did their best with the tools they had. I do not blame them for this, I can now thank them for their bravery and hold them in their pain. I have understood the impact of migration does not occur in a vacuum and impact the entire family. Often, we suffer in silence without realizing that share in the pain, on different levels and different experiences but within this pain, through vulnerability and compassion we can understand our experiences better.

The concept of *Mas de una Mama*/More than one Mother, did not form until my adulthood, when I reframed this aching experience as not the loss of a mother but the gaining of a network of women who cared for me. My life was influenced by my grandmother and sisters who helped shape me but also by the women in my parents' new community, other women who also understood the difficulty in parenting across nations. In a way this recreated a system of caregiving I once had in Mexico with extended family and taught me the importance to building community and reestablishing connections.

Finding quality time as a family was also an important in the process of feeling reunited. The purpose of our migration was to be together as a family, but the pace of our new life left very little time for family togetherness. My parents grueling work schedule left little time to see them during the week and not as rarely available as I desired. As children it was easier to make time for a trip to the park or play outside with my parents. No matter how tired they were, even for a few minutes they tried. However, quality required significant effort to ensure this took place the older the children got and as the need of the family grew. For my family, this made mealtime and pick up from school very important, it was the only time we had for ourselves in a busy day. As teenager, I regrettably did not appreciate it as I should. My desire to fit in with friends and get assimilated to this new lifestyle prompted me to have less meals with my family and more time with friends without noticing how important this time was for my parents. Our family had to relearn how to become a family, how to spend time together, explore how we individually viewed connection, love and care. I see this to be an ongoing practice that will shift as our lives continues to develop. What we have found to bring us together is Sunday meals where we intentionally share laughs and allow ourselves to just be.

My life has been deeply impacted by my migration experience and my connection to my community. I witnessed the necessity for competent bilingual/bicultural Latinx psychologists across the lifespan from my own experience and my family when we recently arrived. I observed how limited support existed, particularly when considering Latinx representation, language diversity, and health providers who understand the strengths and complexities of experiences in underserved and marginalized communities. For me a crucial part of my identity was to maintain my Spanish monolingual abilities. Unfortunately, due to impactful experiences of discouragement by prejudicial educators who, caused me to intentionally deny and halt my Spanish speaking ability. I started to turn away from my language. In return, shame and guilt of losing my native tongue creeped in, turning me further away from my connection to Mexico. I became less optimistic that I could relearn my language, however, my mother's encouragement to use my education as service to the community, was the encouragement I needed to keep trying. At moments when I stumbled and stuttered over my words and my insecurities grew, I continued trying. I am still learning, I am still trying, but I have regained my bilingual ability. I have viewed regaining my native tongue as my resistance to the theme of separation and loss. I came to a state which had an evident anti-immigrant sentiment, something a child could observe by our need to be secretive of my nationality and increasing urgency to assimilate an American identity. However, I found guidance and encouragement by my many mothers, the stories of my family and my parents migration plight to keep going.

My journey to where I am now started with my parent's desire to give us a better future and bring our family together. I often felt a pressure to produce for my parents as a repayment for all their effort and struggle. Always working towards the next goal, never feeling that it was enough to compensate them for their selfless journey. Yet, I have arrived at a realization, that we as a family have simultaneously brought fruit to our parents' labor. Their desire was not only to give us a better future and be physically together but truly be a family and live our lives feeling fulfilled. We are actively making up for the time lost, healing our individual and collective wounds of migration. Migration has always been part of my lineage and through these conversations we hold, I hope we can continue to take steps to heal intergenerational harm cause by migration and grow the compassion we feel for each other. The migration experiences of families vary and should not be generalized but I view my experiences as waves of complexities that can be experienced all at once individually and collectively within the same household, like forces pulling and pushing. By taking a compassionate view of my experience, through my lens as a child and now as an adult, I see the fruit of our parent's labor, finally we can be a family, together at last, recovering from the past, appreciating the present and staying engaged in our collective future.

RECOMMENDATIONS

The testimonios shared in this chapter have been pulled together through ongoing conversations held at the dinner table and at the comfort level of each writer. However, through our writing we are able to conceptualize common themes that are present in these narratives. Below we will provide recommendations for mental health providers, community member and readers to consider exploring when working with Latinx immigrant communities.

Un Paso Adelante (A Step Forward)

Pre-Migration

Each writer described the complexity of their pre-migration experiences which varied based on level of power and decision making held at that time. For the father, as a young unmarried and fatherless man, his decision to migrate presented as an opportunity to seek financial advancement not seen as a possibility in his country of origin and to escape ongoing system of oppression witnessed through generations. For the mother, she went in search of her husband, to render aid while he recovered from an injury. She did not have intentions of ever migrating but circumstances outside her control propelled her journey. Finally, the daughters' pre-migration experiences were products of the decisions made for them by their parents. Exploring pre-migration experiences are essential to have a deeper understanding of the individual and family's experience of their country of origin. Ongoing exploration of historical and social political climate of their country is required to understand ongoing impact on individual and influence for migrating. This includes economic stability, access to social mobility, education, healthcare, war, and seeking safety to mention a few.

Additionally, the role of power to make this decision are important to process particularly when considering younger children who migrate to join family or are unable to migrate with family. Processing the impact of migration on those who are not necessary being included in the decision-making process of life altering events should be considered.

Furthermore, exploring the family connection to migration within their county or origin can provide insight to messages received before settling to the United States. This may highlight meaning making of the journey and provide information of sources of strength. For the father and mother in this chapter, migration has occurred in their respective families before their journey to the United States, as their parents come to the city from a rural town in Mexico. As implied by the first author of this chapter, previous messages of migration allowed him to view this process as a form of surviving, a journey he took as needed. Similarly, it is recommended that the impact of circular migration be assessed. In the father's narrative the writer speaks of circular migration being part of his life before becoming a father and husband, part of his identity as a young man. He found this approach of migration to come out of necessity and be temporary until he could provide for his family.

Importantly, it is recommended that pre-migration trauma be assessed from a trauma informed lens. For some, trauma could be witness in the tragic and ever-present loss of life, during the migration journey. Witnessing such traumatic experiences may go unprocessed for long periods of time until finding a mental health provider who is bilingual and connects to the client.

The Journey

Although everyone's experience varies, particularly when you consider the documentation status on arrival. It is imperative that these disclosures are approached through a trauma-informed lens as they are potentially sources of unresolved trauma that may have not been shared with others, including family. For the authors, opening about their migration stories, specifically this section of their journey, has developed throughout the years, building towards the level of comfort in the disclosure. Mental health providers should consider the potential exposure to sexual assault, over exposure to elements, near death experiences, human trafficking, vicarious trauma and survivor guilt during the process of the journey. The impact of these experiences can deeply affect the mental health of individuals and families who migrate.

Finding New Connections in Our New Home

All authors describe the isolating experiences when arriving to the United States and a desire to recreate connections with new communities and support systems. Creation of connections can be particularly difficult if families resettle in geographic areas that are culturally isolating versus areas that have an abundance of culture and language that resonates with the individual. For example, individuals who migrate to a regional area that has an anti-immigrant sentiment may experience many layers of trauma as they experience ongoing structural limits of access to care and education. This experience can provide obstacles when attempting to create connections but also amplify the importance of these connections when navigating new challenging systems. For some individuals who migrate, they arrive to extended families who can provide housing, potential employment and an overall a great sense of grounding that will be beneficial to their resettling. In the experience of the authors, they did not have extended family who were able to provided that level of support and arrived in a region of the South-East that had an ongoing anti-immigrant sentiment. However, by resettling in an urban community with a growing Latinx immigrant population, the authors found connections through local Latinx grocery stores and Spanish speaking churches. These connections continue to grow as social interactions expanded.

Inner Ruptures

In experiences where connections where not as easily created, writers provide an insight to the inner fragmentation felt while efforts to be connected to their new surroundings and new community become difficult to form. It is recommended to consider the impact these ruptures can have on within group conflict, the view of connection with a larger Latinx community, the understanding of being accepted and perceived forms of strengths brought by these interactions. In the father's narrative, the writer alludes to a shock, felt when he reflected in his experience once arriving to the United States "As I reflect on my experience in this country (United States) there was no home cook meals by my mother, there was no real comfort here, there was a man here or there who appeared to be Hispanic, but they didn't want to speak Spanish. The local business I encountered were Black, Asian or White own." The writer expresses a lack of familiarity in his surroundings, his attempt to connect with the surrounding Latinx individuals, only to encounter a differential in their desire to not speak their language, a common and constant thread of his life prior to migration. The writer describes these experiences as a further disconnection with the existing community in the United States, being distinct from the areas and connections he frequented in his home countries. Considerations should be placed on the views of being accepted at arrive within the larger American community but also the acceptance from the existing Latinx community. While attending to ruptures experienced, it is also recommended that focus be place on strengths approaches while navigating these interactions such as learning to adapt to ever changing surroundings and engaging with other cultures while retaining individuals' values and cultural identity.

 The middle child/daughter writer describes anti-Black racism within her Latinx community and the difficulty to name this racism, while being made aware by the children of those who survived the violence towards Mexican immigrants who arrive to their region of Georgia prior to the 1996 in predominantly Black communities. The "unspoken divide amongst Mexicans and African Americans" noted by the writer, alludes to her experience with Mexican peers of being discouraged to socialize with African American classmates and ultimately lead to being outcast and made feel distant from the Mexican community for deciding to interact outside her cultural group. However, learning to lean on her adaptability and usage of language to name the anti-Black racism and solidarity within the Mexican immigrant community. The writer also refers to her ongoing ability to use resources at her grasp, to learn and teach the complex history of violence in her community and recognizing the influence of Black and Mexican culture have in her region. Through her personal commitment learn she is teaching others in her community, including elders to learn tolerance to others, name anti-Black racism and find commonality between both communities, a message that is particularly important for her children to understand.

Grief, Loneliness, Uncertainty, and Growth

Along with feeling isolated in a new country, the authors described a sense of feeling alone in their grief as they dealt with processing their migration experience. Although it is apparent many of the authors experienced a similarity of concerns, they did not process this as a collective experience. Through the author's narratives we see the theme of grief in the of connection to land, connection with family, death of friends and family during migration process among other forms of loss. It is recommended that mental health providers be attentive to the possible presentation of grief and loss in individuals who migrate and explore coping skills to deal with the loneliness experienced. Another presentation of this theme is seen in the presence of uncertainty across the authors experience. The authors described an uncertainty in their decision to take the initial migration journey, ambiguity on how long this journey will take and vagueness of when they will return to their homeland. Another recommendation to consider is the anxiety provoking nature of the uncertainty of migration. As mentioned by some authors a prevailing sense of enduring with the grief, loneliness and uncertainty became normalized and difficult to identify as an area of concern, making it more imperative to consider.

Access to Bilingual and Bicultural Mental Health Services

The most notable recommendation shared by all authors was the necessity to have access to social services that would assist in resettling process, including mental health services in Spanish that are culturally responsive and from a strength perspective. Authors expressed the need to process migration, adjustment and family communication with mental health providers. The authors shed light to the limited providers and social services offered in Spanish that are culturally responsive in the South-East at the time of their arrival. Like the author's experience, many readers may also be aware and facing a shortage and the ever-growing need of Latinx Spanish speaking providers. Beyond dedication to training bilingual and culturally responsive mental health providers there should also be structural implication to prevent burn-out of these providers. Other consideration should be the benefits and positive implications of language courses, access to health care and supportive education systems.

Post-Migration Psychological Growth

Optimistically and from a strength perspective the writers provide a reframe of effort made by all members of the Cardenas Bautista family to address their individual and collective harm encountered during the migration journey. In working with other immigrant families who have paid a heavy price for a chance of a better future, the writers provided a different mind frame that encourages to view the importance of addressing and rebuilding ruptures but most importantly using the time and conditions provided to honor the legacy and strength of their family through collective healing.

APPENDIX

The Descendance of an Old Ancient: A Father's Testimony

Mario Cárdenas Villanueva

I never thought that I could share my story, but my family has a long-standing history of migration, even before my own journey to the North. I was born in the population/community of San Miguel Enyege, Municipality of Ixtlahuaca, town of Masagua, you can say that I was raised with the presence of my father, he often would visit, in my home I had my mother and siblings. I'm the second to last of seven siblings and our responsibility was to attend school until we could [with the resources allowed] and work. During one occasion, I left classes and I asked for a ride on a truck, [I rode in the truck bed]. As I attempted to get of the truck [bed], my foot got trapped and I was dragged by this tuck. That day, I lost part of my scalp. Due to this accident, I was hospitalized for a year and upon being discharged, my parents [and family] migrated to the Estado de Mexico, with our cows and pigs. Attempting to survive in a *Colonia* [an urban densely populated neighbor, poor infrastructure built on mountain side] was difficult. I started to work hard [as our] most needed necessities such as [access to] water, electricity, sewage and school [were being developed and meet]. To help ourselves financially, my parents established a [corner] store and I took care of my cows and would attend school. With my spare time I would restock the store with merchandise brought in public transportation. I remember having to carry sacks of potatoes, boxes of bananas, tomatoes, and orange sacks and everything was in bulk. The years passed by and my brothers got married, and the store eventually ended. The cows were sold, and my life became very pressured by the urbanization of our zone. My means allowed me to study until the sixth grade and I started to work in a car parts factory.

There was no ability to overcome or advance, law enforcement would harass the youth. We were always being arrested and beaten. [The year] 1980 was a difficult year, like what we see now. All of my friends we in the colonia and out of all my friends there was one friend, may he rest in peace, [who] had traveled to Houston, Texas. He invited me to come along for the opportunity of a better future. I was always ready to work, since in my childhood I have always worked. I tried to come without my mother's permission given that I was her right hand for everything, and I knew that she would not want me come. I left nonetheless, on my way as I exited the bus terminal of Mexico City to Matamoros, my mother, without me knowing caught up to me in the avenue and with a loud yell she told me:

My mother said: "Where do you think you're going Mario!?"

I answered: "To the United States, I plan to work"

My mother pleaded: "Please return!"

I said: "No, I have to go"

My mother said (with a longing voice): "May God accompany you, my son."

Un Paso Adelante (A Step Forward)

    In our first trip we arrived to Matamoros with the border of Brownsville, Texas. Our journey took two days and one night, we walked, hopped on a train and caught a truck. I finally arrived in Houston, and I earned my living as day laborer. Three months later, with much effort, I sent my mother $300 USD. At this time the exchange rate of the dollar was 12 Pesos. My mother sent word back that she saved my earnings in my bank account.

    As I reflect on my experience in this country (the United States) it was not one like being at home with mama's cooking. There was no comfort, there was one or another man who physically appeared to be Hispanic, but they did not want to speak Spanish. The local businesses I frequented were Black, Asian or White owned. I worked in a restaurant, cleaning tables from 9:00am-12:00pm and my form of transportation was a bike. No one bothered me. It was very different than my country. All the men lived alone, and I was alone. When I returned to the United States I had a clearer vision, there were opportunities for a better future and to help my brothers. But just as there were possibilities there were also great tragedies. On my way back, I experienced something horrible. I lost my friend to the Rio Grande in Matamoros; may he rest in peace.

    I returned to Mexico, and I contained my courtship and then married my love, Silvia, My Chivis. We built our house, with two rooms and one bathroom. The money I had ran out after building the house and getting married. So I went back to Houston, Texas and I worked for sessions for a year and a half. And that is how I traveled back and forth to Mexico. I had three beautiful daughters, Eva, Gaby and Eli. They have always given me much strength in my life. Strength to not see obstacles. Although every time I would have to say goodbye they would cry, I also cried but, on the bus, alone for hours. This part of my life is filled with many sad memories, feeling so empty, loneliness, sadness but at the end we powered through, drew strength and live the acceptance that immigrating from one another country to another is very devastating and dangerous. But we do it for the love of our family and our family is what gives us the strength that we need.

    At the time, arriving to Georgia I realized how access to basic English classes could help me as support and integrate. It would have help me having access to a psychologies or therapist, therapy in Spanish, but at that time there was not anybody. Normally we take on a rhythm, that live is isolating, walk onward, work and overcome. But the reality is having your family with you is most important. Life is about overcoming and surviving, but one cannot forget, that live can be more than surviving. Before my family arrived to Georgia, I believed to have everything, but was not complete. When my wife arrived, it was a rebirth, a reinforcement. After great effort and because of God my daughters arrived. It was something profound my life became complete. Our family being separated was difficult, but you try not to acknowledge it. I had forgotten my suffering. But, being together as a family you are found with a deep happiness, energy and through all of the support you feel strengthen. You realize what was missing. My family's arrival felt like childhood, sharing with everyone.

A Step Forward: A Mother's Testimony

Manuela Silvia Bautista Gil

"In life, decisions are made that we do not understand at that moment why we do them: but as time passes, we discover why we did it."

Un Paso Adelante (A Step Forward)

Manuela Silvia Cardenas is my married name, my name is Manuela Silvia Bautista Gil and I'm 56 years old, my husband Mario Cardenas and our three daughters Eva María Cardenas, Gabriela E. Cardenas and Elizabeth Cardenas Bautista. I have been in the United States for 28 years, I arrived May 22, 1995, I entered through San Isidro California, I came on a religious pilgrimage from a church of my place of origin in Mexico and by May 24th, I found myself in Atlanta Georgia, the place I arrived and continue to reside.

What was the reason that made me migrate to this country, the majority of the people do it to find a better future, for financial necessities, due to war, or political reasons but my story was different. I never envisioned it as a future plan, all I knew was that my husband was already in the United States, worked and earnings were sent as remittance to support us. After a predetermined time, he would return and be with us for a brief period of time and he would return. This was our system of life that we carried, a life that I became accustomed to, but I did not realize that this was not correct, that this was not a marriage, that this was not a family and overall that this was not healthy for my daughters and us as a couple, but we had necessities in our family and my husband was in search of an opportunity and that opportunity was in the United States.

In February 1995, while my husband was in Atlanta, while working in construction he suffered an accident which left him in a bad condition, his accident was the fall from approximately two floors where he fell on his back over some containers. This left him with an injury on his back on his spine. I became aware of what occurred and from there the reason for migrating to the United States began. This news made me think of my reality, extreme ideas came to mind: What to do? How could I go see him? How could I leave my daughters? They were so young, Eva 7 years old, Gaby 5 years old and Eli 2 years old. How could I leave them? If things were not good with their father. What would I tell them? What explication would I give them for leaving? They were so young, would they understand? What if something happens to me, and my return is delayed? Many unanswered questions went through my mind. I spoke to my parents, and they supported me, that was a good start. Thank God the father of my parish granted me permission to be a part of the group of pilgrims that were going to California, in the pilgrimage of our Lady of the Rosary of Talpa and I was able to enter [the country] without facing those great risks that our migrant bother/sisters face.

My reason, my motive, my necessity was to find and help with the health and rehabilitation of my husband, the father of my daughters. Be able to tell them that their father was well and soon will return to be with them. In my life that was the most difficult decision, to leave my daughters, I was not a good mother, but I loved them in my way, with what I had, to my capacity to provide for them and made a decision, I made it decision because I had to, but did not make it because I wanted to.

The first three years were the most difficult and draining of my life, in a foreign country without family, only my husband and me, without friends, a language I did not speak, a different culture, without documents to work and under constant anguish to not have freedom, exhausting jobs and poorly paid due to not knowing how to drive to find better employment, anguish knowing my daughters were so far away, needing financial support and not being able to communicate with them with the frequency needed, due to low earnings, having to pay rent, water, electricity, gas groceries and having to send money to them, month to month having to minimize as much possible. On many occasions only one meal for my husband and me for that day. Frustration from going to doctor with my husband and not being able to express his health conditions, not having time to rest, waiting for my husband's health to soon improve, his recovery to start working, it was difficult but thank God experienced and overcome.

Un Paso Adelante (A Step Forward)

What were my expectations. I remember when I left my country, I did not expect anything, I only wanted to arrive to know the true state of my husband's health and to see what I could do for him, knowing that it would not be good, that I will face hard moments, but preparing for it.

The reality of what happened was severe since when I arrived, Mario was in bad conditions, he lived with some friends, but in poor conditions, in a small room with a couch as his bed, everything was in poor condition while he was dealing with his back pain. The first thing I thought was: his home situation is making his condition worst and we need to change all of this. I was thinking this situation is making his condition worst; we need to change it. I was thankful that it was not as bad as thought, thankful to God he could move, with pain and difficulty but he could do it.

When I arrived in this country, I had to immediately work and there was no time to wait. My connection was through labor I could produce, integrated myself in their culture through work, I did not have the opportunity to do it any other way. What I admired was the order, capacity, and effort given at these jobs, at that time I was always unskilled labor, I worked as a housekeeper, it was very exhausting work, my respect for all those workers [who face] such difficult conditions. Heavy labor and poor wages and there you stayed. I worked cleaning hotel kitchens, cleaning buffet restaurants, cleaning houses and as a waitress. In those jobs there were always safety meetings, conversations about employee needs, your work hours were respected, if your worked extra hours you were compensated with overtime. This are things we do not see in my country. In the places I worked [in my country], I was an office secretary, there you witness the preference, unhealthy work environment, the need to seek favors from your superior, poor paying wages, no respect of your work hours, they were abusive. [Back in the US] when I worked here, my job did not require a certification, and based on my situation it made me think what the work environment would be in other jobs that did require certifications? The few times I went to the doctor or another office for services I realized how different the environment was, how employees were treated. I then understood that this country had good points in their culture and for me this is due to the access of education people have. I understand that in every country there are people who cannot access education but what I have seen is the more education becomes accessible more of a possibility for social mobility. During my experience here, I saw an independent culture and the possibilities for opportunities for those who wanted it. In Mexico, I feel ashamed what I'm about to share, but in my experience those in my country with the access to education or most educated believe that they deserve everything and look down on those that do not have an education. In the US what I have experienced is people give you respect, attention without considering your appearance or education level. This treatment encourages employees, you are treated with respect, you can work and even if you're unkept you will be treated well. In my experience those with authority use it fairly, there might be examples otherwise but what I saw in comparison to what I lived in Mexico it was very different. I learned from my co-workers and the culture here, everyone had different values and principals which we were taught in my home, I will never change those, I will carry those teachings with me and hope that my daughters and future generations will conserve. Family is very important that should be preserved and kept together, along with their principles and values, that should never be lost.

The education in this country also forms part of my culture, and this impacted me when I realized the importance in allowing all children to attend the most basic levels of school. To know that the most basic level of education provided to every child goes up to high school was surprising to me. Since when I was growing up, having access to education was very difficult financially, school since kindergarten had to be paid, everything from tuition, uniforms, materials and if you could not afford any part of this then you would not get an education. If someone could complete elementary school this was viewed as an accomplishment, completing middle school and high school was very difficult to accomplish.

When I became aware of the access of education here, my dream became something else. I now wanted my daughters to get to this country and be educated and achieve what they wanted. This dream, kept me going during every moment of sadness, feeling hopeless, during solitude, during moments of anxiety, I would always tell myself that one day we would be reunited, and we will start our lives together in this place of opportunities. When I ask myself if I lost or gain something leaving my country, I say: Yes, I lost valuable time with my daughters during their childhood, the familiarity with my family, and my daughters did not have that familiarity with their cousins, uncles, they lost that love from their grandparents, I also lost my paternal last name "Bautista" at the moment of becoming naturalized by the immigration department, it was not easy for me, my last name is who I am. This is something I had to do so I could bring my parents over [to the US] when I became a citizen. Even though I lost my last name, I give God thanks for the opportunity it provided my daughters, to be in this country, be educated and reach their goals. They are doing just that. This allowed us to be together like a family and that our future generation be born in this country. That the effort of our labor be seen in their fruits, we can support our family and community. In this way we can advance and reach our goals.

There are experiences that I still need to process but I have tried to teach and share my experiences. Expressing that every person has value and needs to be respected without mattering their situation, we all have the same rights and that we also need to respect the rights of others and adapt to what we are presented with. Without losing our presence, who I am, my being. I also learned to feel proud of my roots, where I come from, my family, my origin, and transmit this all to my generations, the values and principals born in my home and transmitted in my home. This are values that should be maintain with us and within us. My culture who I am and what I represent. Every time I get to see my daughters and husband, I feel very proud of each of them, for what they have accomplished, and I thank God for everything I have lived and experienced.

"The family will always be united

Without mattering the distance that exist

Since in all our hearts

All of our souls maintained united"

For a mother it was difficult to start the family process in a new country, with a different language, culture, and over all to be allowed to educate and guide my children. We often have customs or our own teachings from our mother on how to parent, and at times those teaching take us down the wrong path.

It is important to considered that we were educated to respect, provide, accept and be content with what life provides. As for what was freely elected, rarely we were given the option to choose, that we can change our life path, better our situation, even if it meant to end what we had to have another option and begin anew. This is what my generation taught, new generations have changed a bit, but our school of thought remains the same.

Un Paso Adelante (A Step Forward)

We need to feel supported, understood and overall to believe in ourselves and have confidence in us. When I started the new process with my daughter in this country, I would have liked to have support with information in Spanish. To know about counseling services, educational opportunities for my children, options for schools, through the state or private institutions. To better understand what opportunities my children could have like scholarships, know about government aid and to know if a child is experiencing an emotional concern to know what support for individual and family services [were available]. In addition, have better connections with school systems so we can better support our children. We worked more than 8 hours a day and even then, we found some time to interact with our children mainly through school. I would have found a group setting helpful to discuss our necessities as parents. I emphasize the relationship with children and education because I view educating our youth as the base of our future of our society, I have witness youth being lost because they lack guidance, the home is important, but their safety and education gives our children the opportunity to reach their dreams. Many times, the reality is that we make decisions that lead us to not continue, because they feel misunderstood, by educators, friends or members of their own family. This is the reality for many and should be changed to have a positive impact in our generations. If the parents of a family feel supported and included with our generations, we have a good future. In our country education is not viewed with the same importance, the government in our country has no interest and maybe for that reason we conform, if my child studies or not, but here thanks to God, they have basic education until High School, and for us to see our children finish high school without realizing that this is just the start of our children's education journey. Our children can reach more, that is what we as mothers and fathers should encourage our children to do, there educational advancement, because they can accomplish this.

Lastly, it would be helpful to have tools needed to change or better our perspective to see the future of our children and to feel that we can do something for them and not to become frustrated for feeling that we haven't done right by them.

One step forward, for however small it may be, make a big difference.

Chapter 14
From Silos to Integration:
Healthcare, Politics, and Transformation

Jhokania De Los Santos
Philips, USA

Pierluigi Mancini
Multicultural Development Institute, Inc., USA

Amelia Hoyle Miller
Best Within You Therapy & Wellness, USA

ABSTRACT

This chapter introduces integrated behavioral healthcare and why it shows promise to be effective in Latinx populations. While the field is shifting rapidly toward an integrated care model, discussions on cultural factors and how they interplay with integrated care are substantially lacking. This chapter attempts to fill this gap and provide understanding of the current socio-political landscape, outline integrated care application when treating Latinxs with eating disorders, and briefly summarize key strategies to consider when part of an effective IBHC team that promotes patient-centered culturally-responsive care.

INTRODUCTION

Despite the growth of behavioral health services in the United States (U.S.), persistent disparities in racial and ethnic minority populations' access to behavioral health continue to exist. Studies consistently report Latinxs' underutilization of mental health services (Keyes et al., 2012; Alegría et al., 2002; Harris et al., 2005), which lead to Latinxs being less likely to receive guideline congruent care, and rely more often on primary care services (Cabassa, et al., 2008). Primary care settings have become the entryway of mental health services for many Latinx people, increasing the relevance of culturally competent, integrated physical and mental health care (Talen et al., 2005). As the field continues to shift and adjust to the current socio-political landscape, discussions on cultural factors and how they interplay with in-

DOI: 10.4018/978-1-6684-4901-1.ch014

tegrated behavioral care are severely lacking. This calls us to contemplate, why is this so, and how can we improve cultural considerations to enhance Latinx behavioral health services?

This chapter attempts to fill this gap and provide practical solutions to the issues Latinxs experience, as it relates to disparities in behavioral health care utilization and quality of care. The authors have years of experience in integration on the ground; together they combine the perspectives of primary care clinicians, behavioral health clinicians, health system leaders, health service researchers, and practice transformation experts with steps on how to make integrated behavioral health care (IBHC) work. We will demonstrate how IBHC is well-positioned to treat behavioral health disparities among Latinxs, use specific examples contextualizing eating disorder treatment, with particular attention focusing on interprofessional collaboration, and most importantly, empowering the patient to be the expert.

What Is Integrated Behavioral Health Care?

IBHC is the systematic coordination of physical and behavioral health. Both behavioral and physical health problems often occur at the same time and treating both may yield the best results. This is particularly true where there are major disparities in overall health status and barriers to accessing services. Populations of color appear to benefit equally using this approach. The focus of IBHC is to reduce stigma and service utilization barriers by embedding mental health professionals into the fabric of the primary care team. The team works together under one roof, allowing for a one-stop shop approach, facilitating access for patients and their families, and providing patient-centered, and cost-effective care for a defined population (Brewer, 2021).

According to the National Quality Forum (2010), care coordination has been defined as "a function that helps ensure that the patient's needs and preferences for health services and information sharing across people, functions, and sites are met over time" (p. 2). Within an integrated approach, patients are placed at the center of care, while physicians and mental health providers work together to ensure patient's biopsychosocial needs and preferences for services are met. This concentrated effort has been made by the World Health Organization to achieve integrated behavioral health within the health sector, especially in primary care settings. Some of the major concerns that prompt IBHC include "the need to close the treatment gap for mental health disorders, increasing access for patients, making care affordable and cost-effective, and improving better outcomes at both the patient and community level" (Zubatsky et al., 2018, p. 645).

The alarming reality of today's current healthcare system is that there is a potential for patients to fall through the cracks, especially in one that has been fragmented for a very long time, and one that operates with a silo mentality with little to no collaboration or implementation. What typically perpetuates this fragmentation is the carved-out funding streams, separate medical records, along with the different training and practices providers have obtained. While the call to integrate behavioral health and primary care to better serve patients has resonated broadly, there are still significant barriers to ensure success, especially vulnerable populations, such as Latinxs, immigrants, refugees and even the uninsured. We must then ask ourselves, how are they being included in this transition to integrated health care?

Immigrants are often defined as a "vulnerable population," with increased risk for poor physical, psychological, and social health outcomes and inadequate health care. Vulnerability is shaped by many factors, including political and social marginalization and a lack of socioeconomic and societal resources. Currently, due to the changing landscape with regard to immigration enforcement over the last two decades, undocumented Latinx people face challenges that threaten to impact their psychological and emotional well-being (APA, 2012). Following the passage of the Illegal Immigration Reform and Immigration Responsibility Act of 1996, and the creation of the Immigration and Customs Enforcement (ICE) agency after the attacks of September 11, 2001, detentions and deportation activity has increased substantially. Due to the harsh sociopolitical climate, undocumented Latinxs living in the U.S. are often confronted with discrimination, prejudice, hate crimes, and anti-immigration laws (Arredondo et al., 2014). These challenges significantly threaten to impact Latinxs' psychological and emotional well-being and engender internalized stigma at the interpersonal and individual level, which has been associated with psychological distress and depressive symptoms (Viruell-Fuentes et al., 2012).

Because Latinx people are the fastest growing ethnic group and are currently the largest minority group, it is important to recognize how culture may influence the health behaviors of patients as well as how they are treated by healthcare professionals. In a culturally diverse society, healthcare disparities among individuals from different ethnic, racial, and economic groups may be in part a function of cultural differences between a healthcare system primarily based on Anglo cultural assumptions and the population it serves (Roosa et al., 2002). This incongruence between culturally diverse patients and the delivery of healthcare services based on mainstream cultural assumptions may lead to negative interactions, unequal quality of care, and perceptions of discrimination on the part of the ethnic minority and low SES individuals (Smedley et al., 2003). Lanesskog and Piedra (2016) note that tensions and misunderstandings are common when immigrants engage with healthcare systems that are designed for English speakers familiar with American culture and systems of care. Over time, these structures can affect the quality-of-care immigrants and refugees receive, further contributing to health disparities. Thus, a responsive integrated system would be beneficial to tend to immigrant health care needs based on varying levels of acculturation, pre- and post-migration experiences, citizenship status, and settlement context (Lanesskog & Piedra, 2016).

One innovation to address the evident need to generate greater awareness of the role of ethnicity in the provision of appropriate health services is the integration of behavioral health and primary care for patients with mental and physical health comorbidities. Primary care goes beyond physicians, and instead, demonstrates the power of interdisciplinary teams working together to effectively treat patients. Primary care is "the provision of integrated, accessible health care services by physicians and their health care teams who are accountable for addressing a large majority of personal health care needs, developing a sustained partnership with patients, and practicing in the context of family and community" (AAFP, 2017). Notably, primary care is cost-effective, individualized, and team-based, to ensure the highest quality of services within healthcare, and is known to have similarities with integrated behavioral health. Common factors like cost-effective healthcare services that are person-centered create a base through which IBHC has been developed. Primary care and IBHC serve the same objective, which is to: improve health for the whole person (*What Is Integrated Behavioral Health Care (IBHC)? | the Academy*, n.d.). Therefore, adopting an integrated health care system helps realize the goals and the objectives of primary care.

Policy Matters: The Intersection of Policy and Care

Several factors have made adopting integrated behavioral health into primary care difficult. Some of the main barriers that have hindered the adoption of integrated health care models include vulnerable populations, patient and family factors, comorbidities, provider factors, financing and costs, and organizational issues (Grazier et al., 2016). Notably, efforts have been made to eliminate most of the barriers to achieving the desired level of primary care in the health sector. Some solutions to the identified challenges include prioritizing vulnerable populations, extending community collaboration, using team approaches that include the patient and family, diversifying funding streams, and using data-driven policies and practices (Grazier et al., 2016). Primary care proves to be a good solution, as it focuses on improving the health of individuals through using health systems developed within each state, while incorporating culturally and linguistically responsive modalities. However, not every state considers Latinx, immigrant and refugee communities and their unique needs in planning and implementing integration.

For effective policies to be established within healthcare, there must be significant levels of collaboration between practice and policy. Before IBHC was adopted, primary care focused on integrating and coordinating different players within the health sector to achieve the desired outcomes. According to the World Health Organization, the policies and practices that should be initiated within IBHC should be comprehensive, equitable, coordinated, continuous, holistic, preventive, empowering, goal-oriented, respectful, collaborative, co-produced, endowed with rights and responsibilities, governed through shared accountability, evidence-informed, led by whole-system thinking, and ethical (WHO, 2018). These tenets make up the policy part of integrated behavioral health care and primary care. The challenge, however, comes with the implementation of the policy.

Actualizing IBHC has been a challenge within healthcare, as governments struggle to systematically create payment models that incentivize providers to routinely engage in behavioral health care (Zubatsky et al., 2018). Based on the demand levels for primary health care workers and the finances required to initiate and realize IBHC, it has not been easy to implement. The U.S. has been experiencing shortages of nurses, psychiatrists, psychologists and professional counselors, which has created additional barriers, especially for patients who speak languages other than English. Furthermore, issues of diversity, equity, and inclusivity have been major impediments. The stigma associated with IBHC has also been a challenge in practicing integration in healthcare. The public needs to be educated about the idea of IBHC in a culturally and linguistically responsive manner. Stakeholders should also address the issue of diversity, equity, and policy within healthcare to ensure that the practice is embraced. Therefore, allowing for an effective approach that guides the practice of IBHC while identifying the challenges and suggesting possible solutions.

Social, Political, Immigrant Determinants of Health

The social element of health covers both the economic and social policies within the political spheres of governments. Latinxs are disproportionately affected by poor conditions of daily life, shaped by structural and social position factors (cultural values, income, education, occupation, and social support systems, including health services), known as social determinants of health. Focusing on social determinants of health has become a central element amongst efforts to advance health equity. Thus, ensuring that Latinxs have access to high-quality health care is important, but so is focusing on policy and systems change and using a wide variety of approaches to support health equity is essential. Society and politics have a complex relationship that traverses the entire sector within the government. Immigrants form part of the society and should play a role in the decision-making process by influencing the government's policies on their health issues, unfortunately this is not the case. Horner (2021) notes that policymakers should make it a point to address policies that disregard the well-being of immigrants, through explicit exclusion or by addressing the many fears that are inhibiting benefit access.

A country's policy regarding immigrant intake should cater to the basic human rights as chartered by the United Nations. In essence, policies devised by governments should aim to cover the interests of every citizen, be it an immigrant or a native citizen, and thus work to reduce disparities in access to healthcare. The socio-economic gap within society has been a concern to governments, but unfortunately, little has been done to bridge the gap to ensure that access to healthcare is possible for every individual regardless of ethnicity.

As indicated earlier, a significant majority of studies have shown that Latinxs are less likely to seek treatment, have less access to treatment, receive fewer services (Wells et al., 2001), and are less likely to report overall satisfaction with treatment (Tonigan, 2003; Wells et al., 2001). These inconsistencies may be attributable to regional variations; however, untreated mental health issues are a significant part of the larger health equity problem in the U.S. Equity is one of the main political determinants of health, in which governments work toward achieving healthcare. Raine and colleagues (2016) define equity as fairness and justice and imply that everyone should have an equal opportunity to attain their full potential for health or the use of health care.

Raine and colleagues (2016) note that the future of health equity starts and ends with the political determinants of health, and thus, the government represents the political sphere of health. The political determinants of health are typically the main contributors to the inequities within the health sector. The disparities are propagated through established systems of discrimination that marginalize ethnic minority communities and geographical areas. The government has the power to influence change in such places through improving healthcare and security, encouraging and embracing diversity, providing civic education about health, and practicing inclusivity. The government can also ensure equitable distribution of resources and opportunities to every citizen to ensure that everyone enjoys quality healthcare. Therefore, the issues surrounding equity within healthcare are of paramount importance, and it greatly influences the government as it is a political determinant of health.

Dawes (2020) makes an engaging and important contribution to the health equity discourse, and defines political determinants of health as involving "the systematic process of structuring relationships, distributing resources, and administering power, operating simultaneously in ways that mutually reinforce or influence one another to shape opportunities that either advance health equity or exacerbate health inequities" (p. 97). He argues that political determinants of health create the social drivers——including poor environmental conditions, inadequate transportation, unsafe neighborhoods, and lack of healthy food options——that affect all other dynamics of health. It also affects immigrants' health and access to healthcare. Dawes (2020) recalls the fear and concern related to the Trump administration's controversial plan to add a citizenship question to the 2020 census, in a move that threatened to further disenfranchise immigrants and minority residents, had it not been blocked by the Supreme Court.

Dawes (2020) also describes the backlash against the Affordable Care Act and efforts to undermine other programs and policies focused on addressing health inequities. Even rumors of policy changes like the public charge rule can cause problems. "Public charge" is a ground of inadmissibility, which are reasons that a person could be denied a green card, visa, or admission into the U.S. In deciding whether to grant applicants a green card or a visa, an immigration officer must decide whether that person is likely to become dependent on certain government benefits in the future, which would make them a "public charge." It is not a test that applies to everyone, not even to all those applying for green cards. Rumors of this and other policies send immigrant communities into hiding and in fear of using services that they may very well be eligible for and keeping them away from health service providers.

Certain governments across the world initiate health policies and agendas such as universal health coverage. Notably, the government is the primary financer of healthcare services. Governments finance health care by "mobilizing the necessary resources through public budgets and other contributive mechanisms, pooling resources allocated to health development, guiding the process of resource allocation and purchasing health services from various providers" (Regional Committee for the Eastern Mediterranean, 2006, p. 6). Therefore, the government is the main player and a significant stakeholder within the health sector. Kickbusch (2015) notes that health is often a political choice, and politics lends itself to be an ongoing struggle for power among competing interests. Political determinants of health cover and analyze how different power constellations, institutions, processes, interests, and ideological positions affect health within other political systems and cultures and at varying levels of governance (Kickbusch, 2015). Given the enormous importance of health to a government, it must ensure that each of its citizens enjoys health benefits. Thus, most health determinants depend on political action as they create a basis for human rights and citizenship (Kickbusch, 2015). Factors such as social, political, and immigrant determinants of health, equity, reducing disparities, and practice are influenced by the political determinants of health.

Policies: A Root Cause of Racial Health Inequities

Political determinants of health help shape practice within health care. Governments define the healthcare sector by making policies that make healthcare delivery possible. Changing tax legislation, consumer protection and employment regulations, and insurance mandates are all elements in the political sphere that have an impact on healthcare. Health disparities prompted by global issues like race, ethnicity, social-economic classes, and other disparities within the health sector can be combated by the government if the necessary policies are implemented by the right agencies (Haines et al., 2004). In order to make equitable policies, we must confront racism, which requires not only changing attitudes, but also transforming and dismantling the policies and institutions that undergird the U.S. racial hierarchy (Bailey et al., 2021). Bailey and colleagues (2021) strongly express that "dismantling structural racism's impact on health care is not an issue of a 'few bad apples'; we must reflect on the way our everyday, accepted practices reify race - that is treat the social construct of race as an intrinsic biologic difference - thereby exemplifying and contributing to a broader system of structural racism" (p. 771). More steps are needed by the government to ensure that the policies proposed are implemented at all levels and in all sectors within healthcare. Dawes (2020) recommends the development of health equity task forces that can identify and address inequities in our governments, engage in collaborative efforts among public health spheres, and lay the groundwork for a sustainable future toward health equity.

For Latinx communities the issue is compounded, the microaggressions that exist in healthcare toward Latinx immigrant and refugee communities contribute to the delay in implementing culturally and linguistically responsive services. It is ironic that today we are seeing the consequences of the previous administration's lowering of immigrant and refugee numbers allowed to enter the U.S., that left us with a shortage of workers in all industries but in particular, in the healthcare sector. In fact, immigration has slowed in the U.S. between 2019 and 2021 amidst the spread of COVID-19, along with policy changes, leaving the labor force about 1.6 million workers smaller than it would have been if it had stayed on its pre-pandemic trend (Goldman Sachs, 2022). Flooded health-care facilities have underlined the urgency for international health-care workers to fill workforce needs, however, getting an interview at the U.S. consulate has been in a holding pattern, constraining the ability of health-care workers to fill those in-demand jobs. Unfortunately, there's been little progress addressing these barriers to employment in the U.S. Biden's administration would have to reverse restrictive policies that former President Trump put in place, in order to remove bureaucratic roadblocks, which includes rescinding the federal government's pandemic-era border policy and ramping up the U.S. refugee resettlement capacity. If the government doesn't address the staffing shortage, the natural consequence is continued healthcare disparities, and a system that moves away from culturally responsive care.

In considering how to promote health and health equity, there are several initiatives that seek to shape policies and practices in non-health sectors. Within the healthcare system, there are multi-payer federal and state initiatives as well as Medicaid-specific initiatives focused on addressing social needs. These include models under the Center for Medicare and Medicaid Innovation, Medicaid delivery system and payment reform initiatives, and options under Medicaid.

Universal healthcare coverage is acknowledged by the World Health Organization as a political choice (Kittelsen et al., 2019), and thus, health should be accessed by every individual within a country. Nonetheless, disparities within healthcare are common in almost every country. Healthy People 2020 defines a health disparity as:

A particular type of health difference that is closely linked with social, economic, and/or environmental disadvantage. Health disparities adversely affect groups of people who have systematically experienced greater obstacles to health based on their racial or ethnic group; religion; socioeconomic status; gender; age; mental health; cognitive, sensory, or physical disability; sexual orientation or gender identity; geographic location; or other characteristics historically linked to discrimination or exclusion. (p. 28)

The threats caused by inequalities within the health sector are grave and often result in the fatality of minority group members. Notably, disparities within the health sector have long-lasting effects on the mental and physical health of the affected populations. Differences are notable in the issues relating to diversity, inclusivity, and equity within the health sector. The disparities within the health sector have been propagated and magnified by the social-economic difference and discrimination experienced by ethnic minority group members. Discrimination due on the basis of race and ethnicity has been a major impediment to bridging the disparities. The government has a crucial role to play when it comes to reducing inequalities within the health sector. There is evidence that health systems which successfully address equity share several broad features such as, aiming for universal coverage, integrating social determinants approaches, measuring and monitoring inequities in health to address them, and leadership that encourage intersectoral action across governmental departments to promote population health (World Health Organization, 2013). Provisions of healthcare to every citizen by making healthcare facilities culturally responsive through a diversified work environment are some of the solutions to eliminate the disparities.

One solution is to address the social determinants of health for Latinxs, immigrant and refugee communities. These determinants refer to non-medical factors determined by social and economic systems and inequalities that have important effects on health. They are the conditions in which people are born, grow, live, work, and age and are mostly responsible for health inequities. Immigrants in particular are at a great risk of suffering from health disparities due to social factors like poverty that impact their lives (Chang, 2019).

Access to food – nutritious food, specifically – is regarded as a key social determinant of health that has a direct impact on a patient's wellbeing. Individuals who cannot afford or obtain quality food rich in vitamins run the risk of developing chronic illnesses or exacerbating illnesses they may already have. Limited access to food can also have a domino effect on other social determinants or medical issues. Children who are food insecure may experience more difficulty focusing on school, which may stunt their educational attainment and ultimately harm their chances of success (Health, 2019). The relationship with food is built at an early age, and a lack of nutrition information, along with lack of access to healthy foods may lead to developing eating disorders, a condition that is frequently overlooked in Latinx communities.

INTEGRATED HEALTH AND EATING DISORDER TREATMENT

We now shift to examining eating disorder treatment for Latinx patients to illustrate the intersection of health disparities, policies, and integrative health. While research on the prevalence of eating disorders for Latinx patients continues to be scarce, some research suggests elevated rates of Binge Eating Disorder and Bulimia Nervosa for Latinas, while further reporting that the rates of treatment utilization are "exceedingly low" (Perez et al., 2016; Alegria et al., 2007). This portion of the chapter will focus on a holistic and strengths-based approach to eating disorder treatment, including the benefits of integrated health care/healthcare teams, culturally relevant assessment, barriers to seeking treatment, costs of these barriers, and person-centered treatment planning. By exploring integrated health through the lens of eating disorders for Latinx patients, we may better understand the impact of incorporating individual strengths, support networks and cultural values as a culturally responsive approach to mental health and health treatment.

A Team Approach to Treatment of Eating Disorders

Coordination of a healthcare team is invaluable in the treatment of eating disorders. The ideal treatment team would include patient, patient support system, therapist, primary care provider, registered dietician, and psychiatrist (Walsh et al., 2000). These team members would engage in consistent and effective communication to track progress of the patient and address barriers. Trust would be established and fostered between team members to provide holistic and impactful patient care with the patient's goals at the center of the team process.

Patients with eating disorders may be unaware of the need for this team and perhaps even reluctant in having providers take a systematic approach to treatment when experiencing their own ambivalence regarding change (Abbate-Daga et al., 2013). It is likely that the patient may only share their concerns with their primary care or mental health provider, necessitating culturally competent assessment of eating concerns by these providers, as well as providing a bridge to some configuration of integrated care. While the team listed above would be ideal, for someone with limited resources, their primary care provider may serve several of these roles, providing medication management and food planning, and would coordinate with a mental health provider regarding care.

However, research suggests that physicians and mental health providers may experience an inclination towards racial stereotyping when assessing for eating concerns. Latinas are less likely to receive a recommendation or referral for eating disorder evaluation and care, despite a lack of difference in eating disorder symptoms (Becker, Franko, Speck & Herzog, 2003; Palmer, 2007). Providers may fail to recognize and treat individuals with eating disorders who do not present with the traditional symptomology based on the experiences of white women (Gilbert, 2003; Palmer, 2007). As Talleyrand (2012) stated, "traditional screening and counseling approaches used to examine and treat women's eating disorder symptoms may not necessarily capture the unique sociocultural experiences of women of color" (p. 271). Melinda[1] a research participant, described talking to her primary care provider about her eating disorder, during a period of intense restriction, but noted feeling dismissed by her provider because of her body type. She recalled being told by her provider that she was a "curvy girl" and "would be fine" (Hoyle, 2019). By failing to assess symptomology in a culturally responsive way, patients may be denied necessary treatment for life-threatening mental health concerns.

Barriers to Receiving Treatment of Eating Disorders

While emphasis in the literature has been placed on the lower rates of help seeking for Latinx patients (Alegria et al., 2007), it is imperative that integrative health teams reflect and respond to the significant barriers for patients in receiving holistic treatment. These may include affordability/lack of insurance, few Spanish speaking therapists and Latinx therapists, limited materials for psychoeducation in Spanish, distance and time limitations in accessing a team of providers, and citizenship status (Bridges et al., 2012; Sanchez et al., 2012). Patients may also experience justifiable distrust towards White providers at treatment centers and the individualized nature of western medicine (Edward & Hines-Martin, 2016). For immigrant communities, there may not only be fears around the lack of understanding of the experience of immigration, but also fear of using services (Hoyle, 2019). Furthermore, language barriers may contribute to patients feeling disempowered in the therapy process by being unable to use language that is reflective of their experience (Hoyle, 2019)

The costs of these barriers can be significant and life-threatening for patients. For example, someone with Anorexia Nervosa, these barriers may contribute to misdiagnosis, delay in diagnosis, and poor quality of care. A delay in diagnosis for someone battling an eating disorder may be a matter of life and death. When most healthcare systems are designed for white, American, English speaking, middle-to-upper class men and women, every aspect of referral, help-seeking and treatment must be adapted to address barriers and provide meaningful change for clients.

MOVING FORWARD

Recommendations for Providers and Policy

With these barriers and costs in mind, how can the current integrated health care systems be adapted to meet these needs and how do we support culturally congruent providers in the creation of these institutions? When only 9% of those who earn their doctorates in psychology identify as Latinx, the inclusion of Latinx clinicians in the field is of utmost importance (U.S. Department of Education, 2012). An increase of Latinx clinicians can only occur as educational systems support, both emotionally and financially, the inclusion of Latinx students in master's and doctoral programs in psychology, counseling, and social work.

Patients should have availability and access to work with clinicians who fit their demographic preferences. Few studies have attempted to link patients' beliefs about racism in the healthcare system with how Latinxs use and experience health care, however, a study conducted by Chen and colleagues (2005) identified that Latinxs perceive racism in the healthcare system, and are more likely to prefer a Latinx physician. For these patients, racial beliefs and preferences may affect the quality of their interaction with their physician, and may be a factor in racial disparities in health care (Chen et al., 2005). It is important to shed light that not all minority patients want or need minority clinicians, however, it is possible that patients with strong racial preferences who are in race-discordant relationships may trust their clinician

Table 1.

Culturally Responsive Treatment Components	Example
Financial Access to Treatment	Access to insurance benefits for treatment, sliding scale options; For eating concerns, scholarship opportunities (including financial assistance and housing)
Culturally Responsive Assessment for Eating Concerns	First and foremost, assessing for eating disorders and eating concerns with all Latinx patients, recognizing that eating disorders are safety concerns and an area some patients may be hesitant to disclose without prompting from providers; Utilizing assessment tools for eating concerns valid for use with Latinx patients, including Eating Disorder Examination Questionnaire, Body Esteem Scale, Sociocultural Attitudes Towards Appearance Questionnaire, and Body Shape Questionnaire (Franko et al., 2012)
Awareness of Latinx Culture	Asking questions and trying to understand cultural experiences; Doing research outside of patient interactions (i.e. not relying on patient to "teach" provider); Avoiding making assumptions about cultural values
Reconnecting with Cultural Values	Inclusion of Latinx cultural values (as appropriate) including religion and food; For eating disorder treatment, understanding the role food plays in the family and reconnecting with cultural foods as part of the healing process (See above regarding not generalizing about cultural values); Recognizing and responding to potential treatment barriers, such as food deserts and lack of access to nutritious foods
Incorporating Value of Family Connectedness through Family Interventions	Using family therapy as an opportunity for growth for supportive others in awareness, knowledge and skills; Examples include giving family members the opportunity to ask questions to the provider prior to family therapy; Offering tailored psychoeducation to the family to foster familial connection
Incorporating Value of Family Connectedness Through Individual Interventions	Understanding when the patient's support system does not have the foundation of understanding around a mental health concern, particularly for eating disorders such as Anorexia Nervosa (i.e. recognizing that Anorexia is rarely discussed in Latinx families and discussing how to explain the disorder to patients' families); In individual therapy, discussing and preparing for conversations with support system
Having an Open and Transparent Approach to Treatment	Provider appropriately demonstrating affect and mirroring the patient's emotional experience as a sign of understanding; When a patient is experiencing a sense of isolation when battling a mental health concern, such as an eating disorder, the provider sharing their genuine emotional response can assist the patient in feeling "seen." Providers may also use self-disclosure in a constructive and client-focused way.

less, be less likely to follow up with clinicians' recommendations, may not understand their clinician, and may be less likely to develop a collaborative therapeutic relationship (Chen et al., 2005). These findings from Chen's study (2005) help to illuminate the role of patients' beliefs and preferences with their physician and satisfaction with the care they receive. Thus, when there is racial/ethnic concordance, a Latinx clinician may be able to understand the patient's cultural values and co-create culturally responsive interventions. Working with a Latinx clinician in an integrated health setting may further lead to bilingual communication with support systems and important discussions with clinicians around roles, expectations, and boundaries in the family. Furthermore, patients may feel that their clinician can relate or understand their cultural values, as well as experiences of marginalization.

Culturally responsive treatment may also include financial access to treatment, awareness of Latinx culture, and an open and transparent approach to therapy. Key components to person-centered access and treatment planning can be found in Table 1.

In summary, Latinx patients in integrated health settings may appreciate an open and transparent approach to therapy, as well as awareness of Latinx culture. Many Latinxs have a strong sense of *dignidad* (pride), which can result in being too proud to seek help, and if Latinxs are unable to establish *confianza* (trust) with their clinicians, they are unlikely to return for treatment (Barrera & Longoria, 2018). Thus, it's imperative that clinicians who provide behavioral health care to Latinxs understand these cultural concepts. Patients may also value when their therapists have encountered or understand the experience of feeling marginalized or othered in U.S. society. This ability to relate may be especially powerful when working with Latinx clinicians. Significant progress must be made to recruit and prioritize Latinx students and clinicians, particularly those who specialize in eating disorder treatment, as Latinxs "deserve a diverse, multidisciplinary, bilingual and bicultural behavioral workforce" (Chapa & Acosta, 2010, p. 4). Formal bilingual training programs in psychology and social work can offer the kind of coursework, field experience, and clinical supervision that will prepare future clinicians to work with Latinx populations (Clouse & Delgado-Romero, 2008). Programs designed to assist bilingual clinicians in becoming equally competent at providing services in English and Spanish, include coursework in professional and technical Spanish, language and psychological variables in interviews and assessments with Latinxs, Spanish-language professional communication skills, sociocultural foundations of counseling Latinxs, normal family development processes across cultures, and theories of multicultural counseling (Delgado-Romero et al., 2012). These training opportunities that are interwoven into the curriculum are great efforts to increase the representation of Spanish-speaking clinicians, and better equip the workforce to enhance interdisciplinary approaches to service delivery, collaboration, and continuity of care.

COLLABORATION AND BEYOND

As we have come to learn, the IBHC approach has plenty to offer and has the strength to bring forth close collaboration and communication between patients, families, providers and the larger healthcare system. Because primary care settings have become the entryway of IBHC, the benefits of implementing culturally competent responsive care, includes patient satisfaction, quality of care, improved access to services, and lower overall healthcare costs (Jongen et al., 2018). The increasing involvement of various providers in care delivery, has brought forth a level of improved collaboration that effectively allows providers to address the "whole person" while ensuring smooth movement of patients across services (Gold et al., 2017).

The integration of behavioral health services into primary health care requires the effective sharing of tasks among members of the integrated care team. The team works together with the patient to ensure connectivity, alignment and collaboration. Transformations toward integrated care require a good understanding of the various dimensions of integration, which in effect calls for the development of a comprehensive overview of the team composition. Focusing on the function, rather than title or previous role of team members ensures that all sharing of tasks are delivered to provide effective patient care. A formal team-building process is heavily encouraged, as it can help members understand and identify everyone's function on the team. Common roles on the integrated team include those shown in Figure 1.

INTEGRATED CARE TEAM INTRODUCTION

It is imperative to introduce and explain the concept of integrated care, so that the patient understands how the team of providers work behind the scenes to deliver care in the primary care setting. One of

Figure 1. Common Roles on the integrated team

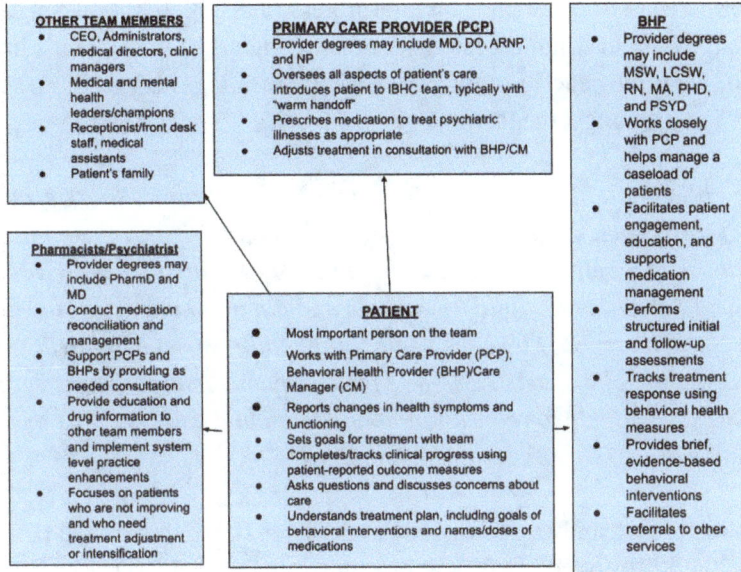

the best and most common ways to do this is to introduce the patient to the Behavioral Health Provider (BHP) during the "warm handoff" exchange. But this may vary, depending on whom the patient may see first. The key information that should be shared with the patient regarding this team-based approach includes informing the patient that they are an integral member of the team; one treatment plan will be utilized to support patient-centered goals; patient's PCP will oversee all aspects of patient care at the clinic; patient's team will be in frequent contact with one another to keep track of progress and provide counseling.

BREAKDOWN PROFESSIONAL SILOS

If you step into most healthcare facilities today, it is likely that you might notice that each provider typically operates within its own distinct silo. Unfortunately, the silo method contributes to a disconnect between providers and patients, contributing to the lack of information between groups in the healthcare system. Federal and state governments are seeking ways to break down silos that hinder the delivery of high quality, efficient services (Ewing & Tobler, 2014). Nowhere is this more evident than with the silos between physical health and behavioral health. IBHC however, has the potential to improve quality, improve patients' health, by successfully implementing an integrated system that streamlines and allows for one healthcare team or health entity to treat the "whole person."

Effective communication is central to breaking down silos. When information can seamlessly be shared between providers and patients, high-quality shared care is practiced, which leads to increased patient satisfaction and implementation, to a truly integrated behavioral health system. In this author's dissertation, the theme "interprofessional collaboration and teamwork" (De Los Santos, 2020) was present, as participants reported the importance of multiple healthcare providers from different professional backgrounds working together alongside patients. Providers recounted how interprofessional collaboration is the practice of approaching patient care from a team-based perspective. One participant, a nurse practitioner, shared their experience on interprofessional collaboration, specifically, their use of the electronic medical record to communicate with other members of the patient's integrated care team. This participant also shares the benefits of interprofessional meetings serving as an avenue of discussing treatment plans and goals amongst the team.

I love being able to collaborate. I love getting messages from therapists too, because sometimes your patients will tell therapists something that they won't tell us. Or if I start them on a new medication I love getting the feedback and being able to talk about that. I love the [Integrated Mental and Physical Care Team] meetings. I think it's so helpful to sit down and put all of our heads together. You know with having the pharmacists in there. So, I love the behavioral health aspect and having social workers here onsite, and I love having the pharmacists onsite. I mean any medication questions. You know, [names pharmacists] are always available for consultation and that's the amazing part that most people don't have working in primary care (De Los Santos, 2020, p. 61).

Nearly all providers in this study discussed the benefits of IBHC, and noted being overwhelmingly satisfied with having the ability to collaborate interprofessionally on site (De Los Santos, 2020). Further research has also explored provider perspectives on having a behavioral health provider within their collaborative team, agreeing that behavioral health providers help patients by reducing patient distress, improve patient's abilities to cope, assist primary care providers with providing better patient care, and lower primary care providers stress (Butler et al., 2011; Miller-Matero et al., 2016). We created a table with key strategies to consider when focusing on strengthening collaboration within team members of the IBHC team.

PATIENT ENGAGEMENT=PATIENT EMPOWERMENT

As we continue to remember to keep the patient front and center, and as the most important member of the team, it is evident that the concept of patient-centered care is an essential aspiration of high-quality health care systems. The Institute of Medicine (2001) defines patient-centered care as "care that is respectful of and responsive to individual patient preferences, needs, and values." We advocate very strongly on the relationship between the patient and the IBHC team, as it results in improved care processes and health outcomes, including the ability of the patient to survive and thrive.

In De Los Santos's study (2020), one of the most powerful findings was how providers were not educating undocumented patients about what integrated care is. The patients in the study defined integrated care in a way that indicated a lack of knowledge about the concept. However, patients were still able to perceive when integration and coordination were happening. Furthermore, providers in the study shared the perception that a majority of their undocumented patients had no desire to partake in decision-making in regards to their treatment, justifying paternalistic practices (De Los Santos, 2020). De Los Santos (2020) importantly highlights the number of factors presumed to exacerbate undocumented patients' acquiescence to providers' decisions, including a lack of thorough understanding of the U.S. healthcare system, their treatment, or the role of providers (Casas & Cabrera, 2011). Notably, many Latinx patients may also have low self-perceptions of their social status, which are likely to be reinforced by the power imbalance inherent in the patient provider relationship.

Table 2.

Key Strategies	Example
Sharing Goals	All team members collaboratively work toward understanding and agreeing to focus on the patient's goals for the treatment plan. These goals help to establish a shared language and vision for providers working together, and leads to clarification of roles and responsibilities in delivery of care.
Building Mutual Trust	Close interpersonal ties between providers can act as an effective mechanism to build mutual trust and respect within a partnership. This type of partnership develops over time through team building and meetings, as well as shared understanding of concepts of care. Creating a safe space to allow providers to share patient success stories and challenges can strengthen team members' commitment to sharing care.
Refining Workflow	As the team identifies the patient's needs, monitors treatment outcomes and makes adjustments, clinical workflows can be refined to improve integrated care delivery and conduct additional problem solving as needed (i.e. follow up with patients during routine primary care appointments and schedule as needed integrated appointments)
Agreeing on Communication Strategy	Reach an agreement on communication strategy, including in-person communication, electronic communication, or using the electronic medical record. Consider frequent huddles to facilitate prompt team communication around patients and organizing team priorities.

Patient-centeredness has long been recognized as a desirable attribute within the healthcare industry. Advocates of patient centered care honor patient's preferences, needs, values, apply a biopsychosocial perspective versus a biomedical perspective, and build a strong alliance between patient and provider (Greene et al., 2012). Patients are at the center of integrated care, and health systems need to support and empower them to successfully navigate the integrated care system. For the Latinx patient experience of IBHC to improve, we must consider all of interactions that take place within the healthcare system, particularly those who are undocumented. Research has found that patients who are empowered in regards to their health and healthcare are most successful at navigating the healthcare system (Arnold, 2007). Patient involvement in programs to educate them about the care they are receiving has been found to be positively associated with positive patient outcomes and increased satisfaction with care in patients of diverse socioeconomic backgrounds (Grieger et al., 2000; Kaplan et al.,2004; Stewart et al., 1995; White, 2012). When patients are involved in patient-empowerment training, patients are provided with skills and knowledge that will enable them to take charge of their health. Such empowerment trainings are needed, given that disempowerment has been identified as a significant health risk factor, especially for disadvantaged populations like racial/ethnic minorities (Bergsma, 2004).

Improving patient engagement in their own care should be a main priority for providers, with the goal of improving health care delivery, quality and efficacy (Hibbard, Mahoney, Stock, & Tusler, 2007; Hibbard & Cunningham, 2008; Fitzsimons & Fuller, 2002). Research suggests that patient engagement levels differ by race and ethnicity (Hibbard, Greene, & Overton, 2013), with Latinxs demonstrating lower engagement levels compared to whites (Cunningham, Hibbard, & Gibbons, 2011). Evidence suggests that culturally tailored community-based patient education programs (Alegría, Sribney, Perez, et al., 2009), and programs targeted to reduce language barriers can effectively engage minorities in their own care, and eventually improve population health of underserved minorities. Therefore, it is critical for providers to have a comprehensive understanding of how to enhance patient engagement, particularly among Latinxs, to improve health and reduce health disparities (Alegria et al, 2014).

Active patient involvement and engagement is crucial for good integrated care. When team members are successful at working directly with the patient to develop the treatment plan, this approach helps to foster the patients' commitment to the plan. Successful efforts play a role in providing patients with information and tools to enable them to take greater control over their own health, and promote a sense of personal and interpersonal control, as well as address social, political, and legal factors that influence valued social roles, and outcomes such as health care decision making and treatment choices (Gutiérrez & Ortega, 1991; Rappaport, 1987; Solomon, 1976).

To that end, patient-centered culturally responsive health care includes an arrangement of teaching patients personal empowerment skills and strategies for impacting the healthcare system to meet their needs. Furthermore, teaching clinic providers and office staff members interpersonal skills that foster patient empowerment, and promoting the use of patient comment boxes for patients to provide feedback to providers, staff, overall health care system, and health care researchers on the quality of health care they experience (Tucker, 2007). Patient empowerment training can be provided by behavioral health providers as well as by other professionals and community health workers trained to provide this training. It is imperative however, that the trainers include some individuals of similar cultural backgrounds to be represented among the patients being trained.

CONCLUSION

This chapter has been a long answer to the question, "What is integrated behavioral healthcare?" It is our hope that as you finish reading this chapter, you'll have a general definition, you'll understand the roles of your teammates, and specifically know how to make integrated behavioral healthcare work. The evidence of benefit to people in integrated behavioral healthcare settings compels considerations of how to get it done. Therefore, with these points in mind, you can retain responsiveness to published literature and definitions while navigating realistically in your settings to enhance behavioral health in Latinx populations, reduce healthcare disparities, and provide more inclusive and culturally attuned care. Integrated behavioral healthcare centers on putting patients first, improving health outcomes and empowering the patient. If executed well, integrated behavioral healthcare can address the fragmented and inadequate nature of care for Latinx people who experience common systemic barriers, while helping them regain control over their health

REFERENCES

AAFP. (2017). *Primary Care.* https://www.aafp.org/about/policies/all/primary-care.html https://www.ncbi.nlm.nih.gov/pmc/articles/PMC5890504/

Abbate-Daga, G., Amianto, F., Delsedime, N., De-Bacco, C., & Fassino, S. (2013). Resistance to treatment in eating disorders: A critical challenge. *BMC Psychiatry, 13,* 294. doi:10.1186/1471-244X-13-294 PMID:24199620

Alegria, M., Canino, G., Rios, R., Vera, M., Calderon, J., Rusch, D., & Ortega, A. N. (2002). Inequalities in use of specialty mental health services among Latinos, African Americans, and non-White Latinos. *Psychiatric Services (Washington, D.C.), 53,* 1547–1555. doi:10.1176/appi.ps.53.12.1547 PMID:12461214

Alegría, M., Chatterji, P., Wells, K., Cao, Z., Chen, C., Takeuchi, D., & Meng, X.-L. (2008). Disparity in depression treatment among racial and ethnic minority populations in the United States. [PubMed: 18971402]. *Psychiatric Services (Washington, D.C.)*, *59*(11), 1264–1272. doi:10.1176/ps.2008.59.11.1264 PMID:18971402

Alegría, M., Mulvaney-Day, N., Torres, M., Polo, A., Cao, Z., & Canino, G. (2007). Prevalence of psychiatric disorders across Latino subgroups in the United States. *American Journal of Public Health*, *97*(1), 68–75. doi:10.2105/AJPH.2006.087205 PMID:17138910

Alegría, M., Sribney, W., Perez, D., Laderman, M., & Keefe, K. (2009). The role of patient activation on patient–provider communication and quality of care for US and foreign born Latino patients. *Journal of General Internal Medicine*, *24*(3), 534–541. doi:10.100711606-009-1074-x PMID:19842003

Alegria, M., Woo, M., Cao, Z., Torres, M., Meng, X. L., & Striegel-Moore, R. (2007). Prevalence and correlates of eating disorders in Latinos in the United States. *The International Journal of Eating Disorders*, *40*(Suppl), S15–S21. 1 doi:0.1002/eat.2040

American Psychological Association. (2017). *Multicultural guidelines: An ecological approach to context, identity, and intersectionality*. Retrieved from: http://www.apa.org/about/policy/multicultural-guidelines.pdf

Bailey, Z. D., Feldman, J. M., & Bassett, M. T. (2021). How structural racism works—Racist policies as a root cause of US racial health inequities. *The New England Journal of Medicine*, *384*(8), 768–773. doi:10.1056/NEJMms2025396 PMID:33326717

Becker, A. E., Franko, D. L., Speck, A., & Herzog, D. B. (2003). Ethnicity and differential access to care for eating disorder symptoms. *International Journal of Eating Disorders*, *33*(2), 205–212. doi:10.1002/eat.10129 PMID:12616587

Brewer, B. (2021). *What is Integrated Health? Models & Systems For Healthcare Innovation*. Mhaonline. https://www.mhaonline.com/blog/integrated-behavioral-health

Bridges, A. J., Andrews, A. R. III, & Deen, T. L. (2012). Mental health needs and service utilization by Hispanic immigrants residing in mid-southern United States. *Journal of Transcultural Nursing*, *23*(4), 359–368. doi:10.1177/1043659612451259 PMID:22802297

Butler, M., Kane, R. L., McAlpine, D., Kathol, R., Fu, S. S., Hagedorn, H., & Wilt, T. (2011). Does integrated care improve treatment for depression? A systematic review. *The Journal of Ambulatory Care Management*, *34*(2), 113–125. doi:10.1097/JAC.0b013e31820ef605 PMID:21415610

Cabassa, L. J., Zayas, L. H., & Hansen, M. C. (2006). Latino adults' access to mental health care: A review of epidemiological studies. *Administration and Policy in Mental Health*, *33*(3), 316–330. doi:10.100710488-006-0040-8 PMID:16598658

Chang, C. (2019). Social Determinants of Health and Health Disparities Among Immigrants and their Children. *Current Problems in Pediatric and Adolescent Health Care, 49*(1), 23-30. https://www.sciencedirect.com/science/article/pii/S1538544218301755 doi:10.1016/j.cppeds.2018.11.009

Chapa, T., & Acosta, H. (2010). *Movilizandonos por nuestro futuro: Strategic development of a mental health workforce for Latinos—Consensus statements and recommendations*. Retrieved from http://minorityhealth.hhs.gov/Assets/pdf/Checked/1/MOVILIZANDONOS_POR_NUESTRO_FUTURO_CONSENSUS_REPORT2010.pdf

Chen, F. M., Fryer, G. E., Phillips, R. L., Wilson, E., & Pathman, D. E. (2005). Patients' beliefs about racism, preferences for physician race, and satisfaction with care. *Annals of Family Medicine*, *3*(2), 138–143. doi:10.1370/afm.282 PMID:15798040

Cunningham, P. J., Hibbard, J., & Gibbons, C. B. (2011). Raising low 'patient activation'rates among Hispanic immigrants may equal expanded coverage in reducing access disparities. *Health Affairs*, *30*(10), 1888–1894. doi:10.1377/hlthaff.2009.0805 PMID:21976331

Dawes, D. (2020). *The political determinants of health*. Johns Hopkins University Press.

De Los Santos, J. (2020). *Under one roof: The experiences of undocumented Latinx patients and providers navigating integrated care* [Unpublished doctoral dissertation]. University of Georgia.

Delgado-Romero, E. A., Espino, M., Werther, E., & Gonzalez, M. J. (2012). Building infrastructure through training of bilingual mental health providers. In L. P. Buki & L. M. Piedra (Eds.), *Haciendo camino al andar: Creating infrastructures for Latino mental health* (pp. 99–116). Springer.

Edward, J., & Hines-Martin, V. (2016). Examining perceived barriers to healthcare access for Hispanics in a southern urban community. *Journal of Hospital Administration*, *5*(2), 101–108. doi:10.5430/jha.v5n2p102

Ewing, J., & Tobler, L. (2014, November 12). *Quashing the Silos and Getting to Integrated Health Care*. NCSL. https://www.ncsl.org/blog/2014/11/12/quashing-the-silos-and-getting-to-integrated-health-care.aspx

Fitzsimons, S., & Fuller, R. (2002). Empowerment and its implications for clinical practice in mental health: A review. *Journal of Mental Health (Abingdon, England)*, *11*(5), 481–499. doi:10.1080/09638230020023

Franko, D. L., Jenkins, A., Roehrig, J. P., Luce, K. H., Crowther, J. H., & Rodgers, R. F. (2012). Psychometric properties of measures of eating disorder risk in Latina college women. *International Journal of Eating Disorders*, *45*(4), 592–596. doi:10.1002/eat.20979 PMID:22271562

Gilbert, S. (2003). Eating disorders in women of color. *Clinical Psychology: Science and Practice*, *10*(4), 444–455. doi:10.1093/clipsy.bpg045

Gold, S. B., Green, L. A., & Peek, C. J. (2017). From our practices to yours: Key messages for the journey to integrated behavioral health. *Journal of the American Board of Family Medicine*, *30*(1), 25–34. doi:10.3122/jabfm.2017.01.160100 PMID:28062814

Goldman Sachs. (2022, May 31). *Could immigration solve the US worker shortage?* Retrieved September 4, 2022, from https://www.goldmansachs.com/insights/pages/could-immigration-solve-the-us-worker-shortage.html

Grazier, K. L., Smiley, M. L., & Bondalapati, K. S. (2016). Overcoming Barriers to Integrating Behavioral Health and Primary Care Services. *Journal of Primary Care & Community Health, 7*(4), 242–248. doi:10.1177/2150131916656455 PMID:27380923

Greene, S. M., Tuzzio, L., & Cherkin, D. (2012). A framework for making patient-centered care front and center. *The Permanente Journal, 16*(3), 49–53. doi:10.7812/TPP/12-025 PMID:23012599

Haines, A., Kuruvilla, S., & Borchert, M. (2004). *Policy and Practice Theme Papers Bridging the implementation gap between knowledge and action for health.* https://www.who.int/bulletin/volumes/82/10/724.pdf

Harris, K. M., Edlund, M. J., & Larson, S. (2005). Racial and ethnic differences in the mental health problems and use of mental health care. *Medical Care, 43*(8), 775–784. doi:10.1097/01.mlr.0000170405.66264.23 PMID:16034291

Healthy People 2030. Office of Disease Prevention and Health Promotion. (n.d.). *Health Equity.* U.S. Department of Health and Human Services. https://health.gov/healthypeople/priority-areas/health-equity-healthy-people-2030

Hibbard, J. H., & Cunningham, P. J. (2008). *How engaged are consumers in their health and health care, and why does it matter?* (Vol. 8). Center for Studying Health System Change.

Hibbard, J. H., Greene, J., & Overton, V. (2013). Patients with lower activation associated with higher costs; delivery systems should know their patients' 'scores'. *Health Affairs, 32*(2), 216–222. doi:10.1377/hlthaff.2012.1064 PMID:23381513

Hibbard, J. H., Mahoney, E. R., Stock, R., & Tusler, M. (2007). Do increases in patient activation result in improved self-management behaviors? *Health Services Research, 42*(4), 1443–1463. doi:10.1111/j.1475-6773.2006.00669.x PMID:17610432

Horner, K. (2021, November 16). *Immigration Status: A Political Determinant of Health.* Gender Policy Report.

Hoyle, A. (2019). *Treatment for anorexia nervosa with latinx clients: a qualitative inquiry* [Unpublished doctoral dissertation]. University of Georgia.

Institute of Medicine (US) Committee on Quality of Health Care in America. (2001). *Crossing the quality chasm: a new health system for the 21st century.* National Academies Press.

Jongen, C., McCalman, J., & Bainbridge, R. (2018). Health workforce cultural competency interventions: A systematic scoping review. *BMC Health Services Research, 18*(1), 1–15. doi:10.118612913-018-3001-5 PMID:29609614

Keyes, K. M., Martins, S. S., Hatzenbuehler, M. L., Blanco, C., Bates, L. M., & Hasin, D. S. (2012). Mental health service utilization for psychiatric disorders among Latinos living in the United States: The role of ethnic subgroup, ethnic identity, and language/social preferences. *Social Psychiatry and Psychiatric Epidemiology, 47*(3), 383–394. doi:10.100700127-010-0323-y PMID:21290097

Kickbusch, I. (2015). The political determinants of health--10 years on. *BMJ, 350*(2), h81–h81. doi:10.1136/bmj.h81

Kittelsen, S. K., Fukuda-Parr, S., & Storeng, K. T. (2019). Editorial: The political determinants of health inequities and universal health coverage. *Globalization and Health, 15*(S1). doi:10.1186/s12992-019-0514-6

Lanesskog, D., & Piedra, L. (2016). *Integrated Health Care for Latino Immigrants and Refugees: What Do They Need?* doi:10.1007/978-3-319-42533-7_2

Palmer, L. C. (2007). Crossing the color line: Emerging realities about eating disorders and treatment with women of color. *Journal of Feminist Family Therapy, 19*(4), 21–41. doi:10.1300/J086v19n04_02

Perez, M., Ohrt, T. K., & Hoek, H. W. (2016, November). Prevalence and treatment of eating disorders among Hispanics/Latino Americans in the United States. *Current Opinion in Psychiatry, 29*(6), 378–382. doi:10.1097/YCO.0000000000000277 PMID:27648780

Raine, R., Or, Z., Prady, S., & Bevan, G. (2016). *Evaluating health-care equity.* NIHR Journals Library. https://www.ncbi.nlm.nih.gov/books/NBK361257/

Regional Committee for the Eastern Mediterranean. (2006). *Fifty-third Session Original: Arabic Agenda item 7 (a) The role of government in health development.* https://applications.emro.who.int/docs/EM_RC53_Tech.Disc.1_en.pdf

Sanchez, K., Chapa, T., Ybarra, R., & Martinez, O. N. (2012). Eliminating disparities through the integration of behavioral health and primary care services for racial and ethnic minority populations, including individuals with limited English proficiency: A literature review report. United States Department of Health and Human Services, Office of Minority Health.

Talen, M. R., Fraser, J. S., & Cauley, K. (2005). Training Primary Care Psychologists: A Model for Predoctoral Programs. *Professional Psychology, Research and Practice, 36*(2), 136–143. doi:10.1037/0735-7028.36.2.136

Talleyrand, R. M. (2012). Disordered eating in women of color: Some counseling considerations. *Journal of Counseling and Development, 90*(3), 271–280. doi:10.1002/j.1556-6676.2012.00035.x

U.S. Department of Education, National Center for Education Statistics, Integrated Postsecondary Education Data System (IPEDS). (1984-2012). *Completion surveys* [Data files and dictionaries]. Retrieved from https://nces.ed.gov/ipeds/datacenter/DataFiles.aspx

U.S. Department of Health and Human Services. (2001). *Mental health: Culture, race, and ethnicity—A supplement to mental health: A report of the surgeon general.* Author.

Walsh, J. M., Wheat, M. E., & Freund, K. (2000). Detection, evaluation, and treatment of eating disorders. *Journal of General Internal Medicine, 15*(8), 577–590. doi:10.1046/j.1525-1497.2000.02439.x PMID:10940151

What Is Integrated Behavioral Health Care (IBHC)? (n.d.). Retrieved April 2, 2022, from https://integrationacademy.ahrq.gov/products/behavioral-health-measures-atlas/what-is-ibhc

WHO. (2018). *Integrating health services Brief.* https://www.who.int/docs/default-source/primary-health-care-conference/linkages.pdf

World Health Organization. (2013). *Closing the health equity gap: policy options and opportunities for action*. Available at: https://www.cdc.gov/nchhstp/socialdeterminants/docs/who-closing-health-equity-gap-policyopportunities-.pdf

Zubatsky, M., Edwards, T. M., Wakabayashi, H., & Ivbijaro, G. (2018). Integrated behavioural health in primary care across the world: Three countries, three perspectives. *Family Practice, 35*(6), 645–648. doi:10.1093/fampra/cmy034 PMID:29741628

ENDNOTE

[1] A pseudonym

Chapter 15
Gaining Access and Treatment Equity (GATE):
A Framework for Culturally Responsive Clinical Care

Ana Julia Bridges
University of Arkansas, USA

ABSTRACT

Despite often similar or higher prevalence rates of many psychiatric disorders, Latinxs residing in the continental US are significantly less likely to seek needed clinical care than ethnic majority group members. This inequality creates or exacerbates mental health disparities. Here, the authors provide a framework for understanding barriers Latinxs may face to accessing and receiving culturally-responsive mental healthcare. The gaining access and treatment equity (GATE) model articulates four major barriers: perceived need, internal barriers, external barriers, and clinical/procedural barriers. Increasing mental health equity for Latinxs will require attending to all four levels. The authors articulate how clinics have used the GATE model to expand the reach of services.

GAINING ACCESS AND TREATMENT EQUITY (GATE): A FRAMEWORK FOR CULTURALLY RESPONSIVE CLINICAL CARE

Despite similar or higher rates of psychiatric disorders, most Latinxs are less likely to seek mental health care than ethnic majority group members (Alegría et al., 2008; SAMHSA, 2020; Young et al., 2001). Even when care is sought, Latinxs are less likely to remain in treatment and, consequently, to obtain good therapeutic outcomes (Cabassa et al., 2006; Olfson et al., 2009). However, engaging fully in treatment results in comparably beneficial outcomes for Latinxs and non-Latinxs alike (e.g., Horrell, 2008; Miranda et al., 2005; Sue, 1988; Tonigan, 2003). Inequities in mental health care use create or exacerbate mental health disparities in Latinxs. Here, I provide a framework for understanding the barriers Latinxs

DOI: 10.4018/978-1-6684-4901-1.ch015

face when accessing needed mental health care, illustrating the application of this framework in two Latinx-serving behavioral health clinics.

Health Disparities

A health disparity is defined as significant differences in disease incidence, prevalence, or burden (e.g., mortality rates) in a particular subgroup as compared to the general population (US Public Law 106-525, 2000). A health disparity is not the same as a health difference. To illustrate this distinction using a somewhat ridiculous example, one can accurate note that men experience prostate problems at a much higher rate than women. However, this difference in disease prevalence rate would not be seen as evidence of a health disparity among men and women, given women lack a prostate. Instead, what is concerning is a difference born of *avoidable* health inequities (Graham, 2004). Health status inequities are variations in the disease prevalence and burden between population sub-groups, while health care inequities are differences in access to or availability of healthcare services (National Academies of Sciences, Engineering, and Medicine, 2017).

According to the World Health Organization (WHO, 2018), avoidable inequities in health status and healthcare access between groups of people arise from inequalities in social and economic conditions. These conditions and their effects on people's lives determine a group's risk of illness. For instance, children living in older housing units with lead paint are at elevated risk of brain damage, learning, and behavior problems (CDC, 2022), while migrant farmworkers working in close proximity to fertilizers, pesticides, and chemicals are at increased risk of infectious diseases, respiratory conditions, and cancer (Hansen & Donohoe, 2003). Social and economic conditions also are related to the actions people take to prevent or treat illness when it occurs. Are preventive medical services easily accessible? Does the person have access to health insurance or affordable medications? Is the community supportive of help-seeking (St. Arnault & Woo, 2018)? The National Institutes of Health (HealthyPeople.gov, 2022) notes health disparities adversely affect groups of people who have systematically experienced discrimination or exclusion. These characteristics include race or ethnicity, as well as other aspects of social identity (gender, gender identity, sexual orientation, religion), socioeconomic status (educational attainment, employment status, income, health insurance), ability (cognitive, sensory, physical), and geographic region. The conditions that give rise to unequal social and economic conditions between groups are called social determinants of health (US Department of Health and Human Services, 2022).

Across many social determinants of health, Latinxs show a disadvantage (Figure 1). For instance, Latinxs are less likely to have completed high school, more likely to be unemployed, living in poverty, and uninsured, less likely to own two or more vehicles per household, and less likely to have basic health literacy skills compared to non-Latinx Whites[1]. Although differences in health equity appear to be largely born out of economic differences among groups (and certainly increased personal wealth improves health), even when comparing within income brackets, Latinxs show poorer self-rated health status (Robert Wood Johnson Foundation, 2008).

Mental Health Disparities

National epidemiological studies suggest Latinxs are at similar or even lower risk for many common mental health disorders as majority group members (Alegria et al., 2009; Cabassa et al., 2006). For instance, rates of depressive disorders, anxiety disorders, and substance use disorders tend to be lower

Figure 1.

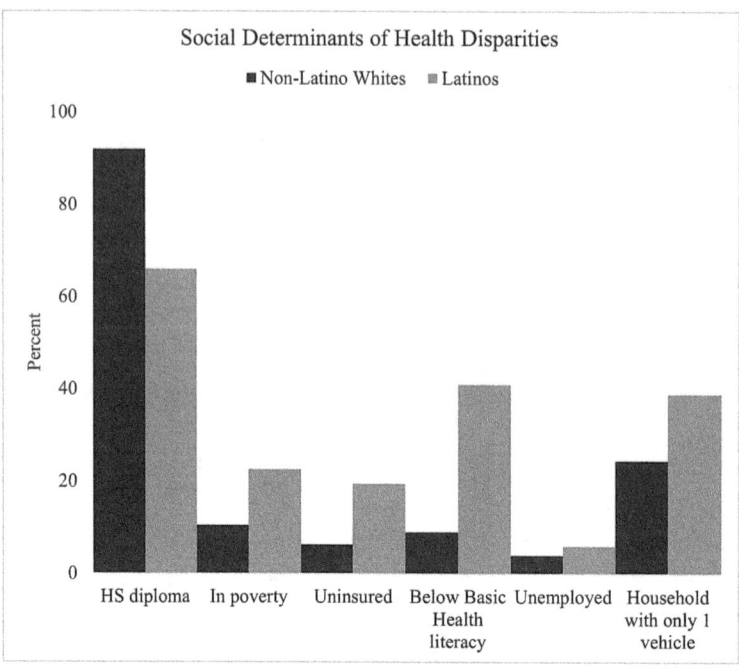

in Latinxs in general and Latinx immigrants in particular compared to non-Latinx Whites (Alegria et al., 2009). However, some specific symptoms of psychiatric problems are more likely to be endorsed by Latinxs, including internalizing symptoms such as feelings of worthlessness or hopelessness, sadness, and serious psychological distress (CDC, 2018). .

Mental health disparities become more pronounced when narrowing the focus to just people who meet criteria for a psychiatric disorder. For instance, only one-third of Latinxs meeting criteria for a major depressive disorder sought psychiatric care in the past year (Alegria et al., 2008). A review of national epidemiological studies concludes that, compared to non-Latinx Whites with psychiatric disorders, Latinxs with psychiatric disorders are less likely to use specialty mental health services, more likely to rely on the medical sector to obtain mental health care, more likely to delay seeking services, less likely to receive guideline-congruent care once services are sought and, perhaps not surprisingly, less satisfied with the care they do receive (Cabassa et al., 2006). They are also more likely to drop out of treatment (CDC, 2015).

THE GAINING ACCESS AND TREATMENT EQUITY (GATE) MODEL

Numerous theoretical models have been developed to understand how and why people seek care for health conditions. These models include the theory of planned behavior (Ajzen, 1991), the health belief model (Rosenstock, 1974), the health care utilization model (Andersen, 1995), and the cultural determinants of help seeking model (St. Arnault, 2009). According to the theory of planned behavior (Ajzen, 1991), attitudes, subjective norms, and self-efficacy influence behavioral intentions which, in turn, influences actual help-seeking behavior. The health belief model (Rosenstock, 1974) explains help seeking as a function of individual and environmental factors that influence perceived need and access to services. The model also includes individuals' health behaviors and outcomes of help seeking, such as evaluated need and satisfaction with services. The health care utilization model (Andersen, 1995) sees help seeking as arising from individual perceptions of the illness (susceptibility, severity), demographic factors, and cues to action (which include symptoms or pain); these all influence perceived need. Demographic and sociopsychological variables also influence the relative pros and cons of help seeking. The combination of pros/cons and perceived need then influence the likelihood of someone engaging in a health-related behavior or action. The cultural determinants of help seeking model was developed specifically for understanding help seeking for health-related problems in minority populations and includes information about the social context and dynamics that influence help seeking and how culture may influence the interpretation of symptoms (St. Arnault, 2009).

The above models vary in their complexity (from relatively simple to highly complex) and their focus (from quite narrow to very broad). However, as a framework for understanding psychiatric care specifically, they tend to be limited by: (a) a focus on medical health care rather than mental health care; (b) a focus on taking one specific health care action (e.g., screening for tuberculosis) versus on help seeking generally; (c) a lack of cultural considerations critical to understanding differences in help seeking for people of color; and/or (d) a lack of attention to what happens *after* the person seeks care (i.e., components of the care delivery itself that may contribute to health disparities).

In response, I propose a framework for understanding mental health help seeking that integrates components of other models while simplifying and describing the nature of barriers that can interfere with successful treatment outcomes. The *Gaining Access and Treatment Equity* (GATE) model describes the process of help seeking as a series of steps (Figure 2). Barriers at earlier steps are theorized to interfere with subsequent steps and, ultimately, benefitting from mental-health help-seeking behavior. The steps of help seeking, according to the GATE model, are: perceiving a need for care, overcoming internal barriers, overcoming structural barriers, and overcoming possible clinical or procedural barriers. Each is described below.

Perceived Need

The mental health help-seeking process begins with the perception that something is wrong (or less than optimal), that what is wrong is a problem for the person, and that symptoms are unlikely to remit on their own without some sort of intervention (Mojtabai et al., 2002). If a person does not perceive they have a psychiatric problem (e.g., depression), they will not seek care. Relatedly, if a person does not perceive themselves as *susceptible* to a problem (e.g., posttraumatic stress following a traumatic event), they are also unlikely to seek care. Finally, perceiving the illness/condition or its consequences to be no big deal (e.g., symptoms are not seen as creating problems in work, family, or other important domains of life), or that the problems are temporary and will go away with time, then that person will not move forward with seeking care.

Internal Barriers

Once a person perceives the need for psychiatric care, then the next step is navigating internal barriers. Internal barriers include beliefs and attitudes about both the symptoms and the sources of help. Although oftentimes lumped in with perceived need (Mojtabai et al., 2002), I find it conceptually useful to con-

Figure 2.

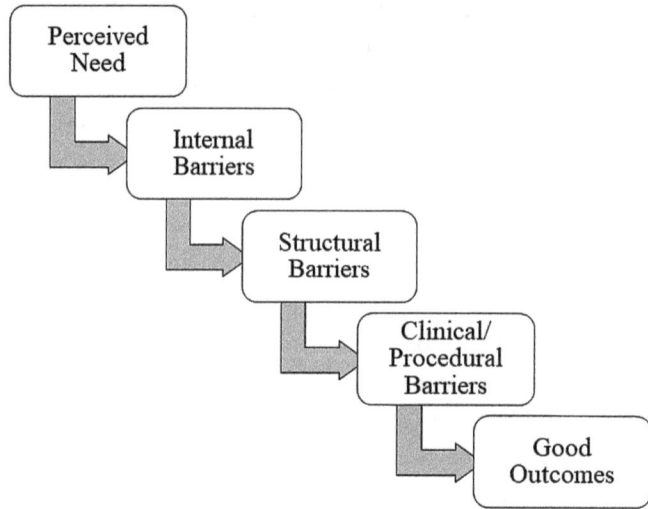

sider internal barriers as a second step in the help-seeking process. Once individuals believe they have a problem that is unlikely to improve without help (i.e., they have a perceived need for care), internal barriers can facilitate or impede help-seeking. One example of an internal barrier is the stigma someone may hold about psychiatric symptoms or helping services. Examples of stigma can include feelings of shame, being concerned of how others will view the person, and beliefs that mental health help seeking is only appropriate for people who are "*loco*"—i.e., crazy. A second example of an internal barrier is an attitude, such as holding negative attitudes towards therapy. Internal barriers can also include some cultural values, such as believing that one should not disclose personal struggles to others, especially people outside of the family, or that seeking help is a sign of weakness.

When in this stage, the individual may consider multiple ways of dealing with problems, not just seeking therapy. Indeed, therapy is often the last place people look for help, once other helping methods have been exhausted (Cabassa & Zayas, 2007). For each potential helping resource, the individual must balance the perceived benefits of treatment with perceived costs. Some of the benefits a person might anticipate they will get from seeking help include beliefs that the treatment is appropriate for that illness/ailment, and that one would *personally* benefit from the treatment, and confidence in the provider's skills. However, these benefits must be weighed in the context of possible conflicting values or beliefs. Values or beliefs that may conflict, as described above, include stigma about the condition or about needing help, cultural values of stoicism or machismo, or even a lack of self-efficacy that one is capable of changing. If the internal calculus favors cons of help seeking relative to pros, the individual will not progress further.

External Barriers

Even once the person has made the decision to seek help, external barriers can thwart the best of intentions. Not having a clinic nearby means people may not get care they need. Even if a clinic is nearby, if it is not within walking distance or on a major public transportation route, if the person lacks a car or other form of transportation, or if the person faces mobility issues, then care may not be sought

(SAMHSA, 2015). Probably the most common reason people do not seek needed care is because of prohibitive costs and, relatedly, a lack of health insurance (Bridges et al., 2012). Other things that can interfere with help-seeking include clinics only offering appointments during hours that conflict with work or other obligations (e.g., only 9 AM – 5 PM hours), a lack of childcare options, and even long waiting lists or delays before an open appointment time is available (SAMHSA, 2015). For immigrants in particular, fear of the consequences of seeking care (such as worries about deportation) can present an additional external barrier.

Clinical/Procedural Barriers

Navigated all prior barriers to seeking care is not enough to reduce mental health disparities. Attention must also be paid to clinical or procedural practices that may sustain inequitable outcomes among vulnerable groups. For instance, even if someone believes they have a problem that requires help, believes the pros of seeking help are greater than the cons, and can navigate structural barriers to make an initial appointment, they may find the help lacking in ways that lead to premature termination of services or less efficacious treatment outcomes (Benish et al., 2011; Vasquez, 2007). Clinical or procedural barriers are varied; all focus on the context of mental health care itself—what is happening in the therapy room. For example, if a client is unable to access a therapist who speaks her preferred language, she may have to conduct sessions in a non-preferred language. Speaking in a non-preferred language can interfere with therapy since therapists literally use their words to help people heal from psychiatric challenges. If a client cannot express herself precisely because she is speaking in a second language, or if she cannot fully understand the nuance of the English words and phrases that the therapist is speaking, it is reasonable to assume therapy will be less effective. Indeed, Griner & Smith (2006) found therapy provided in the client's native language was twice as effective as therapy in a second language. While using an interpreter can be helpful so that both client and therapist are able to use their preferred language to communicate, untrained interpreters can interfere with quality therapy (Paone & Malott, 2008). Even trained interpreters may struggle with the nuance of translating into diverse dialects or may be efficient at translating words, but not at providing context or cultural brokering (Chang et al., 2021). Clients who have low literacy may also experience clinical barriers to good mental health care if, for instance, they are provided with bulky reading materials that are not easily comprehended. Worse yet, many clients may be denied any psychoeducational materials at all because they are only available in English (Pastrana et al., 2017). Clinical barriers also can occur if standardized assessment instruments are not available in the client's preferred language or if they were not normed on populations that are like the client. Inappropriately normed assessment instruments can result in a client being misdiagnosed. Finally, clinical barriers can occur because of prejudice or biases the clinician may hold, which could result in therapeutic microaggressions or improper care (Owen et al., 2014).

Unlike other types of health behaviors, such as receiving a cancer screening, most psychiatric care requires *continued* engagement with the health service provider for clinical change to occur. This means that we must attend to the clinical or procedural barriers a person encounters when accessing care that interferes with treatment engagement and retention. For example, if someone attends a first therapy appointment but the provider does not speak the person's preferred language and if there is a lack of interpreters, the person has encountered a clinical barrier that will thwart continued help-seeking at that location. Similarly, if important paperwork such as policies on confidentiality are not available in the person's native language, this is a clinical barrier that can interfere with a patient obtaining services (and being asked to sign a consent form one does not understand is a violation of psychologists' code of ethics). A therapist may interact with a client in a manner that is perceived as culturally insensitive or even rude or racist—clearly, this will result in a client (rightly) discontinuing services before being helped. In fact, such an interaction may actually *harm* a patient and may exacerbate health disparities. As noted above, another common clinical barrier occurs when a clinic lacks symptom measures and other assessment tools are properly translated and normed for populations like that of the client. Finally, therapeutic approaches do not match the client's beliefs about the nature of their difficulties (such as asking someone to challenge a "cognitive distortion" rather than helping with addressing a role conflict or a curse) can be a clinical barrier. Importantly, clinical barriers increase the likelihood that a person will drop out of treatment prematurely (or will be less engaged with treatment), ultimately resulting in fewer benefits of help seeking.

ADDRESSING GATE BARRIERS: EXAMPLES FROM TWO CLINICS

The GATE model serves as an organizational framework for clinics interested in serving diverse populations that tend not to access mental health resources, and how they can expand their services thoughtfully and fruitfully. Below I describe how two clinics, one stand-alone specialty mental health clinic and one primary care clinic, incorporated components of the GATE model to promote their services to Latinx Spanish-speaking residents of their respective geographic areas. One clinic, *la Clinica in La K'ech,* is in a southeastern state (Delgado-Romero et al., 2021). The other, *Community Clinic,* is in a mid-southern state (Bridges & Anastasia, 2016). Both clinics provide mental health care services and are at least in part staffed by psychology graduate students completing external practicum placements and supervised by licensed psychologists. At *Community Clinic,* mental health services are also provided by full-time behavioral health consultants, mostly licensed clinical social workers.

Addressing Perceived Need

General strategies that enhance a person's perceived need for services include media campaigns that raise awareness of mental health conditions, receiving a psychiatric diagnosis from a medical provider, hearing of someone else's experiences that mirror one's own, taking a diagnostic screening test, or even recognizing (or being told) that one's symptoms are interfering with important life roles. Providers at *la Clinica in La K'ech* and *Community Clinic* attend local festivals geared towards the Latinx community. At these festivals, they have booths/tents or tables where they provide psychoeducational materials related to mental health concerns. Materials are provided in English and Spanish. Both clinics have also engaged with local media, such as Spanish language newspapers, radio stations, and even appeared in podcasts and conducted workshops to disseminate information about the clinic's services and psychoeducation on mental health concerns. Both clinics work with other agencies to understand the mental health needs of the community (e.g., local domestic violence shelters, school boards, non-profit centers) and work to ensure these organizations are aware of the services provided by the clinics. Furthermore, at *Community Clinic* any member of the medical team can make a referral to behavioral health on behalf of the patient, thereby eliminating the need for the patient to perceive a need for mental health services. Indeed, as I point out in subsequent sections, integrated behavioral health care may be particularly compelling for addressing most of the steps in the GATE model and is therefore a promising approach to reducing health disparities (Bridges et al., 2014).

Addressing Internal Barriers

Interventions such as psychoeducation, campaigns to shift norms and expectations, open discussions with others who have had the condition, prior positive experiences with the mental health system, and motivational enhancement can be beneficial to address stigma and other attitudinal barriers people may face when considering seeking mental health care. In addition to the strategies described above that generally enhance perceived need through media campaigns and psychoeducation, our clinics have tried to increase the visibility of services as a way to normalize help-seeking in Latinx communities. For instance, members of *la Clinica in La K'ech* participate in an annual holiday parade. They create a float promoting *la Clinica,* thus promoting the view that mental health care is appropriate for Latinxs. At these community events, people can seek a brief consultation with a mental health care provider who can then help the potential client determine whether mental health care services are appropriate. A brief assessment and psychoeducation, including motivational interviewing, can help reduce stigma and attitudinal barriers to care. Similarly, at *Community Clinic,* mental health care providers can meet briefly with primary care patients while they are waiting for their medical appointments. These meetings often take place right in the medical exam room and the provider, whose title is *behavioral health consultant* rather than *psychologist, therapist,* or *counselor,* is introduced as one member of the medical team. The thought is that by embedding providers in primary care, the stigma of specialty mental health care is reduced. Another strategy used by *la Clinica in LaK'ech* is to work closely with paraprofessionals, or *promotores*. These are members of the Latinx community who receive special training in mental health. Because they are a trusted and an integral part of the Latinx community, *promotores* can link members of their community to needed services. In addition, both *la Clinica in LaK'ech* and *Community Clinic* have diverse bilingual providers featured on their websites, and websites are in both Spanish and English. *La Clinica in LaK'ech*'s website emphasizes the Latinx heritage shared among providers and care recipients.

Addressing External Barriers

Efforts to address structural barriers include expanding services through satellite clinics or mobile health care teams, advocating for increased health care benefits and insurance coverage for populations the clinic hopes to serve, training and increasing the mental health care workforce, using paraprofessionals for some components of mental health care, extending clinic hours of operation, and advocating for increased federal and state funding for community health and mental health care clinics (Bridges & Lindly, 2008). Immigration reform would certainly help with bringing people in need out of the shadows and into the health care system. In the meantime, clinic policies on record-keeping that do not require social security numbers or other sensitive information can reduce the potential risks of harm to patients. Notably, these efforts will require significant advocacy efforts on the part of psychologists and other mental health care allies.

Mental health care providers at both *la Clinica in LaK'ech* and *Community Clinic* try to reduce structural barriers by attending to language, location of services, cost of services, access to appointments, and advocacy. For instance, both clinics have websites in English and Spanish. At *Community Clinic,* staff members (e.g., front office staff who answer phones) and many medical assistants are bilingual so that when a person calls for an appointment, they are able to speak to someone right away who understands their language. While nearly all clinicians at *la Clinica in LaK'ech* speak Spanish, many behavioral health consultants at *Community Clinic* do not. Therefore, *Community Clinic* uses bilingual behavioral health case managers and/or a telephonic interpretation service to provide services in the patient's preferred language. Assessment and psychoeducation materials are similarly available in the person's preferred language, and both clinics maintain a virtual repository of Spanish-language resources that can be readily accessed by clinicians and shared with clients/patients. Recognizing that childcare can be a barrier to maintaining mental health care appointments, *la Clinica in LaK'ech* provides free childcare for clients who may need it. Both clinics provide services for free and do not require insurance coverage. At *la Clinica in LaK'ech,* all sessions are free. At *Community Clinic,* sessions are free if the patient is seeing a graduate clinician, and very affordable (e.g., $10/session) if seeing a licensed provider. In addition, because graduate student clinicians are providing services in both locations and are therefore obtaining needed training experiences that advance their degrees, the services are sustainable. Both clinics are located along major public transportation routes and in locales that are already familiar to and frequently accessed by Latinxs: *la Clinica in LaK'ech* operates out of a church that houses services for the Latinx community, while *Community Clinic* is the top provider of medical care services for Latinxs in their community. Both clinics have an easy referral system and avoid extensive intake processes, so people can get into care quickly. At *Community Clinic,* same-day appointments are available for established medical patients. In both clinics, care is taken to avoid requiring documentation that could put clients in legal jeopardy, such as legal status. Finally, graduate student clinicians and supervising psychologists at both clinics have been involved in local, state, and national advocacy to promote the expansion of health care and other reforms that would reduce stress and increase wellness in Latinxs.

Addressing Clinical/Procedural Barriers

Clinics can continue efforts to ensure people remain in therapy once they are finally able to access it by overcoming the prior barriers. Specific strategies that the mental health field in general undertakes include: the development and validation of measures for use with diverse populations, the adaptation of evidence-based treatments for diverse communities, the effort to train professionals in cultural competence and intentional recruitment of bilingual and bicultural students into mental health disciplines, and the employment of bilingual support staff to enhance linguistically-appropriate services. In our clinics, we have bilingual psychologists providing supervision to graduate students who see Spanish-speaking clients/patients. By opening these behavioral health clinics, both sites have seen an increase in the number of Latinx graduate students who matriculate into their associated doctoral programs. Both clinics also embed community-based research into their students' training, promoting cultural competence and disseminating findings to the larger field of mental health care scholars. At *Community Clinic,* brief assessments are provided in the patient's preferred language, using instruments validated in that language, such as the Patient Health Questionnaire-9 (e.g., Merz et al., 2011) and the Generalized Anxiety Disorders Questionnaire-7 (e.g., Mills et al., 2014). At *la Clinica in LaK'ech,* providers regularly engage in Spanish-language supervision, case consultation, and presentations to ensure they have practice in communicating ideas and concepts in the patient's preferred language. Both clinics regularly incorporate discussions of multiculturalism, social determinants of health, self-care, and culturally-informed case conceptualization into supervision to enhance the competence and responsiveness of clinicians. It is our belief that by attending to the diverse barriers Latinx patients face when trying to access mental health care, we are having a measurable, positive impact on our communities.

CONCLUSION AND FUTURE DIRECTIONS

A call for "rebooting" psychotherapy has been issued before (Kazdin & Blasé, 2011) with the clear understanding that simply doing things as we have traditionally done them is insufficient for reducing the burden of mental health in general, and for people of color in particular. The focus of much of these rebooting efforts has been on how we can increase access to care. However, unlike in the movie *Field of Dreams* (1989), to really impact the burden of psychiatric conditions in vulnerable and underserved communities requires us to do more than just "build it"- we need to understand all of the barriers to mental health care access these communities face. In this chapter, I articulated a framework for organizing the considerable knowledge we have accumulated about help-seeking. The GATE model is conceptualized as a series of stages. Successful navigation through *each* stage is thought to be critical for reducing mental health care disparities.

Moving forward, it will be important to apply the GATE model to help-seeking research to see whether the progressive and ordered nature of these stages comports with how people experience care access. It will also be useful to determine which components of the GATE model are most strongly associated with help-seeking so we can direct our efforts to reducing disparities there. For example, if perceived need accounts for the bulk of the variance in help-seeking, greater attention to individual and community-based interventions that increase perceived need would be critical and perhaps more important than efforts to change stigma or to modify a particular treatment. In contrast, if structural barriers account for most of the variance in help-seeking, advocacy and attention to when, where, and how care is delivered will be central to reducing disparities. Attention to novel methods of mental health service delivery, such as telehealth or primary care integration, may also be warranted, especially if these novel approaches have the potential to address multiple components of the GATE model.

REFERENCES

Ajzen, I. (1991). The theory of planned behavior. *Organizational Behavior and Human Decision Processes*, 50(2), 179–211. doi:10.1016/0749-5978(91)90020-T

Alegría, M., Chatterji, P., Wells, K., Cao, Z., Chen, C., Takeuchi, D., Jackson, J., & Meng, X. (2008). Disparity in depression treatment among racial and ethnic minority populations in the United States. *Psychiatric Services (Washington, D.C.)*, 59(11), 1264–1272. doi:10.1176/ps.2008.59.11.1264 PMID:18971402

Andersen, R. M. (1995). Revisiting the behavioral model and access to medical care: Does it matter? *Journal of Health and Social Behavior*, 36(1), 1–10. doi:10.2307/2137284 PMID:7738325

Benish, S. G., Quintana, S., & Wampold, B. E. (2011). Culturally adapted psychotherapy and the legitimacy of myth: A direct-comparison meta-analysis. *Journal of Counseling Psychology*, 58(3), 279–289. doi:10.1037/a0023626 PMID:21604860

Bridges, A. J., & Anastasia, E. (2016). Enhancing and improving treatment engagement with Hispanic patients. In W. O'Donohue & L. Benuto (Eds.), *Enhancing Behavioral Health in Hispanic Populations: Eliminating Disparities Through Integrated Behavioral and Primary Care* (pp. 125–143). Springer International Publishing. doi:10.1007/978-3-319-42533-7_8

Bridges, A. J., Andrews, A. R. III, & Deen, T. L. (2012). Mental health needs and service utilization by Hispanic immigrants residing in mid-southern United States. *Journal of Transcultural Nursing, 23*(4), 359–368. doi:10.1177/1043659612451259 PMID:22802297

Bridges, A. J., Andrews, A. R. III, Pastrana, F. A., Villalobos, B. T., Cavell, T. A., & Gomez, D. (2014). Does integrated behavioral health care reduce mental health disparities for Hispanics? Initial findings. *Journal of Latina/o Psychology, 2*(1), 37–53. doi:10.1037/lat0000009 PMID:25309845

Bridges, A. J., & Lindly, E. (2008). Service utilization and case management. In Workgroup on Adapting Latino Services (Ed.), Adaptation guidelines for serving Latino children and families affected by trauma (pp. 53-56). Chadwick Center for Children and Families.

Cabassa, L. J., & Zayas, L. H. (2007). Latino immigrants' intentions to seek depression care. *The American Journal of Orthopsychiatry, 77*(2), 231–242. doi:10.1037/0002-9432.77.2.231 PMID:17535121

Cabassa, L. J., Zayas, L. H., & Hansen, M. C. (2006). Latino adults' access to mental health care: A review of epidemiological studies. *Administration and Policy in Mental Health, 33*(3), 316–330. doi:10.100710488-006-0040-8 PMID:16598658

Centers for Disease Control and Prevention. (2018). *National Health Interview Survey: Tables of Summary Health Statistics.* Retrieved from https://www.cdc.gov/nchs/nhis/SHS/tables.htm

Centers for Disease Control and Prevention. (2022). *Childhood lead poisoning prevention program.* Retrieved from https://www.cdc.gov/nceh/lead/default.htm

Chang, D. F., Hsieh, E., Somerville, W. B., Dimond, J., Thomas, M., Nicasio, A., Boiler, M., & Lewis-Fernández, R. (2021). Rethinking interpreter functions in mental health services. *Psychiatric Services (Washington, D.C.), 72*(3), 353–357. doi:10.1176/appi.ps.202000085 PMID:32988324

Delgado-Romero, E. A., Mahoney, G. E., Muro-Rodriguez, N., Atilano, R., Cardenas-Bautista, E., De Los Santos, J., Duran, M., Espinoza, L., Fuentes, J., Gomez, S., Ingram, R., Jiminez-Ruiz, J., Monroig, M., Mora-Ozuna, C., Ordaz, A. C., Rappaport, B., Suazo-Padilla, K., & Vazquez, M. S. (2021). *Clinica In Lak'ech:* The establishment of a practicum site to integrate practice, advocacy, and research with Latinx clients. *The Counseling Psychologist, 49*(7), 987–1012. doi:10.1177/00110000211025270

Graham, H. (2004). Social determinants and their unequal distribution: Clarifying policy understandings. *The Milbank Quarterly, 82*(1), 101–124. doi:10.1111/j.0887-378X.2004.00303.x PMID:15016245

Griner, D., & Smith, T. B. (2006). Culturally adapted mental health intervention: A meta-analytic review. *Psychotherapy (Chicago, Ill.), 43*(4), 531–548. doi:10.1037/0033-3204.43.4.531 PMID:22122142

Hansen, E., & Donohoe, M. (2003). Health issues of migrant and seasonal farmworkers. *Journal of Health Care for the Poor and Underserved, 14*(2), 153–164. doi:10.1353/hpu.2010.0790 PMID:12739296

HealthyPeople.gov. (2022). *Disparities*. Retrieved from http://www.healthypeople.gov/2020/about/disparitiesAbout.aspx

Horrell, S. C. V. (2008). Effectiveness of cognitive-behavioral therapy with adult ethnic minority clients: A review. *Professional Psychology, Research and Practice, 39*(2), 160–168. doi:10.1037/0735-7028.39.2.160

Merz, E. L., Malcarne, V. L., Roesch, S. C., Riley, N., & Sadler, G. R. (2011). A multigroup confirmatory factor analysis of the Patient Health Questionnaire-9 among English- and Spanish-speaking Latinas. *Cultural Diversity & Ethnic Minority Psychology, 17*(3), 309–316. doi:10.1037/a0023883 PMID:21787063

Mills, S. D., Fox, R. S., Malcarne, V. L., Roesch, S. C., Champagne, B. R., & Sadler, G. R. (2014). The psychometric properties of the Generalized Anxiety Disorder-7 Scale in Hispanic Americans with English or Spanish language preference. *Cultural Diversity & Ethnic Minority Psychology, 20*(3), 463–468. doi:10.1037/a0036523 PMID:25045957

Miranda, J., Bernal, G., Lau, A., Kohn, L., Hwang, W. C., & LaFromboise, T. (2005). State of the science on psychosocial interventions for ethnic minorities. *Annual Review of Clinical Psychology, 1*(1), 113–142. doi:10.1146/annurev.clinpsy.1.102803.143822 PMID:17716084

Mojtabai, R., Olfson, M., & Mechanic, D. (2002). Perceived need and help-seeking in adults with mood, anxiety, or substance use disorders. *Archives of General Psychiatry, 59*(1), 77–84. doi:10.1001/archpsyc.59.1.77 PMID:11779286

National Academies of Sciences, Engineering, and Medicine. (2017). *Communities in action: Pathways to health equity*. Washington, DC: The National Academies Press. doi:10.17226/24624

Olfson, M., Mojtabai, R., Sampson, N. A., Hwang, I., Druss, B., Wang, P. S., Wells, K. B., Pincus, H. A., & Kessler, R. C. (2009). Dropout from outpatient mental health care in the United States. *Psychiatric Services (Washington, D.C.), 60*(7), 898–907. doi:10.1176/ps.2009.60.7.898 PMID:19564219

Owen, J., Tao, K. W., Imel, Z. E., Wampold, B. E., & Rodolfa, E. (2014). Addressing racial and ethnic microaggressions in therapy. *Professional Psychology, Research and Practice, 45*(4), 283–290. doi:10.1037/a0037420

Paone, T. R., & Malott, K. M. (2008). Using interpreters in mental health counseling: A literature review and recommendations. *Journal of Multicultural Counseling and Development, 36*(3), 130–142. doi:10.1002/j.2161-1912.2008.tb00077.x

Pastrana, F. A., Bridges, A. J., Villalobos, B. T., Dueweke, A. R., & Rodriguez, J. H. (2017). Cognitive behavioral therapy tools for clients with limited functional literacy. *Behavior Therapist, 40*(4), 137–145.

Robert Wood Johnson Foundation. (2008). *Income is linked with health regardless of racial or ethnic group*. Retrieved from http://www.commissiononhealth.org/PDF/inchlthxeg.pdf

Rosenstock, I. M. (1974). The Health Belief Model and Preventive Health Behavior. *Health Education Monographs, 2*(4), 354–386. doi:10.1177/109019817400200405

St. Arnault, D. (2009). Cultural determinants of help seeking: A model for research and practice. *Research and Theory for Nursing Practice, 23*(4), 259–278. doi:10.1891/1541-6577.23.4.259 PMID:19999745

St. Arnault, D., & Woo, S. (2018). Testing the influence of cultural determinants on help-seeking theory. *The American Journal of Orthopsychiatry, 88*(6), 650–660. doi:10.1037/ort0000353 PMID:30179023

Substance Abuse and Mental Health Services Administration. (2015). *Racial/ethnic differences in mental health service use among adults.* HHS Publication No. SMA-15-4906. Rockville, MD: Author.

Substance Abuse and Mental Health Services Administration. (2020). *Results from the 2019 National Survey on Drug Use and Health: Mental Health Detailed Tables.* Retrieved from https://www.samhsa.gov/data/report/2019-nsduh-detailed-tables

Sue, S. (1988). Psychotherapeutic services for ethnic minorities: Two decades of research findings. *The American Psychologist, 43*(4), 301–308. doi:10.1037/0003-066X.43.4.301 PMID:3289427

Tonigan, J. S. (2003). Project match treatment participation and outcome by self-reported ethnicity. *Alcoholism, Clinical and Experimental Research, 27*(8), 1340–1344. doi:10.1097/01.ALC.0000080673.83739.F3 PMID:12966335

US Department of Health and Human Services. (2022). *Social determinants of health.* Retrieved from https://health.gov/healthypeople/priority-areas/social-determinants-health

Vasquez, M. J. T. (2007). Cultural difference and the therapeutic alliance: An evidence-based analysis. *The American Psychologist, 62*(8), 878–885. doi:10.1037/0003-066X.62.8.878 PMID:18020774

World Health Organization. (2018). *Health inequities and their causes.* Retrieved from https://who.int/news-room/facts-in-pictures/detail/health-inequities-and-their-causes

Young, A. S., Klap, R., Sherbourne, C. D., & Wells, K. B. (2001). The quality of care for depressive and anxiety disorders in the United States. *Archives of General Psychiatry, 58*(1), 55–61. doi:10.1001/archpsyc.58.1.55 PMID:11146758

ENDNOTE

[1] While comparisons are often made between Latinx and non-Latinx Whites in research and epidemiological studies, I do not mean to imply that non-Latinx Whites are the "standard" against which to compare the health and well-being of Latinxs. Instead, the statistics I cite in this chapter are used to illustrate how privileges afforded to some groups can result in health inequities for non-privileged members of the society.

Chapter 16
From Surviving to Thriving:
Future Directions

Eckart Werther
Clayton State University, USA

Jhokania De Los Santos
Philips, USA

Brooke Rappaport
Tennessee State University, USA

Ammy E. Sena
University of Georgia, USA

Cristalis Capielo Rosario
Arizona State University, USA

Edward A. Delgado-Romero
University of Georgia, USA

ABSTRACT

The authors of this book are part of a diverse network of scholars and practitioners with expertise in various aspects of Latinx psychology and mental health. They share a similar purpose of expanding the pipeline of Latinx counselors and psychologists to collectively create a just and healthy society for all Latinxs. This chapter reflects on the common linkages and underdeveloped areas among the chapters. Future directions for Latinx mental health are presented and include but are not limited to the incorporation of liberatory frameworks and interdisciplinary approaches.

FROM SURVIVING TO THRIVING: FUTURE DIRECTIONS

As we finish this book, the U.S. midterm elections of 2022 are heating up. Latinx people in the U.S. have

DOI: 10.4018/978-1-6684-4901-1.ch016

once again become the target of political attack ads, and the focus of pundits that speculate about how Latinx people will vote in this and the next (2024 presidential) election. Latinx people find themselves at the center of political discourse, paradoxically both as scapegoats and courted for votes at the same time. In a highly visible political stunt Latinx immigrants were used as political pawns by the governors of Florida and Texas (Henderson, 2022; Montoya-Galvez, 2022). Latinx asylum seekers were deceived with promises of nonexistent opportunities and then transported to northern "sanctuary cities" like Chicago and Martha's Vineyard (Sandoval et al., 2022). These political stunts problematize the status of asylum seekers, in this case from Venezuela, as a public charge to literally be dumped elsewhere. Among the thousands of asylum seekers who have been caught up in these recent political stunts include many buses filled with children (ABC7 New York, 2022; Jorgenson, 2022). These recent acts are reminiscent of the "Reverse Freedom Rides" during the 1960's when white segregationists and racist organizations devised the plan to bus African Americans to northern "liberal" cities under false pretenses (Brockell &Tillman, 2022; Simon & Emanuel, 2022; Webb, 2004). These cruel and inhumane tactics are rooted in racist, white nationalistic, and white supremacy ideologies that have permeated the social fabric of this country (GALE, ND).

These acts against immigrants and asylum seekers are used to gain political capital and threaten the mental health of Latinx people in several ways. First, by dehumanizing immigrants and asylum seekers as problematic and disruptors of law and order, all Latinx people may potentially be seen as invasive and a threat to the economic stability of the U.S. In the 1980's the Cuban freedom flotillas were also portrayed as an invasion of the U.S. by criminal, communist and dark-skinned Cubans (Stephens, 2021). The constant stereotyping and dehumanization of immigrants can erode empathy for immigrants, asylum seekers, and the issues that impact them. Second, in response to constant portrayals of immigrants as not human and a threat to life in the U.S., Latinx people may instead align themselves with the oppressor. That is, they may choose to identify as white and adopt anti-immigrant and anti-Latinx sentiments. This insidious process of assimilation where culture of origin practices is sacrificed while white dominant culture norms are adopted can rob Latinxs from their history and impact their mental health. Dehumanizing other human beings, internalizing negative stereotypes, and within group fragmentation that takes place because of internalized oppression among Latinx people is not conducive to mental health (Friere, 1970; Duran et al., 2008; Comas-Diaz, 2012; Capielo Rosario et al., 2019).

This book is a critical look at Latinx mental health from the lens of research, practice, education, and personal accounts. Each chapter has examined the historical and contemporary context of Latinx people within an intersectional framework of identities and systems. That is, none of us hold only one identity, rather we are a dynamic mix of salient aspects of ourselves that interact with systems of oppression. Likewise, the systems that Latinxs navigate, and their oppressive nature are also intersectional and dynamic. These oppressive systems are embedded within the structural, institutional, community and individual levels of U.S. society and have a detrimental impact on the wellbeing of Latinx persons (Torres et al, 2022). Oppressive practices are evident in educational policies, immigration laws and practices, judicial policies, political rhetoric, healthcare inequalities, housing, and banking.

Each chapter has focused on a particular aspect of Latinx identity and attempted to inclusively represent the many manifestations of *Latinidad*. For example, in the Latinx feminist chapters, the authors are careful to examine the intersectional identities of Latinx feminists who operate within broad frameworks such as the feminist movement, which has historically excluded them. It is critical for Latinx people to reject simplistic, reductionistic, and stereotypical notions of who Latinx people are, who they can be, or what they can achieve in high-stakes arenas such as education, healthcare, and policy.

We propose that a thriving framework for Latinx people, Latinx mental health, and Latinx psychology includes a deliberate embrace of the richness and diversity of Latinx life in the U.S. Although we may choose to discover and emphasize our commonalities, there are many layers of complexity, distinctiveness, and unique historical context that coexists simultaneously within broad categories. This embrace of a messy, constantly changing, and evolving dynamic culture runs counter to the foundations of U.S. mainstream psychology, which was based on the medical model of illness and sought to control and predict human behavior (Guthrie, 2004, Tomicic & Berardi, 2018). To do so, human experience must be measured in discrete categories and intersectional variables are often reduced to "noise" in the data. The search for universal principles of human experience unintentionally serves the aims of colonization and domination of people who deviate from expected norms.

In this book many authors have highlighted the need for resistance to colonization and attempts to commodify or assimilate Latinx values. Often these attempts are collectively referred to as decolonization. In other words, reimagine a Latinx psychology that is delinked from white and oppressive power dynamics and frameworks. Although many of the mental health fields have progressively adopted a multicultural and social justice orientation over the last several decades, the inclusion of Latinx people and perspectives has been slow to materialize. For example, within the field of psychology, Latinxs are underrepresented in doctoral training programs, only make up 5% of those in academia or in the general U.S. psychology workforce, and only about 13% of doctoral degrees in psychology were awarded to Latinxs (APA, 2016; Delgado-Romero, et al., 2018). Specific examples of student or faculty resistance in academia around Latinx issues are rare, and we encourage Latinx scholars to connect with contemporary and historical examples of Latinx resistance, but also to continue to articulate what that resistance might look like and how that might challenge the practice, teaching, research, and training of mental health professions. One such example of resistance and redefinition is the work of many of the authors of this book in creating and developing a Spanish-language psychological clinic, *la Clinica En LaK'ech* (Delgado-Romero et al., 2021; Delgado-Romero et al., 2018). *La Clinica* challenges many of the norms of psychological training at a predominantly white training program by adopting a community focus, offering free services, being staffed by Latinx and bilingual trainees in psychology and social work, and collaborating with medical, education and legal providers. Clinical case staffing were conducted in Spanish, critical and liberatory frameworks in therapy are the first line of treatment and the clinicians view themselves as part of the community rather than outsiders. The work of *la Clinica* disrupted both the traditional training found at a predominantly white institution and challenged the notion of what accessible mental health service entailed to serve a population of Spanish speaking, largely undocumented and uninsured clients. Clinicians desired to decolonize the practice of therapy with Latinx people, and other examples of resistance and redefinition of psychology need to be shared.

MAIN THEMES AND FUTURE CONSIDERATIONS IN LATINX MENTAL HEALTH

Besides capturing the richness of different Latinx experiences, our critical analysis also highlights several common themes across our stories. Throughout the chapters we see examples of resiliency, resistance, value created from within, culture as an asset, community centeredness, and need for interdisciplinary work. Below we summarize these themes and how we believe they relate to the future of Latinx mental health.

Resiliency and Theoretical Frameworks

Latinx people thrive in the U.S. despite having to navigate and overcome discriminatory immigration and law enforcement practices, and disparities in the social, health, employment, and educational sectors. A paradigm shift is necessary within the mental health fields to move away from a pathological and deficit-based perspective, and move toward a strength-based perspective when working with Latinxs. Strength-based perspectives should integrate Latinx ethnocultural norms that contribute to resiliency practices and how Latinxs have navigated oppressive elements in society with cultural, regional and historical context.

Cultural resiliency displayed by members of the Latinx community as they navigate the various challenges in the U.S. are often linked to Latinx cultural values and practices. Ethnocultural variables such as the use of native language, *familismo*, collectivistic norms, and biculturalism can "insulate" and "buffer" Latinxs from the detrimental effects of mental health stressors in the U.S. Given their protective qualities, we believe that it is prudent for mental health practitioners and researchers alike to better understand how these factors operationalize contextually in the lives of Latinxs. A better understanding of how these cultural buffers operate could help enhance culturally informed interventions for Latinxs in the U.S.

For these reasons the authors encourage mental health practitioners and scholars to begin familiarizing themselves with Latinx specific frameworks that have been proposed. One example would be Gonzalez (2020) who introduced a model of Latinx resiliency that aims to understand the sources of resiliency for Latinxs across various contexts (e.g., home, education, community and vocational). The model offers a linear and nonlinear framework to understand how cultural values contribute to the resiliency of Latinxs and emphasizes the role that cultural values, behaviors, and knowledge contribute to resiliency. The model supports a "non-deficit, asset-based approach" (Gonzalez, 2020, p.793) that focuses on the unique lived experiences of Latinxs in the U.S. Although this model was developed in an educational context, their findings are applicable to the issues we have highlighted within Latinx mental health.

Adames and colleagues (2017) also identified coping strategies that Latinxs have developed to overcome oppressive experiences. These strategies include: determination, *esperanza* (hope), adaptability, strong work ethic, connectedness to others, collective emotional expression, and resistance. They propose that for Latinxs, having knowledge about these factors and internalizing them can serve a protective function as they navigate oppressive structures in U.S. society. The reader will note we have addressed these experiences in our chapters, but more examples, research and best practice guidelines would be useful.

The following conceptual frameworks are provided for readers as examples of emerging perspectives and areas of further inquiry. These frameworks focus on aspects of resistance and liberation: Centering Race and Ethnicity in Latinx Identity (Adames & Chavez-Dueñas, 2017), Ethnopolitical Psychology (Comas-Diaz, 2000), Framework for Hispanic Health (Borrell, 2005), Intersectionality in Psychotherapy (Adames et al. 2018), Healing Ethno and Racial Trauma (Chavez-Dueñas et al. 2019) and the Radical healing framework for people of color (French et al., 2020). Each of these frameworks call attention to the need to understand Latinx mental health and wellbeing from an intersectional and sociopolitical perspective. They also call on us to bear witness to community challenges, their assets, and ways of resisting, and build solidarity across communities to promote anti-racism and anti-colonial change.

In addition to the development and adoption of strength based and culturally informed frameworks, a larger scale liberation movement is necessary within the mental health fields. The liberation discussion that follows will focus on the field of psychology, but the authors want to be clear that each mental health discipline can adopt similar efforts.

Liberation as a Pathway

To do liberation psychology requires first, to liberate psychology - Ignacio Martín-Baró (1994)

A commitment to a social justice agenda includes addressing social inequalities, their influences on behavior, and striving for work towards a change in institutions and systems that perpetuate injustice and inequities. It is in this very commitment and the research and practice that gives psychologists momentum to pursue the quest for social change by an ethic that emphasizes liberating psychology. Dominant/mainstream psychology still needs to be liberated, as it is still firmly Eurocentric, heteronormative, linear, and even perceived as universal. If dominant psychology was truly universal, then Latinx psychology would not be necessary. Another way to consider this statement is to think about a psychologist who looks at a non-Western culture through Western glasses. It is very likely that the psychologist may fail to notice important aspects of the non-Western culture since the schema for recognizing them has not been provided by their science. Dominant psychology has remained conspicuously insensitive to intra- as well as inter-cultural variations, and has attempted to develop objective, decontextualized and universal theories of human behavior by excluding the subjective aspects of human functioning (i.e., consciousness, agency, meaning, and goals).

If psychologists decontextualize the experiences of clients, they cause harm, as they end up preventing recognition of potential sources of healing and promote the internalization of individuals' struggles as 'self-issues' when really, they are natural responses to structural inequality. For example, problem-based diagnoses tend to ignore the client's complex contexts by encouraging an individualistic rather than an ecological understanding of clients. As clinicians, psychologists should pay attention to elements of a person's life—cultural, social, political, ethnic, spiritual, and economic—and how these factors contribute to sustain, and shape a person's struggles. If they are attentive to these factors, psychologists can help indicate important resources that can help toward positive transformation as well as problem solving.

The trajectory of the term "Latinx" as a discursive marker of inclusivity and diversity is heavily valued on being sensitive to diversity and engaged in social justice. Martín-Baró, a Spanish-born Jesuit priest trained in psychology, devoted his career to making psychology speak to the community as well as to the individual, and it is our hope that throughout readings, the reader has felt safe to expand on their perspective on oppression, power, and liberation. Martín-Baró's (1994) call for liberation psychology centered on the idea that psychology should be more context-based and focus on people's problems, and that one should view oppression as the interaction of intrapsychic factors with systemic factors, such as sociopolitical injustice (Comas-Díaz, Hall, & Neville, 2019). Notably, liberation psychologists foster awareness of discrimination and inequality, fortify individuals' strengths, affirm cultural identities, and promote change to attenuate human suffering and improve people's lives (Martín-Baró, 1994; Montero & Sonn, 2009).

The psychology of liberation movement has been a catalyst for collective and individual change in communities, and recent political developments are making its powerful, transformative ideas more relevant than ever before. One cannot mention Martín-Baró without the Brazilian Paulo Freire (1970, 2005), who developed the pedagogy of the oppressed, and suggested that the oppressed carry an internalized oppressor, which needs liberation. Freire (1970) identified certain traits that complement the traits of the dominant group and that serve to help sustain the circumstances of their disadvantage. These traits of the oppressed include: powerlessness, division, prevention from realizing their full human potential, internalization of the oppressor's consciousness, behaving in ways according to the prescribed norms of the dominant group, and unawareness of being manipulated and exploited (Butts & Rich, 2015). On the contrary, those who are privileged and act as oppressors have the following traits: powerful, failure to recognize others as human, use of power to sustain self-interests, hegemonic viewpoints, and exploitations and manipulation of the oppressed without apology (Butts & Rich, 2015). These complementary characteristics of the oppressor and oppressed groups exist because of systematic conditions inherent in the social structure that sustain injustice.

In following liberation psychology's value of inclusivity, it is encouraged that psychologists understand structural discrimination; utilize affirmative, strength-based, gender, and culturally relevant interventions; engage in promoting agency and critical consciousness; understand sociopolitical contexts; use indigenous and complementary alternative healing, when appropriate; and work to change institutional, systemic, and global discrimination. In working together, engaging in radical humility, and practicing authentic collaboration, we as a collective can work toward challenging and dismantling anti-Blackness, racial oppression, and white supremacy.

Liberation psychology emphasizes the collective well-being, consciousness of social injustices and resistance to the normalization of discrimination and oppression. Psychologists should always be mindful of how they can cause harm, especially when they fail to attend to clients by not developing collaborative and or participatory relationships. Psychologists should find time to routinely ask clients what matters most to them in their experience of illness and treatment. In finding out what matters most to clients, psychologists build an elective affinity to the client, empower clients to be experts in their own experience, and demystify how systems work. Through these approaches, psychologists constantly work to understand what their positionality could symbolize to clients, and support clients to recognize and make meaning of their experiences and the ways parts of themselves may have been fragmented through harmful relationships with people and systems

In strengthening a commitment to liberation psychology, psychologists can transform themselves in order to transform the discipline. Psychologists must unlearn what they learned during their training. Instead, they can cultivate reflexivity, enhance our critical awareness, and become vessels of healing and social justice.

No matter your theoretical or professional orientation, liberation psychology can be incorporated into your work. When you begin to include and really value the information received from the people you work with, you welcome and are open to different worldviews. Your commitment to diversity, equity, and inclusion will be as meaningful as your action.

Community Centeredness

In various chapters, authors discussed the centrality of community in the lives of Latinx individuals. For example, Chapter 4 on *campesinos*, discusses the role of "deep community networks" in the lives of farmworkers for survival and resistance against racism and institutional oppression. Another example is observed in chapter 3 on LGBTQ+ Latinx communities which highlights the importance of community in resiliency building for members of this community. This inherent value is not only a source for external needs but is also one that has allowed Latinx communities to move from survival and coping to healing. Here we highlight again the value of Latinx culturally informed Frameworks such as the HEART

(Healing Ethno and Racial Trauma) model that incorporates the strengthening communities as part of the clinical recommendation in helping Latinx clients heal (Chavez-Duenas et al., 2019).

Although a value the predates colonialism for Latinx individuals, community has only recently been accepted as vital in mainstream (Western) psychological science (Comas-Diaz, 2012; DeAngelis, 2008). We see this through recent scientific developments on suicidality which emphasizes the importance of social supports and connectedness as a protective factor (Jahangard et al., 2020). Similarly, we see this in neuroscientific "developments" on the hormone oxytocin, a chemical which popular media has called the "love hormone" because it is released when people engage in things such as bonding, trust or safety, and hugs (Olff et al., 2013). Some of these studies have found that when experiencing stressors, humans release oxytocin, which is human' biology's way of letting us know we need connection to reduce stress (Olff et al., 2013). Neuroscientific research is now looking at oxytocin and its potential for assisting individuals with various psychiatric disorders such as autism, depression, and anxiety (Gordon et al., 2013; Olff et al., 2013); Sippel et al., 2017). In this instance it appears that research has caught up with the traditional Latinx cultural value of community and is recognizing it as legitimate antidote to suffering.

Value Created From Within

While external sources of professional validation such as financial success, awards, special recognitions, titles, publications, or membership in professional societies are all notable accomplishments, internal sources of validation cannot be undervalued. We encourage Latinx mental health professionals and academics to recognize the value of internal sources of validation that are rooted in our cultural practices and norms, connection to family and community, knowledge, skills, and lived experiences. These internal sources of strength and validation might often go unconsidered in professional settings and may also be misunderstood or misconstrued by peers. As an example, for some Latinxs, their connections and devotion to family can be misinterpreted as being enmeshment or dependency. For those Latinxs who are native Spanish speakers or who grow up bilingual, speaking with an accent or not speaking in standard English could be perceived as one being less competent.

Our skills, lived experiences, interests, curiosities, perspectives, and contributions in professional settings are valuable and additive and should not be minimized. We (Latinx mental health professionals) play a significant role in addressing the underserved needs of our communities and developing the theoretical models to inform practice with the Latinx community. Developing an appreciation for these contributions and internal sources should be nurtured and emphasized throughout training and during the early years of a Latinx's professional career. Professors, mentors, supervisors, and supportive peers/communities are instrumental in creating these supportive networks and environments where these internal sources can be valued, understood, and supported.

The low numbers of Latinxs within the psychology, human services, and mental health pipelines results in an underrepresentation of providers, academics, and scholars who are of Latinxs background or that have interest in the Latinx community. Given the current low numbers, it is vital for those of us who have successfully navigated these pipelines to support and facilitate the success of early career Latinx professionals and those with a vested interested in serving the Latinx community. Early career professionals, particularly those who are first generation or that come from marginalized backgrounds, could benefit greatly from guidance and mentorship on topics such as applying and interviewing for jobs, negotiating employment offers, applying for licensure, engaging in other post-graduation/early career processes, and establishing healthy work-life boundaries. Examples of such efforts include the student programming at the 2022 National Latinx Psychological Association's conference. Topics that are part of the student program include how to apply to graduate school, a discussion about postdocs and fellowships, a leadership academy, and a session about the psychology internship application process.

Those of us who have obtained positions of power within academic institutions or industry must work towards leveling the playing field for future Latinx mental health professionals. Within academic settings for example, working towards removing the GRE for graduate admissions requirements would be one method of eliminating a barrier for Latinx students wanting to pursue graduate study. Helms and Dupree (2021) noted the way in which the GRE serves to keep out students of color from graduate training; removing this standardized test would allow us to continue to fill the pipeline with more Latinx scholars, who because of various systemic barriers, may not thrive when taking an exam like the GRE.

We must also aim to make psychological knowledge more consumable and easier to access. Currently, a large portion of the research that is published in psychology and other related disciplines is done so in journals that sit behind paywalls. One must have access via individual or institutional membership or pay to access the journal articles. This practice keeps knowledge boxed in and only accessible to certain people with resources. We believe that open access of published materials makes it more impactful and of greater use to society (Fuentes et al., 2022).

Interdisciplinary Approach

As some authors in this book have highlighted, none of the mental health or social service disciplines (e.g., psychology, psychiatry, social work, counseling, marriage and family, human services) have been able to independently address the mental health needs of the Latinx community. Disparities continue to exist despite attempts within each field to address cultural competency and to increase the representation of Latinxs within their ranks. The National Academy of Sciences (2005) stated that an interdisciplinary and collaborative approach is warranted when solutions to problems are beyond the scope of a single discipline. More interdisciplinary and collaborative training, research, and treatment efforts are needed to better prepare the mental health workforce to meet the mental health needs of U.S. Latinxs.

Treatment settings should facilitate the communication and interaction of all members of the treatment team. Given the benefits of utilizing interdisciplinary approaches to enhance mental health services (Schultz, Walker et al., 2014), many of the authors in this book are aware of settings that do not value interdisciplinary collaboration when serving the Latinx community. In many examples, despite working with the same clients and in the same treatment system, providers in some settings were not allotted time during work hours to meet or discuss cases with each other. Authors have also observed in certain treatment settings where time allotted for clinical supervision came secondary to "billable hours." Providers who value interdisciplinary collaboration in these types of professional environments are often required to use personal time to meet with colleagues. This should not be the case and we encourage treatment facilities, community mental health centers, private practices, and non-profit agencies to reconsider such arrangements. All business decisions made in treatment settings should always consider client welfare, relevant professional ethical guidelines as well as local or state laws. We must resist the urge to place profits above quality of care.

Graduate training programs should strive to offer opportunities for trainees to work outside of their disciplinary silos. Ways this can be accomplished includes respective training programs partnering with other graduate programs and community service providers to develop practicum sites that offer interdisciplinary training experiences focused on the Latinx community. For example, in addition to serving the local Latinx community *la Clinica* also serves as an interdisciplinary practicum site. The staff is comprised of doctoral students from Counseling Psychology, Clinical Psychology, and Social Work. Practicum students are supervised by two Latinx licensed psychologists. *La Clinica* also collaborates with the School of Law and the immigration law clinic. Trainees at *la Clinica* are provided with culturally and linguistically competent supervision, mentorship, and training experiences; afforded the opportunity to staff and conceptualize cases from multiple disciplinary perspectives; and gain experiences collaborating with legal experts on immigration related cases. These interdisciplinary experiences model early for those in training the value of collaborating outside of one's discipline.

CONCLUSION

The authors of this book are part of a diverse network of scholars and practitioners with expertise in various aspects of Latinx psychology and mental health. We are an example of what a successful student pipeline can produce. While most of us have been trained as counseling psychologists and are alumni of the same training program, there are authors from other institutions and disciplines. But we share a similar purpose, expanding the pipeline of Latinx counselors and psychologists so that we can collectively create a just and healthy society for all Latinxs. The alumni from the program have gone on to research and practice around the U.S. and Latin America.

Some of the authors are currently finishing their respective doctoral or masters level training, some are completing post-doctoral fellowships and/or licensure processes. Others serve in academic, leadership, supervisory, or clinical capacities. Those of us who have navigated these academic and professional spaces, remain connected to our training program, mentors, and network of current graduate students through scholarship, collaborative projects, and involvement in national organizations. We collectively recognize that we each play an instrumental role in shaping the future of Latinx mental health. We also acknowledge that this effort is only possible because of those that came before us and opened the door to educational opportunities. This book represents our collective commitment and gratitude to our communities. We hope that it has inspired readers to commit themselves to improving the state of Latinx mental health.

REFERENCES

ABC7 New York. (2022, August 31). *More buses carrying asylum seekers arrive in NYC from Texas.* https://abc7ny.com/nyc-asylum-seekers-buses-texas/12179735/

Adames, H. Y., & Chavez-Dueñas, N. Y. (2017). *Cultural foundations and interventions in Latino/a mental health: History, theory, and within group differences*. Routledge.

APA. (2016). *2015 APA Survey of Psychology Health Service Providers.* https://www.apa.org/workforce/publications/15-health-service-providers

Brockell, G., & Tillman, J. (2022, September 16). 'Reverse Freedom Rides': An echo of Martha's Vineyard migrant flights 60 years ago. *The Washington Post*. https://www.washingtonpost.com/history/2022/09/16/reverse-freedom-rides-marthas-vineyard-desantis/

Butts, J., & Rich, K. L. (2015). *Philosophies and theories for advanced nursing practice* (2nd ed.). Jones & Bartlett Learning.

Capielo Rosario, C., Schaefer, A., Ballesteros, J., Rentería, R., & David, E. (2019). A caballo regalao no se le mira el colmillo: Colonial mentality and Puerto Rican depression. *Journal of Counseling Psychology, 66*(4), 396–408. doi:10.1037/cou0000347 PMID:30998052

Chavez-Dueñas, N. Y., Adames, H. Y., Perez-Chavez, J. G., & Salas, S. P. (2019). Healing ethno-racial trauma in Latinx immigrant communities: Cultivating hope, resistance, and action. *The American Psychologist, 74*(1), 49–62. doi:10.1037/amp0000289 PMID:30652899

Comas-Diaz, L. (2012). *Multicultural care: A clinicians guide to cultural competence.* American Psychological Association. doi:10.1037/13491-000

Comas-Díaz, L., Hall, G. N., & Neville, H. (2019). Introduction to the special issue: Racial trauma, theory, research and healing. *The American Psychologist, 74*, 1–5. doi:10.1037/amp0000442 PMID:30652895

DeAngelis, T. (2008). The two faces of oxytocin. *APA Monitor, 39*(2), 30. https://www.apa.org/monitor/feb08/oxytocin

Delgado-Romero, E. A., De Los Santos, J., Raman, V., Merrifield, J., Vazquez, M., Monroig, M., Cárdenas-Bautista, E., & Durán, M. (2018). Caught in the Middle: Bilingual Mental Health Counselors as Language Brokers. *Journal of Mental Health Counseling, 40*(4), 341–352. doi:10.17744/mehc.40.4.06

Delgado-Romero, E. A., Mahoney, G. E., Muro-Rodriguez, N., Atilano, R., Cardenas-Bautista, E., De Los Santos, J., Duran, M., Espinoza, L., Fuentes, J., Gomez, S., Ingram, R., Jiminez-Ruiz, J., Monroig, M., Mora-Ozuna, C., Ordaz, A. C., Rappaport, B., Suazo-Padilla, K., & Vazquez, M. S. (2021). *Clinica In Lak'ech:* The establishment of a practicum site to integrate practice, advocacy, and research with Latinx clients. *The Counseling Psychologist*–Special Issue, the Integration of Practice, Advocacy, and Research in Counseling Psychology. *The Counseling Psychologist, 49*(7), 987–1012. doi:10.1177/00110000211025270

Duran, E., Firehammer, J., & Gonzalez, J. (2008). Liberation psychology as the path toward healing cultural soul wounds. *Journal of Counseling and Development, 86*(3), 288–295. doi:10.1002/j.1556-6678.2008.tb00511.x

Freire, P. (1970). *Pedagogy of the oppressed.* Continuum.

Freire, P. (2005). *Education for critical consciousness.* Continuum.

French, B. H., Lewis, J. A., Mosley, D. V., Adames, H. Y., Chavez-Dueñas, N. Y., Chen, G. A., & Neville, H. A. (2020). Toward a psychological framework of radical healing in communities of color. *The Counseling Psychologist, 48*(1), 14–46. doi:10.1177/0011000019843506

Fuentes, M.A., Zelaya, D.G., Delgado-Romero, E.A. & Butt, M. (in press). Open science: Friend, foe or both to an antiracist psychology? *Psychological Review.* doi:10.1037/rev0000386

Gale. (n.d.). *History of Hate in America Collections.* https://www.gale.com/primary-sources/political-extremism-and-radicalism/collections/history-of-hate

Gonzalez, E. (2020). Foreword: Understanding Latina/o resilience. *International Journal of Qualitative Studies in Education: QSE, 33*(8), 791–795. doi:10.1080/09518398.2020.1783016

Gordon, I., Vander Wyk, B. C., Bennett, R. H., Cordeaux, C., Lucas, M. V., Eilbott, J. A., Zagoory-Sharon, O., Leckman, J. F., Feldman, R., & Pelphrey, K. A. (2013). Oxytocin enhances brain function in children with autism. *Psychology and Cognitive Sciences: Open Journal, 110*(52), 20953–20958. doi:10.1073/pnas.1312857110 PMID:24297883

Guthrie, R. V. (2004). *Even the Rat was White: A Historical View of Psychology*. Allyn & Bacon.

Helms, J. E., & Dupree, K. C. (2021). Elimination of the GRE Could Be Counseling Psychology's Rejection of Anti-Black Racism. In C. Davis III (Chair), *Big Ideas in Counseling Psychology: Uprooting Anti-Blackness*. APA Division 17 Virtual Symposium. https://www.youtube.com/watch?v=0Y0y2j59vi8

Henderson, T. (2022, August 23). *GOP Governors Bus Migrants to Blue Cities, but Many Exit in Red States*. Stateline. https://www.pewtrusts.org/en/research-and-analysis/blogs/stateline/2022/08/23/gop-governors-bus-migrants-to-blue-cities-but-many-exit-in-red-states

Jahangard, L., Shayganfard, M., Ghiasi, F., Salehi, I., Haghighi, M., Ahmadpanah, M., Sadeghi Bahmani, D., & Brand, S. (2020). Serum oxytocin concentrations in current and recent suicide survivors are lower than in healthy controls. *Journal of Psychiatric Research, 128*, 75–82. doi:10.1016/j.jpsychires.2020.05.014 PMID:32535343

Jorgenson, J. (2022, August 17). *City working to enroll children of asylum seekers in public schools*. Spectrum News. https://www.ny1.com/nyc/all-boroughs/education/2022/08/17/city-working-to-enroll-children-of-asylum-seekers-in-public-schools

Martín-Baró, I. (1994). *Writings for a liberation psychology: Ignacio Martín-Baró* (A. Aron & S. Corne, Eds. & Trans.). Harvard University Press.

Montero, M., & Sonn, C. C. (Eds.). (2009). *Psychology of liberation: Theories and applications*. Springer.

Montoya-Galvez, C. (2022, September 16). *GOP Govs. Ron DeSantis, Greg Abbott send migrants to Martha's Vineyard and vice president's residence*. CBS News. https://www.cbsnews.com/news/ron-desantis-flies-texas-florida-migrants-marthas-vineyard-kamala-harris-residence/

National Academy of Sciences, National Academy of Engineering, and Institute of Medicine. (2005). *Facilitating Interdisciplinary Research*. The National Academies Press. doi:10.17226/11153

Olff, M., Frijling, J. L., Kubzansky, L. D., Bradley, B., Ellenbogen, M. A., Cardoso, C., Bartz, J. A., Yee, J. R., & van Zuiden, M. (2013). The role of oxytocin in social bonding, stress regulation and mental health: An update on the moderating effects of context and interindividual differences. *Psychoneuroendocrinology, 38*(9), 1883–1894. doi:10.1016/j.psyneuen.2013.06.019 PMID:23856187

Sandoval, E., Jordan, M., Mazzei, P., & Goodman, J. D. (2022, October 4). The Story Behind DeSantis's Migrant Flights to Martha's Vineyard. *The New York Times*. https://www.nytimes.com/2022/10/02/us/migrants-marthas-vineyard-desantis-texas.html

Simon, S., & Emanuel, G. (2022, September 17). *Before migrants were sent to Martha's Vineyard, there were the "Reverse Freedom Rides"*. NPR. https://www.npr.org/2022/09/17/1123629655/60-years-before-migrants-were-sent-to-marthas-vineyard-there-were-the-reverse-fr

Sippel, L. M., Allington, C. E., Pietrzak, R. H., Harpaz-Rotem, I., Mayes, L. C., & Olff, M. (2017). Oxytocin and Stress-related Disorders: Neurobiological Mechanisms and Treatment Opportunities. *Chronic Stress, 1*. Advance online publication. doi:10.1177/2470547016687996 PMID:28649672

Stephens, A. M. (2021). Making Migrants "Criminal": The Mariel Boatlift, Miami, and U.S. Immigration Policy in the 1980s. *Anthurium, 17*(2), 4. doi:10.33596/anth.439

Tomicic, A., & Berardi, F. (2018). Between past and present: The sociopsychological constructs of colonialism, coloniality and postcolonialism. *Integrative Psychological & Behavioral Science, 52*(1), 152–175. doi:10.100712124-017-9407-5 PMID:29063442

Torres, S. A., Sosa, S. S., Flores Toussaint, R. J., Jolie, S., & Bustos, Y. (2022). Systems of Oppression: The Impact of Discrimination on Latinx Immigrant Adolescents' Well-Being and Development. *Journal of Research on Adolescence, 32*(2), 501–517. doi:10.1111/jora.12751 PMID:35365889

Webb, C. (2004). A Cheap Trafficking in Human Misery: The Reverse Freedom Rides of 1962. *Journal of American Studies, 38*(2), 249–271. doi:10.1017/S0021875804008436

Compilation of References

AAFP. (2017). *Primary Care*. https://www.aafp.org/about/policies/all/primary-care.html https://www.ncbi.nlm.nih.gov/pmc/articles/PMC5890504/

Abadía-Rexach, B. I. (2021). Adolfina Villanueva Osorio, Presente. *NACLA Report on the Americas*, *53*(2), 174–180. doi:10.1080/10714839.2021.1923222

Abalos, D. T. (2002). *The Latino Male: A Radical Redefinition*. Lynne Rienner Publishers.

Abbate-Daga, G., Amianto, F., Delsedime, N., De-Bacco, C., & Fassino, S. (2013). Resistance to treatment in eating disorders: A critical challenge. *BMC Psychiatry*, *13*, 294. doi:10.1186/1471-244X-13-294 PMID:24199620

Abbott, J. Y., & Geraths, C. (2021). Modern Masculinities: Resistance to Hegemonic Masculinity in Modern Family. *Journal of Contemporary Rhetoric*, *11*(1/2), 36–56.

ABC7 New York. (2022, August 31). *More buses carrying asylum seekers arrive in NYC from Texas*. https://abc7ny.com/nyc-asylum-seekers-buses-texas/12179735/

Abrego, L. J., & Hernández, E. (2021). 13.# FamiliesBelongTogether: Central American Family Separations from the 1980s to 2019. In Critical Dialogues in Latinx Studies (pp. 173-185). New York University Press.

Abreu, R. L., & Gonzalez, K. A. (2020). Redefining collectivism: Family and community among sexual and gender diverse people of color and indigenous people: Introduction to the special issue. *Journal of GLBT Family Studies*, *16*(2), 107–110. doi:10.1080/1550428X.2020.1736038

Abreu, R. L., Gonzalez, K. A., Capielo Rosario, C., Lockett, G. M., Lindley, L., & Lane, S. (2021). "We are our own community": Immigrant Latinx transgender people community experiences. *Journal of Counseling Psychology*, *68*(4), 390–403. Advance online publication. doi:10.1037/cou0000546 PMID:33983757

Abreu, R. L., Gonzalez, K. A., Capielo Rosario, C., Pulice-Farrow, L., & Rodríguez, M. M. D. (2020). "Latinos have a stronger attachment to the family": Latinx fathers' acceptance of their sexual minority children. *Journal of GLBT Family Studies*, *16*(2), 192–210. doi:10.1080/1550428X.2019.1672232

Adames, H. Y., & Chavez-Dueñas, N. Y. (2017). *Cultural foundations and interventions in Latino/a mental health: History, theory, and within group differences*. Routledge.

Adames, H. Y., & Chavez-Dueñas, N. Y. (2017). *Cultural foundations and interventions in Latino/a mental health: History, theory, and within-group differences*. Routledge.

Adames, H. Y., Chavez-Dueñas, N. Y., & Jernigan, M. M. (2021). The fallacy of a raceless Latinidad: Action guidelines for centering Blackness in Latinx psychology. *Journal of Latina/o Psychology*, *9*(1), 26–44. doi:10.1037/lat0000179

Adames, H., & Chavez-Duenas, N. (2017). *Cultural foundations and interventions in latino/a mental health history, theory and within group differences*. Taylor & Francis.

Adames, H.Y., Chavez-Dueñas, N.Y., & Jernigan, M.M. (2021). The fallacy of a raceless Latinidad: Action guidelines for centering Blackness in Latinx psychology. *Journal of Latina/o Psychology, 9*(1), 1–19.

Addis, M. E., & Cohane, G. H. (2005). Social scientific paradigms of masculinity and their implications for research and practice in men's mental health. *Journal of Clinical Psychology, 61*(6), 633–647. doi:10.1002/jclp.20099 PMID:15732091

Addis, M. E., & Mahalik, J. R. (2003). Men, masculinity, and the contexts of help seeking. *The American Psychologist, 58*(1), 5–14. doi:10.1037/0003-066X.58.1.5 PMID:12674814

Agricultural Health Study. (2019). https://aghealth.nih.gov/about/

Ai, A. L., Pappas, C., & Simonsen, E. (2015). Risk and protective factors for three major mental health problems among Latino American men nationwide. *American Journal of Men's Health, 9*(1), 64–75. doi:10.1177/1557988314528533 PMID:24707037

Ajzen, I. (1991). The theory of planned behavior. *Organizational Behavior and Human Decision Processes, 50*(2), 179–211. doi:10.1016/0749-5978(91)90020-T

Alegria, M., Woo, M., Cao, Z., Torres, M., Meng, X. L., & Striegel-Moore, R. (2007). Prevalence and correlates of eating disorders in Latinos in the United States. *The International Journal of Eating Disorders, 40*(Suppl), S15–S21. 1 doi:0.1002/eat.2040

Alegria, M., Canino, G., Rios, R., Vera, M., Calderon, J., Rusch, D., & Ortega, A. N. (2002). Inequalities in use of specialty mental health services among Latinos, African Americans, and non-White Latinos. *Psychiatric Services (Washington, D.C.), 53*, 1547–1555. doi:10.1176/appi.ps.53.12.1547 PMID:12461214

Alegría, M., Chatterji, P., Wells, K., Cao, Z., Chen, C., Takeuchi, D., & Meng, X. L. (2008). Disparity in depression treatment among racial and ethnic minority populations in the United States. [PubMed: 18971402]. *Psychiatric Services (Washington, D.C.), 59*(11), 1264–1272. doi:10.1176/ps.2008.59.11.1264 PMID:18971402

Alegría, M., Mulvaney-Day, N., Torres, M., Polo, A., Cao, Z., & Canino, G. (2007). Prevalence of psychiatric disorders across Latino subgroups in the United States. *American Journal of Public Health, 97*(1), 68–75. doi:10.2105/AJPH.2006.087205 PMID:17138910

Alegría, M., Sribney, W., Perez, D., Laderman, M., & Keefe, K. (2009). The role of patient activation on patient–provider communication and quality of care for US and foreign born Latino patients. *Journal of General Internal Medicine, 24*(3), 534–541. doi:10.100711606-009-1074-x PMID:19842003

Amadiume, I. (1987). *Male daughters, female husbands: Gender and sex in an African society*. Zed Books Ltd.

American Psychological Association. (2015). Guidelines for psychological practice with transgender and gender nonconforming people. *The American Psychologist, 70*(9), 832–864. doi:10.1037/a0039906 PMID:26653312

American Psychological Association. (2017). *Multicultural guidelines: An ecological approach to context, identity, and intersectionality*. Retrieved from: http://www.apa.org/about/policy/multicultural-guidelines.pdf

American Psychological Association. (2020). *Demographics of U.S. Psychology Workforce* [Interactive data tool]. http://www.apa.org/workforce/data-tools/demographics.aspx

American Psychological Association. (2021). *Guidelines for psychological practice with sexual minority persons*. Retrieved from www.apa.org/about/policy/psychological-practice-sexual-minority-persons.pdf

Compilation of References

Andersen, R. M. (1995). Revisiting the behavioral model and access to medical care: Does it matter? *Journal of Health and Social Behavior, 36*(1), 1–10. doi:10.2307/2137284 PMID:7738325

Anderson, M. A., Malhotra, A., & Non, A. L. (2021). Could routine race-adjustment of spirometers exacerbate racial disparities in COVID-19 recovery? *The Lancet. Respiratory Medicine, 9*(2), 124–125. doi:10.1016/S2213-2600(20)30571-3 PMID:33308418

Anthony, M., Nichols, A. H., & Del Pilar, W. (2021, December 21). A look at degree attainment among Hispanic women and men and how COVID-19 could deepen racial and gender divides. *The Education Trust*. Retrieved May 8, 2022, from https://edtrust.org/resource/a-look-at-degree-attainment-among-hispanic-women-and-men-and-how-covid-19-could-deepen-racial-and-gender-divides/

Anzaldúa, G. (2002). now let us shift... the path of conocimiento... inner work, public acts. In G.E. Anzaldúa & A. L. Keating (Ed.), This bridge we call home: Radical visions for transformation (pp. 540-578). New York, NY: Routledge.

Anzaldúa, G. (2002). Now let us shift... the path of conocimiento... inner work, public acts. In G.E. Anzaldúa & A. L. Keating (Ed.), This bridge we call home: Radical visions for transformation (pp. 540-578). New York, NY: Routledge.

Anzaldúa, G. (1987). *Borderlands/La Frontera: The new mestiza*. Aunt Lute Books.

Anzaldúa, G. (2007). *Borderlands : the new mestiza = La frontera* (3rd ed.). Aunt Lute Books.

Anzaldúa, G. (2007). *Borderlands/ La Frontera: The New Mestiza*. Aunt Lute Books.

Anzaldúa, G. E. (1987). *Borderlands/La Frontera: The New Mestiza*. Aunt Lute.

Anzaldúa, G., & Keating, A. (2015). *Light in the Dark/Luz en lo Oscuro: Rewriting Identity, Spirituality, Reality*. Duke University Press.

APA. (2016). *2015 APA Survey of Psychology Health Service Providers*. https://www.apa.org/workforce/publications/15-health-service-providers

Arciniega, G. M., Anderson, T. C., Tovar-Blank, Z. G., & Tracey, T. J. G. (2008). Toward a Fuller Conception of Machismo: Development of a Traditional Machismo and Caballerismo Scale. *Journal of Counseling Psychology, 55*(1), 19–33. doi:10.1037/0022-0167.55.1.19

Arcury, T. A., Laurienti, P. J., Chen, H., Howard, T. D., Barr, D. B., Mora, D. C., Summers, P., & Quandt, S. A. (2016). Organophosphate pesticide urinary metabolites among Latino immigrants: North Carolina farmworkers and fon-farmworkers compared. *Journal of Occupational and Environmental Medicine, 58*(11), 1079–1086. doi:10.1097/JOM.0000000000000875 PMID:27820757

Arcury, T. A., & Quandt, S. A. (2020). *Latinx farmworkers in the eastern united states: Health, safety, and justice*. Springer International Publishing. doi:10.1007/978-3-030-36643-8

Arellano-Morales, L., Roesch, S. C., Gallo, L. C., Emory, K. T., Molina, K. M., Gonzalez, P., Penedo, F. J., Navas-Nacher, E. L., Teng, Y., Deng, Y., Isasi, C. R., Schneiderman, N., & Brondolo, E. (2015). Prevalence and Correlates of Perceived Ethnic Discrimination in the Hispanic Community Health Study/Study of Latinos Sociocultural Ancillary Study. *Journal of Latina/o Psychology, 3*(3), 160–176. doi:10.1037/lat0000040 PMID:26491624

Arevalo, I., So, D., & McNaughton-Cassill, M. (2016). The role of collectivism among Latino American college students. *Journal of Latinos and Education, 15*(1), 3–11. doi:10.1080/15348431.2015.1045143

Arnett, J. J. (2016). Life stage concepts across history and cultures: Proposal for a new field on indigenous life stages. *Human Development, 59*(5), 290–316. doi:10.1159/000453627

Arredondo, P. (2002). Mujeres Latinas—Santas y Marquesas. *Cultural Diversity & Ethnic Minority Psychology*, *8*(4), 308–319. doi:10.1037/1099-9809.8.4.308 PMID:12416317

Arredondo, P. (2010). In J. G. Ponterotto, J. M. Casas, L. A. Suzuki, & C. M. Alexander (Eds.), *Handbook of Multicultural Counseling* (3rd ed., pp. 38–44). Sage.

Arredondo, P. (2018). Latinx immigrants set the stage for 2050. In *Latinx Immigrants* (pp. 1–13). Springer. doi:10.1007/978-3-319-95738-8_1

Arredondo, P., Gallardo-Cooper, M., Delgado-Romero, E. A., & Zapata, A. L. (2014). *Culturally responsive counseling with Latinas/os*. John Wiley & Sons.

Arredondo, P., Toporek, R. L., Pack Brown, S., & Jones, J. (1996). Operationalization of the Multicultural Counseling Competencies. *Journal of Multicultural Counseling and Development*, *24*(1), 42–78. doi:10.1002/j.2161-1912.1996.tb00288.x

Arredondo, P., & Tovar-Blank, Z. G. (2014). Multicultural competencies: A dynamic paradigm for the 21st century. In F. T. L. Leong, L. Comas-Díaz, G. C. Nagayama Hall, V. C. McLoyd, & J. E. Trimble (Eds.), APA handbook of multicultural psychology: Vol. 2. *Applications and training* (pp. 19–34). American Psychological Association. doi:10.1037/14187-002

Arrizón, A. (2008). Latina subjectivity, sexuality and sensuality. *Women & Performance*, *18*(3), 189–198. doi:10.1080/07407700802495928

Asad, A., & Clair, M. (2017). Racialized legal status as a social determinant of health. *Social Science & Medicine*, *199*, 19–28. doi:10.1016/j.socscimed.2017.03.010 PMID:28359580

Avalos, R. (2011). *Lost leader in history: The transforming and empowering partnership of Dolores Huerta & César Chávez*. https://csulb-dspace.calstate.edu/bitstream/handle/10211.14/3/Rebecca%20Avalos.pdf?sequence=1

Avila, L. (2022, June 29). It's time to retire toxic ride-or-die culture. In *Hot Girl Somos*. Refinery29. https://www.refinery29.com/en-us/2022/06/11027589/marianismo-ride-or-die-culture-toxic

Azmitia, M. (2021). Latinx Adolescents' Assets, Risks, and Developmental Pathways: A Decade in Review and Looking Ahead. *Journal of Research on Adolescence*, *31*(4), 989–1005. doi:10.1111/jora.12686 PMID:34820953

Baams, L., Grossman, A. H., & Russell, S. T. (2015). Minority stress and mechanisms of risk for depression and suicidal ideation among lesbian, gay, and bisexual youth. *Developmental Psychology*, *51*(5), 688–696. doi:10.1037/a0038994 PMID:25751098

Babich, E., & Batalova, J. (2021). *Immigrants from the Dominican Republic in the United States*. Migration Policy Institute. Retrieved from https://www.migrationpolicy.org/article/dominican-immigrants-united-states-2019

Baez, A., & Hernandez, D. (2001). Complementary spiritual beliefs in the Latino community: The interface with psychotherapy. *The American Journal of Orthopsychiatry*, *71*(4), 408–415. doi:10.1037/0002-9432.71.4.408 PMID:11822213

Bailey, Z. D., Feldman, J. M., & Bassett, M. T. (2021). How structural racism works—Racist policies as a root cause of US racial health inequities. *The New England Journal of Medicine*, *384*(8), 768–773. doi:10.1056/NEJMms2025396 PMID:33326717

Balbuena, A. (2018). El debate sobre el aborto y las tres causales: La cuestión de la autonomía de la mujer [The Debate on Abortions and the Three grounds; The Issue of Woman's Anatomy]. *Perspectivas*, *2*(18), 1–8.

Baldwin, J., & DeSouza, E. (2001). Modelo de Maria and machismo: The social construction of gender in Brazil. *Interamerican Journal of Psychology*, *35*(1), 9–29.

Balsam, K. F., Molina, Y., Beadnell, B., Simoni, J., & Walters, K. (2011). Measuring multiple minority stress: The LGBTQ+ People of Color Microaggressions Scale. *Cultural Diversity & Ethnic Minority Psychology*, *17*(2), 163–174. doi:10.1037/a0023244 PMID:21604840

Balsam, K. F., Molina, Y., Blayney, J. A., Dillworth, T., Zimmerman, L., & Kaysen, D. (2015). Racial/ethnic differences in identity and mental health outcomes among young sexual minority women. *Cultural Diversity & Ethnic Minority Psychology*, *21*(3), 380–390. doi:10.1037/a0038680 PMID:25642782

Basurto, L. E. (2020, October 22). *Why we should be talking about mental health among Latinx communities*. Urban Institute. Retrieved May 1, 2022, from https://www.urban.org/urban-wire/why-we-should-be-talking-about-mental-health-among-latinx-communities

Beatty, T., Hill, A., Martin, P., & Rutledge, Z. (2020). Covid-19 and farm workers: Challenges facing. *California Agriculture*, *23*(5), 2–4.

Beauregard, C. (2020). Being in between: Exploring cultural bereavement and identity expression through drawing. *Journal of Creativity in Mental Health*, *15*(3), 292–310. doi:10.1080/15401383.2019.1702131

Becker Herbst, R., Sabet, R. F., Swanson, A., Suarez, L. G., Marques, D. S., Ameen, E. J., & Aldarondo, E. (2018). "They were going to kill me": Resilience in unaccompanied immigrant minors. *The Counseling Psychologist*, *46*(2), 241–268. doi:10.1177/0011000018759769

Becker, A. E., Franko, D. L., Speck, A., & Herzog, D. B. (2003). Ethnicity and differential access to care for eating disorder symptoms. *International Journal of Eating Disorders*, *33*(2), 205–212. doi:10.1002/eat.10129 PMID:12616587

Benish, S. G., Quintana, S., & Wampold, B. E. (2011). Culturally adapted psychotherapy and the legitimacy of myth: A direct-comparison meta-analysis. *Journal of Counseling Psychology*, *58*(3), 279–289. doi:10.1037/a0023626 PMID:21604860

Bermúdez, J. M., & Bermúdez, S. (2002). Altar-making with Latino families: A narrative therapy perspective. *Journal of Family Psychotherapy*, *13*(3/4), 329–347. doi:10.1300/J085v13n03_06

Bernal, D. D. (2002). Critical race theory, Latino critical theory, and critical raced-gendered epistemologies: Recognizing students of color as holders and creators of knowledge. *Qualitative Inquiry*, *8*(1), 105–126. doi:10.1177/107780040200800107

Bernal, D. D., Elenes, C. A., & Godinez, F. E. (Eds.). (2006). *Chicana/Latina education in everyday life: Feminista perspectives on pedagogy and epistemology*. Suny Press.

Bernstein, A. (2003). Waking up from the American dream. *Business Week*, *1*, 54-58.

Berrios-Miranda, M. (2004). Salsa music as expressive liberation. *Centro Journal*, *16*(2), 158–173.

Berry, J. W. (1997). Immigration, acculturation, and adaptation. *Applied Psychology*, *46*(1), 5–34. doi:10.1111/j.1464-0597.1997.tb01087.x

Biglieri, P. (2020). Ni Una Menos—Not One Woman Less: How Feminism Could Become a Popular Struggle. *Baltic Worlds*, *13*(1), 64–66.

Bishop, M., Mallory, A. B., Gessner, M. K., Frost, D. M., & Russell, S. T. (2021). School-based sexuality education experiences across three generations of sexual minority people. *Journal of Sex Research*, *58*(5), 648–658. doi:10.1080/00224499.2020.1767024 PMID:32486928

Bockting, W., & Coleman, E. (2016). Developmental stages of the transgender coming-out process: Toward an integrated identity. In R. Ettner, S. Monstrey, & E. Coleman (Eds.), Principles of transgender medicine and surgery (2nd ed., pp. 137–158). Routledge/Taylor & Francis Group.

Bockting, W., Barucco, R., LeBlanc, A., Singh, A., Mellman, W., Dolezal, C., & Ehrhardt, A. (2020). Sociopolitical change and transgender people's perceptions of vulnerability and resilience. *Sexuality Research & Social Policy*, *17*(1), 162–174. doi:10.100713178-019-00381-5 PMID:32742526

Boe, J. L., Maxey, V. A., & Bermudez, J. M. (2018). Is the closet a closet? Decolonizing the coming out process with Latin@ adolescents and families. *Journal of Feminist Family Therapy*, *30*(2), 90–108. doi:10.1080/08952833.2018.1427931

Bolivar, A. (2021). "This Pussy Actually Grabs Back": A Trans Latina Expansion of "Pussy." *Frontiers*, *42*(2), 1–23. doi:10.1353/fro.2021.0020

Bonner-Prado, J., Mulay, P. R., Kasner, E. J., Bojes, H. K., & Calvert, G. M. (2018). Acute pesticide-related illness among farmworkers: Barriers to reporting to public health authorities. *Journal of Agromedicine*, *22*(4), 395–405. doi:10.1080/1059924X.2017.1353936 PMID:28762882

Borrell, L. N. (2009). Race, ethnicity, and self-reported hypertension: Analysis of data from the national health interview survey, 1997-2005. *American Journal of Public Health*, *99*(2), 313–320. doi:10.2105/AJPH.2007.123364 PMID:19059869

Boss, P. (1999). *Ambiguous loss: learning to live with unresolved grief*. Harvard University Press.

Bowleg, L. (2008). When Black+ lesbian+ woman¹ Black lesbian woman: The methodological challenges of qualitative and quantitative intersectionality research. *Sex Roles*, *59*(5-6), 312–325. doi:10.100711199-008-9400-z

Boyle, K. (2019). # MeToo, Weinstein and feminism. In # MeToo, Weinstein and Feminism (pp. 1-20). Palgrave Pivot.

Bradley, D. (1984). Novelist Alice Walker Telling the Black Woman's Story. *New York Times Magazine*, *8*, 24-37.

Breslow, A. S., Brewster, M. E., Velez, B. L., Wong, S., Geiger, E., & Soderstrom, B. (2015). Resilience and collective action: Exploring buffers against minority stress for transgender individuals. *Psychology of Sexual Orientation and Gender Diversity*, *2*(3), 253–265. doi:10.1037gd0000117

Brewer, B. (2021). *What is Integrated Health? Models & Systems For Healthcare Innovation*. Mhaonline. https://www.mhaonline.com/blog/integrated-behavioral-health

Brewer, R. M. (2020). Black Feminism and Womanism. In N. A. Naples (Ed.), *Companion to Feminist Studies*. doi:10.1002/9781119314967.ch6

Bridges, A. J., & Lindly, E. (2008). Service utilization and case management. In Workgroup on Adapting Latino Services (Ed.), Adaptation guidelines for serving Latino children and families affected by trauma (pp. 53-56). Chadwick Center for Children and Families.

Bridges, A. J., & Anastasia, E. (2016). Enhancing and improving treatment engagement with Hispanic patients. In W. O'Donohue & L. Benuto (Eds.), *Enhancing Behavioral Health in Hispanic Populations: Eliminating Disparities Through Integrated Behavioral and Primary Care* (pp. 125–143). Springer International Publishing. doi:10.1007/978-3-319-42533-7_8

Bridges, A. J., Andrews, A. R. III, & Deen, T. L. (2012). Mental health needs and service utilization by Hispanic immigrants residing in mid-southern United States. *Journal of Transcultural Nursing*, *23*(4), 359–368. doi:10.1177/1043659612451259 PMID:22802297

Compilation of References

Bridges, A. J., Andrews, A. R. III, Pastrana, F. A., Villalobos, B. T., Cavell, T. A., & Gomez, D. (2014). Does integrated behavioral health care reduce mental health disparities for Hispanics? Initial findings. *Journal of Latina/o Psychology*, *2*(1), 37–53. doi:10.1037/lat0000009 PMID:25309845

Brockell, G., & Tillman, J. (2022, September 16). 'Reverse Freedom Rides': An echo of Martha's Vineyard migrant flights 60 years ago. *The Washington Post*. https://www.washingtonpost.com/history/2022/09/16/reverse-freedom-rides-marthas-vineyard-desantis/

Brumbaugh-Johnson, S. M., & Hull, K. E. (2019). Coming out as transgender: Navigating the social implications of a transgender identity. *Journal of Homosexuality*, *66*(8), 1148–1177. doi:10.1080/00918369.2018.1493253 PMID:30052497

Bryant-Davis, T., & Comas-Díaz, L. (2016). Womanist and mujerista psychologies: Voices of fire, acts of courage (T. Bryant-Davis & L. Comas-Díaz, Eds.). American Psychological Association. doi:10.1037/14937-000

Budge, S. L., Chin, M. Y., & Minero, L. P. (2017). Trans individuals' facilitative coping: An analysis of internal and external processes. *Journal of Counseling Psychology*, *64*(1), 12–25. doi:10.1037/cou0000178 PMID:28068128

Budiman, A. (2020). *Key findings about U.S. immigrants*. Pew Research Center. Retrieved from https://www.pewresearch.org/fact-tank/2020/08/20/key-findings-about-u-s-immigrants/

Burgos, G., Rivera, F. I., & Garcia, M. A. (2017). Contextualizing the relationship between culture and Puerto Rican health: Towards a place-based framework of minority health disparities. *Centro Journal*, *29*(3), 36–73.

Butler, M., Kane, R. L., McAlpine, D., Kathol, R., Fu, S. S., Hagedorn, H., & Wilt, T. (2011). Does integrated care improve treatment for depression? A systematic review. *The Journal of Ambulatory Care Management*, *34*(2), 113–125. doi:10.1097/JAC.0b013e31820ef605 PMID:21415610

Butts, J., & Rich, K. L. (2015). *Philosophies and theories for advanced nursing practice* (2nd ed.). Jones & Bartlett Learning.

Caba, M., Mallory, A. B., Simon, K. A., Rathus, T., & Watson, R. J. (2022). Complex Outness Patterns Among Sexual Minority Youth: A Latent Class Analysis. *Journal of Youth and Adolescence*, *51*(4), 746–765. doi:10.100710964-022-01580-x PMID:35150376

Cabassa, L. J. (2007). Latino Immigrant Men's Perceptions of Depression and Attitudes Toward Help Seeking. *Hispanic Journal of Behavioral Sciences*, *29*(4), 492–509. doi:10.1177/0739986307307157

Cabassa, L. J., & Zayas, L. H. (2007). Latino immigrants' intentions to seek depression care. *The American Journal of Orthopsychiatry*, *77*(2), 231–242. doi:10.1037/0002-9432.77.2.231 PMID:17535121

Cabassa, L. J., Zayas, L. H., & Hansen, M. C. (2006). Latino adults' access to mental health care: A review of epidemiological studies. *Administration and Policy in Mental Health*, *33*(3), 316–330. doi:10.100710488-006-0040-8 PMID:16598658

Cabrera, N. J., Alonso, A., & Chen, Y. (2021). Parenting contributions to Latinx children's development in the early years. *The Annals of the American Academy of Political and Social Science*, *696*(1), 158–178. doi:10.1177/00027162211049997

Cade, J. (2013). Policing the immigration police: ICE prosecutorial discretion and the fourth amendment. *Columbia Law Review Sidebar*, *113*, 182–183.

Cade, J. (2020). "Water is life!" (and speech!): Death dissent, and democracy in the borderlands. *Indiana Law Journal (Indianapolis, Ind.)*, *96*(1), 267–272.

Calavita, K. (2010). *Inside the state: The bracero program, immigration, and the I.N.S.* Academic Press.

California office of environmental health hazard assessment. (2019). *Heat-Related Mortality and Morbidity.* https://oehha.ca.gov/epic/impacts-biological-systems/heat-related-mortality-and-morbidity

Call, J. B., & Shafer, K. (2018). Gendered Manifestations of Depression and Help Seeking Among Men. *American Journal of Men's Health, 12*(1), 41–51. doi:10.1177/1557988315623993 PMID:26721265

Calvillo, J. E., & Bailey, S. R. (2015). Latino religious affiliation and ethnic identity. *Journal for the Scientific Study of Religion, 54*(1), 57–78. doi:10.1111/jssr.12164

Capielo Rosario, C., Schaefer, A., Ballesteros, J., Rentería, R., & David, E. (2019). A caballo regalao no se le mira el colmillo: Colonial mentality and Puerto Rican depression. *Journal of Counseling Psychology, 66*(4), 396–408. doi:10.1037/cou0000347 PMID:30998052

Captari, L. E., Hook, J. N., Hoyt, W., Davis, D. E., McElroy, H. S. E., & Worthington, E. L. (2018). Integrating clients' religion and spirituality within psychotherapy: A comprehensive meta-analysis. *Journal of Clinical Psychology, 74*(11), 1938–1951. doi:10.1002/jclp.22681 PMID:30221353

Cardona, B., & Softas-Nall, L. (2010). Family therapy with Latino families: An interview with Patricia Arredondo. *The Family Journal, 18*(1), 73–77. doi:10.1177/1066480709356543

Cardoso, J. B., & Thompson, S. J. (2010). Common Themes of Resilience among Latino Immigrant Families: A Systematic Review of the Literature. *Families in Society, 91*(3), 257–265. doi:10.1606/1044-3894.4003

Carillo, K. J. (2021). Mexico's first liberated city commemorates its founding. *Jstor Daily.* https://daily.jstor.org/mexicos-yanga-commenorates-founding/

Carlo, G., Murry, V. M., Davis, A. N., Gonzalez, C. M., & Debreaux, M. L. (2022). Culture-Related Adaptive Mechanisms to Race-Related Trauma Among African American and US Latinx Youth. *Adversity and Resilience Science*, 1-13.

Castañeda-Sound, C. L., Martinez, S., & Durán, J. E. (2016). Mujeristas and social justice: La lucha es la vida. In T. Bryant-Davis & L. Comas-Díaz (Eds.), *Womanist and mujerista psychologies: Voices of fire, acts of courage* (pp. 237–259). American Psychological Association. doi:10.1037/14937-011

Castellanos, J., White, J. L., & Franco, V. (2022). *Riding the academic freedom train: A Culturally responsive, multigenerational mentoring model.* Stylus Publishing.

Castillo, L. G., Perez, F. V., Castillo, R., & Ghosheh, M. R. (2010). Construction and initial validation of the Marianismo Beliefs Scale. *Counselling Psychology Quarterly, 23*(2), 163–175. doi:10.1080/09515071003776036

Causadias, J. M., Vitriol, J. A., & Atkin, A. L. (2018). Do we overemphasize the role of culture in the behavior of racial/ethnic minorities? Evidence of a cultural (mis) attribution bias in American psychology. *The American Psychologist, 73*(3), 243–255. doi:10.1037/amp0000099 PMID:29355353

Centers for Disease Control and Prevention. (2018). *National Health Interview Survey: Tables of Summary Health Statistics.* Retrieved from https://www.cdc.gov/nchs/nhis/SHS/tables.htm

Centers for Disease Control and Prevention. (2022). *Childhood lead poisoning prevention program.* Retrieved from https://www.cdc.gov/nceh/lead/default.htm

Cerdeña, J. P., Rivera, L. M., & Spak, J. M. (2021). Intergenerational trauma in Latinxs: A scoping review. *Social Science & Medicine, 270*, 113662. doi:10.1016/j.socscimed.2020.113662

Cerezo, A. (2020). Expanding the reach of Latinx psychology: Honoring the lived experiences of sexual and gender diverse Latinxs. *Journal of Latina/o Psychology, 8*(1), 1–6. doi:10.1037/lat0000144

Cerezo, A., Cummings, M., Holmes, M., & Williams, C. (2020). Identity as resistance: Identity formation at the intersection of race, gender identity, and sexual orientation. *Psychology of Women Quarterly, 44*(1), 67–83. doi:10.1177/0361684319875977 PMID:32194296

Cerezo, A., Morales, A., Quintero, D., & Rothman, S. (2014). Trans migrations: Exploring life at the intersection of transgender identity and immigration. *Psychology of Sexual Orientation and Gender Diversity, 1*(2), 170–180. doi:10.1037gd0000031

Cervantes, A., Fernandez, I. T., & Carmona, J. F. (2019). Nosotros importamos (we matter): The use of testimonios with Latino male adolescents in group counseling. *Journal of Creativity in Mental Health, 14*(2), 181–192. doi:10.1080/15401383.2019.1568941

Cha, B. S., Enriquez, L. E., & Ro, A. (2019). Beyond access: Psychosocial barriers to undocumented students' use of mental health services. *Social Science & Medicine, 233*, 193–200. doi:10.1016/j.socscimed.2019.06.003 PMID:31212126

Chandra, A., Scott, M. M., Jaycox, L. H., Meredith, L. S., Tanielian, T., & Burnam, A. (2009). Racial/ethnic differences in teen and parent perspectives toward depression treatment. *The Journal of Adolescent Health, 44*(6), 546–553. doi:10.1016/j.jadohealth.2008.10.137

Chang, C. (2019). Social Determinants of Health and Health Disparities Among Immigrants and their Children. *Current Problems in Pediatric and Adolescent Health Care, 49*(1), 23-30. https://www.sciencedirect.com/science/article/pii/S1538544218301755 doi:10.1016/j.cppeds.2018.11.009

Chang, C. W., & Biegel, D. E. (2018). Factors affecting mental health service utilization among Latino Americans with mental health issues. *Journal of Mental Health (Abingdon, England), 27*(6), 552–559. doi:10.1080/09638237.2017.1385742 PMID:28980838

Chang, D. F., Hsieh, E., Somerville, W. B., Dimond, J., Thomas, M., Nicasio, A., Boiler, M., & Lewis-Fernández, R. (2021). Rethinking interpreter functions in mental health services. *Psychiatric Services (Washington, D.C.), 72*(3), 353–357. doi:10.1176/appi.ps.202000085 PMID:32988324

Chang, S. C., Singh, A. A., & Dickey, L. m. (2018). *A Clinician's Guide to Gender-Affirming Care: Working with Transgender and Gender Nonconforming Clients*. New Harbinger Publications.

Chapa, T., & Acosta, H. (2010). *Movilizandonos por nuestro futuro: Strategic development of a mental health workforce for Latinos—Consensus statements and recommendations*. Retrieved from http://minorityhealth.hhs.gov/Assets/pdf/Checked/1/MOVILIZANDONOS_ POR_NUESTRO_FUTURO_CONSENSUS_REPORT2010.pdf

Chaplin, T. M., Cole, P. M., & Zahn-Waxler, C. (2005). Parental socialization of emotion expression: Gender differences and relations to child adjustment. *Emotion (Washington, D.C.), 5*(1), 80–88. doi:10.1037/1528-3542.5.1.80 PMID:15755221

Chapman-Hilliard, C., & Adam-Bass, V. (2016). A conceptual framework for utilizing Black history knowledge as a path to psychological liberation for Black youth. *The Journal of Black Psychology, 42*(6), 479–507. doi:10.1177/0095798415597840

Charleswell, C. (2014, October 17). *Latina Feminism: National and Transnational Perspectives*. Retrieved July 01, 2016, from http://www.hamptoninstitute.org/latina-feminism.html#.V4klOJMrLfZ

Chavez-Dueñas, N. Y., & Adames, H. Y. (2021). Intersectionality Awakening Model of Womanista: A transnational treatment approach for Latinx women. *Women & Therapy, 44*(1-2), 83–100. doi:10.1080/02703149.2020.1775022

Chavez-Dueñas, N. Y., Adames, H. Y., & Organista, K. C. (2014). Skin-color prejudice and within-group racial discrimination: Historical and current impact on Latino/a populations. *Hispanic Journal of Behavioral Sciences, 36*(1), 3–26. doi:10.1177/0739986313511306

Chavez-Duenas, N. Y., Adames, H. Y., & Perez-Chavez, J. G. (2022). Anti-colonial futures: Indigenous Latinx women healing from the wounds of racial-gendered colonialism. *Women & Therapy*, *45*(2-3), 191–206. Advance online publication. doi:10.1080/02703149.2022.2097593

Chavez-Dueñas, N. Y., Adames, H. Y., Perez-Chavez, J. G., & Salas, S. P. (2019). Healing ethno-racial trauma in Latinx immigrant communities: Cultivating hope, resistance, and action. *The American Psychologist*, *74*(1), 49–62. doi:10.1037/amp0000289 PMID:30652899

Chen, F. M., Fryer, G. E., Phillips, R. L., Wilson, E., & Pathman, D. E. (2005). Patients' beliefs about racism, preferences for physician race, and satisfaction with care. *Annals of Family Medicine*, *3*(2), 138–143. doi:10.1370/afm.282 PMID:15798040

Cheng, J. K. Y., & Sue, S. (2014). Addressing cultural and ethnic minority issues in the acceptance and mindfulness movement. In A. Masuda (Ed.), *Mindfulness and acceptance in multicultural competency: A contextual approach to sociocultural diversity in theory and practice* (pp. 21–37). New Harbinger Publications, Inc.

Chen, S. H., Kennedy, M., & Zhou, Q. (2012). Parents' expression and discussion of emotion in the multilingual family: Does language matter? *Perspectives on Psychological Science*, *7*(4), 365–383. doi:10.1177/1745691612447307 PMID:26168473

Chiang, L., Hunter, C. D., & Yeh, C. J. (2004). Coping attitudes, sources, and practices among Black and Latino college students. *Adolescence*, *39*, 793–815. PMID:15727415

Cho, H., Kim, I., & Velez Ortiz, D. (2014). Factors Associated with Mental Health Service Use Among Latino and Asian Americans. *Community Mental Health Journal*, *50*(8), 960–967. Advance online publication. doi:10.100710597-014-9719-6 PMID:24659219

Chow, A. R. (2020). These Afro-Latino actors are pushing back against erasure in Hollywood. *Time*. https://time.com/5889072/afro-latino-actors-roundtable/

Chung, R. C. Y., Bemak, F., & Sánchez, R. O. (2022). Latinx adolescent migrant challenges in reuniting with family members. *International Review of Psychiatry (Abingdon, England)*, 1–10. doi:10.1080/09540261.2022.2072192

Cianelli, R., Ferrer, L., & McElmurry, B. J. (2008). HIV prevention and low-income Chilean women: Machismo, marianismo and HIV misconceptions. *Culture, Health & Sexuality*, *10*, 297–306.

Cokley, K., Hall-Clark, B. N., & Hicks, D. (2011). Ethnic Minority-Majority Status and Mental Health: The Mediating Role of Perceived Discrimination. *Journal of Mental Health Counseling*, *33*(3), 243–263. doi:10.17744/mehc.33.3.u1n011t020783086

Colectiva Feminista en Construcción. (2020a). *La Manifiesta*. https://www.scribd.com/document/263057948/La-Manifiesta-Colectiva-Feminista-en-Construccion

Colectiva Feminista en Construcción. (2020b, March 6). *Manifiesto antirracista de la Colectiva Feminista en Construcción* [Anti-Racist Manifesto of the Feminist Collective in Consrutction]. https://www.todaspr.com/manifiesto-antirracista-de-la-colectiva-feminista-en-construccion/

Coles, S. M., & Pasek, J. (2020). Intersectional invisibility revisited: How group prototypes lead to the erasure and exclusion of Black women. *Translational Issues in Psychological Science*, *6*(4), 1–11. doi:10.1037/tps0000256

Collins, P. H. (1986). Learning from the outsider within: The sociological significance of Black feminist though. *Social Problems*, *33*(6), S14–S32. doi:10.2307/800672

Collins, P. H. (1989). The Social Construction of Black Feminist Thought. *Signs (Chicago, Ill.)*, *14*(4), 745–773. doi:10.1086/494543

Collins, P. H. (2017). The Difference That Power Makes: Intersectionality and Participatory Democracy. *Investigaciones Feministas*, *8*(1), 19–39. doi:10.5209/INFE.54888

Comas-Díaz, L. (2008). Latino psychospitituality. In K. J. Schneider (Ed.), Existential-integrative psychotherapy: Guideposts to the core of practice (pp. 100–109). Routledge/Taylor & Francis Group.

Comas-Díaz, L. (1988). Feminist therapy with Hispanic/Latina women: Myth or reality? *Women & Therapy*, *6*(4), 39–61. doi:10.1300/J015V06N04_06

Comas-Díaz, L. (2000). An ethnopolitical approach to working with people of color. *The American Psychologist*, *55*(11), 1319–1325. doi:10.1037/0003-066X.55.11.1319 PMID:11280941

Comas-Díaz, L. (2006). Latino healing: The integration of ethnic psychology into psychotherapy. *Psychotherapy (Chicago, Ill.)*, *43*(4), 436–453. doi:10.1037/0033-3204.43.4.436 PMID:22122135

Comas-Diaz, L. (2008). 2007 Carolyn Sherif award address: Spirita: Reclaiming womanist sacredness into feminism. *Psychology of Women Quarterly*, *32*(1), 13–21. doi:10.1111/j.1471-6402.2007.00403.x

Comas-Díaz, L. (2012). *Multicultural care: A clinician's guide to cultural competence*. American Psychological Association. doi:10.1037/13491-000

Comas-Díaz, L. (2016). Mujerista psychospirituality. In T. Bryant-Davis & L. Comas-Díaz (Eds.), *Womanist and mujerista psychologies: Voices of fire, acts of courage* (pp. 149–169). American Psychological Association. doi:10.1037/14937-007

Comas-Diaz, L. (2020). Afro-Latinxs: Decolonization, healing and liberation. *Journal of Latina/o Psychology*, *9*(1), 65–75. doi:10.1037/lat0000164

Comas-Díaz, L., & Bryant-Davis, T. (2016). Conclusion: Toward global womanist and mujerista psychologies. In T. Bryant-Davis & L. Comas-Díaz (Eds.), *Womanist and Mujerista Psychologies: Voices of Fire, Acts of Courage* (pp. 277–290). American Psychological Association. doi:10.1037/14937-013

Comas-Díaz, L., Hall, G. N., & Neville, H. A. (2019). Racial trauma: Theory, research, and healing: Introduction to the special issue. *The American Psychologist*, *74*(1), 1–5. doi:10.1037/amp0000442 PMID:30652895

Combahee River Collective. (1995). Combahee River Collective statement. In B. Guy-Sheftall (Ed.), *Words of fire: An anthology of African American feminist thought* (pp. 232–240). New Press.

Connell, R. W., & Messerschmidt, J. W. (2005). Hegemonic Masculinity: Rethinking the Concept. *Gender & Society*, *19*(6), 829–859. doi:10.1177/0891243205278639

Conrad, D. (2015). Education and social innovation: The youth uncensored project—A case study of youth participatory research and cultural democracy in action. *Canadian Journal of Education/Revue Canadienne de L'éducation*, *38*(1), 1-25.

Conrad, B. K. (2006). Neo-institutionalism, social movements, and the cultural reproduction of a mentalité: Promise keepers reconstruct the Madonna/Whore complex. *The Sociological Quarterly*, *47*(2), 305–331. doi:10.1111/j.1533-8525.2006.00047.x

Conroy, S. (2022). Narrative Matters: Encanto and intergenerational trauma. *Child and Adolescent Mental Health*, *27*(3), 309–311. Advance online publication. doi:10.1111/camh.12563 PMID:35394693

Consideration of deferred action for childhood arrivals (DACA). (2022, April 12). USCIS. Retrieved May 1, 2022, from https://www.uscis.gov/DACA

Consoli, A. J., Bunge, E., Oromendia, M. F., & Bertone, A. (2018). Argentines in the United States: Migration and Continuity. In *Latinx Immigrants* (pp. 15–32). Springer. doi:10.1007/978-3-319-95738-8_2

Cordero, A. L.Colegio de Abogados de Puerto Rico. (1979). *Cerro Maravilla: Estudio Del Informe Del Departamento De Justicia* [Cerro Maravilla: Study of the Department of Justive Report]. Colegio de Abogados de Puerto Rico.

Corntassel, J. J. (2003). An activist posing as an academic? *American Indian Quarterly*, *27*(1/2), 160–171. doi:10.1353/aiq.2004.0029

Cotter, E. W., & Jones, N. (2020). A review of Latino/Latinx participants in mindfulness-based intervention research. *Mindfulness*, *3*(3), 529–553. doi:10.100712671-019-01266-9

Courtenay, W. (2000). Constructions of masculinity and their influence on men's wellbeing: A theory of gender and health. *Social Science & Medicine*, *50*(10), 1385–1401. doi:10.1016/S0277-9536(99)00390-1 PMID:10741575

Covarrubias, R., Valle, I., Laiduc, G., & Azmitia, M. (2019). "You never become fully independent": Family roles and independence in first-generation college students. *Journal of Adolescent Research*, *34*(4), 381–410. doi:10.1177/0743558418788402

COVID-19 Farmworker Study (COFS). (2020). *Preliminary Data Brief*. https://cirsinc.org/wp-content/uploads/2021/08/EN-COFS-Preliminary-Data-Brief_FINAL.pdf

Crenshaw, K. (1991). Mapping the margins: Intersectionality, identity politics and violence against women of color. *Stanford Law Review*, *43*(6), 1241–1299. doi:10.2307/1229039

Crisóstomo Tejada, V. (2021). La Colectiva Feminista en Construcción: Puerto Rico's antiracist & feminist movement [The Feminist Collective under Construction: Puerto Rico's antiracist & feminist movement]. *Review of Education, Pedagogy & Cultural Studies*, *43*(5), 398–418. doi:10.1080/10714413.2021.1970466

Cross, W. E., Jr., Parham, T. A., & Helms, J. E. (1991). The stages of Black identity development: Nigrescence models. Black Psychology, 3, 319–338.

Cross, W. E. (1971). Toward a psychology of black liberation: The negro-to-black conversion experience. *Black World*, *20*, 13–27.

Cross, W. E. (2016). *Disjunctive: Social Injustice, black identity, and the normality of black people. In The Oxford Handbook of Social Psychology and Social Justice*. Oxford University Press.

Cross, W. E. Jr, & Vandiver, B. J. (2001). Nigrescence theory and measurement: Introducing the Cross Racial Identity Scale (CRIS). In J. G. Ponterotto, J. M. Casas, L. A. Suzuki, & C. M. Alexander (Eds.), *Handbook of multicultural counseling* (pp. 371–393). Sage Publishers.

Cuellar, M. G. (2019). Creating Hispanic-Serving Institutions (HSIs) and emerging HSIs: Latina/o college choice at 4-year institutions. *American Journal of Education*, *125*(2), 231–258. doi:10.1086/701250

Cunningham, P. J., Hibbard, J., & Gibbons, C. B. (2011). Raising low 'patient activation'rates among Hispanic immigrants may equal expanded coverage in reducing access disparities. *Health Affairs*, *30*(10), 1888–1894. doi:10.1377/hlthaff.2009.0805 PMID:21976331

D'Augelli, A. R. (1994). Identity development and sexual orientation: Toward a model of lesbian, gay, and bisexual development. *Human Diversity: Perspectives on People in Context.*, *486*, 312–333.

Daby, M., & Moseley, M. W. (2021). Feminist Mobilization and the Abortion Debate in Latin America: Lessons from Argentina. *Politics & Gender*, 1–35. doi:10.1017/S1743923X20000197

Danieli, Y. (2007). Assessing trauma across cultures from a multigenerational perspective. In J. P. Wilson & C. S.-K. Tang (Eds.), *Cross-cultural assessment of psychological trauma and PTSD* (pp. 65–89). Springer. doi:10.1007/978-0-387-70990-1_4

Dass-Brailsford, P. (2007). A practical approach to trauma: Empowering interventions. *Sage (Atlanta, Ga.)*.

DataUSA. (2017). *DataUSA: Counselors*. https://datausa.io/profile/soc/211010/#demographics

Davidson, B. (2014). *West Africa before the colonial era: A history to 1850*. Routledge. doi:10.4324/9781315840369

Davis, J. M., & Liang, C. T. H. (2015). A test of the mediating role of gender role conflict: Latino masculinities and help-seeking attitudes. *Psychology of Men & Masculinity*, *16*(1), 23–32. doi:10.1037/a0035320

Dawes, D. (2020). *The political determinants of health*. Johns Hopkins University Press.

De Los Santos Upton, S. (2019). Nepantla activism and coalition building: Locating identity and resistance in the cracks between worlds. *Women's Studies in Communication*, *42*(2), 135–139. doi:10.1080/07491409.2019.1605232

De Los Santos, J. (2020). *Under one roof: The experiences of undocumented Latinx patients and providers navigating integrated care* [Unpublished doctoral dissertation]. University of Georgia.

de Onís, K. (2015). Lost in Translation: Challenging (White, Monolingual Feminism's) <Choice> with Justicia Reproductiva. *Women's Studies in Communication*, *38*(1), 1–19. doi:10.1080/07491409.2014.989462

de Sant'Anna Machado, T., & Perry, K. K. Y. (2021). Translation of "The Black Woman: A Portrait". *Feminist Anthropology*, *2*(1), 38–49. doi:10.1002/fea2.12031

Deaderick, L. (2022). A White reggaeton artist was named 'Afro-Latino artist of the year' and that's a problem. *The San Diego Union-Tribune*. https://www.sandiegouniontribune.com/columnists/story/2022-01-09/a-white-reggaeton-

DeAngelis, T. (2008). The two faces of oxytocin. *APA Monitor*, *39*(2), 30. https://www.apa.org/monitor/feb08/oxytocin

Del Rincon, F. (2016, August 29). ¿Juan Gabriel es gay? "Lo que se ve, no se pregunta", dijo [Is Juan Gabriel Gay? "What is seen, is not asked," he said] [Video]. CNN. https://cnnespanol.cnn.com/video/cnnee-conclusiones-entrevista-juan-gabriel-fernando-del-rincon-2002-p3/

del Valle, L. E., & Alvelo, J. (1996). Perception of post traumatic stress disorder symptoms by children of Puerto Rican Vietnam veterans. *Puerto Rico Health Sciences Journal*, *15*(2), 101–106. doi:10.4135/9781452204123

Delgado-Romero, E. A., Lau, M. Y., & Shullman, S. L. (2012). The Society of Counseling Psychology: Historical values, themes, and patterns viewed from the American Psychological Association presidential podium. In N. A. Fouad (Ed.), APA handbook of counseling psychology (Vol. 1, pp. 3–29). American Psychological Association.

Delgado-Romero, E. A., De Los Santos, J., Raman, V., Merrifield, J., Vazquez, M., Monroig, M., Cárdenas-Bautista, E., & Durán, M. (2018). Caught in the Middle: Bilingual Mental Health Counselors as Language Brokers. *Journal of Mental Health Counseling*, *40*(4), 341–352. doi:10.17744/mehc.40.4.06

Delgado-Romero, E. A., Espino, M., Werther, E., & Gonzalez, M. J. (2012). Building infrastructure through training of bilingual mental health providers. In L. P. Buki & L. M. Piedra (Eds.), *Building Infrastructures for Latino Mental Health*. Springer.

Delgado-Romero, E. A., Espino, M., Werther, E., & Gonzalez, M. J. (2012). Building infrastructure through training of bilingual mental health providers. In L. P. Buki & L. M. Piedra (Eds.), *Haciendo camino al andar: Creating infrastructures for Latino mental health* (pp. 99–116). Springer.

Delgado-Romero, E. A., & Hernandez, C. A. (2002). Empowering Hispanic students through student organizations: Competencies for faculty advisors. *Journal of Hispanic Higher Education, 1*(2), 144–157. doi:10.1177/1538192702001002004

Delgado-Romero, E. A., Mahoney, G.-E., Muro-Rodriguez, N. J., Atilano, R., Cárdenas Bautista, E., De Los Santos, J., Durán, M. Y., Espinoza, L., Fuentes, J., Gomez, S. N., Ingram Estevez, R. E., Jimenez-Ruiz, J., Monroig Garcia, M. M., Mora-Ozuna, C. J., Ordaz, A. C., Rappaport, B., Suazo-Padilla, K., & Vazquez, M. (2021). La Clinica In LaK'ech : Establishing a practicum site integrating practice, advocacy, and research with Latinx clients. *The Counseling Psychologist, 49*(7), 987–1012. doi:10.1177/00110000211025270

Delgado-Romero, E. A., Merrifield, J., & Werther, E. (2015, Fall). Latina/o Psychologists: Who decides who we are? *Latina/o. Psychology Today, 2*, 22–25.

Delgado-Romero, E. A., & Romero-Shih, A. (2016). Patricia Arredondo: Creating a pathway for cultural empowerment. Legacies and Traditions Forum. *The Counseling Psychologist, 44*(8), 1212–1253. doi:10.1177/0011000016683943

Delgado-Romero, E. A., Singh, A. A., & De Los Santos, J. (2018). Cuéntame: The promise of qualitative research with Latinx populations. *Journal of Latina/o Psychology, 6*(4), 318–328. doi:10.1037/lat0000123

Delgado-Romero, E. A., Unkefer, E. N. S., Capielo, C., & Crowell, C. N. (2017). El que oye consejos, llega a viejo: Examining the published life narratives of U.S. Latino/a psychologists. *Journal of Latina/o Psychology, 5*(3), 127–141. doi:10.1037/lat0000071

Delgado-Romero, E. A., & Werther, E. (2012). Hispanic Psychologists. In R. DelCampo & D. M. Blancero (Eds.), *Hispanics @ Work: A Collection of Research, Theory and Application* (pp. 177–188). Nova Science Publishers.

Delgado-Romero, E. A., & Werther, E. (2012). Hispanic Psychologists. In R. DelCampo & D. M. Blancero (Eds.), *Hispanics at Work: A Collection of Research, Theory, and Application* (pp. 177–188). Nova Science Publishers.

Delucio, K., Morgan Consoli, M. L., & Israel, T. (2020). Lo que se ve no se pregunta: Exploring nonverbal gay identity disclosure among Mexican American gay men. *Journal of Latina/o Psychology, 8*(1), 21–40. doi:10.1037/lat0000139

Delucio, K., Villicana, A. J., & Biernat, M. (2022). Verbal disclosure and mental health among gay Latino and gay white men. *The Counseling Psychologist, 50*(2), 241–274. doi:10.1177/00110000211051325

Dillon, F. R., De La Rosa, M., & Ibañez, G. E. (2013). Acculturative stress and diminishing family cohesion among recent Latino immigrants. *Journal of Immigrant and Minority Health, 15*(3), 484–491. doi:10.100710903-012-9678-3 PMID:22790880

Doak, R. S. (2008). *Dolores Huerta: Labor Leader and Civil Rights Activist*. Capstone.

Domínguez-Rebollar, R., & Acevedo-Polakovich, I. D. (2021). Factors and interventions that foster success of Latinx students in public community colleges: A theory-driven systematic review and content analysis of psychological research. *Journal of Hispanic Higher Education*.

Donner, P. (2021, August). *Fatalismo beliefs as a oderator of the relationship between financial stress, depression, anxiety, and life satisfaction among Latinx college students*. Texas Tech University Libraries. https://ttu-ir.tdl.org/handle/2346/87843

Dorner, L. M., Orellana, M. F., & Jiménez, R. (2008). "It's one of those things that you do to help the family" language brokering and the development of immigrant adolescents. *Journal of Adolescent Research, 23*(5), 515–543. doi:10.1177/0743558408317563

Douglas, K. B. (1993). Womanist theology: What is its relationship to Black theology? *Black Theology*, 290–299.

Dreby, J. (2006). Honor and virtue: Mexican parenting in the transnational context. *Gender & Society*, *20*(1), 32–59. doi:10.1177/0891243205282660

Dueñas, M., & Gloria, A. M. (2017). ¿Pertenezco a esa universidad?: The mediating role of belonging for collective self-esteem and mattering for Latin@ undergraduates. *Journal of College Student Development*, *58*(6), 891–906. doi:10.1353/csd.2017.0070

Duran, M.Y. (2022). *"Las luchonas" that feed you: Campesinas in the central valley of California*. Academic Press.

Duran, D. (1967). *Historia de las Indias de la Nueva España e Islas de la Tierra Firme* [History of the Indies of New Spain and the Islands of Tierra Firme]. Porrua.

Duran, E., Firehammer, J., & Gonzalez, J. (2008). Liberation psychology as the path toward healing cultural soul wounds. *Journal of Counseling and Development*, *86*(3), 288–295. doi:10.1002/j.1556-6678.2008.tb00511.x

Dwyer, S. C., & Buckle, J. L. (2009). The space between: On being an insider-outsider in qualitative research. *International Journal of Qualitative Methods*, *8*(1), 54–63. doi:10.1177/160940690900800105

Eagly, A. H., Eaton, A., Rose, S. M., Riger, S., & McHugh, M. C. (2012). Feminism and psychology: Analysis of a half-century of research on women and gender. *The American Psychologist*, *67*(3), 211–230. doi:10.1037/a0027260 PMID:22369245

Eagly, I. (2010). Prosecuting immigration. *Northwestern University Law Review*, *104*(4).

Eaton, A. A., & Rios, D. (2017). Social challenges faced by queer Latino college men: Navigating negative responses to coming out in a double minority sample of emerging adults. *Cultural Diversity & Ethnic Minority Psychology*, *23*(4), 457–467. doi:10.1037/cdp0000134 PMID:28252982

Edward, J., & Hines-Martin, V. (2016). Examining perceived barriers to healthcare access for Hispanics in a southern urban community. *Journal of Hospital Administration*, *5*(2), 101–108. doi:10.5430/jha.v5n2p102

Engle, J. (2007). Postsecondary access and success for first-generation college students. *American Academic*, *3*(1), 25-48.

Escovar, E. L., Craske, M., Roy-Byrne, P., Stein, M. B., Sullivan, G., Sherbourne, C. D., Bystritsky, A., & Chavira, D. A. (2018). Cultural influences on mental health symptoms in a primary care sample of Latinx patients. *Journal of Anxiety Disorders*, *55*, 39–47. doi:10.1016/j.janxdis.2018.03.005 PMID:29576380

Estevez, R. (2022). *"Talk about resilient: We just don't give up": The risk and resilience experiences of Latinx trans and nonbinary individuals* [Dissertation, University of Georgia]. ProQuest Dissertations and Theses Global.

Evans, J., Blye, F., Oliffe, J., & Gregory, D. (2011). Health, illness, men and masculinities (HIMM): A theoretical framework for understanding men and their health. *The Journal of Men's Health*, *8*(1), 7–15. doi:10.1016/j.jomh.2010.09.227

Ewing, J., & Tobler, L. (2014, November 12). *Quashing the Silos and Getting to Integrated Health Care*. NCSL. https://www.ncsl.org/blog/2014/11/12/quashing-the-silos-and-getting-to-integrated-health-care.aspx

Falicov, C. J. (2019). Transnational journeys. In M. McGoldrick & K. Hardy (Eds.), *Revisioning culture, race and class in family therapy* (3rd ed., pp. 108–122). Guilford Press.

Fanon, F. (1967). *Black skins, White masks*. Grove.

Farreras, I. G. (2014). Clara Harrison Town and the origins of the first institutional commitment law for the "feebleminded": Psychologists as expert diagnosticians. *History of Psychology*, *17*(4), 271–281. doi:10.1037/a0036123 PMID:24885000

Fernández, J. (2019). *The young lords: A radical history*. UNC Press Books.

Fisher, P., & Goodley, D. (2007). The linear medical model of disability: Mothers of disabled babies resist with counter-narratives. *Sociology of Health & Illness*, *29*(1), 66–81. doi:10.1111/j.1467-9566.2007.00518.x PMID:17286706

Fitzsimons, S., & Fuller, R. (2002). Empowerment and its implications for clinical practice in mental health: A review. *Journal of Mental Health (Abingdon, England)*, *11*(5), 481–499. doi:10.1080/09638230020023

Flanagin, A., Frey, T., Christiansen, S. L., & Bauchner, H. (2021). The reporting of race and ethnicity in medical and science journals: Comments invited. *Journal of the American Medical Association*, *325*(11), 1049–1052.

Flores, J. (2009). *The diaspora strikes back: Caribeno tales of learning and turning*. Routledge.

Flores, J., & Jimenez Roman, M. (2009). Triple-consciousness? Approaches to Afro-Latino culture in the United States. *Latin American and Caribbean Ethnic Studies*, *4*(3), 319–328.

Flores, T. (2021). "Latinidad is canceled": Confronting an anti-Black construct. *Latin American and Latinx Visual Culture*, *3*(3), 58–79.

Forehand, E. S. (2012). *Multiple identities: The intersection of womanism and ethnicity in a diverse sample of women* [Unpublished doctoral dissertation]. The University of Georgia, Athens, GA.

Fortuna, L., Álvarez, K., Ramos Ortiz, Z., Wang, Y., Mozo Alegría, X., Cook, B., & Alegría, M. (2016). Mental health, migration stressors and suicidal ideation among Latino immigrants in Spain and the United States. *European Psychiatry*, *36*, 15–22. doi:10.1016/j.eurpsy.2016.03.001 PMID:27311103

Franco, M. (2019). *What Racial Discrimination Will Look Like in 2060*. https://blogs.scientificamerican.com/voices/what-racial-discrimination-will-look-like-in-2060/

Franklin, A. J. (1999). Invisibility syndrome, and racial identity development in psychotherapy, and counseling African American men. *The Counseling Psychologist*, *27*(6), 761–793.

Franklin, A. J., & Boyd-Franklin, N. (2000). Invisibility syndrome: A clinical model of the effects of racism on African-American males. *Journal of Orthopsychiatry*, *70*(1), 33–41.

Frankl, V. E. (1962). *Man's search for meaning: an introduction to logotherapy*. Beacon Press.

Franko, D. L., Jenkins, A., Roehrig, J. P., Luce, K. H., Crowther, J. H., & Rodgers, R. F. (2012). Psychometric properties of measures of eating disorder risk in Latina college women. *International Journal of Eating Disorders*, *45*(4), 592–596. doi:10.1002/eat.20979 PMID:22271562

Freire, P. (2000). *Pedagogy of the oppressed* (30th ed.). Continuum.

Freire, P. (2005). *Education for critical consciousness*. Continuum Publishing.

French, B. H., Lewis, J. A., Mosley, D. V., Adames, H. Y., Chavez-Duenas, N. Y., Chen, G. A., & Neville, H. A. (2020). Toward a psychological framework of radical healing in communities of color. *The Counseling Psychologist*, *48*(1), 14–46.

Friedman, B. D., & Allen, K. N. (2011). Systems theory. *Theory & Practice in Clinical Social Work*, *2*(3), 3-20.

Fuentes, M.A., Zelaya, D.G., Delgado-Romero, E.A. & Butt, M. (in press). Open science: Friend, foe or both to an antiracist psychology? *Psychological Review*. doi:10.1037/rev0000386

Fuentes, M. A., Reyes-Portillo, J. A., Tineo, P., Gonzalez, K., & Butt, M. (2021). Skin color matters in the Latinx community: A call for action in research, training, and practice. *Hispanic Journal of Behavioral Sciences*, *43*, 32–58.

Fukuyama, M. A., & Reid, A. D. (1996). The politics and poetry of multiculturalism. *Journal of Multicultural Counseling and Development*, *24*(2), 82–88. doi:10.1002/j.2161-1912.1996.tb00291.x

Fuller, B., & García Coll, C. (2010). Learning from Latinos: Contexts, families, and child development in motion. *Developmental Psychology*, *46*(3), 559–565. doi:10.1037/a0019412 PMID:20438170

Fuller, N. (1995). *Acerca de la polaridad marianismo machismo. Lo femenino y lo masculino: Estudios sociales sobre las identidades de género en América Latina*. Third World Editions & Ediciones Uniandes.

Funk, C., & Lopez, M. H. (2022). *A brief statistical portrait of U.S. Hispanics.* PEW Research Center. Retrieved from https://www.pewresearch.org/science/2022/06/14/a-brief-statistical-portrait-of-u-s-hispanics/

Gale. (n.d.). *History of Hate in America Collections.* https://www.gale.com/primary-sources/political-extremism-and-radicalism/collections/history-of-hate

Gallardo, L. H., & Batalova, J. (2021). *Venezuelan immigrants in the United States*. Migration Policy Institute. Retrieved from https://www.migrationpolicy.org/article/venezuelan-immigrants-united-states-2018

Galvan, T., & Gudino, O. (2019). Understanding Latinx youth mental health disparities by problem type: The role of caregiver culture. *Psychological Services*, *18*(1), 116–123. Advance online publication. doi:10.1037er0000365 PMID:31192675

Garcia, E. (2021). Blending the gender binary: The machismo-marianismo dyad as a coping mechanism. *Honors Project*, 23.

Garcia, M. (2016). Cesar Chavez and the united farm workers movement. *Oxford Research Encyclopedia of American History*. https://oxfordre.com/americanhistory/view/10.1093/acrefore/9780199329175.001.0001/acrefore-9780199329175-e-217

Garcia-Colon, I. (2008). *Calining equality: Puerto Rican farmworkers in western New York*. CUNY Academic Works.

Garcini, L. M., Rosenfeld, J., Kneese, G., Bondurant, R. G., & Kanzler, K. E. (2022). Dealing with distress from the COVID-19 pandemic: Mental health stressors and coping strategies in vulnerable Latinx communities. *Health & Social Care in the Community*, *30*(1), 284–294. doi:10.1111/hsc.13402 PMID:33894080

Garfield, C. F., Abbott, C., Rutsohn, J., & Penedo, F. (2018). Hispanic Young Males' Mental Health From Adolescence Through the Transition to Fatherhood. *American Journal of Men's Health*, *12*(5), 1226–1234. doi:10.1177/1557988318765890 PMID:29577835

Garvey, M., Mobley, S. D. Jr, Summerville, K. S., & Moore, G. T. (2019). Queer and Trans Students of Color: Navigating Identity Disclosure and College Contexts. *The Journal of Higher Education (Columbus)*, *90*(1), 150–178. doi:10.1080/00221546.2018.1449081

Garza, Y., & Bratton, S. (2005). School-based child centered play therapy with Hispanic children: Outcomes and cultural consideration. *International Journal of Play Therapy*, *14*(1), 51–80. doi:10.1037/h0088896

Gast, J., Peak, T., & Hunt, A. (2020). Latino health behavior: An exploratory analysis of health risk and health protective factors in a community sample. *American Journal of Lifestyle Medicine*, *14*(1), 97–106. doi:10.1177/1559827617716613 PMID:31903089

Gates, H.L. (Presenter, Writer) & Pollack, R. (Director, Producer). (2011). *Black in Latin America* [Film Series]. PBS Distribution.

Gattamorta, K., & Quidley-Rodriguez, N. (2018). Coming out experiences of Hispanic sexual minority young adults in South Florida. *Journal of Homosexuality*, *65*(6), 741–765. doi:10.1080/00918369.2017.1364111 PMID:28771094

Georgia Farmworker Health Program. (2019). *Georgia farmworker health program needs assessment. Center for Public Health Practice and Research.* Georgia Southern University.

Germán, M., Gonzales, N. A., & Dumka, L. (2009). Familism Values as a Protective Factor for Mexican-origin Adolescents Exposed to Deviant Peers. *The Journal of Early Adolescence*, *29*(1), 16–42. doi:10.1177/0272431608324475 PMID:21776180

Gilbert, S. (2003). Eating disorders in women of color. *Clinical Psychology: Science and Practice*, *10*(4), 444–455. doi:10.1093/clipsy.bpg045

Gil, R. M., & Vasquez, C. I. (1996). *The Maria paradox*. Perigee.

Gil, R. M., & Vazquez, C. I. (2014). *The Maria paradox: How Latinas can merge old world traditions with new world self-esteem*. Open Road Media.

Ginorio, A., Guttierrez, L., Cauce, A. M., & Acosta, M. (1995). The psychology of Latinas. In C. Travis (Ed.), *Feminist perspectives on the psychology of women* (pp. 89–108). American Psychological Association.

Gloria, A. M., & Robinson Kurpius, S. E. R. (1996). The validation of the Cultural Congruity Scale and the University Environment Scale with Chicano/a students. *Hispanic Journal of Behavioral Sciences*, *18*(4), 533–549. doi:10.1177/07399863960184007

Gobat, M. (2013). The Invention of Latin America: A Transnational History of Anti-Imperialism, Democracy, and Race. *The American Historical Review*, *118*(5), 1345–1375. doi:10.1093/ahr/118.5.1345

Godreau, I., & Bonilla, Y. (2021). Nonsovereign racecraft: How colonialism, debt, and disaster are transforming Puerto Rican racial subjectivities. *American Anthropologist*, *123*, 509–525. doi:10.1111/aman.13601

Goforth, A. N., Pham, A. V., Chun, H., Castro-Olivo, S. M., & Yosai, E. R. (2016). Association of acculturative stress, Islamic practices, and internalizing symptoms among Arab American adolescents. *School Psychology Quarterly*, *31*(2), 198–212. doi:10.1037pq0000135 PMID:27243243

Goldman Sachs. (2022, May 31). *Could immigration solve the US worker shortage?* Retrieved September 4, 2022, from https://www.goldmansachs.com/insights/pages/could-immigration-solve-the-us-worker-shortage.html

Gold, S. B., Green, L. A., & Peek, C. J. (2017). From our practices to yours: Key messages for the journey to integrated behavioral health. *Journal of the American Board of Family Medicine*, *30*(1), 25–34. doi:10.3122/jabfm.2017.01.160100 PMID:28062814

Gomez, R. (2020). Success is being an example: Trajectories and notions of success among Latinx faculty, staff, and students in academia. *Journal of Latinos and Education*, *19*(3), 258–276. doi:10.1080/15348431.2018.1507909

Gonzales, R. G., Suárez-Orozco, C., & Dedios-Sanguineti, M. C. (2013). No Place to Belong: Contextualizing Concepts of Mental Health Among Undocumented Immigrant Youth in the United States. *The American Behavioral Scientist*, *57*(8), 1174–1199. doi:10.1177/0002764213487349

Gonzalez, L. (1988). *Por un feminismo afro-latino-americano* [For an Afro-Latin American feminism]. Retrieved from https://edisciplinas.usp.br/pluginfile.php/271077/mod_resource/content/1/Por%20um%20feminismo%20Afro-latino-americano.pdf

Gonzalez. (2009). *Mujeres of the Young Lords*. https://www.colorlines.com/articles/mujeres-young-lords

González-Burchard, E., Borrell, L. N., Choudhry, S., Naqvi, M., Tsai, H. J., Rodriguez-Santana, J. R., Chapela, R., Rogers, S. D., Mei, R., Rodriguez-Cintron, W., Arena, J. F., Kittles, R., Perez-Stable, E. J., Ziv, E., & Risch, N. (2005). Latino populations: A unique opportunity for the study of race, genetics, and social environment in epidemiological research. *American Journal of Public Health*, *95*(12), 2161–2168. doi:10.2105/AJPH.2005.068668 PMID:16257940

Gonzalez, C., Early, J., Gordon-Dseagu, V., Mata, T., & Nieto, C. (2021). Promoting Culturally Tailored mHealth: A Scoping Review of Mobile Health Interventions in Latinx Communities. *Journal of Immigrant and Minority Health*, *23*(5), 1065–1077. doi:10.100710903-021-01209-4 PMID:33988789

Gonzalez, E. (2020). Foreword: Understanding Latina/o resilience. *International Journal of Qualitative Studies in Education: QSE*, *33*(8), 791–795. doi:10.1080/09518398.2020.1783016

Gonzalez, L. (1979). Primavera Para As Rosas Negras [Spring for Black Roses]. *Diáspora Africana. Editora Filhos da África*, *2018*, 103–8.1.

Gonzalez, L. M., Stein, G. L., Prandoni, J. I., Eades, M. P., & Magalhaes, R. (2015). *Perceptions of Undocumented Status and Possible Selves Among Latino/a Youth*. The Counseling. doi:10.1177/0011000015608951

Gonzalez, S. (2022). Jotería Pedagogy. In K. K. Strunk & A. S. Shelton (Eds.), *Encyclopedia of Queer Studies in Education* (pp. 316–319). BRILL. doi:10.1163/9789004506725

Goodman, R. D. (2013). The transgenerational trauma and resilience genogram. *Counselling Psychology Quarterly*, *26*(3-4), 386–405. doi:10.1080/09515070.2013.820172

Gordon, I., Vander Wyk, B. C., Bennett, R. H., Cordeaux, C., Lucas, M. V., Eilbott, J. A., Zagoory-Sharon, O., Leckman, J. F., Feldman, R., & Pelphrey, K. A. (2013). Oxytocin enhances brain function in children with autism. *Psychology and Cognitive Sciences: Open Journal*, *110*(52), 20953–20958. doi:10.1073/pnas.1312857110 PMID:24297883

Gould. (1996). Space, time and the human being. *International Social Science Journal*, *48*(150), 449–460. doi:10.1111/j.1468-2451.1996.tb00099.x

Graham, H. (2004). Social determinants and their unequal distribution: Clarifying policy understandings. *The Milbank Quarterly*, *82*(1), 101–124. doi:10.1111/j.0887-378X.2004.00303.x PMID:15016245

Gray, N. N., Mendelsohn, D. M., & Omoto, A. M. (2015). Community connectedness, challenges, and resilience among gay Latino immigrants. *American Journal of Community Psychology*, *55*(1-2), 202–214. doi:10.100710464-014-9697-4 PMID:25576015

Grazier, K. L., Smiley, M. L., & Bondalapati, K. S. (2016). Overcoming Barriers to Integrating Behavioral Health and Primary Care Services. *Journal of Primary Care & Community Health*, *7*(4), 242–248. doi:10.1177/2150131916656455 PMID:27380923

Greene, S. M., Tuzzio, L., & Cherkin, D. (2012). A framework for making patient-centered care front and center. *The Permanente Journal*, *16*(3), 49–53. doi:10.7812/TPP/12-025 PMID:23012599

Greenfield, P. M., & Quiroz, B. (2013). Context and culture in the socialization and development of personal achievement values: Comparing Latino immigrant families, European American families, and elementary school teachers. *Journal of Applied Developmental Psychology*, *34*(2), 108–118. doi:10.1016/j.appdev.2012.11.002

Griffith, D. M., Gilbert, K. L., Bruce, M. A., & Thorpe, R. J. Jr. (2016). Masculinity in men's health: Barrier or portal to healthcare? In J. J. Heidelbaugh (Ed.), *Men's health in primary care* (pp. 19–31). Springer. doi:10.1007/978-3-319-26091-4_2

Grimm, R. T. (2002). *Notable American philanthropists: Biographies of giving and volunteering*. Greenwood Publishing Group.

Griner, D., & Smith, T. B. (2006). Culturally adapted mental health intervention: A meta-analytic review. *Psychotherapy (Chicago, Ill.)*, *43*(4), 531–548. doi:10.1037/0033-3204.43.4.531 PMID:22122142

Grosso Richins, L., Hansen-Thomas, H., Lozada, V., South, S., & Stewart, M. A. (2021). Understanding the power of Latinx families to support the academic and personal development of their children. *Bilingual Research Journal, 44*(3), 1–20. doi:10.1080/15235882.2021.1998806

Grzywacz, J. G., Hovey, J. D., Seligman, L. D., Arcury, T. A., & Quandt, S. A. (2006). Evaluating short-form versions of the CES-D for measuring depressive symptoms among immigrants from Mexico. *Hispanic Journal of Behavioral Sciences.* doi:10.1177/0739986306290645

Guild, A., & Figueroa, I. (2018). The neighbors who feed us: Farmworkers and government policy- challenges and solutions. *Policy Review, 13,* 31.

Guthrie, R. V. (2004). *Even the rat was white: A historical view of psychology* (2nd ed.). Pearson/Allyn & Bacon.

Guthrie, R. V. (2004). *Even the Rat was White: A Historical View of Psychology.* Allyn & Bacon.

Guthrie, R. V. (2004). *Even the rat was White: A historical view of psychology.* Pearson/Allyn and Bacon.

Gutierrez, D., Gonzalez, C., & Seshadri, G. (2022). We are the unicorns: Exploring experiences of Latina graduate women utilizing an intersectional Latino/a critical theory framework. *Peace and Conflict, 28*(1), 130–139. doi:10.1037/pac0000595

Guzmán, J. R., & Medeiros, M. A. (2020). Damned if you drive, damned if you don't: Meso-level policy and im/migrant farmworker tactics under a regime of Immobility. *Human Organization, 79*(2), 130–139. https://doi.org/10.17730/1938-3525.79.2.130

Haines, A., Kuruvilla, S., & Borchert, M. (2004). *Policy and Practice Theme Papers Bridging the implementation gap between knowledge and action for health.* https://www.who.int/bulletin/volumes/82/10/724.pdf

Hall, N. (2018, April 23). *Argentina and "Los Desparecidos."* International Federation of Social Workers. https://www.ifsw.org/argentina-and-los-desaparecidos/

Hall, W. D. (2016). *Masculine ideology in adolescent male relationships: a quantitative study* [Master's Thesis]. Smith College, Northampton, MA. https://scholarworks.smith.edu/theses/1691

Hall, C. C. I. (1997). Cultural malpractice: The growing obsolescence of psychology with the changing U.S. population. *The American Psychologist, 52*(6), 642–651. doi:10.1037/0003-066X.52.6.642 PMID:9229997

Hall, G. C. N., Yip, T., & Zárate, M. A. (2016). On becoming multicultural in a monocultural research world: A conceptual approach to studying ethnocultural diversity. *The American Psychologist, 71*(1), 40–51. doi:10.1037/a0039734 PMID:26766764

Hammerback, J. C., & Jensen, R. J. (1998). *The rhetorical career of Cesar Chavez.* Texas A&M University Press.

Hamp, A., Stamm, K., Lin, L., & Christidis, P. (2016). *2015 APA survey of psychology health service providers.* American Psychological Association. https://www.apa.org/workforce/publications/15-health-service-providers/

Hansen, E., & Donohoe, M. (2003). Health issues of migrant and seasonal farmworkers. *Journal of Health Care for the Poor and Underserved, 14*(2), 153–164. doi:10.1353/hpu.2010.0790 PMID:12739296

Hardin, M. (2002). Altering masculinities: The Spanish conquest and the evolution of the Latin American machismo. *International Journal of Sexuality and Gender Studies, 7*(1), 1–22. doi:10.1023/A:1013050829597

Harris, K. M., Edlund, M. J., & Larson, S. (2005). Racial and ethnic differences in the mental health problems and use of mental health care. *Medical Care, 43*(8), 775–784. doi:10.1097/01.mlr.0000170405.66264.23 PMID:16034291

Harrison, F. V. (2004). Global apartheid, environmental degradation, and women's activism for sustainable well-being: A conceptual and theoretical overview. *Urban Anthropology and Studies of Cultural Systems and World Economic Development*, *33*(1), 1–35.

Haskie-Mendoza, S., Serrata, J. V., Escamilla, H., & Jaimes, C. (2021). Xinachtli: A Healing-Informed, Gendered, and Culturally Responsive Approach with System-Involved Latinas. *Latinas in the Criminal Justice System: Victims, Targets, and Offenders*, *18*, 315–332. doi:10.18574/nyu/9781479804634.003.0015

Healthy People 2030. Office of Disease Prevention and Health Promotion. (n.d.). *Health Equity*. U.S. Department of Health and Human Services. https://health.gov/healthypeople/priority-areas/health-equity-healthy-people-2030

HealthyPeople.gov. (2022). *Disparities*. Retrieved from http://www.healthypeople.gov/2020/about/disparitiesAbout.aspx

Hegewisch, A., & Mefferd, E. (2022, March 9). *Gender wage gaps remain wide in year two of the pandemic*. IWPR. Retrieved May 8, 2022, from https://iwpr.org/iwpr-publications/fact-sheet/gender-wage-gaps-remain-wide-in-year-two-of-the-pandemic/

Helms, J. E., & Dupree, K. C. (2021). Elimination of the GRE Could Be Counseling Psychology's Rejection of Anti-Black Racism. In C. Davis III (Chair), *Big Ideas in Counseling Psychology: Uprooting Anti-Blackness*. APA Division 17 Virtual Symposium. https://www.youtube.com/watch?v=0Y0y2j59vi8

Helms, J. E. (1990). *Black and white racial identity: Theory research, and practice*. Greenwood Press.

Helms, J. E., & Cook, D. A. (1999). *Using race and culture in counseling and psychotherapy: Theory and process*. Allyn and Bacon.

Henderson, T. (2022, August 23). *GOP Governors Bus Migrants to Blue Cities, but Many Exit in Red States*. Stateline. https://www.pewtrusts.org/en/research-and-analysis/blogs/stateline/2022/08/23/gop-governors-bus-migrants-to-blue-cities-but-many-exit-in-red-states

Hendricks, M. L., & Testa, R. J. (2012). A conceptual framework for clinical work with transgender and gender nonconforming clients: An adaptation of the Minority Stress Model. *Professional Psychology, Research and Practice*, *43*(5), 460–467. doi:10.1037/a0029597

Henrich, J. (2020). *The WEIRDest people in the world: How the West became psychologically peculiar and particularly prosperous*. Farrar, Straus and Giroux.

Hernández Castillo, R. A. (2010). The emergence of indigenous feminism in Latin America. *Journal of Women in Culture and Society*, *35*(3), 539–545. doi:10.1086/648538

Hernandez, E. D. (2016). Cultura Joteria: The Ins and Outs of Latina/o Popular Culture. In F. L. Aldama (Ed.), *The Routledge Companion to Latina/o Popular Culture* (pp. 291–300). Routledge.

Herrera, L. J. P., & Obregón, N. (2018). Challenges facing Latinx ESOL students in the Trump era: Stories told through testimonios. *Journal of Latinos and Education*, *19*(4), 383–391. doi:10.1080/15348431.2018.1523793

Herrera, N., & Gloria, A. M. (2021). Latina Students' Post-IPV Healing: A Bodymindspirit Approach Using the ELLA-SANA Model. *Women & Therapy*, 1–20. doi:10.1080/02703149.2021.1982537

Hibbard, J. H., & Cunningham, P. J. (2008). *How engaged are consumers in their health and health care, and why does it matter?* (Vol. 8). Center for Studying Health System Change.

Hibbard, J. H., Greene, J., & Overton, V. (2013). Patients with lower activation associated with higher costs; delivery systems should know their patients' 'scores'. *Health Affairs*, *32*(2), 216–222. doi:10.1377/hlthaff.2012.1064 PMID:23381513

Hibbard, J. H., Mahoney, E. R., Stock, R., & Tusler, M. (2007). Do increases in patient activation result in improved self-management behaviors? *Health Services Research*, *42*(4), 1443–1463. doi:10.1111/j.1475-6773.2006.00669.x PMID:17610432

Higgins Neyland, M. K., & Bardone-Cone, A. M. (2017). Tests of escape theory of binge eating among Latinas. *Cultural Diversity & Ethnic Minority Psychology*, *23*(3), 373–381. doi:10.1037/cdp0000130 PMID:27831694

Hill, C. M., Williams, E. C., & Ornelas, I. J. (2019). Help Wanted: Mental Health and Social Stressors Among Latino Day Laborers. *American Journal of Men's Health*, *13*(2). Advance online publication. doi:10.1177/1557988319838424 PMID:30880547

Hofferth, S. L., & Moon, U. J. (2016). How do they do it? The immigrant paradox in the transition to adulthood. *Social Science Research*, *57*, 177–194. doi:10.1016/j.ssresearch.2015.12.013 PMID:26973039

Hoffman, K. M., Trawalter, S., Axt, J. R., & Oliver, M. N. (2016). Racial bias in pain assessment and treatment recommendations, and false beliefs about biological differences between blacks and whites. *Proceedings of the National Academy of Sciences*, *113*(16), 4296-4301.

Holloway-Friesen, H. (2021). The role of mentoring on Hispanic graduate students' sense of belonging and academic self-efficacy. *Journal of Hispanic Higher Education*, *20*(1), 46–58. doi:10.1177/1538192718823716

Hoogasian, R. O., & Gloria, A. M. (2015). The healing powers of a patron espiritual: Latina/o clinicians' understanding and use of spirituality and ceremony in psychotherapy. *Journal of Latina/o Psychology*, *3*(3), 177–192. doi:10.1037/lat0000045

Hook, J. N., Captari, L. E., Hoyt, W., Davis, D. E., McElroy, S. E., & Worthington, E. L. Jr. (2019). Religion and spirituality. In J. C. Norcross & B. E. Wampold (Eds.), *Psychotherapy relationships that work: Evidence-based therapist responsiveness* (pp. 212–263). Oxford University Press. doi:10.1093/med-psych/9780190843960.003.0008

Hooks, B. (1984). *Black women shaping feminist theory*. ProQuest Information and Learning.

Hordge-Freeman, E. & Loblack, A. (2021). "Cops only see the brown skin, they could care less where it originated": Afro-Latinx perceptions of the #BlackLivesMatter movement. *Sociological Perspectives*, *64*(4), 518-535. doi: 107.171/077/30173112124124020996611135

Horner, K. (2021, November 16). *Immigration Status: A Political Determinant of Health*. Gender Policy Report.

Horrell, S. C. V. (2008). Effectiveness of cognitive-behavioral therapy with adult ethnic minority clients: A review. *Professional Psychology, Research and Practice*, *39*(2), 160–168. doi:10.1037/0735-7028.39.2.160

Howard, G. S. (1986). *Dare we develop a human science?* Academic Publications.

Howard, G. S. (1991). Culture tales. A narrative approach to thinking, cross-cultural psychology, and psychotherapy. *The American Psychologist*, *46*(3), 187–197. doi:10.1037/0003-066X.46.3.187 PMID:2035929

Hoyle, A. (2019). *Treatment for anorexia nervosa with latinx clients: a qualitative inquiry* [Unpublished doctoral dissertation]. University of Georgia.

Huang, Y. T., & Chan, R. C. (2022). Effects of sexual orientation concealment on well-being among sexual minorities: How and when does concealment hurt? *Journal of Counseling Psychology*, *69*(5), 630–641. Advance online publication. doi:10.1037/cou0000623 PMID:35696152

Huq, N., Stein, G. L., & Gonzalez, L. M. (2016). Acculturation Conflict Among Latino Youth: Discrimination, Ethnic Identity, and Depressive Symptoms. *Cultural Diversity & Ethnic Minority Psychology*, *22*(3), 377–385. doi:10.1037/cdp0000070 PMID:26460666

Hurley, K. D., Huscroft-D'Angelo, J., Trout, A., Griffith, A., & Epstein, M. (2014). Assessing parenting skills and attitudes: A review of the psychometrics of parenting measures. *Journal of Child and Family Studies*, *23*(5), 812–823. doi:10.100710826-013-9733-2

Hursh, D., & Martina, C. A. (2003). Neoliberalism and Schooling in the US: How state and federal government education policies perpetuate inequality. *The Journal for Critical Education Policy Studies*, *1*(2). http://www.jceps.com

Hurtado, A. (1997). Understanding multiple group identities: Inserting women into cultural transformations. *The Journal of Social Issues*, *53*(2), 299–328. doi:10.1111/j.1540-4560.1997.tb02445.x

Hurtado, A., & Sinha, M. (2008). More than men: Latino feminist masculinities and intersectionality. *Sex Roles*, *59*(5), 337–349. doi:10.100711199-008-9405-7

Hwahng, S. J., Allen, B., Zadoretzky, C., Barber, H., McKnight, C., & Des Jarlais, D. (2018). Alternative kinship structures, resilience and social support among immigrant trans Latinas in the USA. *Culture, Health & Sexuality*, *21*(1), 1–15. doi:10.1080/13691058.2018.1440323 PMID:29658825

Imperialism in Latin America. (n.d.). Retrieved May 11, 2022, from https://web-clear.unt.edu/course_projects/HIST2610/content/06_Unit_Six/19_lesson_nineteen/06_imp_lat_am.htm

IndígenaH. (2020). https://www.herenciaindigena.com/

Institute of Medicine (US) Committee on Quality of Health Care in America. (2001). *Crossing the quality chasm: a new health system for the 21st century*. National Academies Press.

Instituto Nacional de Estadística Guatemala. (2022). *Censo de Población* [Publication Census]. Retrieved from https://www.ine.gob.gt/ine/

Instituto Nacional de Estadísticas y Censos (INEC). (2015). *Estadística de Etnicidad en Censos, Encuestas de Hogares, y Registros Administrativos* [Ethnicity Statistics in Censuses, Household Surveys and Administrative Records]. Retrieved from https://www.inei.gob.pe/media/dme/17.MarleneHaro.pdf

Isasi-Díaz, A. M. (2002). Lo cotidiano: A key element of mujerista theology. *Journal of Hispanic/Latino Theology*, *10*(1), 5–17.

Ishikawa, R. Z., Cardemil, E. V., & Falmagne, R. J. (2010). Help seeking and help receiving for emotional distress among Latino men and women. *Qualitative Health Research*, *20*(11), 1558–1572. doi:10.1177/1049732310369140 PMID:20448272

Jahangard, L., Shayganfard, M., Ghiasi, F., Salehi, I., Haghighi, M., Ahmadpanah, M., Sadeghi Bahmani, D., & Brand, S. (2020). Serum oxytocin concentrations in current and recent suicide survivors are lower than in healthy controls. *Journal of Psychiatric Research*, *128*, 75–82. doi:10.1016/j.jpsychires.2020.05.014 PMID:32535343

James, S. E., & Salcedo, B. (2017). 2015 U.S. Transgender Survey: Report on the Experiences of Latino/a Respondents. National Center for Transgender Equality and TransLatin@ Coalition.

Jamil, O. B., Harper, G. W., & Fernandez, M. I. (2009). Sexual and ethnic identity development among gay–bisexual–questioning (GBQ) male ethnic minority adolescents. *Cultural Diversity & Ethnic Minority Psychology*, *15*(3), 203–214. doi:10.1037/a0014795 PMID:19594249

Jarrett, N. C., Bellamy, C. D., & Adeyemi, S. A. (2007). Men's Health Help-Seeking and Implications for Practice. *American Journal of Health Studies*, *22*(2), 88–95.

Jayawardene, S. M., & McDougal, S. III. (2017). Francis Cress Welsing's contributions to Africana studies epistemology. *Journal of Black Studies*, *48*(1), 43–56.

Jimenez Roman, M., & Flores, J. (2010). *The Afro-Latin@ reader: History and culture in the United States*. Duke University Press.

Jongen, C., McCalman, J., & Bainbridge, R. (2018). Health workforce cultural competency interventions: A systematic scoping review. *BMC Health Services Research*, *18*(1), 1–15. doi:10.118612913-018-3001-5 PMID:29609614

Jordan, M. (2020). *Farmworkers, mostly undocumented, become 'essential' during pandemic*. https://www.nytimes.com/2020/04/02/us/coronavirus-undocumented-immigrant-farmworkers-agriculture.html

Jordan, K. (2004). The Color-Coded Timeline Trauma Genogram. *Brief Treatment and Crisis Intervention*, *4*(1), 57–70. Advance online publication. doi:10.1093/brief-treatment/mhh005

Jorgenson, J. (2022, August 17). *City working to enroll children of asylum seekers in public schools*. Spectrum News. https://www.ny1.com/nyc/all-boroughs/education/2022/08/17/city-working-to-enroll-children-of-asylum-seekers-in-public-schools

Justice, F. (2013). *Exposed and ignored: How pesticides are endangering our nation's farmworkers*. https://kresge.org/sites/default/files/Exposed-and-ignored-Farmworker-Justice-KF.pdf

Kassem, N., Rum, Y., & Perry, A. (2022). To feel and talk in a language of conflict: Distinct emotional experience and expression of bilinguals among disadvantaged minority members. *Journal of Multilingual and Multicultural Development*.

Keating, A., & Anzaldúa, G. (1993). Writing, Politics, and las Lesberadas: Platicando con Gloria Anzaldúa. *Frontiers*, *14*(1), 105–130. doi:10.2307/3346563

Kennedy, A., & Moorhead, A. (2022). Help-seeking and masculinity in opposition: A quantitative study investigating the potential of coaching to increase men's engagement in help-seeking. *The Coaching Psychologist*, *17*(2).

Keyes, K. M., Martins, S. S., Hatzenbuehler, M. L., Blanco, C., Bates, L. M., & Hasin, D. S. (2012). Mental health service utilization for psychiatric disorders among Latinos living in the United States: The role of ethnic subgroup, ethnic identity, and language/social preferences. *Social Psychiatry and Psychiatric Epidemiology*, *47*(3), 383–394. doi:10.100700127-010-0323-y PMID:21290097

Kickbusch, I. (2015). The political determinants of health--10 years on. *BMJ*, *350*(2), h81–h81. doi:10.1136/bmj.h81

Kittelsen, S. K., Fukuda-Parr, S., & Storeng, K. T. (2019). Editorial: The political determinants of health inequities and universal health coverage. *Globalization and Health*, *15*(S1). doi:10.1186/s12992-019-0514-6

Koech, J. M., Sostre, J. P., Lockett, G. M., Gonzalez, K. A., & Abreu, R. L. (2022). Resisting by Existing: Trans Latinx Mental Health, Well-Being, and Resilience in the United States. In *Latinx Queer Psychology* (pp. 43–67). Springer. doi:10.1007/978-3-030-82250-7_4

Kolker, A. F. (2020). *Unauthorized immigrants' eligibility for COVID-19 relief benefits: In brief*. https://www.everycrsreport.com/files/20200507_R46339_881c6255f6f0c398207472c97e2846375e3a7505.pdf

Kuper, L. E., Wright, L., & Mustanski, B. (2018). Gender identity development among transgender and gender nonconforming emerging adults: An intersectional approach. *International Journal of Transgenderism*, *19*(4), 436–455. doi:10.1080/15532739.2018.1443869

Lanesskog, D., & Piedra, L. (2016). *Integrated Health Care for Latino Immigrants and Refugees: What Do They Need?* doi:10.1007/978-3-319-42533-7_2

Latinas/xs Summary. Intersections of Our Lives. (2021). Retrieved August 1, 2022, from https://intersectionsofourlives.org/wp-content/uploads/2021/07/ISOOL_Fact-Sheet-SummarLat a-final.pdf

Lawton, K. E., & Gerdes, A. C. (2014). Acculturation and Latino adolescent mental health: Integration of individual, environmental, and family influences. *Clinical Child and Family Psychology Review, 17*(4), 385–398. doi:10.100710567-014-0168-0 PMID:24794635

Lee, C. C. (2019). *Multicultural issues in counseling : new approaches to diversity* (5th ed.). American Counseling Association.

Lenz, A. S., Gómez Soler, I., Dell'Aquila, J., & Uribe, P. M. (2017). Translation and cross-cultural adaptation of assessments for use in counseling research. *Measurement & Evaluation in Counseling & Development, 50*(4), 224–231. doi:10.1080/07481756.2017.1320947

Levant, R. F., Hall, R. J., Weigold, I. K., & McCurdy, E. R. (2016). Construct validity evidence for the Male Role Norms Inventory-Short Form: A structural equation modeling approach using the bifactor model. *Journal of Counseling Psychology, 63*(5), 534–542. doi:10.1037/cou0000171 PMID:27598043

Levant, R. F., & Richmond, K. (2007). A review of research on masculinity ideologies using the Male Role Norms Inventory. *Journal of Men's Studies, 15*(2), 130–146. doi:10.3149/jms.1502.130

Levant, R. F., Wimer, D. J., & Williams, C. M. (2011). An evaluation of the psychometric properties of the Health Behavior Inventory-20 (HBI- 20) and its relationships to masculinity and attitudes towards seeking psychological help among college men. *Psychology of Men & Masculinity, 12*, 26–41. doi:10.1037/a0021014

Lewis, A. (2020). *Krewe Du Kanaval honors the Haitian roots of New Orleans.* NPR. https://www.npr.org/sections/world-cafe/2020/02/12/804873908/krewe-du-kanaval-honors-the-haitian-roots-of-new-orleans

Lewis, P., & Simpson, R. (2010). *Introduction: Theoretical insights into the practices of revealing and concealing gender within organizations.* Academic Press.

Liang, C. T. H., Salcedo, J., & Miller, H. A. (2011). Perceived racism, masculinity ideologies, and gender role conflict among Latino men. *Psychology of Men & Masculinity, 12*(3), 201–215. doi:10.1037/a0020479

Lifton, R. J. (2000). *The Nazi doctors: Medical killing and the psychology of genocide.* Basic Books.

Lindinger-Sternart, S. (2015). Help-seeking behaviors of men for mental health and the impact of diverse cultural backgrounds. *International Journal of Social Science Studies, 3*(1), 1–6. doi:10.11114/ijsss.v3i1.519

Lin, L., Stamm, K., & Christidis, P. (2018). How diverse is the psychology workforce? *Monitor on Psychology, 49*(2). https://www.apa.org/monitor/2018/02/datapoint

Liou, D. D., Martinez, J. A. L., & Rotheram-Fuller, E. (2021). Latinas at a Hispanic-serving institution: Resilient resistance affirming race–gender expectancies for college attainment. *Journal of Diversity in Higher Education.* Advance online publication. doi:10.1037/dhe0000340

Liu, W. M. (2005). The study of men and masculinity as an important multicultural competency consideration. *Journal of Clinical Psychology, 61*(6), 685–697. doi:10.1002/jclp.20103 PMID:15732087

Lollar, K. (2015). Strategic Invisibility: Resisting the Inhospitable Dwelling Place. *The Review of Communication, 15*(4), 298–315. https://doi.org/10.1080/15358593.2015.1116592

Lomash, E. F., Brown, T. D., & Galupo, M. P. (2018). "A whole bunch of love the sinner hate the sin": LGBTQ microaggressions experienced in religious and spiritual context. *Journal of Homosexuality*, *66*(10), 1495–1511. doi:10.1080/00918369.2018.1542204 PMID:30475163

Lombana, Y. (2021). Possibilities and challenges in providing psychotherapeutic interventions to meet the needs of the Latinx population in the United States. *Genealogy*, *5*(1), 12. doi:10.3390/genealogy5010012

Lopez, M. H., & Moslimani, M. (2022). *Latinos See US as Better Than Place of Family's Ancestry for Opportunity, Raising Kids, Health Care Access*. Pew Research Center. Retrieved from https://www.pewresearch.org/race-ethnicity/2022/01/20/latinos-see-u-s-as-better-than-place-of-familys-ancestry-for-opportunity-raising-kids-health-care-access/

Lopez, M. H., Gonzalez-Barrera, A., & López, G. (2017). *Hispanic identity fades across generations as immigrant connections fall away*. Pew Research Center. Retrieved from https://www.pewresearch.org/hispanic/2017/12/20/hispanic-identity-fades-across-generations-as-immigrant-connections-fall-away/

Lopez, M. H., Krogstad, J. M., & Passel, J. S. (2021). *Who is Hispanic?* Pew Research Center. Retrieved from https://www.pewresearch.org/fact-tank/2021/09/23/who-is-hispanic/

López, B. G., Lezama, E., & Heredia, D. Jr. (2019). Language brokering experience affects feelings toward bilingualism, language knowledge, use, and practices: A qualitative approach. *Hispanic Journal of Behavioral Sciences*, *41*(4), 481–503. doi:10.1177/0739986319879641

López, R. M., Valdez, E. C., Pacheco, H. S., Honey, M. L., & Jones, R. (2020). Bridging silos in higher education: Using Chicana feminist participatory action research to foster Latina resilience. *International Journal of Qualitative Studies in Education: QSE*, *33*(8), 872–886. doi:10.1080/09518398.2020.1735566

Lorde, A. (1988). *A burst of light*. Firebrand Books.

Lozada, C. (2022, July 2). Perspective | how three major abortion rulings reveal a fractured culture. *The Washington Post*. Retrieved September 3, 2022, from https://www.washingtonpost.com/outlook/2022/07/01/roe-casey-dobbs-abortion-supreme-court/

Lozano, A., Salinar, C. Jr, & Orozco, R. C. (2021). Constructing meaning of the termLatinx: A trioethnography through Pláticas. *International Journal of Qualitative Studies in Education: QSE*, 1–18. Advance online publication. doi:10.1080/09518398.2021.1930251

Loza, O., Beltran, O., & Mangadu, T. (2017). A qualitative exploratory study on gender identity and the health risks and barriers to care for transgender women living in a US–Mexico border city. *International Journal of Transgenderism*, *18*(1), 104–118. doi:10.1080/15532739.2016.1255868

Luedke, C. L. (2019). "Es como una familia": Bridging emotional support with academic and professional development through the acquisition of capital in Latinx student organizations. *Journal of Hispanic Higher Education*, *18*(4), 372–388. doi:10.1177/1538192717751205

Lugones, M. (2008). The coloniality of gender. *Worlds & Knowledge Otherwise*, 1–17.

Lu, Y., He, Q., & Brooks-Gunn, J. (2020). Diverse experience of immigrant children: How do separation and reunification shape their development? *Child Development*, *91*(1), e146–e163. doi:10.1111/cdev.13171

Machado-Casas, M. (2012). Pedagogías del camaleón/Pedagogies of the chameleon: Identity and strategies of survival for transnational indigenous Latino immigrants in the US South. *The Urban Review*, *44*(5), 534–550. doi:10.100711256-012-0206-5

Mahalik, J. R., Locke, B. D., Ludlow, L. H., Deimer, M. A., Scott, R. P. J., Gottfried, M., & Freitas, G. (2003). Development of the Conformity to Masculine Norms Inventory. *Psychology of Men & Masculinity*, *4*(1), 3–25. doi:10.1037/1524-9220.4.1.3

Maiorana, J. (2021). *Yolanda Guzmán (1943-1965)*. https://www.blackpast.org/global-african-history/people-global-african-history/yolanda-guzman-1943-1965/

Maldonado, A., Preciado, A., Buchanan, M., Pulvers, K., Romero, D., & D'Anna-Hernandez, K. (2018). Acculturative stress, mental health symptoms, and the role of salivary inflammatory markers among a Latino sample. *Cultural Diversity & Ethnic Minority Psychology*, *24*(2), 277–283. doi:10.1037/cdp0000177 PMID:29154561

Marks, A. K., Ejesi, K., & García Coll, C. (2014). Understanding the US immigrant paradox in childhood and adolescence. *Child Development Perspectives*, *8*(2), 59–64. doi:10.1111/cdep.12071

Marques, L., Eustis, E. H., Dixon, L., Valentine, S. E., Borba, C. P. C., Simon, N., Kaysen, D., & Wiltsey-Stirman, S. (2016). Delivering cognitive processing therapy in a community health setting: The influence of Latino culture and community violence on posttraumatic cognitions. *Psychological Trauma: Theory, Research, Practice, and Policy*, *8*(1), 98–106. doi:10.1037/tra0000044 PMID:25961865

Marrun, N. A. (2018). "My mom seems to have a *dicho* for everything!": Family engagement in the college success of Latina/o students. *Journal of Latinos and Education*, *19*(1), 164–180. doi:10.1080/15348431.2018.1489811

Martín-Baró, I. (1994). *Writings for a liberation psychology*. Harvard University Press.

Martín-Baró, I. (1994). *Writings for a liberation psychology: Ignacio Martín-Baró* (A. Aron & S. Corne, Eds. & Trans.). Harvard University Press.

Martin, D., & Shaw, D. (2021). Chilean and Transnational Performances of Disobedience: LasTesis and the Phenomenon of Un violador en tu camino. *Bulletin of Latin American Research*, *40*(5), 712–729. doi:10.1111/blar.13215

Martinez, R. (2020). Hispanic Men's Perceptions About Depression and Attitudes Toward Mental Health Treatment. *UC Merced Undergraduate Research Journal*, *12*(1). Retrieved from https://escholarship.org/uc/item/93x0104f doi:10.5070/M4121046071

Martinez, A. (2018). Pathways to the professoriate: The experiences of first-generation Latino undergraduate students at Hispanic serving institutions applying to doctoral programs. *Education Sciences*, *8*(1), 32. doi:10.3390/educsci8010032

Martinez, C. R. Jr, McClure, H. H., & Eddy, J. M. (2009). Language brokering contexts and behavioral and emotional adjustment among Latino parents and adolescents. *The Journal of Early Adolescence*, *29*(1), 71–98. doi:10.1177/0272431608324477 PMID:19898605

Martinez, J. M. (2000). *Phenomenology of Chicana experience and identity: Communication and transformation in praxis*. Rowman and Littleðeld.

Martinez, M. (2019). Toxic masculinity: An outcome of colonialism and its effects on the Latinx/Chicanx LGBTQ+ community. *McNair Research Journal SJSU*, *15*(1), 6. doi:10.31979/mrj.2019.1506

Martinez, M. (2021). Toxic Masculinity: An Outcome of Colonialism and its Effects on the Latinx/ Chicanx LGBTQ+ Community. *McNair Research Journal SJSU*, *17*(11). Advance online publication. doi:10.31979/mrj.2021.1711

Martinez, M. A. (2013). (Re) considering the role familismo plays in Latina/o high school students' college choices. *High School Journal*, *97*(1), 21–40. doi:10.1353/hsj.2013.0019

Martinez, M. E. (2008). *Genealogical fictions: Limpieza de sangre, religion and gender in colonial Mexico*. Stanford University Press.

Mastro, D., Behm-Morawitz, E., & Ortiz, M. (2007). The Cultivation of Social Perceptions of Latinos: A Mental Models Approach. *Media Psychology*, *9*(2), 347–365. doi:10.1080/15213260701286106

Matsuno, E., & Israel, T. (2018). Psychological interventions promoting resilience among transgender individuals: Transgender resilience intervention model (TRIM). *The Counseling Psychologist*, *46*(5), 632–655. doi:10.1177/0011000018787261

Mayes, A. (2014). *The mulatto republic: Class, race and Dominican national identity*. University Press of Florida.

Mazzula, S. L., & Sanchez, D. (2021). The state of Afrolatinxs in Latinx psychological research: Findings from a content analysis from 2009 to 2020. *Journal of Latina/o Psychology*, *9*(1), 8–25.

McConnell, E. A., Janulis, P., Phillips, I., Truong, R., & Birkett, M. (2018). Multiple minority stress and LGBTQ+ community resilience among sexual minority men. *Psychology of Sexual Orientation and Gender Diversity*, *5*(1), 1–12. doi:10.1037gd0000265 PMID:29546228

McCurdy, S. A., Stoecklin-Marois, M. T., Tancredi, D. J., Hennessy-Burt, T. E., & Schenker, M. B. (2015). Region of birth, sex, and reproductive health in rural immigrant latino farmworkers: The MICASA study: Reproductive health in Latino farmworkers. *The Journal of Rural Health*, *31*(2), 165–175. https://doi.org/10.1111/jrh.12083

McLaughlin, K. A., & Lambert, H. K. (2017). Child Trauma Exposure and Psychopathology: Mechanisms of Risk and Resilience. *Current Opinion in Psychology*, *14*, 29–34. doi:10.1016/j.copsyc.2016.10.004 PMID:27868085

McLeod, S. A. (2019, July 30). *Qualitative vs. quantitative research*. Simply Psychology. https://www.simplypsychology.org/qualitative-quantitative.html

Meca, A., Gonzales-Backen, M., Davis, R., Rodil, J., Soto, D., & Unger, J. B. (2020). Discrimination and Ethnic Identity: Establishing Directionality among Latino/a Youth. *Developmental Psychology*, *56*(5), 982–992. doi:10.1037/dev0000908 PMID:32105119

Meca, A., Moreno, O., Cobb, C., Lorenzo-Blanco, E. I., Schwartz, S. J., Cano, M. A., Zamboanga, D. L., Gonzales-Backen, M., Szapocznik, J., Unger, J. B., Baezconde-Garbanati, L., & Soto, D. W. (2021). Directional effects in cultural identity: A family systems approach for immigrant Latinx families. *Journal of Youth and Adolescence*, *50*(5), 965–977. doi:10.100710964-021-01406-2 PMID:33599938

Medina, L., & Gonzales, M. R. (Eds.). (2019). *Voices from the Ancestors: Xicanx and Latinx spiritual expressions and healing practices*. University of Arizona Press. doi:10.2307/j.ctvq4c07x

Meierotto, L., & Som Castellano, R. L. (2019). A case study of transitions in farming and farm labor in southwestern Idaho. *Journal of Agriculture, Food Systems, and Community Development*, *8*(4), 111–123. doi:10.5304/jafscd.2019.084.008

Mejia, A. P., Quiroz, O., Morales, Y., Ponce, R., Chavez, G. L., & Torre, E. O. Y. (2013). From madres to mujeristas: Latinas making change with Photovoice. *Action Research*, *11*(4), 301–321. doi:10.1177/1476750313502553

Meléndez, E., & Hinojosa, J. (2017). *Estimates of Post-Hurricane Maria Exodus from Puerto Rico*. Retrieved from https://centropr.hunter.cuny.edu/research/data-center/research-briefs/estimates-post-hurricane-maria-exodus-puerto-rico

Menakem, R. (2021). *My grandmother's hands: Racialized trauma and the pathway to mending our hearts and Bodies*. Penguin Books.

Mendez, L. O., & Cortina, K. S. (2021). Within Group Ethnic Diversity in Latinx Psychological Research: A Publication Analysis. *Hispanic Journal of Behavioral Sciences*, *43*(1-2), 114–130. doi:10.1177/0739986321996478

Mendoza-Álvarez, C., & Espino-Armendáriz, S. (2018). A critical approach to gender identities in the "Muxe" case. *Humanities and Social Sciences*, *6*(4), 130–136. doi:10.11648/j.hss.20180604.16

Menjívar, C. (2006). Liminal legality: Salvadoran and Guatemalan immigrants' lives in the United States 1. *American Journal of Sociology*, *111*(4), 999–1037. doi:10.1086/499509

Mercado Jones, R. (2019). Dolores: The Silenced Cofounder of the United Farm Workers. *Women & Language*, *1*, 105.

Merz, E. L., Malcarne, V. L., Roesch, S. C., Riley, N., & Sadler, G. R. (2011). A multigroup confirmatory factor analysis of the Patient Health Questionnaire-9 among English- and Spanish-speaking Latinas. *Cultural Diversity & Ethnic Minority Psychology*, *17*(3), 309–316. doi:10.1037/a0023883 PMID:21787063

Meyer, I. H. (1995). Minority stress and mental health in gay men. *Journal of Health and Social Behavior*, *36*(1), 38–56. doi:10.2307/2137286 PMID:7738327

Meyer, I. H. (2003). Prejudice, social stress, and mental health in lesbian, gay, and bisexual populations: Conceptual issues and research evidence. *Psychological Bulletin*, *129*(5), 674–697. doi:10.1037/0033-2909.129.5.674 PMID:12956539

Meyer, I. H. (2015). Resilience in the study of minority stress and health of sexual and gender minorities. *Psychology of Sexual Orientation and Gender Diversity*, *2*(3), 209–213. doi:10.1037gd0000132

Meza Lazaro, Y., & Bacio, G. A. (2021). Determinants of mental health outcomes among transgender Latinas: Minority stress and resilience processes. *Psychology of Sexual Orientation and Gender Diversity*. Advance online publication. doi:10.1037gd0000545

Mibilishaka, A., Ray, M., Hall, J., & Wilson, I. P. (2020). 'No toques mi pelo' (don't touch my hair): Decoding Afro-Cuban identity politics through hair. *African and Black Diaspora: An International Journal*, *13*(1), 114–126.

Mills, S. D., Fox, R. S., Malcarne, V. L., Roesch, S. C., Champagne, B. R., & Sadler, G. R. (2014). The psychometric properties of the Generalized Anxiety Disorder-7 Scale in Hispanic Americans with English or Spanish language preference. *Cultural Diversity & Ethnic Minority Psychology*, *20*(3), 463–468. doi:10.1037/a0036523 PMID:25045957

Miranda, J., Bernal, G., Lau, A., Kohn, L., Hwang, W. C., & LaFromboise, T. (2005). State of the science on psychosocial interventions for ethnic minorities. *Annual Review of Clinical Psychology*, *1*(1), 113–142. doi:10.1146/annurev.clinpsy.1.102803.143822 PMID:17716084

Mirandé, A. (2018). Hombres y machos: Masculinity and Latino culture [Men and Males: Masculinity and Latino Culture]. Routledge. doi:10.4324/9780429500008

Mirandé, A. (2011). The Muxes of Juchitan: A preliminary look at transgender identity and acceptance. *Cal. W. Int'l LJ*, *42*(2), 509–540.

Miville, M. L., Arredondo, P., Consoli, A., Santiago-Rivera, A., Delgado-Romero, E. A., Fuentes, M., Domenech Rodriguez, M., Field, L., & Cervantes, J. (2017). Liderazgo/Leadership Through Cultural Lenses: The National Latina/o Psychological Association. *The Counseling Psychologist*, *45*, 830–856. doi:10.1177/0011000016668413

Miville, M. L., Calle, C. Z., Mendez, N., & Borenstein, J. (2018). Colombians in the United States: History, values, and challenges. In *Latinx Immigrants* (pp. 53–73). Springer. doi:10.1007/978-3-319-95738-8_4

Miville, M. L., Constantine, M. G., Baysden, M. F., & So-Lloyd, G. (2005). Chameleon Changes: An Exploration of Racial Identity Themes of Multiracial People. *Journal of Counseling Psychology*, *52*(4), 507–516. doi:10.1037/0022-0167.52.4.507

Miville, M. L., & Ferguson, A. D. (2014). Intersections of race-ethnicity and gender on identity development and social roles. In M. L. Miville & A. D. Ferguson (Eds.), *Handbook of race-ethnicity and gender in psychology*. Springer. doi:10.1007/978-1-4614-8860-6_1

Miville, M. L., Mendez, N., & Louie, M. (2017). Latina/o Gender Roles: A content analysis of empirical research from 1982 to 2013. *Journal of Latina/o Psychology*, 5(3), 173–194. doi:10.1037/lat0000072

Mize, R. L., & Swords, A. C. S. (2011). *Consuming Mexican labor from the bracero program to NAFTA*. University of Toronto Press.

Moe, J. L. (2016). Wellness and distress in LGBTQ populations: A meta-analysis. *Journal of LGBT Issues in Counseling*, 10(2), 112–129. doi:10.1080/15538605.2016.1163520

Mojtabai, R., Olfson, M., & Mechanic, D. (2002). Perceived need and help-seeking in adults with mood, anxiety, or substance use disorders. *Archives of General Psychiatry*, 59(1), 77–84. doi:10.1001/archpsyc.59.1.77 PMID:11779286

Moll, L. C., Amanti, C., Neff, D., & Gonzalez, N. (1992). Funds of knowledge for teaching: Using a qualitative approach to connect homes and classrooms. *Theory into Practice*, 31(2), 132–141. doi:10.1080/00405849209543534

Molock, S. D., & Parchem, B. (2020). The impact of COVID-19 on college students from communities of color. *Journal of American College Health*, 1–7. PMID:33502970

Montero, M., & Sonn, C. C. (Eds.). (2009). *Psychology of liberation: Theories and applications*. Springer.

Montoya, C., & Seminario, M. G. (2022). Guerreras y Puentes: The theory and praxis of Latina(x) activism. *Politics, Groups & Identities*, 10(2), 171–188. doi:10.1080/21565503.2020.1821233

Montoya-Galvez, C. (2022, September 16). *GOP Govs. Ron DeSantis, Greg Abbott send migrants to Martha's Vineyard and vice president's residence*. CBS News. https://www.cbsnews.com/news/ron-de-santis-flies-texas-florida-migrants-marthas-vineyard-kamala-harris-residence/

Mora, A. M., Lewnard, J. A., Kogut, K., Rauch, S. A., Hernandez, S., Wong, M. P., Huen, K., Chang, C., Jewell, N. P., Holland, N., Harris, E., Cuevas, M., Eskenazi, B., Camacho, J., Casillas, G., Castro, C., de Vere, M. J., Flores, L., ... Zepeda, L. (2021). Risk factors associated with SARS-CoV-2 infection among farmworkers in Monterey County, California. *JAMA Network Open*, 4(9). doi:10.1001/jamanetworkopen.2021.24116

Moradi, B., & Grzanka, P. R. (2017). Using intersectionality responsibly: Toward critical epistemology, structural analysis, and social justice activism. *Journal of Counseling Psychology*, 64(5), 500–513. doi:10.1037/cou0000203 PMID:29048196

Moraga, C. (1997). La guera. *Critical White studies: Looking behind the mirror*, 471-474.

Moraga, C. (2019). *Native country of the heart: A memoir*. Farrar, Straus and Giroux.

Moraga, C., & Anzaldúa, G. (Eds.). (1981). *This bridge called my back: Writings by radical women of color*. SUNY Press.

Mora, J. K. (2002). Caught in a policy web: The impact of education reform on Latino education. *Journal of Latinos and Education*, 1(1), 29–44. doi:10.1207/S1532771XJLE0101_3

Morales, A., & Pérez, O. F. R. (2020). Marianismo. The Wiley Encyclopedia of Personality and Individual Differences: Clinical, Applied, and Cross-Cultural Research, 247-251.

Morales, A., & Wang, K. T. (2018). The relationship among language brokering, parent–child bonding, and mental health correlates among Latinx college students. *Journal of Mental Health Counseling*, 40(4), 316–327. doi:10.17744/mehc.40.4.04

Compilation of References

Morales, E. (2013). Latino lesbian, gay, bisexual, and transgender immigrants in the United States. *Journal of LGBT Issues in Counseling*, 7(2), 172–184. doi:10.1080/15538605.2013.785467

Morgan, M., Pigg, E. N., Consoli, A., Pavone, D., & Meza, D. (2021). Like a chameleon: Resilience among self-identified latinx mixed adults. *Revista Interamericana de Psicología. Interamerican Journal of Psychology*, 55(1), e988–e988. doi:10.30849/ripijp.v55i1.988

Morner, M. (1967). *Race mixture in the history of Latin America*. Little Brown and Company.

Morrell, R. (1998). Of boys and men: Masculinity and gender in Southern African studies. *Journal of Southern African Studies*, 24(4), 605–630. doi:10.1080/03057079808708593

Moschetti, R. V., Plunkett, S. W., Efrat, R., & Yomtov, D. (2018). Peer Mentoring as Social Capital for Latina/o College Students at a Hispanic-Serving Institution. *Journal of Hispanic Higher Education*, 17(4), 375–392. doi:10.1177/1538192717702949

Moullin, J. C., Dickson, K. S., Stadnick, N. A., Albers, B., Nilsen, P., Broder-Fingert, S., Mukasa, B., & Aarons, G. A. (2020). Ten recommendations for using implementation frameworks in research and practice. *Implementation Science Communications*, 1(1), 1-12.

Muñoz, M. (2017). *10 Reasons Why Colonialism Strengthened Rape Culture In Latinx Communities*. Everyday Feminism. Retrieved May 6, 2022, from https://everydayfeminism.com/2017/07/colonialism-latinx-rape-culture/

Munroe, E. (2013). Feminism: A fourth wave? *Political Insight*, 22-25.

Murphy, S. L., Kochanek, K. D., Xu, J. Q., & Arias, E. (2021). Mortality in the United States, NCHS Data Brief, no 427. Hyattsville, MD: National Center for Health Statistics. icon. doi:10.15620/cdc:112079external

Myers, H. F., Wyatt, G. E., Ullman, J. B., Loeb, T. B., Chin, D., Prause, N., Zhang, M., Williams, J. K., Slavich, G. M., & Liu, H. (2015). Cumulative burden of lifetime adversities: Trauma and mental health in low-SES African Americans and Latino/as. *Psychological Trauma: Theory, Research, Practice, and Policy*, 7(3), 243–251. doi:10.1037/a0039077 PMID:25961869

Nash, J. C. (2019). *Black feminism reimagined: After intersectionality*. Duke University Press. doi:10.1215/9781478002253

National Academies of Sciences, Engineering, and Medicine. (2017). *Communities in action: Pathways to health equity*. Washington, DC: The National Academies Press. doi:10.17226/24624

National Academy of Sciences, National Academy of Engineering, and Institute of Medicine. (2005). *Facilitating Interdisciplinary Research*. The National Academies Press. doi:10.17226/11153

National Agricultural Worker Survey. (2018). https://www.dol.gov/sites/dolgov/files/ETA/naws/pdfs/NAWS_Research_Report_13.pdf

National Agricultural Worker Survey. (2022). https://www.dol.gov/sites/dolgov/files/ETA/naws/pdfs/NAWS%20Research%20Report%2016.pdf

National Center for Education Statistics. (2016). *The condition of education 2016, characteristics of postsecondary faculty*. https://nces.ed.gov/fastfacts/display.asp?id=61

National Employment Law Project, National Immigration Law Center, & OSH Law Project. (2020). *FAQ: Immigrant workers' rights and COVID-19 -- a resource for Workers and Their Advocates*. https://s27147.pcdn.co/wp-content/uploads/FAQ-immigrant-workers-rights-COVID-19-resource-v-2020-04-10.pdf

National Hispanic and Latino MHTTC. (2019, October 28). *Complicated grief: Cultural considerations when working with loss in Hispanic and Latino Students and their families.* https://mhttcnetwork.org/centers/national-hispanic-and-latino-mhttc/product/complicated-grief-cultural-considerations-when

National Latinx Psychological Association. (2020). Ethical guidelines of the National Latinx Psychological Association. *Journal of Latina/o Psychology, 8*(2), 101–111. doi:10.1037/lat0000151

National Museum Liverpool. (2022). *West Africa.* https://www.liverpoolmuseums.org.uk/history-of-slavery/west-africa

Negron-Muntaner, F., Abbas, C., Figueroa, L., & Robson, S. (2014). *The Latino media gap: A report on the state of Latinos in U.S. media.* The Center for the Study of Ethnicity and Race Columbia University.

Ngai, M. M. (2004). *Impossible subjects: Illegal aliens and the making of modern america.* Princetion University Press.

Nguyen, C. M., Liu, W. M., Hernandez, J. O., & Stinson, R. (2012). Problem-solving appraisal, gender role conflict, help-seeking behavior, and psychological distress among men who are homeless. *Psychology of Men & Masculinity, 13*(3), 270–282. doi:10.1037/a0025523

Nielsen, M., Haun, D., Kärtner, J., & Legare, C. H. (2017). The persistent sampling bias in developmental psychology: A call to action. *Journal of Experimental Child Psychology, 162*, 31–38. doi:10.1016/j.jecp.2017.04.017 PMID:28575664

Nieto-Phillips, J. M. (2004). *The language of blood: The making of Spanish-American identity in New Mexico.* The University of New Mexico Press.

NLPA. (2018). *Ethical guidelines national Latina/o psychological association.* https://www.nlpa.ws/assets/docs/ethical%20guidelines%20nlpa_adopted%20jan%201st.pdf

Noe-Bustamante, L. (2019). *Key Facts About U.S. Hispanics and Their Diverse Heritage.* Pew Research Center. https://www.pewresearch.org/fact-tank/2019/09/16/key-facts-about-u-s-hispanics/

Noe-Bustamante, L. (2020). *Key facts about U.S. hispanics and their diverse heritage.* Pew Research Center. Retrieved from https://www.pewresearch.org/fact-tank/2019/09/16/key-facts-about-u-s-hispanics/

Noe-Bustamante, L., Gonzalez-Barrera, A., Edwards, K., Mora, L., & Lopez, M. H. (2021). *Majority of Latinos Say Skin Color Impacts Opportunity in America and Shapes Daily Life.* Pew Research Center. https://www.pewresearch.org/hispanic/2021/11/04/majority-of-latinos-say-skin-color-impacts-opportunity-in-america-and-shapes-daily-life/

Noe-Bustamante, L., González-Barrera, A., Edwards, K., Mora, L., & López, M. H. (2021). *Majority of Latinos Say Skin Color Impacts Opportunity in America and Shapes Daily Life.* Pew Research Center. Retrieved from https://www.pewresearch.org/hispanic/2021/11/04/majority-of-latinos-say-skin-color-impacts-opportunity-in-america-and-shapes-daily-life/

Nosotros a las 8. (2022, March 8). *Abinader reafirma su apoyo al aborto en las tres causales* [Abinader reaffirms his support for abortion on all three grounds] [Video]. Youtube. https://www.youtube.com/watch?v=R3uH-c_rL8g

Noyola, N., Sánchez, M., & Cardemil, E. V. (2020). Minority stress and coping among sexual diverse Latinxs. *Journal of Latina/o Psychology, 8*(1), 58–82. doi:10.1037/lat0000143

Nuñez, A., González, P., Talavera, G. A., Sanchez-Johnsen, L., Roesch, S. C., Davis, S. M., Arguelles, W., Womack, V. Y., Ostrovsky, N. W., Ojeda, L., Penedo, F. J., & Gallo, L. C. (2016). Machismo, Marianismo, and Negative Cognitive-Emotional Factors: Findings From the Hispanic Community Health Study/Study of Latinos Sociocultural Ancillary Study. *Journal of Latina/o Psychology, 4*(4), 202–217. doi:10.1037/lat0000050 PMID:27840779

O'Neil, J. M. (1990). Assessing men's gender role conflict. In D. Moore & F. Leafgren (Eds.), *Problem-solving strategies and interventions for men in conflict* (pp. 23–38). American Association for Counseling and Development.

O'Neil, J. M. (2008). Summarizing 25 years of research on men's gender role conflict using the gender role conflict scale: New research paradigms and clinical implications. *The Counseling Psychologist*, *36*(3), 358–445. doi:10.1177/0011000008317057

O'Neil, J. M., Helms, B. J., Gable, R. K., David, L., & Wrightsman, L. S. (1986). Gender-Role Conflict Scale: College men's fear of femininity. *Sex Roles*, *14*(5-6), 335–350. doi:10.1007/BF00287583

Ojeda, L., & Piña-Watson, B. (2014). Caballerismo may protect against the role of machismo on Mexican day laborers' self-esteem. *Psychology of Men & Masculinity*, *15*(3), 288–295. doi:10.1037/a0033450

Olff, M., Frijling, J. L., Kubzansky, L. D., Bradley, B., Ellenbogen, M. A., Cardoso, C., Bartz, J. A., Yee, J. R., & van Zuiden, M. (2013). The role of oxytocin in social bonding, stress regulation and mental health: An update on the moderating effects of context and interindividual differences. *Psychoneuroendocrinology*, *38*(9), 1883–1894. doi:10.1016/j.psyneuen.2013.06.019 PMID:23856187

Olfson, M., Mojtabai, R., Sampson, N. A., Hwang, I., Druss, B., Wang, P. S., Wells, K. B., Pincus, H. A., & Kessler, R. C. (2009). Dropout from outpatient mental health care in the United States. *Psychiatric Services (Washington, D.C.)*, *60*(7), 898–907. doi:10.1176/ps.2009.60.7.898 PMID:19564219

Olita, I. (2018, January 29). *The Third Gender* [Video]. The Atlantic. https://www.theatlantic.com/video/index/551738/muxes-mexico-third-gender/

Ornelas, I., Fung, W., Gabbard, S., & Carroll, D. (2021). *Findings from the national agricultural workers survey (NAWS) 2017–2018: A demographic and employment profile of United States farmworkers*. The U.S. Department of Labor. https://wdr.doleta.gov/research/FullText_Documents/ETAOP2021-22%20NAWS%20Research%20Report%2014%20(2017-2018)_508%20Compliant.pdf

Orozco, R. C., Gonzalez, S., & Duran, A. (2021). Centering Queer Latinx/a/o Experiences and Knowledge: Guidelines for Using Jotería Studies in Higher Education Qualitative Research. *Journal Committed to Social Change on Race and Ethnicity*, *7*(1), 117–148. doi:10.15763/issn.2642-2387.2021.7.1.117-148

Ortega, A. N., Feldman, J. M., Canino, G., Steinman, K., & Alegría, M. (2006). Co-occurrence of mental and physical illness in US Latinos. *Social Psychiatry and Psychiatric Epidemiology*, *41*(12), 927–934. doi:10.100700127-006-0121-8 PMID:17013767

Ortega, A. N., Rosenheck, R., Alegría, M., & Desai, R. A. (2000). Acculturation and the lifetime risk of psychiatric and substance use disorders among Hispanics. *The Journal of Nervous and Mental Disease*, *188*(11), 728–735. doi:10.1097/00005053-200011000-00002 PMID:11093374

Owen, J., Drinane, J., Tao, K. W., Adelson, J. L., Hook, J. N., Davis, D., & Fookune, N. (2017). Racial/ethnic disparities in client unilateral termination: The role of therapists' cultural comfort. *Psychotherapy Research*, *27*(1), 102–111. doi:10.1080/10503307.2015.1078517 PMID:26390171

Owen, J., Tao, K. W., Imel, Z. E., Wampold, B. E., & Rodolfa, E. (2014). Addressing racial and ethnic microaggressions in therapy. *Professional Psychology, Research and Practice*, *45*(4), 283–290. doi:10.1037/a0037420

Owens, L. R. (2020). *Love and rage: The path of liberation through anger*. North Atlantic Books.

Pager, D., & Shepherd, H. (2008). The Sociology of Discrimination: Racial Discrimination in Employment, Housing, Credit, and Consumer Markets. *Annual Review of Sociology*, *34*(1), 181–209. doi:10.1146/annurev.soc.33.040406.131740 PMID:20689680

Palmeiro, C. (2018). The Latin American Green Tide: Desire and Feminist Transversality. *Journal of Latin American Cultural Studies*, *27*(4), 561–564. doi:10.1080/13569325.2018.1561429

Palmer, L. C. (2007). Crossing the color line: Emerging realities about eating disorders and treatment with women of color. *Journal of Feminist Family Therapy*, *19*(4), 21–41. doi:10.1300/J086v19n04_02

Paone, T. R., & Malott, K. M. (2008). Using interpreters in mental health counseling: A literature review and recommendations. *Journal of Multicultural Counseling and Development*, *36*(3), 130–142. doi:10.1002/j.2161-1912.2008.tb00077.x

Paredes, T. M., & Parchment, T. M. (2021). The Latino father in the postnatal period: The role of egalitarian masculine gender role attitudes and coping skills in depressive symptoms. *Psychology of Men & Masculinity*, *22*(1), 113–123. doi:10.1037/men0000315

Parmenter, J. G., Galliher, R. V., Wong, E., & Perez, D. (2021). An intersectional approach to understanding LGBTQ+ people of color's access to LGBTQ+ community resilience. *Journal of Counseling Psychology*, *68*(6), 629–641. doi:10.1037/cou0000578 PMID:34398620

Parra, C. J. R. (2019). Healing through parenting: An intervention delivery and process of change model developed with low-income Latina/o immigrant families. *Family Process*, *58*(1), 34–52. doi:10.1111/famp.12429 PMID:30786004

Passel, J. S., Lopez, M. H., & Cohn, D. (2022). *U.S. Hispanic population continued its geographic spread in the 2010's*. Pew Research Center. https://www.pewresearch.org/fact-tank/2022/02/03/u-s-hispanic-population-continued-its-geographic-spread-in-the-2010s/

Passel, J. S., & D'Vera Cohn, D. (2008). *US population projections, 2005-2050*. Pew Research Center.

Pastrana, A. J. Jr. (2015). Being out to others: The relative importance of family support, identity and religion for LGBT Latina/os. *Latino Studies*, *13*(1), 88–112. doi:10.1057/lst.2014.69

Pastrana, F. A., Bridges, A. J., Villalobos, B. T., Dueweke, A. R., & Rodriguez, J. H. (2017). Cognitive behavioral therapy tools for clients with limited functional literacy. *Behavior Therapist*, *40*(4), 137–145.

Paulsen, E. (n.d.). *Covid-19 mental health facts - american psychiatric association*. Retrieved May 1, 2022, from https://www.psychiatry.org/File%20Library/Psychiatrists/APA-COVID-19-Mental-Health-Facts-Hispanics.pdf

Paulus, D. J., Tran, N., Gallagher, M. W., Viana, A. G., Bakhshaie, J., Garza, M., Ochoa-Perez, M., Lemaire, C., & Zvolensky, M. J. (2019). Examining the indirect effect of posttraumatic stress symptoms via emotion dysregulation on alcohol misuse among trauma-exposed Latinx in primary care. *Cultural Diversity & Ethnic Minority Psychology*, *25*(1), 55–64. doi:10.1037/cdp0000226 PMID:30714767

Pedrotti, J. T., & Burnes, T. R. (2016). The new face of the field: Dilemmas for diverse early-career psychologists. *Training and Education in Professional Psychology*, *10*(3), 141–148. doi:10.1037/tep0000120

Pelaez Lopez, A. (2018). *The X in Latinx is a wound, not a trend*. Color Bloq's X Collection. Retrieved May 11, 2022, from https://www.colorbloq.org/article/the-x-in-latinx-is-a-wound-not-a-trend

Perez, M., Ohrt, T. K., & Hoek, H. W. (2016, November). Prevalence and treatment of eating disorders among Hispanics/Latino Americans in the United States. *Current Opinion in Psychiatry*, *29*(6), 378–382. doi:10.1097/YCO.0000000000000277 PMID:27648780

Pérez, O. F. R., & Morales, A. (2020). Machismo. In B. J. Carducci, C. S. Nave, J. S. Mio, & R. E. Riggio (Eds.), *The Wiley Encyclopedia of Personality and Individual Differences*. doi:10.1002/9781118970843.ch305

Perry, V. M., & Sias, S. M. (2018). Ethical concerns when supervising Spanish-English bilingual counselors: Suggestions for practice. *The Journal of Counselor Preparation and Supervisor*, *11*(1), 10.

Pew Research Center. (2014, May 7). *The Shifting Religious Identity of Latinos in the United States*. Pew Research Center. https://www.pewresearch.org/religion/2014/05/07/the-shifting-religious-identity-of-latinos-in-the-united-states/

Pew Research Center. (2021). *Majority Latinos say skin color impacts opportunity in America and shapes daily life*. https://www.pewresearch.org/hispanic/2021/11/04/majority-of-latinos-say-skin-color-impacts-opportunity-in-america-and-shapes-daily-life/

Pew Research Center. (2022). *About 6 million U.S. adults identify as Afro-Latino*. https://www.pewresearch.org/fact-tank/2022/05/02/about-6-million-u-s-adults-identify-as-afro-latino/

Piña-Watson, B., Gonzalez, I. M., & Manzo, G. (2019). Mexican-descent adolescent resilience through familismo in the context of intergeneration acculturation conflict on depressive symptoms. *Translational Issues in Psychological Science*, *5*(4), 326–334. doi:10.1037/tps0000210

Pineda Santiago, I. (2021). *Intraducibles*. Libro Intraducibles. Retrieved from https://intraducibles.org/libro/

Pinto, K. M., & Coltrane, S. (2013). Understanding structure and culture in the division of household labor for Mexican immigrant families. In S. S. Chuang & C. S. Tamis-LeMonda (Eds.), Gender Roles in Immigrant Families (pp. 43–62). Springer New York. https://doi.org/10.1007/978-1-4614-6735-9_4.

Pizarro, C. (2021). Children with unspeakable trauma: Unaccompanied minors and family separations. *Play Therapy*, *16*(3), 20–23.

Placeres, V., & Ordaz, A. C. (2021). Religion and spiritual concerns to consider when using mindfulness interventions with Latinx/Hispanic clients. *Journal of Psychology and Christianity*, *40*(2), 143–150.

Placido, S. I. (2017). *A Global Vision: Dr. Ana Livia Cordero and the Puerto Rican Liberation Struggle, 1931-1992* [Doctoral dissertation]. Harvard University, Graduate School of Arts & Sciences.

Polanski, P. J. (2003). Spirituality in supervision. *Counseling and Values*, *47*(2), 131–141. doi:10.1002/j.2161-007X.2003.tb00230.x

Popescu, I. (2021). Memorialization and Escraches: Ni Una Menos and the Documentation of Feminicidio in Argentina. *The Latin Americanist*, *65*(3), 367–392. doi:10.1353/tla.2021.0024

Poston, W. C. (1990). The biracial identity development model: A needed addition. *Journal of Counseling and Development*, *69*(2), 152–155. doi:10.1002/j.1556-6676.1990.tb01477.x

Postsecondary National Policy Institute. (2021). *Factsheets: Women in Higher Education*. https://pnpi.org/women-in-higher-education/

Postsecondary National Policy Institute. (2022). *Factsheets: Men of Color*. https://pnpi.org/men-of-color/

Potochnick, S. R., & Perreira, K. M. (2010). Depression and Anxiety among First-Generation Immigrant Latino Youth: Key Correlates and Implications for Future Research. *The Journal of Nervous and Mental Disease*, *198*(7), 470–477. doi:10.1097/NMD.0b013e3181e4ce24 PMID:20611049

Pousadela, I. (2021). *#BLM beyond the US: Anti-racist struggles in Latin America*. Open Democracy. https://www.opendemocracy.net/en/democraciaabierta/blm-beyond-the-us-anti-racist-struggles-in-latin-america/

Presser. (1969). The role of sterilization in controlling Puerto Rican fertility. *Population Studies*, *23*(3), 343–361. doi:10.1080/00324728.1969.10405290

Prilleltensky, I. (1997). Values, assumptions, and practices: Assessing the moral implications of psychological discourse and action. *The American Psychologist*, *52*(5), 517–535.

Project South. (2020, September 14). Retrieved July 31, 2022, from https://projectsouth.org/wp-content/uploads/2020/09/OIG-ICDC-Complaint-1.pdf

Proulx, J., Croff, R., Oken, B., Aldwin, C. M., Fleming, C., Bergen-Cico, D., & Noorani, M. (2018). Considerations for research and development of culturally relevant mindfulness interventions in American minority communities. *Mindfulness*, *9*(2), 361–370. doi:10.100712671-017-0785-z PMID:29892321

Przeworski, A., & Piedra, A. (2020). The role of the family for sexual minority Latinx individuals: A systematic review and recommendations for clinical practice. *Journal of GLBT Family Studies*, *16*(2), 211–240. doi:10.1080/1550428X.2020.1724109

Quintero, D., Cerezo, A., Morales, A., & Rothman, S. (2015). Supporting transgender immigrant Latinas: The case of Erika. In *Gendered journeys: Women, migration and feminist psychology* (pp. 190–205). Springer. doi:10.1057/9781137521477_9

Raeff, C., Greenfield, P. M., & Quiroz, B. (2000). Conceptualizing interpersonal relationships in the cultural contexts of individualism and collectivism. *New Directions for Child and Adolescent Development*, *2000*(87), 59–74. doi:10.1002/cd.23220008706 PMID:10763567

Raine, R., Or, Z., Prady, S., & Bevan, G. (2016). *Evaluating health-care equity*. NIHR Journals Library. https://www.ncbi.nlm.nih.gov/books/NBK361257/

Ramirez, E. (2017). Unequal socialization: Interrogating the Chicano/Latino (a) doctoral education experience. *Journal of Diversity in Higher Education*, *10*(1), 25–38. doi:10.1037/dhe0000028

Ramos, G., Ponting, C., Bocanegra, E., Chodzen, G., Delgadillo, D., Rapp, A., Escovar, E., & Chavira, D. (2021). Discrimination and Internalizing Symptoms in Rural Latinx Adolescents: The Protective Role of Family Resilience. *Journal of Clinical Child and Adolescent Psychology*, 1–14. doi:10.1080/15374416.2021.1923018 PMID:34038290

Ramos-Zayas, A. Y., & Rúa, M. M. (Eds.). (2021). *Critical Dialogues in Latinx Studies: A Reader*. NYU Press. doi:10.18574/nyu/9781479805198.001.0001

Ranft, E. (2013). Connecting intersectionality and Nepantla to resist oppressions: A feminist fiction approach. *Women, Gender, and Families of Color*, *1*(2), 207–223. doi:10.5406/womgenfamcol.1.2.0207

Rappaport, B. (2019). *Exploring the experiences of Latina feminists in psychology: navigating intersecting identities, understanding Latina feminism, and implications for allies* (Publication No. 9949333998202959) [Doctoral dissertation, University of Georgia]. https://getd.libs.uga.edu/pdfs/rappaport_brooke_s_201908_phd.pdf

Regional Committee for the Eastern Mediterranean. (2006). *Fifty-third Session Original: Arabic Agenda item 7 (a) The role of government in health development*. https://applications.emro.who.int/docs/EM_RC53_Tech.Disc.1_en.pdf

Reif, L. L. (1986). Women in Latin American Guerrilla Movements: A Comparative Perspective. *Comparative Politics*, *18*(2), 147–169. doi:10.2307/421841

Rendón, J. A. G. (2008). *Mestizaje lingüístico en los Andes: génesis y estructura de una lengua mixta* [Linguistic Miscegenation in the Andes: Genesis and Structure of a Mixed Language]. Editorial Abya Yala.

Resick, P. A., & Schnicke, M. K. (1992). Cognitive processing therapy for sexual assault victims. *Journal of Consulting and Clinical Psychology*, *60*(5), 748–756. https://doi.org/10.1037//0022-006x.60.5.748

Compilation of References

Reversal of Roe vs. Wade Devastating Impact on Latina Health: Joint Statement Illinois Latino Agenda 2.0 and Illinois Unidos. (2022, July 1). Latino Policy Forum. Retrieved August 1, 2022, from https://www.latinopolicyforum.org/news/press-releases/document/SCOTUS-reversal-of-Roe-v.-Wade.pdf

Reyes, J. A., & Elias, M. J. (2011). Fostering social–emotional resilience among Latino youth. *Psychology in the Schools*, *48*(7), 723–737. doi:10.1002/pits.20580

Rimes, K. A., Shivakumar, S., Ussher, G., Baker, D., Rahman, Q., & West, E. (2019). Psychosocial factors associated with suicide attempts, ideation, and future risk in lesbian, gay, and bisexual youth: The youth chances study. *Crisis*, *40*(2), 83–92. doi:10.1027/0227-5910/a000527 PMID:29932021

Rios Casas, F., Ryan, D., Perez, G., Maurer, S., Tran, A. N., Rao, D., & Ornelas, I. J. (2020). "Se vale llorar y se vale reír": Latina immigrants' coping strategies for maintaining mental health in the face of immigration-related stressors. *Journal of Racial and Ethnic Health Disparities*, *7*(5), 937–948. doi:10.100740615-020-00717-7 PMID:32040841

Rivera-Rideau, P. (2015). *Remixing reggaeton: The cultural politics of race in Puerto Rico*. Duke University Press.

Robert Wood Johnson Foundation. (2008). *Income is linked with health regardless of racial or ethnic group*. Retrieved from http://www.commissiononhealth.org/PDF/inchlthxeg.pdf

Robinson, M. (2019). Two-spirit identity in a time of gender fluidity. *Journal of Homosexuality*. PMID:31125297

Roblyer, M. I., Grzywacz, J. G., Suerken, C. K., Trejo, G., Ip, E. H., & Arcury, T. A. (2016). Interpersonal and social correlates of depressive symptoms amoung Latinas in farmworker families living in North Carolina. *Women & Health. Vol.*, *56*(2), 177–193. doi:10.1080/03630242.2015.108664646

Rochin, R. I. (2016). Latinos and Afro-Latino legacy in the United States: History, culture, and issues of identity. *Professional Agricultural Workers Journal*, *3*(2).

Rochlen, A. B. (2005). Men in (and out of) therapy: Central concepts, emerging directions, and remaining challenges. *Journal of Clinical Psychology*, *61*(6), 627–631. doi:10.1002/jclp.20098 PMID:15732139

Rochlen, A. B., Land, L. N., & Wong, Y. J. (2004). Male restrictive emotionality and evaluations of online versus face-to-face counseling. *Psychology of Men & Masculinity*, *5*(2), 190–200. doi:10.1037/1524-9220.5.2.190

Rodriguez, Y. (2014). The triple double: Racially ambiguous Afro-Latino identities in America. *Master of Arts in American Studies Capstones*. Paper 1.

Rodriguez, M. C., & Morrobel, D. (2004). A review of Latino youth development research and a call for an asset orientation. *Hispanic Journal of Behavioral Sciences*, *26*(2), 107–127. doi:10.1177/0739986304264268

Rodriguez, V. J., La Barrie, D. L., Zegarac, M., & Shaffer, A. (2021). A systematic review of parenting scales the literature on measurement invariance/equivalence of parenting scales by race and ethnicity: Recommendations for inclusive parenting research. *Assessment*. Advance online publication. doi:10.1177/10731911211038630

Rodriguez, V. J., Shaffer, A., Are, F., Madden, A., Jones, D. L., & Kumar, M. (2019). Identification of differential item functioning by race and ethnicity in the Childhood Trauma Questionnaire. *Child Abuse & Neglect*, *94*, 104030. doi:10.1016/j.chiabu.2019.104030 PMID:31181398

Rojas-Araúz, B. O. (2021). *Undocumented Healing: Strengths and Resilience from the Shadows* [Doctoral dissertation]. University of Oregon.

Rolnick, A. C. (2019). Resilience and Native girls: A critique. *BYU L. Rev.*, *1407*. https://digitalcommons.law.byu.edu/lawreview/vol2018/iss6/8/

Rosales, R., Figuereo, V., Woo, B., Perez-Aponte, J., & Cano, M. (2018). Preparing to work with Latinos: Latino-focused content in social work master's degree programs. *Journal of Teaching in Social Work*, *38*(3), 251–262. doi:10.1080/08841233.2018.1472175

Rosenstock, I. M. (1974). The Health Belief Model and Preventive Health Behavior. *Health Education Monographs*, *2*(4), 354–386. doi:10.1177/109019817400200405

Rousseau, N. (2013). Historical womanist theory: Re-visioning Black feminist thought. *Race, Gender, & Class*, 191–204.

Ruff, N., Smoyer, A. B., & Breny, J. (2019). Hope, courage, and resilience in the lives of transgender women of color. *Qualitative Report*, *24*(8), 1990–2008. doi:10.46743/2160-3715/2019.3729

Ruiz, P. (2000). *Ethnicity and psychopharmacology* (1st ed.). American Psychiatric Press.

Russell, S. T., Toomey, R. B., Ryan, C., & Diaz, R. M. (2014). Being out at school: The implications for school victimization and young adult adjustment. *The American Journal of Orthopsychiatry*, *84*(6), 635–643. doi:10.1037/ort0000037 PMID:25545431

Saavedra, C. M., & Salazar Pérez, M. (2017). Chicana/Latina Feminist Critical Qualitative Inquiry: Meditations on Global Solidarity, Spirituality, and the Land. *International Review of Qualitative Research*, *10*(4), 450–467. doi:10.1525/irqr.2017.10.4.450

Sacks, V., & Murphey, S. (n.d). *The prevalence of adverse childhood experiences, nationally, by state, and by race or ethnicity*. https://www.childtrends.org/publications/prevalence-adverse-childhood-experiences-nationally-state-race-ethnicity

Saenz, V. B., & Ponjuan, L. (2009). The Vanishing Latino Male in Higher Education. *Journal of Hispanic Higher Education*, *8*(1), 54–89. doi:10.1177/1538192708326995

Sagar-Ouriaghli, I., Godfrey, E., Bridge, L., Meade, L., & Brown, J. (2019). Improving Mental Health Service Utilization Among Men: A Systematic Review and Synthesis of Behavior Change Techniques Within Interventions Targeting Help-Seeking. *American Journal of Men's Health*, *13*(3). doi:10.1177/1557988319857009 PMID:31184251

Salinas, C. Jr. (2017). Transforming academia and theorizing spaces for Latinx in higher education: Voces perdidas and voces de poder. *International Journal of Qualitative Studies in Education: QSE*, *30*(8), 746–758. doi:10.1080/09518398.2017.1350295

Salinas, C. Jr, & Lozano, A. (2019). Mapping and recontextualizing the evolution of the term Latinx: An environmental scanning in higher education. *Journal of Latinos and Education*, *19*(4), 302–315. doi:10.1080/15348431.2017.1390464

Salinas, C., & Lozano, A. (2021). History and evolution of the term Latinx. In E. G. Murillo, D. Delgado Bernal, S. Morales, L. Urrieta, E. Ruiz Bybee, J. Sánchez Muñoz, V. B. Saenz, D. Villanueva, M. Machado-Casas, & K. Espinoza (Eds.), *Handbook of Latinos and Education* (2nd ed., pp. 249–263). Rutledge.

Salsberg, E., Quigley, L., Richwine, C., Sliwa, S., Acquaviva, K., & Wyche, K. (2020). The Social Work Profession; Findings from three years of surveys of new social workers. Fitzhugh Mullan Institute for Health Workforce Equity, The George Washington University.

Samlan, H., Shetty, A., & McWhirter, E. H. (2021). Gender and racial-ethnic differences in treatment barriers among college students with suicidal ideation. *Journal of College Student Psychotherapy*, *35*(3), 272–289. doi:10.1080/87568225.2020.1734133

Sanchez, K., Chapa, T., Ybarra, R., & Martinez, O. N. (2012). Eliminating disparities through the integration of behavioral health and primary care services for racial and ethnic minority populations, including individuals with limited English proficiency: A literature review report. United States Department of Health and Human Services, Office of Minority Health.

Sánchez, B., Salazar, C., & Guerra, J. (2020). "I Feel Like I Have to Be the Whitest Version of Myself": Experiences of Early Career Latina Higher Education Administrators. *Journal of Diversity in Higher Education*. Advance online publication. doi:10.1037/dhe0000267

Sanchez, D. (2021). Introduction to special issue on AfroLatinidad: Theory, research, and practice. *Journal of Latina/o Psychology*, *9*(1), 1–7.

Sanchez, D. (2021). Introduction to special issue on AfroLatinidad: Theory, research, and practice. *Journal of Latina/o Psychology*, *9*(1), 1–7. doi:10.1037/lat0000186

Sandoval, E., Jordan, M., Mazzei, P., & Goodman, J. D. (2022, October 4). The Story Behind DeSantis's Migrant Flights to Martha's Vineyard. *The New York Times*. https://www.nytimes.com/2022/10/02/us/migrants-marthas-vineyard-desantis-texas.html

Sangalang, C. C., Jager, J., & Harachi, T. W. (2017). Effects of maternal traumatic distress on family functioning and child mental health: An examination of Southeast Asian refugee Journal Pre-proof 48 families in the U.S. *Social Science & Medicine*, *184*, 178–186. doi:10.1016/j.socscimed.2017.04.032

Santa-Ramirez, S. (2022). Sink or swim: The mentoring experiences of Latinx PhD students with faculty of color. *Journal of Diversity in Higher Education*, *15*(1), 124–134. doi:10.1037/dhe0000335

Santiago-Rivera, A., Arredondo, P., & Gallardo-Cooper, M. (2002). *Counseling Latinos and La Famila*. Sage.

Santos, S. J., & Reigadas, E. T. (2002). Latinos in Higher Education: An Evaluation of a University Faculty Mentoring Program. *Journal of Hispanic Higher Education*, *1*(1), 40–50. doi:10.1177/1538192702001001004

Schmitz, R. M., Robinson, B. A., Tabler, J., Welch, B., & Rafaqut, S. (2020). LGBTQ+ Latino/a young people's interpretations of stigma and mental health: An intersectional minority stress perspective. *Society and Mental Health*, *10*(2), 163–179. doi:10.1177/2156869319847248

Scholz, S. J. (2013). *Feminism: A beginner's guide*. Retrieved from http://eds.b.ebscohost.com.proxy-remote.galib.uga.edu/eds/ebookviewer/ebook/bmxlYmtfXzkxMDczOV9fQU41?sid=2c2e0ceb-cd4b-4dae-9954-233a8e66916d@sessionmgr102&vid=14&format=EK&rid=4

Schwartz, S. J., & Unger, J. B. (2010). Biculturalism and context: What is biculturalism, and when is it adaptive?: Commentary on Mistry and Wu. *Human Development*, *53*(1), 26–32. doi:10.1159/000268137 PMID:22475719

Schwatken, S. (2011). *Latino/a help-seeking behavior and endorsement of common factors* [Master's Thesis]. Iowa State University, Ames, IA. doi:10.31274/etd-180810-3000

Sellers, R. M., Smith, M. A., Shelton, J. N., Rowley, S. A., & Chavous, T. M. (1998). Multidimensional model of racial identity: A reconceptualization of African American racial identity. *Personality and Social Psychology Review*, *2*, 18–39.

Sengupta, S. (2020). Heat, smoke and covid are battering the workers who feed America. *New York Times*. https://www.nytimes.com/2020/08/25/climate/california-farm-workers-climate-change.html

Serrano-Villar, M., & Calzada, E. J. (2016). Ethnic identity: Evidence of protective effects for young, Latino children. *Journal of Applied Developmental Psychology*, *42*, 21–30. doi:10.1016/j.appdev.2015.11.002 PMID:26778873

Settles, I. H., Buchanan, N. T., & Dotson, K. (2019). Scrutinized but not recognized: (In)visibility and hypervisibility experiences of faculty of color. *Journal of Vocational Behavior*, *113*, 62–74. https://doi.org/10.1016/j.jvb.2018.06.003

Shapiro, F. (2017). *Eye movement desensitization and reprocessing (EMDR) therapy: Basic principles, protocols, and procedures*. Guilford Publications.

Shen, J. J., & Dennis, J. M. (2019). The family context of language brokering among Latino/a young adults. *Journal of Social and Personal Relationships*, *36*(1), 131–152. doi:10.1177/0265407517721379

Shin, R. Q. (2014). The application of critical consciousness and intersectionality as tools for decolonizing racial/ethnic identity development models in the fields of counseling and psychology. In Decolonizing multicultural counseling through social justice. Springer.

Shire, W. (2011). *Home*. Teaching My Mother How to Give Birth.

Silver, P., & Vélez, W. (2017). "Let me go check out Florida": Rethinking Puerto Rican diaspora. *Journal of the Center for Puerto Rican Studies*, *29*(3), 98–125.

Simon, S., & Emanuel, G. (2022, September 17). *Before migrants were sent to Martha's Vineyard, there were the "Reverse Freedom Rides"*. NPR. https://www.npr.org/2022/09/17/1123629655/60-years-before-migrants-were-sent-to-marthas-vineyard-there-were-the-reverse-fr

Simpson. (Eds.). (n.d.). *Revealing and concealing gender: Issues of visibility in organizations*. Palgrave Macmillan.

Singh, A. (2013). Transgender youth of color and resilience: Negotiating oppression and finding support. *Sex Roles*, *68*(11-12), 690–702. doi:10.100711199-012-0149-z

Singh, A. A., Hays, D. G., & Watson, L. S. (2011). Strength in the face of adversity: Resilience strategies of transgender individuals. *Journal of Counseling and Development*, *89*(1), 20–27. doi:10.1002/j.1556-6678.2011.tb00057.x

Singh, A. A., & McKleroy, V. S. (2011). "Just getting out of bed is a revolutionary act" The resilience of transgender people of color who have survived traumatic life events. *Traumatology*, *17*(2), 34–44. doi:10.1177/1534765610369261

Sinha, M. (2017). Colonial masculinity: The 'manly Englishman' and the 'effeminate Bengali' in the late nineteenth century. In *Colonial masculinity*. Manchester University Press. doi:10.7765/9781526123640

Sippel, L. M., Allington, C. E., Pietrzak, R. H., Harpaz-Rotem, I., Mayes, L. C., & Olff, M. (2017). Oxytocin and Stress-related Disorders: Neurobiological Mechanisms and Treatment Opportunities. *Chronic Stress*, *1*. Advance online publication. doi:10.1177/2470547016687996 PMID:28649672

Sladek, M. R., Umaña-Taylor, A. J., Hardesty, J. L., Aguilar, G., Bates, D., Bayless, S. D., Gomez, E., Hur, C. K., Ison, A., Jones, S., Luo, H., Satterthwaite-Freiman, M., & Vázquez, M. A. (2022). "So, like, it's all a mix of one": Intersecting contexts of adolescents' ethnic-racial socialization. *Child Development*, *93*(5), 1284–1303. doi:10.1111/cdev.13756 PMID:35366330

Smith, B. L. (2018, June). *Spanish-speaking psychologists in demand*. Monitor on Psychology. Retrieved April 14, 2022, from https://www.apa.org/monitor/2018/06/spanish-speaking#:~:text=Yet%20there%20are%20only%20about,ago%2C%20according%20to%20Census%20data

Smith, D., & Werther, E. (2017). *Invisible Color: The Continued Lack of Diversity in Professional Psychology*. Poster presented at the Southeastern Psychological Association Annual Conference, Atlanta, GA.

Smith, J., & Spodak, C. (2021). *Black or 'Other'? Doctors may be relying on race to make decisions about your health*. https://www.cnn.com/2021/04/25/health/race-correction-in-medicine-history-refocused/index.html

So Mexican [@somexican]. (2022, July). *Have u thought about this? #somexican via:tiktok/thenosabokidhtx"* [Video]. Instagram. https://www.instagram.com/reel/CgpIvKcj0Cw/?igshid=YmMyMTA2M2Y

Solís, V. (2020). Writing Autohistoria through Conocimiento. In M. Cantú-Sanchez, C. de León- Zepeda, & N. E. Cantú (Eds.), Teaching Gloria E. Anzaldúa: Pedagogy and Practice for Our Classrooms and Communities (pp. 91-111). University of Arizona Press. doi:10.2307/j.ctv1595m67.12

Solorzano, D. G., Ceja, M., & Yosso, T. J. (2000). Critical race theory, racial microaggressions, and campus racial climate: The experience of African American college students. *The Journal of Negro Education*, *69*(1), 60–73.

Southern Poverty Law Center. (2021). *Anti-Immigrant*. https://www.splcenter.org/fighting-hate/extremist-files/ideology/anti-immigrant

Sowards, S. K. (2019). *Sí, ella puede! The rhetorical legacy of Dolores Huerta and the United Farm Workers*. University of Texas Press. doi:10.7560/317662

Sreenivasan, P., Cade, J., & Shahshahani, A. (2021). *Escalating jailhouse immigration enforcement: A report on detainers issued by ICE against persons held by local law enforcement agencies in Georgia, North Carolina, and South Carolina from 2016-2018*. https://www.projectsouth.org/wp-content/uploads/2021/12/120621_Escalating-Jailhouse-Immigration-Enforcement-Report.pdf

St. Arnault, D. (2009). Cultural determinants of help seeking: A model for research and practice. *Research and Theory for Nursing Practice*, *23*(4), 259–278. doi:10.1891/1541-6577.23.4.259 PMID:19999745

St. Arnault, D., & Woo, S. (2018). Testing the influence of cultural determinants on help-seeking theory. *The American Journal of Orthopsychiatry*, *88*(6), 650–660. doi:10.1037/ort0000353 PMID:30179023

Stephens, A. M. (2021). Making Migrants "Criminal": The Mariel Boatlift, Miami, and U.S. Immigration Policy in the 1980s. *Anthurium*, *17*(2), 4. doi:10.33596/anth.439

Stern. (2005). Eugenics and Historical Memory in America. *History Compass*, *3*(1), 1-11. doi:10.1111/j.1478-0542.2005.00145.x

Stone, A. L., Nimmons, E. A., Salcido, R. Jr, & Schnarrs, P. W. (2020). Multiplicity, race, and resilience: Transgender and non-binary people building community. *Sociological Inquiry*, *90*(2), 226–248. doi:10.1111oin.12341

Suárez-Orozco, C., & Suárez-Orozco, M. (2009). Educating Latino immigrant students in the twenty-first century: Principles for the Obama administration. *Harvard Educational Review*, *79*(2), 327–340. doi:10.17763/haer.79.2.231151762p82213u

Substance Abuse and Mental Health Services Administration. (2015). *Racial/ethnic differences in mental health service use among adults*. HHS Publication No. SMA-15-4906. Rockville, MD: Author.

Substance Abuse and Mental Health Services Administration. (2020). *Results from the 2019 National Survey on Drug Use and Health: Mental Health Detailed Tables*. Retrieved from https://www.samhsa.gov/data/report/2019-nsduh-detailed-tables

Sue, S. (1988). Psychotherapeutic services for ethnic minorities: Two decades of research findings. *The American Psychologist*, *43*(4), 301–308. doi:10.1037/0003-066X.43.4.301 PMID:3289427

Sue, S. (1999). Science, ethnicity, and bias: Where have we gone wrong? *The American Psychologist*, *54*(12), 1070–1077. doi:10.1037/0003-066X.54.12.1070 PMID:15332528

Suro, R. (2006). A developing identity: Hispanics in the United States. *Carnegie Reporter*, *3*(4), 1–5.

Szapocznik, J., & Hervis, O. E. (2020). *Brief strategic family therapy*. American Psychological Association. doi:10.1037/0000169-000

Szapocznik, J., & Kurtines, W. M. (1993). Family psychology and cultural diversity: Opportunities for theory, research, and application. *The American Psychologist*, *48*(4), 400–407. doi:10.1037/0003-066X.48.4.400

Talen, M. R., Fraser, J. S., & Cauley, K. (2005). Training Primary Care Psychologists: A Model for Predoctoral Programs. *Professional Psychology, Research and Practice*, *36*(2), 136–143. doi:10.1037/0735-7028.36.2.136

Talleyrand, R. M. (2012). Disordered eating in women of color: Some counseling considerations. *Journal of Counseling and Development*, *90*(3), 271–280. doi:10.1002/j.1556-6676.2012.00035.x

Taylor, Z. E., Ruiz, Y., Nair, N., & Mishra, A. A. (2020). Family support and mental health of Latinx children in migrant farmworker families. *Applied Developmental Science*, 1–18. doi:10.1080/10888691.2020.1800466

Tebbe, E. N., & Moradi, B. (2012). Anti-transgender prejudice: A structural equation model of associated constructs. *Journal of Counseling Psychology*, *59*(2), 251–261. doi:10.1037/a0026990 PMID:22329343

Tello, J., Cervantes, R. C., Cordova, D., & Santos, S. M. (2010). Joven Noble: Evaluation of a culturally focused youth development program. *Journal of Community Psychology*, *38*(6), 799–811. https://doi.org/10.1002/jcop.20396

Telzer, E. H. (2010). Expanding the acculturation gap-distress model: An integrative review of research. *Human Development*, *53*(6), 313–340. doi:10.1159/000322476

Tengan, T. K. (2002). (En) gendering colonialism: Masculinities in Hawai'i and Aotearoa. *Cultural Values*, *6*(3), 239–256. doi:10.1080/1362517022000007194

Testa, R. J., Habarth, J., Peta, J., Balsam, K., & Bockting, W. (2015). Development of the gender minority stress and resilience measure. *Psychology of Sexual Orientation and Gender Diversity*, *2*(1), 65–77. doi:10.1037gd0000081

The Breakfast Club. (2018, January 22). *Amara La Negra discusses being Afro-Latina & the standards of beauty in the entertainment industry* [Radio Broadcast]. Power 105.1FM. https://www.youtube.com/watch?v=0yAiI3Hs-p4

The DREAM act: An overview. (2022, March 7). American Immigration Council. Retrieved May 1, 2022, from https://www.americanimmigrationcouncil.org/research/dream-act-overview

The Latina Feminist Group. (2001). *Telling to live. Latina feminist testimonios*. Duke University Press.

The World Bank. (2018). *Afro-descendants in Latin America: Towards a framework of inclusion*. https://openknowledge.worldbank.org/handle/10986/30201

Thoma, M. E., & Declercq, E. R. (2022). All-Cause Maternal Mortality in the US Before vs During the COVID-19 Pandemic. *JAMA Network Open*, *5*(6), e2219133. Advance online publication. doi:10.1001/jamanetworkopen.2022.19133 PMID:35763300

Thompson, D. (2021). Building and transforming collective agency and collective identity to address Latinx farmworkers' needs and challenges in rural Vermont. *Agriculture and Human Values*, *38*(1), 129–143. https://doi.org/10.1007/s10460-020-10140-7

Tijerina Revilla, A., Nuñez, J., Santillana Blanco, J. M., & Gonzalez, S. (2021). Radical Jotería-Muxerista Love in the Classroom: Brown Queer Feminist Strategies for Social Transformation. In E. G. Murillo, D. Delgado Bernal, S. Morales, L. Urrieta, E. Ruiz Bybee, J. Sánchez Muñoz, V. Sáenz, D. Villanueva, M. Machado-Casas, & K. Espinoza (Eds.), *Handbook of Latinos and Education* (pp. 22–34). Routledge. doi:10.4324/9780429292026-4

Tijerina Revilla, A., & Santillana, J. M. (2014). Jotería Identity and Consciousness. *Aztlán*, *39*(1), 197–179.

Tomicic, A., & Berardi, F. (2018). Between past and present: The sociopsychological constructs of colonialism, coloniality and postcolonialism. *Integrative Psychological & Behavioral Science*, *52*(1), 152–175. doi:10.100712124-017-9407-5 PMID:29063442

Tonigan, J. S. (2003). Project match treatment participation and outcome by self-reported ethnicity. *Alcoholism, Clinical and Experimental Research*, *27*(8), 1340–1344. doi:10.1097/01.ALC.0000080673.83739.F3 PMID:12966335

Torres, M. (2013, March 29). College feminisms: Elementary feminisms: Majoring in English. *The Feministe Wire*. https://thefeministwire.com/2013/03/majoring-in-english/

Torres, N., & Hicks, J.F. (2016). Cultural awareness: Understanding Curanderismo. *Ideas and Research You Can Use: VISTAS 2016*.

Torres, J. B. (1998). Masculinity and gender roles among Puerto Rican men: Adilemma for Puerto Rican men's personal identity. *The American Journal of Orthopsychiatry*, *68*, 16–26. doi:10.1037/h0080266 PMID:9494638

Torres, J. B., Solberg, V. S. H., & Carlstrom, A. H. (2002). The myth of sameness among Latino men and their machismo. *The American Journal of Orthopsychiatry*, *72*(2), 163–181. doi:10.1037/0002-9432.72.2.163 PMID:15792057

Torres, J. M., Alcántara, C., Rudolph, K. E., & Viruell-Fuentes, E. A. (2016). Cross-border ties as sources of risk and resilience: Do cross-border ties moderate the relationship between migration-related stress and psychological distress for latino migrants in the United States? *Journal of Health and Social Behavior*, *57*(4), 436–452. doi:10.1177/0022146516667534 PMID:27803264

Torres, L., Yznaga, S. D., & Moore, K. M. (2011). Discrimination and Latino Psychological Distress: The Moderating Role of Ethnic Identity Exploration and Commitment. *The American Journal of Orthopsychiatry*, *81*(4), 526–534. doi:10.1111/j.1939-0025.2011.01117.x PMID:21977938

Torres-Pagán, L., & Toro-Alfonso, J. (2017). Hegemonic Masculinity as a Key Factor on Health Beliefs and Seeking Help in Puerto Rican Men with Hypertension: A Qualitative Study. *Puerto Rican Journal of Psychology. Revista Puertorriqueña de Psicología*, *28*(1), 134–147.

Torres, S. A., Santiago, C. D., Walts, K. K., & Richards, M. H. (2018). Immigration policy, practices, and procedures: The impact on the mental health of Mexican and Central American youth and families. *The American Psychologist*, *73*(7), 843–854. doi:10.1037/amp0000184 PMID:29504782

Torres, S. A., Sosa, S. S., Flores Toussaint, R. J., Jolie, S., & Bustos, Y. (2022). Systems of Oppression: The Impact of Discrimination on Latinx Immigrant Adolescents' Well-Being and Development. *Journal of Research on Adolescence*, *32*(2), 501–517. doi:10.1111/jora.12751 PMID:35365889

Torres, V. N., Williams, E. C., Ceballos, R. M., Donovan, D. M., & Ornelas, I. J. (2022). Discrimination, acculturative stress, alcohol use and their associations with alcohol-related consequences among Latino immigrant men. *Journal of Ethnicity in Substance Abuse*, 1–16. Advance online publication. doi:10.1080/15332640.2022.2077273 PMID:35634786

Torres, V., Hernández, E., & Martinez, S. (2019). *Understanding the Latinx Experience:Developmental and Contextual Influences* (1st ed.). Stylus Publishing.

Triana, C., Gloria, A. M., & Castellanos, J. (2020). Cultivating success for Latinx undergraduates: Integrating cultural spirituality within higher education. *About Campus: Enriching the Student Learning Experience*, *24*(6), 4–9. doi:10.1177/1086482219896793

Tukachinsky, R., Mastro, D., & Yarchi, M. (2017). The effect of prime time television ethnic/racial stereotypes on Latino and Black Americans: A longitudinal national level study. *Journal of Broadcasting & Electronic Media*, *61*(3), 538–556. doi:10.1080/08838151.2017.1344669

Turner, C. (2002). Women of Color in Academe: Living with Multiple Marginality. *The Journal of Higher Education*, *73*(1), 74–93. doi:10.1080/00221546.2002.11777131

Turner, E. A., & Llamas, J. D. (2017). The role of therapy fears, ethnic identity, and spirituality on access to mental health treatment among Latino college students. *Psychological Services*, *14*(4), 524–530. doi:10.1037er0000146 PMID:29120210

Turner-Trujillo, E., Del Toro, M., & Ramos, A. (2017). *An overview of Latino and Latin American identity*. Getty. Retrieved from https://www.getty.edu/news/an-overview-of-latino-and-latin-american-identity/

Tym, C., McMillion, R., Barone, S., & Webster, J. (2004). *First-generation college students: A literature review. TG*. Texas Guaranteed Student Loan Corporation.

U.S. Census Bureau. (2002). *Measuring America: The Decennial Census from 1790 to 2000*. https://www.census.gov/history/pdf/measuringamerica.pdf

U.S. Census Bureau. (2020). *Educational Attainment, 2020 American Community Survey 5-year estimates.* Retrieved from https://data.census.gov/cedsci/table?q=S1501&tid=ACSST5Y2020.S1501

U.S. Census Bureau. (2020). *Sex by Age (Hispanic or Latino), 2020 American Community Survey 5-Year Estimates*. Retrieved from https://data.census.gov/cedsci/table?q=Hispanic%20by%20sex,%202020&tid=ACSDT5Y2020.B01001I

U.S. Census Bureau. (2021a). *Decennial Census of Population and Housing by Decades Origin Data*. https://www.census.gov/programs-surveys/decennial-census/decade.2010.html

U.S. Census Bureau. (2021b). *Guidance on the Presentation and Comparison of Race and Hispanic Origin Data*. https://www.census.gov/topics/population/hispanic-origin/about/comparing-race-and-hispanic-origin.html

U.S. Department of Education, National Center for Education Statistics, Integrated Postsecondary Education Data System (IPEDS). (1984-2012). *Completion surveys* [Data files and dictionaries]. Retrieved from https://nces.ed.gov/ipeds/datacenter/DataFiles.aspx

U.S. Department of Health and Human Services. (2001). *Mental health: Culture, race, and ethnicity—A supplement to mental health: A report of the surgeon general.* Author.

Umaña-Taylor, A. J., & Updegraff, K. A. (2007). Latino adolescents' mental health: Exploring the interrelations among discrimination, ethnic identity, cultural orientation, self-esteem, and depressive symptoms. *Journal of Adolescence*, *30*(4), 549–567. doi:10.1016/j.adolescence.2006.08.002 PMID:17056105

United Nations. (1948). *The universal declaration for human rights*. https://www.un.org/sites/un2.un.org/files/udhr.pdf

United States Department of Agriculture. (2022). *Farm Labor*. https://www.ers.usda.gov/topics/farm-economy/farm-labor/#:~:text=In2014-16%2C27percent,ofworkerswhoareU.S.

US Department of Health and Human Services. (2022). *Social determinants of health.* Retrieved from https://health.gov/healthypeople/priority-areas/social-determinants-health

Uzogara, E. E. (2019). Gendered Racism Biases: Associations of Phenotypes with Discrimination and Internalized Oppression Among Latinx American Women and Men. *Race and Social Problems*, *11*(1), 80–92. doi:10.100712552-018-9255-z

Uzogara, E. E., Lee, H., Abdou, C. M., & Jackson, J. S. (2014). A comparison of skin tone discrimination among African American men: 1995 and 2003. *Psychology of Men & Masculinity*, *15*(2), 201–212. doi:10.1037/a0033479 PMID:25798076

Valdes, F. (1999). Theorizing "OutCrit" Theories: Coalitional Method and Comparative Jurisprudential Experience-RaceCrits, QueerCrits and LatCrits. *U. Miami L. Rev.*, *53*, 1265–1299.

van der Kolk, B. A. (2014). *The body keeps the score: Brain, mind, and body in the healing of trauma*. Viking.

Vandiver, B., Cross, W.E., Jr., Fhagen-Smith, P.E., Worrell, F., Swim, J., & Caldwell, L. (2000). *The cross-racial identity scale*. Unpublished scale.

Vargas, S. M., Huey, S. J., & Miranda, J. (2020). A critical review of current evidence on multiple types of discrimination and mental health. *The American Journal of Orthopsychiatry*, *90*(3), 374–390. doi:10.1037/ort0000441 PMID:31999138

Vasconcelos, J. (1925). *La raza cósmica. Agencia Mundial de Librería* [The Cosmic Race. World Book Agency]. Retrieved from www.filosofia.org/aut/001/razacos.htm

Vasquez, M. J. T. (2007). Cultural difference and the therapeutic alliance: An evidence-based analysis. *The American Psychologist*, *62*(8), 878–885. doi:10.1037/0003-066X.62.8.878 PMID:18020774

Vasquez-Salgado, Y., Greenfield, P. M., & Burgos-Cienfuegos, R. (2015). Exploring home-school value conflicts: Implications for academic achievement and well-being among Latino first-generation college students. *Journal of Adolescent Research*, *30*(3), 271–305. doi:10.1177/0743558414561297

Vaughan, L. (2020). *Florinda Soriano Muñoz (Mamá Tingó) (1921-1974)*. https://www.blackpast.org/global-african-history/florinda-soriano-munoz-mama-tingo-1921-1974/

Vega, D. (2016). "Why not me?": College enrollment and persistence of high achieving, first-generation Latino college students. *School Psychology Forum*, *10*, 307–320.

Velasquez, R. J., & Burton, M. P. (2004). Psychotherapy of Chicano men. In R. J. Velasquez, L. M. Arrellano, & B. W. McNeill (Eds.), *The handbook of Chicana/o psychology and mental health* (pp. 177–192). Lawrence Erlbaum Associates, Inc.

Velez, B. L., Moradi, B., & DeBlaere, C. (2015). Multiple oppressions and the mental health of sexual minority Latina/o individuals. *The Counseling Psychologist*, *43*(1), 7–38. doi:10.1177/0011000014542836

Villegas, J., Lemanski, J., & Valdéz, C. (2010). Marianismo and machismo: The portrayal of females in Mexican TV commercials. *Journal of International Consumer Marketing*, *22*(4), 327–346. doi:10.1080/08961530.2010.505884

Villenas, S., & Deyhle, D. (1999). Critical race theory and ethnographies challenging the stereotypes: Latino families, schooling, resilience and resistance. *Curriculum Inquiry*, *29*(4), 413–445.

Villicana, A. J., Delucio, K., & Biernat, M. (2016). "Coming out" among gay Latino and gay White men: Implications of verbal disclosure for well-being. *Self and Identity*, *15*(4), 468–487. doi:10.1080/15298868.2016.1156568

Vogel, D. L., Heimerdinger-Edwards, S. R., Hammer, J. H., & Hubbard, A. (2011). "Boys Don't Cry": Examination of the Links between Endorsement of Masculine Norms, Self-Stigma, and Help-Seeking Attitudes for Men from Diverse Backgrounds. *Journal of Counseling Psychology*, *58*(3), 368–382. doi:10.1037/a0023688 PMID:21639615

Von Robertson, R., Bravo, A., & Chaney, C. (2016). Racism and the experiences of Latina/o college students at a PWI (predominantly White institution). *Critical Sociology*, *42*(4-5), 715–735. doi:10.1177/0896920514532664

Vuola, E. (2017). Seriously Harmful For Your Health? Religion, Feminism and Sexuality in Latin America. In M. Althaus-Reid (Ed.), *Liberation Theology and Sexuality* (1st ed., pp. 137–162). Routledge. doi:10.4324/9781351153966-10

Vyas, D. A., Eisenstein, L. G., & Jones, D. S. (2020). Hidden in plain sight— Reconsidering the use of race correction in clinical algorithms. *The New England Journal of Medicine*, *383*(9), 874–882.

Wade, P. (2010). *Race and Ethnicity in Latin America*. Pluto Press. doi:10.26530/OAPEN_625258

Walker, A. (1983). *In Search of Our Mothers' Gardens: Womanist Prose*. Harcourt.

Walsh, J. M., Wheat, M. E., & Freund, K. (2000). Detection, evaluation, and treatment of eating disorders. *Journal of General Internal Medicine*, *15*(8), 577–590. doi:10.1046/j.1525-1497.2000.02439.x PMID:10940151

Walters, A. S., & Valenzuela, I. (2020). More Than Muscles, Money, or Machismo: Latino Men and the Stewardship of Masculinity. *Sexuality and Culture, 24*(3), 967. https://link.gale.com/apps/doc/A621914271/HRCA?u=anon~a27a5c2d&sid=googleScholar&xid=a6f3e8ca

Walters, A. S., & Valenzuela, I. (2019). "To me what's important is to give respect. There is no respect in cheating": Masculinity and Monogamy in Latino Men. *Sexuality & Culture*, *23*(4), 1025–1053. doi:10.100712119-019-09615-5

Webb, C. (2004). A Cheap Trafficking in Human Misery: The Reverse Freedom Rides of 1962. *Journal of American Studies*, *38*(2), 249–271. doi:10.1017/S0021875804008436

Westfield, N. L. (2007). *Dear sisters: A womanist practice of hospitality*. The Pilgrim Press.

What Is Integrated Behavioral Health Care (IBHC) ? (n.d.). Retrieved April 2, 2022, from https://integrationacademy.ahrq.gov/products/behavioral-health-measures-atlas/what-is-ibhc

WHO. (2018). *Integrating health services Brief*. https://www.who.int/docs/default-source/primary-health-care-conference/linkages.pdf

Williams, D. R. (2018). Stress and the Mental Health of Populations of Color: Advancing Our Understanding of Race-related Stressors. *Journal of Health and Social Behavior*, *59*(4), 466–485. doi:10.1177/0022146518814251 PMID:30484715

Williams, D. R., & Mohammed, S. A. (2013). Racism and Health I: Pathways and Scientific Evidence. *The American Behavioral Scientist*, *57*(8), 1152–1173. PMID:24347666

Witzig, R. (1996). The medicalization of race: Scientific legitimization of a flawed social construct. *Annals of Internal Medicine*, *125*(8), 675–679.

Wong, S. J. (2013). Machismo. In K. D. Keith (Ed.), *The Encyclopedia of Cross-Cultural Psychology*. doi:10.1002/9781118339893.wbeccp339

World Health Organization. (2013). *Closing the health equity gap: policy options and opportunities for action*. Available at: https://www.cdc.gov/nchhstp/socialdeterminants/docs/who-closing-health-equity-gap-policyopportunities-.pdf

World Health Organization. (2018). *Health inequities and their causes*. Retrieved from https://who.int/news-room/facts-in-pictures/detail/health-inequities-and-their-causes

Worrell, F. C., Mendoza-Denton, R., & Wang, A. (2019). Introducing a new assessment tool for measuring ethnic-racial identity: The Cross ethnic-racial identity scale–adult (CERIS-A). *Assessment*, *26*(3), 404–418. https://doi.org/10.1177/1073191117698756

Worrell, F. C., Vandiver, B. J., Cross, W. E., & Fhagen, P. E. (2016). *The Cross Ethnic-Racial Identity Scale–Adult (CERIS-A)*. University of California.

Wright, A. (2022). Femicide in Latin America: Reimagining Catholic symbolism in the pursuit of justice. *The Theology Journal of Boston College*, *1*(2), 125–139.

Xiuhtecutli, N., & Shattuck, A. (2021). Crisis politics and US farm labor: Health justice and Florida farmworkers amid a pandemic. *The Journal of Peasant Studies*, *48*(1), 73–98. doi:10.1080/03066150.2020.1856089

Yoshikawa, H. (2011). *Immigrants raising citizens: Undocumented parents and their young children*. Academic Press.

Compilation of References

Young, A. S., Klap, R., Sherbourne, C. D., & Wells, K. B. (2001). The quality of care for depressive and anxiety disorders in the United States. *Archives of General Psychiatry*, *58*(1), 55–61. doi:10.1001/archpsyc.58.1.55 PMID:11146758

Zayas, L. H. (2011). *Latinas attempting suicide: When cultures, families, and daughters collide*. Oxford University Press.

Zerrate, M. C., VanBronkhorst, S. B., Klotz, J., Caraballo, A. A., Canino, G., Bird, H. R., & Duarte, C. S. (2022). Espiritismo and Santeria: A gateway to child mental health services among Puerto Rican families? *Child and Adolescent Psychiatry and Mental Health*, *16*(1), 1–10. doi:10.118613034-022-00439-0 PMID:35016702

Zhou, M. (1997). Segmented assimilation: Issues, controversies, and recent research on the new second generation. *The International Migration Review*, *31*(4), 975–1008. doi:10.1177/019791839703100408 PMID:12293212

Zillman, C. (2018). On equal pay day 2018, there's a troubling trend behind the shrinking gender pay gap. *Fortune*. Retrieved from http://fortune.com/2018/04/10/equal- pay-day-2018-closing-gender-pay-gap/

Zimmerman, M. A. (1990). Toward a theory of learned hopefulness: A structural model analysis of participation and empowerment. *Journal of Research in Personality*, *24*(1), 71–86. doi:10.1016/0092-6566(90)90007-S

Zinnbauer, B. J., Pargament, K. I., Cole, B., Rye, M. S., Butfer, E. M., Belavich, T. G., Hipp, K., Scott, A. B., & Kadar, J. L. (2015). Religion and spirituality: Unfuzzying the fuzzy. *Journal for the Scientific Study of Religion*, *36*(4), 549–564. doi:10.2307/1387689

Zubatsky, M., Edwards, T. M., Wakabayashi, H., & Ivbijaro, G. (2018). Integrated behavioural health in primary care across the world: Three countries, three perspectives. *Family Practice*, *35*(6), 645–648. doi:10.1093/fampra/cmy034 PMID:29741628

About the Contributors

Edward A. Delgado-Romero is the Associate Dean for Faculty and Staff Services in the College of Education. The editor is also a Professor in the Counseling Psychology Doctoral Program in the Department of Counseling and Human Development Services and an affiliate faculty with the Interdisciplinary Qualitative Studies program and the Latin American and Caribbean Studies Institute (LACSI) at UGA. The editor graduated from Rhodes College with an undergraduate degree in Psychology and from the University of Notre Dame with a Ph.D. in Counseling Psychology. The editor completed a predoctoral internship at Michigan State University, worked as an Assistant Clinical Professor at the University of Florida, and an assistant professor at Indiana University Bloomington and joined UGA in 2005. Dr. Delgado-Romero was one of the founding members of the National Latinx Psychological Association (NLPA), a past-president of NLPA (2010), and has been honored with padrino/elder status and the distinguished professional career award from NLPA. The editor has also received a career research award from the Society for the Psychological Study of Race and Ethnicity (Division 45 of APA), an early career award for psychology in the public interest and the Jenny Penny Oliver Award in the Mary Frances Early College of Education. Recently the editor received the Elizabeth Spurlock Beckman Award, a national award that is intended to benefit teachers who have inspired their former students to make a significant contribution to society and was honored with the inaugural UGA First Award (for first generation faculty) and the UGA Engaged Scholar Award in 2021. The editor currently serves on the Board of Directors of the American Association of Hispanics in Higher Education. Dr. Delgado-Romero established a Spanish language psychology clinic, La Clinica In Lak'ech, in 2015. Over the last six years La Clinica has provided over 1,000 hours of therapy to undocumented, mixed-status, uninsured, and Spanish-speaking clients. Under the editor's supervision, over 20 therapists from counseling psychology, counseling, clinical psychology, and social work have provided linguistically and culturally appropriate services free of charge. As an advisor, the editor has mentored close to 50 students to the doctorate, 80% of whom have been people of color or international students. The students have focused their research on a wide array of multicultural areas and the editor has encouraged them to leave communities richer for their presence through community service and active culturally humble participation. A central part of the editor's work is the support and love of family. The editor's wife, Angie Romero-Shih, received her MSW at the school of social work and they have five wonderful children: J., Isa, Nick, Emery, and Gil.

* * *

Manuela Silvia Bautista Gil, originally from Mexico City, has a degree from the Instituto de Programación Bilingüe Estado de México, specializing in bilingual secretarial Programming and Computing,

About the Contributors

a career that expanded over ten years. Manuela migrated to Atlanta, Georgia, twenty-seven years ago and founded Cardenas Servicios Hispanos LLC. The agency's dedication to serving the Hispanic community of the metro Atlanta area has expanded over the years since its foundation in 2003. In collaboration with her daughters, Gabriela and Eva Maria Cárdenas, and her husband Mario Cardenas Villanueva her company and its impact on the community have grown. Manuela takes great pride in the professionalism, determination, and dedication of her company's development. Mainly, Manuel takes pride in the passion she has instilled in her children for serving the Hispanic community in their prospective professional fields. Manuela is an entrepreneur, wife, mother, and grandmother to Izel, Damian, and Amira whom she dedicates her stories of resilience.

Ana Bridges is a licensed clinical psychologist, Professor, and Director of Clinical Training in the Department of Psychological Science at the University of Arkansas. She directs the DREAM lab: Diversity Research and Enhanced Access for Minorities. Her research examines the causes and consequences of mental health service inequities, and she innovates treatment service delivery methods to make care more accessible to underserved and historically marginalized populations. She is a native of Argentina.

Jason A. Cade is Associate Dean for Clinical Programs and Experiential Learning and J. Alton Hosch Professor of Law at the University of Georgia School of Law. As Director of the Community Health Law Partnership Clinic (Community HeLP), Cade teaches law students how to undertake an interdisciplinary approach to the rights and health of immigrants through individual client representation, litigation, and project-based advocacy before administrative agencies and federal courts. Cade's research explores: (1) the role of nonfederal actors and institutions in the modern immigration system, (2) intersections between immigration enforcement and criminal law, and (3) the legal framework for immigration policy activism. He has published in the Northwestern University Law Review, the Washington & Lee Law Review, the Fordham Law Review, the Columbia Law Review Sidebar, the New York University Law Review Online, the UC Davis Law Review, the Indiana Law Journal, and the peer-reviewed interdisciplinary journal Studies in Law, Politics, and Society, among others. Cade's scholarship has been cited in briefs to the U.S. Supreme Court, reprinted in anthologies and practitioner's guides, used in law school curricula, and featured on JOTWELL. In 2022, Cade received the University of Georgia Engaged Scholar Award, a university-level honor bestowed on one tenured faculty member each year whose scholarship and public service accomplishments have significantly advanced progress on issues of public concern. In 2021, he was a co-recipient of the Clinical Legal Education Association's Award for Excellence in a Public Interest Case, in recognition of multi-faceted, collaborative advocacy on behalf of noncitizens alleging medical abuse and retaliation in a Georgia detention center. Cade earned his undergraduate degree from the University of North Carolina at Chapel Hill and his law degree magna cum laude from the Brooklyn Law School. Following law school, he clerked for Judge Steven M. Gold in the Eastern District of New York. As a Skadden Public Interest Fellow at The Door, Cade played a central role in the expansion of New York family court guardianship jurisdiction and was lead counsel or amicus on several state court appeals concerning immigrant juveniles. After a two-year stint in a boutique immigration law firm, Cade served as acting assistant professor at the New York University School of Law, where he taught in the Lawyering Program from 2010 to 2013 and assisted in the Immigrant Rights Clinic.

Cristalís Capielo Rosario was born and raised in Ponce, Puerto Rico. After receiving her doctorate in counseling psychology from the University of Georgia in 2016, she joined the faculty of the Counseling and Counseling and Psychology Department at Arizona State University. Dr. Capielo Rosario's research focuses on understanding the sociopolitical determinants of mental health disparities among Puerto Rican adults and youth living in the United States, particularly Puerto Rican millennial migrants.

Gabriela Cárdenas, B.A., is originally from Estado de Mexico and relocated to South Atlanta in the late 1990s. Gabriela earned a Bachelor of Science in Sociology from Clayton State University. Since completing her degree, Gabriela has channeled the resiliency of her community by assisting first-generation students in navigating systems of education. Gabriela's advocacy work has included the organization and staffing of non-profit DACA workshops for hundreds of first-generation students. These workshops have provided students with the tools to continue their education, career aspirations and enter the workforce. Gabriela has also provided guidance and mentorship to many students. She aspires to continue contributing to the community at large through future advocacy projects. Gabriela values family time and is a dedicated mother, daughter, and sister.

Elizabeth Cárdenas Bautista, M.Ed., identifies as a Mexican woman, inmigrante, who relocated with her family to the Atlanta metropolitan area in the state of Georgia from El Estado de Mexico, Mexico. She is a fifth-year doctoral candidate in the Counseling Psychology program at the University of Georgia and a current Harvard Clinical Fellow completing her predoctoral Psychology Internship in the Latinx Adult Acute Care track at Cambridge Health Alliance. Elizabeth earned a Bachelor of Science in Psychology from Clayton State University and a Master of Education in Community Counseling from the University of Georgia. Elizabeth is a member of the ¡BIEN! Research Team, under the direction of Dr. Edward Delgado-Romero. Nationally, Elizabeth has served as an executive member of the National Latinx Psychological Association (NLPA) within the role of Student Representative. Elizabeth has research and clinical experience in multicultural counseling, Latinx psychology, Liberation psychology, advancement of linguistic diversity in training programs, social justice, and advocacy. In her research, she focuses on addressing the dismantling of systems of oppression, centralizing social justice and political activism while understanding the role of complex trauma, post-traumatic growth, and resiliency in historically and currently marginalized communities. Clinically, she is passionate about providing competent bilingual and accessible mental health services to Latinx immigrant communities in various integrated health care settings and community centers. As a master's and doctoral level clinician, Elizabeth has been instrumental in the expansion of La Clinica In Lak'ech, a bilingual/bicultural clinic that has provided mental health counseling and assessment services to the Latinx immigrant community of Athens, Georgia. Mainly, Elizabeth takes great pride in being a bilingual Latina psychologist in training who seeks to continue supporting the recruitment, development, and retention of Latinx bilingual clinicians in the South-East.

Mario Cárdenas Villanueva originally from Toluca Mexico, proudly completed his elementary education from Escuela Municipio 121, Cuautitlán Izcalli, Estado de México. Mario has resided in Atlanta, Georgia, since 1987, where he worked in construction for fourteen years. Mario's childhood dream was to be near airplanes, and his dream became a reality when he started his career as a Delta employee. Mario has since retired and finds deep satisfaction in accomplishing his dreams and goals. Most importantly, being a dedicated father, grandfather, and husband. Mario dedicates his stories to his wife, daughters, and grandchildren, to whom he is thankful to God.

About the Contributors

Gisela Cruz, MSW, is a social worker and has spent much of her professional career assisting children and families in treatment planning, resource identification, and advocacy in several nonprofit agencies in North Georgia. She has worked with directors, stakeholders, and the community in creating programs needed to aid in mental health, food insecurity, and rebuilding families. In addition, she has provided direct clinical counseling services to mixed-status, uninsured, and Spanish-speaking clients. Her educational background includes a Bachelor of Science from the University of North Georgia and a Master of Social Work from the University of Georgia. She also looks forward to becoming a licensed clinical social worker in the near future.

Jhokania De Los Santos, PhD, is a qualitative research consultant who loves to tackle the big macro level questions when it comes to enhancing healthcare delivery. She is a proud graduate from the University of Georgia, where she received training in counseling psychology, and completed her pre-doctoral internship at the University of Colorado School of Medicine, with an emphasis on integrated primary care. She completed her post doctoral fellowship at Montefiore Medical Center, where she continued her research interests focusing on improving the quality of mental health care delivered to racial/ethnic minorities and examining the implementation of quality improvement interventions. Dr. De Los Santos uses her skills in research to analyze factors affecting healthcare access, while discovering what drives human interaction through different qualitative methodologies and empowering and equipping stakeholders with the skills and tools necessary to make healthcare affordable, safe, effective, equitable, accessible, and patient-centered.

Maritza Y. Duran, PhD, is a Crisis Response Resident at Kaiser Permanente in Richmond, California. Maritza recently completed her APA-accredited internship at the University of California, Berkeley's CAPS. She received her MSW from the University of Michigan and her B.A. from the University of California, Irvine in Chican@/Latin@ Studies and Sociology. Maritza is a APA-Minority Fellow. She is a first-generation college student from McFarland, California and comes from generations of immigrant/migrant farmworkers from Zacatecas, Mx. Her research and bilingual therapeutic work is informed by her experiences growing up in a small immigrant farming community in the Central Valley.

Leslie Espinoza earned a Bachelor of Arts in Psychology with a minor in Spanish from Georgia Southern University. She also completed an MEd in Educational Psychology with an emphasis in Cognition and Development from the University of Georgia. Leslie is now pursuing a doctoral degree in Counseling Psychology at the University of Georgia with an area of emphasis in health psychology. Her clinical interest includes adolescents, students, and women. Her research interest includes Latinx psychology, academic success, racial/ethnic identity, undergraduate education, and historical trauma.

Bekah Estevez (she/her) is an Assistant Professor at Georgia Southern University in the PsyD, Clinical Psychology program. She completed her undergraduate degree in psychology from Berry College (2014), and her master's in Professional Counseling (2016) and PhD in Counseling Psychology (2022) from the University of Georgia. Bekah's teaching interests include multicultural psychology, psychotherapy skills, advocacy, and helping students learn the art and science of psychotherapy grounded in strengths-based, culturally-responsive approaches. Believing in the potential for psychology to attenuate human suffering based in racism, heteronormativity, and other axes of oppression, she works to use her privilege as a white queer cisgender woman to explore the lived experiences of risk and resilience of those living at the intersections of oppressive systems. Broadly, Bekah's research interests include resilience, the impact of intersecting systems of oppression on mental health, best psychotherapy practices for working with the LGBTQ+ community, and bridging scholarly work and practice towards improving the field of psychology's role in mitigating disparate health outcomes experienced in Black and Latinx LGBTQ+ communities. As a clinician, Bekah integrates multicultural counseling theory (MCT) and 3rd wave Cognitive-Behavioral Therapy approaches into her practice. Bekah's approach to the work of psychology is informed by her experiences as a psychotherapist in a variety of settings working mostly with individuals and families from minoritized communities. She is also influenced deeply by the work of liberation-focused psychologists and critical scholars such as Ignacio Martín-Baró, Kimberlé Crenshaw, and Fransico Valdes.

Jacqueline Fuentes is a Xicana first-generation 4th-year doctoral candidate in the Counseling Psychology program at the University of Georgia. She is an APA MFP Predoctoral Fellow and Goizueta Foundation Graduate Scholar. Throughout her practicum and leadership experiences at La Clinica In Lak'Ech, Jacqueline has collaborated to expand language equity, teletherapy mental health, and in the training of mental health providers serving Latinx communities in the Deep South. Before her doctoral studies, Jacqueline served Latinx and African American children and families as a bilingual Spanish child welfare in San Francisco, CA. Professional experiences and support from colegas provided Jacqueline with critical intersectional insight on the realities and stressors families face. Within her roles, she advocated for interdisciplinary advocacy, acknowledgement of intergenerational trauma, and structural violence. She completed her Master in Social Welfare in Children and Families and was a Title IV-E stipend recipient specializing in child welfare at the University of California, Berkeley, in 2016. She was also part of the inaugural class of the Master in Education in Child, Human, and Family Services with a specialization in Prevention Science at the University of Oregon in 2014. Broadly, her research interests focus on structural violence and its impacts on mental health and well-being of children and families, foster youth mental health, expanding decolonial and culturally-rooted sources of healing along with preventative, interdisciplinary, and intersectional mental health interventions.

Marta J. González is a mental health practitioner working with the Latinx community in the San Fernando Valley, California. She obtained a Ph.D. in Counseling Psychology from The University of Georgia and a Master's degree in Counseling with emphasis in Marriage and Family Therapy from California State University, Northridge. Dr. González is also an educator in her community, providing psychoeducational workshops in Spanish and English on mental health topics affecting the Latinx community. Born and raised in Guatemala, she immigrated to the United States as a teenager where she attended High School in Los Angeles, California. Her strong connection with her country of origin has helped her maintain her cultural roots and traditions that have been transferred from one generation to another.

Jocelyn Jimenez-Ruiz is currently a second-year PhD student in the Counseling Psychology program at the University of Georgia. In addition, she has received her Master's of Education in Counseling Psychology from the University of Missouri- Columbia. Jocelyn is a Nicaraguan American, born in Miami, Florida but raised in Buford, GA. She currently provides bilingual therapy services at La Clinica LaK'ech. Jocelyn's interests and experience include working with victims/survivors of domestic abuse,

About the Contributors

individuals with trauma, and depression, and the Latinx community overall. In her free time, Jocelyn greatly enjoys curating her own music playlists, reading, and spending time with family and friends.

Grace-Ellen Mahoney (she/her), Ph.D., is a recent graduate from the University of Georgia Counseling Psychology Ph.D. program, where she worked on the BIEN research team under the advisement of Dr. Edward Delgado-Romero. Grace-Ellen's research interests include multicultural and bilingual counseling and training, cultural responses to grief and loss, and Latinx mental health.

Pierluigi Mancini, PhD, is the President of the Multicultural Development Institute, Inc. He is one of the most sought after national and international consultants and speakers about mental health and substance use disorder, his areas of expertise are cultural and linguistic responsiveness, immigrant behavioral health, social and racial justice, health equity and health disparities. Dr. Mancini founded Georgia's only Latino behavioral health program in 1999 to serve the immigrant population by providing appropriate mental health and addiction treatment and prevention services in English, Spanish and Portuguese. Nationally, he has provided expert content to clients at the local, state, and federal level. Internationally, he has provided consulting in Mexico, Italy, Colombia, Cuba, and Kosovo. He recently led a project to train clinicians in Latin America who are taking care of over 4 million displaced Venezuelans in the region. Dr. Mancini's work addressing Latino underage drinking, suicide and prescription drugs have won a combined six (6) EMMY ® awards. Dr. Mancini has been named one of the 50 Most Influential Latinos in Georgia; honored with the NLPA Star Vega Distinguished Service Award; the UnidosUS (NCLR) - Helen Rodríguez- Trías Award for Health; and the Mental Health America "Heroes in the Fight" Award among others. He serves as the Secretary/Treasurer on the Board of Directors for Mental Health America National, Wellstar Atlanta Regional Medical Center, the Georgia Council on Substance Abuse and R.I. International.

Kiara Manosalvas, MA, (she/her) is a doctoral candidate studying counseling psychology at Teachers College, Columbia University where she works with Dr. Brandon Velez in the Stigma, Identity, and Intersectionality research team. She is currently completing her APPIC internship at the Manhattan VA. Kiara's clinical and research interests broadly include race-based stress and trauma, social justice training in counseling psychology, and womanista/mujerismo psychology. Kiara's ethnic background as an Ecuadorian-Puerto Rican woman deeply informs her passion for uplifting and empowering marginalized communities, especially women of color.

Alyssa Marquez completed her bachelor's degree in psychology at California State Polytechnic University in 2019. Currently, she conducts research at The Semel Institute - UCLA and the Veterans Affair to assess cognition, and brain bases in severe mental illness within the homelessness and veteran community. Alyssa plans on pursuing a PhD in counseling psychology to focus on Latinx mental health.

Jennifer Merrifield, PhD, is a Veteran Care Coordinator for the Veterans Health Administration's LGBTQ+ Health Program. She also serves in her daily role as a Staff Psychologist, Clinical Assistant Professor of Psychiatry, and Outpatient Program Manager at Charlie Norwood Veterans Affairs Medical Center and the Medical College of Georgia. She is dedicated to improving healthcare systems for underserved populations and is often found using her privilege to break down barriers in systems of oppression. Her clinical work includes fostering minority resilience, trauma recovery, addressing LG-

BTQ+ concerns and confronting taboo topics frequently avoided by clinicians and clients. Her research interests include exploring intersectionality of identities, Latinx psychology, Intimate Partner Violence, Civic/Sociopolotical Engagement, Gender Roles, discrimination, racial disparities in mental health and the lived experience of undocumented immigrants living in the U.S.

Amelia Miller, PhD, is a Licensed Psychologist at a private practice in Atlanta, GA. Dr. Miller attended the University of Georgia for her Master's in Professional Counseling before continuing with her PhD in Counseling Psychology. She completed her internship and postdoctoral training at Emory University. Dr. Miller then served as the Embedded Psychologist for the Emory School of Medicine before transitioning to a private practice role in the community. Her research interests include eating disorder treatment for Latinas. Clinically, Dr. Miller specializes in eating concerns and body image from a multicultural feminist lens.

Charmaine Mora-Ozuna is a first-generation, Mexicana from California. She earned her B.A. in Psychology at Georgia State University, where she became the co-founder of the Alpha Pi Chapter of Sigma Lambda Upsilon/ Señoritas Latinas Unidas Sorority Inc. After completing her Master's in Mental Health Counseling at Florida State University, Charmaine pursued her doctoral studies in Counseling Psychology at the University of Georgia. She is a bilingual and bicultural therapist that serves marginalized communities across the lifespan in community mental health clinics (La Clinica in LaK'ech and Mercy Health Center) and hospital settings (The Grady Nia Project). Charmaine's research interests focus on trauma and resilience in the Latinx community. Her dissertation will focus on exploring the healing journey of Latina survivors of domestic violence who receive culturally-competent and interdisciplinary treatment. Charmaine is determined to make a lasting impact on the mental health system by fostering mental health literacy and increasing access to culturally and linguistically relevant services in Georgia. To recharge and pour into herself, Charmaine enjoys spending time with her loved ones, traveling, dancing, and eating!

Nancy Muro-Rodriguez completed her M.Ed. degree in Counseling Psychology at the University of Missouri-Columbia. She began her doctoral program in Counseling Psychology at the University of Georgia in 2019. Her research interests include intergenerational trauma within the Latinx community and caregiver stress for parents with an intellectual disability, and the experience of motherhood. Nancy provides individual bilingual and bicultural therapy with the Latinx community in Athens, GA. Nancy is a mother to her beautiful one year old, Ruben Atilano-Rodriguez III.

Ana Carina Ordaz, hija de inmigrantes Mexicanos, is a bicultural and bilingual Latina therapist. Ana Carina earned her Bachelor of Arts in Psychology and Master's in Clinical Mental Health Counseling from Georgia State University; Ana Carina is a fifth-year doctoral candidate in the Counseling Psychology program at the University of Georgia. She is finishing her second appointment year with the American Psychological Association (APA) Minority Fellowship Program (MFP): Doctoral Fellowship in Mental Health and Substance Abuse Services, funded by a grant from the federal Substance Abuse and Mental Health Services Administration (SAMHSA). Ana Carina has gained experience in counseling centers, community mental health, and hospital settings through her clinical training. She also has training in bilingual play therapy, which she loves using to create spaces of healing and coping for children and families. She will be pursuing her internship at Providence Saint John's Health Center-

About the Contributors

Child and Family Development Center. Her research interests focus on understanding complex trauma and post-traumatic growth within Latinx immigrant communities. More specifically, the pre-, in-transit, and post-immigration narratives of individuals and families in Georgia. Her lived identities and leadership roles have informed her work, and she has also seen first-hand the need to address social and racial injustices within mental health and recovery services. She continues to address and engage in critical dialogue around the need for culturally and linguistically competent behavioral health services. Overall, she is dedicated to serving underrepresented and marginalized communities, and through her work, she hopes to fight the stigma around mental illness one day at a time.

Alexina Pilo completed an M.A. in Mental Health Counseling at Boston College. She began the doctoral program in Counseling Psychology at the University of Georgia in 2020. Her research interests include Latinx college student academic adjustment, psychological well-being, mentorship, healing and perseverance following traumatic events, suicidality, and strength-based interventions. Additionally, she provides counseling to the uninsured Latinx community of Athens in La Clinica in LaK'ech and college students at the Center for Counseling and Personal Evaluation.

Vanessa Placeres received a Ph.D. in Counselor Education and Practice from Georgia State University in addition to master's degrees in Counseling, Marriage and Family Therapy, and School Counseling from California State University, Fresno, and Georgia State University. She is a Licensed Professional Counselor and Certified School Counselor in the state of Georgia in addition to a Registered Play Therapist. She has focused her clinical work on the treatment of children and adolescents and has experience working in community agencies, inpatient rehabilitation centers, and most recently as a high school counselor. Vanessa's research interests include cultural humility, multicultural counseling competence, and school counselor training.

Lucia Quezada, M.A., is a doctoral student in the Counseling Psychology program at the University of Georgia. She is under the advisement of Dr. Edward Delgado-Romero and is a member of the ¡BIENESTAR! Research team.

Brooke Rappaport (she/her), Ph.D., is an assistant professor in the psychology department at Tennessee State University and licensed psychologist in Tennessee. Brooke's research interests revolve around intersectional feminism, ally/accomplice/co-conspirator development, and relational approaches to supervision, training, research, and teaching. As a White woman who holds many privileged identities, Brooke has worked throughout her career to infuse social justice into all aspects of her professional and personal identities. Her research and work related to Latinx populations began as a Spanish minor studying abroad in Buenos Aires and blossomed as a member of Dr. Delgado-Romero's BIEN research team at the University of Georgia.

Inés Rodriguez is a gender non-conforming, Afro-Latine from New York by way of Dominican Republic. Anchored in their purpose, Inés creates healing spaces that reclaim the fullness of our personal, political and cultural identities. As a life-long activist and creative, Inés desired migratory spaces that allowed Black, Queer, Trans, and Immigrant communities to gather freely so they founded Professors ATL, a 36-foot school bus turned mobile community space. This venture is a culmination of many lived experiences, fierce mentorship, and dedicated skill-building and education. Inés completed an 80-hour community trauma-healing intensive in 2016, graduated with their Bachelors and Masters of Social Work from Georgia State University in 2015, and co-founded the Alpha Pi Chapter of Sigma Lambda Upsilon/Señoritas Latinas Unidas Sorority Incorporated in 2012. They love to lay in the sun, hang in trees, and chismear with loved ones.

Madison Rodriguez is a first-generation Mexican American graduate student pursuing a PhD in School Psychology at the University of Georgia. Her research interests include expanding school mental health resources and supporting culturally and linguistically diverse students in academic settings. Madison currently works as a Research Assistant for the Mary Frances Early College of Education. She is a member of the PRISMS Lab in the Educational Psychology department, which focuses on the prevention and intervention of mental health and substance misuse in low-resource minority service schools.

Violeta J. Rodriguez was born in Nicaragua and came to the United States at the age of 9. Violeta is an asylee who grew up in Miami. Violeta moved to Georgia to pursue her PhD in the Department of Psychology. She is now a 5th year student in the Clinical Psychology program, and a Ford Foundation Predoctoral Fellow (2018-2021). Violeta's research has resulted in numerous peer-reviewed manuscripts (90; 22 first author), with several others under review. Broadly, Violeta's research at the University of Georgia has focused on the psychometrics of parenting and family constructs, with an emphasis on making parenting and family measures more representative of diverse families. Violeta's research at the University of Georgia has been recognized and funded by the National Institute of Mental Health, Philanthropic Educational Organization, Psychological Association Division 53 (Society of Clinical Child and Adolescent Psychology), as well as the American Psychological Association of Graduate Students/Psi Chi Junior Scientist Fellowship. Violeta's dissertation will focus on revising and validating the Multidimensional Assessment of Parenting Scale in a racially and ethnically diverse national sample. She will be pursuing a highly competitive internship at the University of Illinois at Chicago's Department of Psychiatry.

Bryan O. Rojas-Araúz is a bilingual bicultural trauma Psychologist and Afro-Latino immigrant of Costa Rican and Panamanian descent. He spent his teenage years in the Bay Area, California, where he became a community organizer and DREAM activist. He received his B.A. in Psychology from San Jose State University and earned his Master's in Counseling in Marriage, Family, and Child Therapy with a dual emphasis in College Counseling at San Francisco State University. He received his doctorate in Counseling Psychology with a Specialization in Spanish Language Psychological Services and Research at the University of Oregon. He has over 10 years of experience providing bilingual mental health services and working with Spanish-speaking communities including children, adults, and families. He is a faculty member in the International Disaster Psychology: Trauma and Global Mental Health program at the University of Denver. His research interests include immigration psychology, DREAMers' mental health, ethnic identity formation, critical consciousness, postsecondary education attainment, and cultural competence development.

Julia Roncoroni is originally from Buenos Aires, Argentina. She has lived in the United States since 2007. She received her doctoral degree in counseling psychology from the University of Florida in 2016. Her pre-doctoral internship was at Harvard Medical School. She has been a faculty member in the Counseling Psychology Department, at the University of Denver (DU), since 2016. She is currently

About the Contributors

an Associate Professor. In the Morgridge College of Education (DU), she leads the Health Disparities Research Lab. She is also passionate about teaching and believes that the classroom can be a uniquely transformative space where students learn to connect theory and practice through experiential learning.

Monica Sanchez earned a Bachelor of Science degree in Psychology with a minor in Woman's and Gender studies from Valdosta State University. She also completed an MEd in Professional Counseling from the University of Georgia. Monica is now pursuing a doctoral degree in Counseling Psychology at the University of Georgia. Her clinical interests include providing bilingual mental health services to Latinx individuals and working with women, children, and families who have experienced traumatic events. Her research interests include trauma work and the Latinx community.

Ammy Sena has over 10 years of experience working with marginalized communities in various settings. She has worked in academic, hospital, residential, and college settings. She received her Bachelor's degree in Psychology and Latin America and Caribbean Studies with a minor in Education from Suffolk University. She also completed her Master's in Mental Health Counseling from Boston College with a certificate in Human Rights and International Justice. Ammy is currently pursuing her Ph.D. in Counseling Psychology from the University of Georgia. There she serves as the Co-Coordinator of La Clinica in LaK'ech, a student-run community clinic that provides free mental health services to the Latinx community of Athens, GA. She also is the instructor of record of ECHD 3030 Diversity and Helping Skills and is the Graduate Teaching Assistant for ECHD 4660/6660 U.S. Latino/a Mental Health: An Introduction. She is the recipient of the American Psychological Association's Interdisciplinary Minority Fellowship, the Graduate Fellowship with the American Association of Hispanics in Higher Education, the Arthur M. Horne Award and the Del Jones Memorial Scholarship. She also recently participated as a Graduate Fellow in the Transnational Dialogues in Afro-Latin and Afro-Latinx Studies program funded by the National Endowment for the Humanities. She is passionate about the mental health and wellness of marginalized communities, specifically Afro-Latinx and Afro-Caribbean persons.

Amanda Shannon has over 14 years of experience in healthcare. She has worked in various culturally diverse organizational environments, including academic, research, medical, and community based settings. Holding a Bachelor's degree in Psychology, with a minor in Biology from North Carolina Central University, she completed post baccalaureate studies in Biology, Spanish, Rehabilitation Psychology, and Behavioral Medicine, and subsequently attained a Master's degree in Clinical Mental Health Counseling from North Carolina Agricultural & Technical State University. Amanda is currently pursuing a Doctoral degree in Counseling Psychology with an emphasis in Clinical Health Psychology from The University of Georgia.

Marjory Vazquez is a Mexican/Salvadorian licensed psychologist in Northern California. She recently opened her own private practice "The Sana House" where she serves Latinas and women of color who have experienced trauma. She also works as a psychologist at Kaiser Permanente Hospital in Richmond, CA. Prior to becoming a licensed psychologist she completed her doctoral studies at the University of Georgia, where she helped start a bilingual clinic and became one of the founders of the clinic now known as La Clinica In Lak'Ech. Her interest focuses on trauma, intimate partner violence, sexual abuse/assault, and decolonizing therapy. Her passion is to work with Latinas and women of color trying to overcome adverse childhood experiences and who are looking to overcome intergenerational trauma.

Eckart Werther, Ph.D., M.S.W., is an Associate Professor in the Department of Psychology at Clayton State University. He is a Licensed Psychologist and a Licensed Clinical Social Worker. He is a 1st generation immigrant and is bilingual (English/Spanish). Eckart has worked extensively in a variety of clinical settings, primarily serving members of the Latinx & African American communities. His areas of interest include applied multicultural competency, ethics, mental health, men's issues, and student mentorship. He earned his B.S.W. from the University of North Alabama, his M.S.W. from Alabama A&M University, and his Ph.D. in Counseling Psychology from the University of Georgia.

Index

A

Acculturation 10-12, 25, 38, 122, 129-130, 141, 162, 169, 184, 186-187, 191, 193, 212, 214, 223, 225-226, 228-229, 250

Acculturative Stress 130, 158, 160, 163, 189-190, 193, 204, 214, 221, 228

Action 11, 29-31, 33-34, 52, 59, 81, 83, 99, 101, 114, 118, 136, 156-157, 168, 177, 179-180, 193, 208, 225, 253-254, 265, 267, 271, 279, 281, 286, 290

Adolescent Development 144, 180, 211-213, 217

Advocacy 11, 37-38, 51, 57-58, 62, 65-67, 84, 91, 109, 129, 168, 176, 182, 191, 206, 208, 220, 222, 275-278, 290

African Diaspora 14-16, 29

Afrodescendientes 14-25, 28-31

Afro-Latinx 14, 33, 88, 92, 95-97, 131, 185

Anti-Blackness 14-15, 17, 80, 92, 97, 212-213, 286, 291

Anzaldúa 78, 82, 87, 90-91, 94, 96-99, 101, 103-107, 111, 115, 118, 121-122, 184, 189, 192-193

Assessment 23, 27, 33, 35, 60, 68-69, 205, 208, 211-212, 217, 220-221, 225, 255, 273-276

Associate Editors 1

B

Borderlands 68, 82, 86, 90, 98-99, 103-104, 107, 115, 118, 184, 193

C

Caballerismo 43, 137-138, 140, 157, 161

Context Of Reception 228

Cultural 1-4, 8, 12, 15-16, 23, 25, 28-31, 34, 38, 40-51, 53-54, 57, 68, 72-75, 77-81, 83-85, 90, 94, 98, 100-101, 110-114, 117-122, 127, 129-130, 133-134, 136-138, 141, 143, 148, 151-156, 159-160, 163, 167, 169, 171-173, 175-176, 178-180, 184, 186-188, 190-193, 196, 198-199, 201-203, 205-206, 208-217, 219-224, 226, 240, 248-251, 255, 257-258, 262, 265, 268, 270-273, 276, 279-281, 284-285, 287-290

Cultural Competence 53, 117, 153-156, 178-179, 193, 268, 276, 290

Cultural Strengths 3-4, 15, 72, 206, 211, 215

Cultural Values 3, 40, 42-43, 45-50, 79, 98, 111, 114, 117, 130, 138, 154, 163, 167, 171-172, 175, 186, 190, 192, 196, 201-203, 206, 212, 214-215, 217, 251, 255, 257, 272, 281, 284

Culturally Responsive 12, 37-38, 47, 51, 80-81, 83, 114, 153, 178, 196, 206, 209, 215, 220, 241, 248, 254-257, 262, 268

Culture 2, 5-6, 9, 11-12, 16, 25, 29, 31-34, 39-41, 44, 47, 49-50, 54, 64, 70, 73, 75-76, 78, 81-82, 87-88, 90, 92, 94, 97, 99, 101, 104-106, 111-114, 116, 118-119, 121, 132-134, 137, 139, 141, 145, 160, 164, 166, 170-172, 176, 179, 182-190, 192, 199, 202-203, 206-209, 212-213, 220, 222-223, 235, 240-241, 244-246, 250, 257, 266, 271, 282-283, 285

D

DACA 59, 165, 168, 176-177, 179

Discrimination and Stereotypes 124, 131

Disparities 3, 11-12, 15, 19-20, 27, 31, 84, 117, 155, 174, 223, 225, 248-250, 252-256, 261-264, 266, 268-271, 273-275, 277-279, 284, 288

Dream Act 165, 168, 181

E

Ethnic Identity 7, 9, 13, 24, 28, 41-42, 45, 48, 54, 83, 85, 87, 90, 104, 111, 129-130, 182, 184, 186-188, 191-192, 213, 223-224, 226, 265

F

Familismo 43, 45, 47-48, 50, 111-113, 117, 122, 130, 141, 154, 170, 180, 190, 201-203, 205-206, 213, 215, 217, 220, 225, 284
Family Mental Health 228
Farmworkers 57-71, 91, 269, 278, 286
Feminism 4, 6, 83, 86-88, 90-91, 93-112, 114, 117-120, 122-123, 209
First-Generation College Student 112, 165, 169
Future Directions 67, 103, 117, 165, 176, 277, 281

G

Gender 6, 19-20, 33, 35, 37-48, 50-52, 54-56, 69-70, 75-76, 78, 87, 89-91, 93-95, 97-100, 102-103, 107, 109, 111-112, 114, 116-118, 120-121, 123-124, 127, 130, 132, 134-141, 146, 154, 156, 158, 160-163, 169, 175, 180-181, 197, 202, 206, 210, 214, 216, 222, 254, 265, 269, 286
Gender Gap 146

H

Health Disparities 11-12, 15, 27, 117, 223, 225, 249-250, 253-255, 261, 263, 268-271, 273-275, 278
Help-Seeking 124, 141, 158-161, 163-164, 256, 268-273, 275, 277, 279-280
Hispanic Serving Institutions 169, 171, 180
History 2-3, 5, 8-9, 11-17, 19, 22, 24-26, 29-35, 62, 67-69, 74, 82, 86-88, 90, 93-95, 99-100, 103, 106, 110, 113, 116, 118, 156, 165, 171-173, 175-176, 185-186, 194, 199, 205, 208, 221, 228-229, 241-242, 282, 289-290
Home Country 5, 112, 182-183, 186, 189, 192
Host Country 182, 186-192

I

Immigrants 4-6, 8, 39, 53, 55, 60, 62, 68-69, 71, 73, 78, 106, 117, 127, 130, 144, 158, 167-168, 182, 184-186, 188-194, 198, 203, 213-214, 221, 224-225, 228, 240, 249-252, 254, 263-264, 266, 270, 273, 278, 282
Immigration 12, 38, 50, 52, 57, 59-61, 65, 68-71, 117, 127, 129, 141, 168, 175, 177, 181, 184-186, 193, 203, 205-206, 212, 216-217, 221, 226, 228-229, 246, 249-250, 252-253, 256, 264-265, 275, 282, 284, 289, 292
Integrative Behavioral Healthcare 248
Intergenerational Trauma 196-198, 201, 203, 205-208, 211-212, 221
Interpersonal 3, 39-40, 70, 93, 117, 180, 196, 198-199, 202-203, 205-206, 212, 250, 262
Intersectionality 13, 27, 37, 39-40, 52-53, 55, 72, 95-97, 100, 102, 105, 107, 115, 119, 175, 187, 191, 205, 209, 263, 284
Interventions 16, 31, 50, 54, 67-68, 72, 84-85, 115, 156, 161, 163, 179, 196, 206, 208, 211-212, 215-216, 218-221, 223, 257, 265, 275, 277, 279, 284, 286, 289
Intrapersonal 39, 196, 198, 204-205, 207
Invisibility 14-17, 19-21, 28, 31-33, 119

L

Latin America 9, 14-21, 23-24, 26, 29-31, 33-35, 59, 77, 85-87, 92, 97, 101-102, 109-110, 116, 120, 123, 134, 164, 182, 184-188, 191-192, 199, 208-209, 289
Latina 2, 15, 31-32, 34, 38-39, 52-53, 55-56, 73, 76, 80-81, 83-84, 86-87, 90, 96-97, 99-100, 102-104, 106-108, 110-112, 115-122, 156-158, 161, 167, 170-171, 178-181, 184, 193, 198, 209, 214, 224-225, 264, 278, 291
Latina Feminism 86, 97, 99, 102-103, 122
Latina Role Models 86, 108
Latinx 1-9, 11-13, 15-16, 19-24, 26, 30-34, 37-55, 58-60, 62, 64-69, 71-74, 76-88, 90, 94-100, 103-108, 110-112, 114-120, 122, 124, 126-139, 141, 143-149, 151-158, 160-161, 163-194, 196-199, 201-226, 228-229, 238, 240-241, 248-251, 253, 255-258, 260-262, 264-265, 268, 270, 274-278, 280-287, 289-290, 292
Latinx Family 43, 112, 141, 211, 216
Latinx Feminism 86, 96, 103, 105-106, 111, 114, 117
Latinx Men 41, 45, 111, 113, 124, 126-127, 129-132, 135-138, 141-142, 146-147, 151-156
Latinx Mental Health 1-4, 7, 54, 182, 198-199, 281-284, 287-289
Latinx Psychology 6-7, 11, 31, 52, 99, 117-118, 124, 156, 281, 283, 285, 289
LGBTQ+ 2, 37-51, 54-56, 74, 76, 110, 116, 160, 209, 286
Liberation 1, 9-10, 14-15, 23-24, 28-32, 51, 74, 78, 80, 83, 89, 94, 96, 98-100, 102, 106, 110, 112, 116, 119, 123, 144, 197, 204, 207, 209, 284-286, 290-291

M

Machismo 47-48, 54, 75-76, 84, 93, 99, 104, 111, 113,

Index

119, 123, 136-141, 157, 161-164, 202, 216, 272
Madrinas 86
Marianismo 47-48, 76, 84, 87, 111, 115, 119, 123, 161, 202, 216
Masculinity 75, 104, 124-125, 130, 134-142, 149, 155-156, 158-164, 209
Mental Health 1-5, 7-9, 11, 14, 16, 22, 31, 39, 42, 44-45, 51, 53-57, 64-69, 72-73, 80-82, 85, 104, 110, 112-113, 115, 124, 126-132, 141-143, 146-147, 154-161, 163-164, 170, 174, 176, 178-180, 182, 186, 191-193, 196, 198-199, 203, 206, 208, 210, 212-214, 220-221, 223-226, 228-229, 236, 238-239, 241, 248-249, 252, 254-256, 262-266, 268-285, 287-291
Mentorship 108, 115, 117, 144, 151, 154-156, 165-167, 169-171, 175, 177, 287, 289
Migration Experiences 228-229, 238
Minority Stress Model 37, 39-40, 54
Mujeres 86, 101, 103, 109, 112, 118
Mujerista 73, 83-84, 94, 96, 99-100, 103-104, 106, 119

N

Nepantla 86, 98, 100, 102-103, 105, 107
Non-Binary 37, 56

P

Pipeline 9, 117, 146, 152, 165, 168-169, 177, 281, 288-289
Politics 12, 17-18, 34, 53, 71, 88, 101, 108, 114, 119-122, 136, 199, 248, 251, 253
Predominantly White Institutions 165, 171

Q

Qualitative Research 53, 67, 103, 114, 120, 122, 158, 178

R

Recommendations 33, 55, 72, 74, 80-81, 127, 149, 152, 211, 217, 224-225, 228-229, 238, 256-257, 264, 279
Resilience 3-4, 6, 8, 29-30, 39-40, 42-43, 46-56, 64, 67, 71, 79, 115, 122, 147, 155, 162, 164, 175, 180, 186, 190, 194-197, 203, 205, 209, 213, 215, 222, 225, 291
Resiliency and Strength 198

S

Sexual Minorities 54
Social Justice 9, 13, 32, 38, 49-50, 55, 64, 80, 99, 109-110, 112, 117, 129, 144, 168, 176, 184, 191, 206, 221, 281, 283, 285-286
Spirituality 17, 30, 39, 49, 72-74, 76-85, 105-106, 118, 122, 201
Strengths-Based 30, 49-51, 114, 117, 207, 211, 213, 255
Survival 1, 18, 26, 29, 73, 78, 90, 95, 125, 137, 194, 201, 204, 206, 212, 215, 286
Systemic 8, 26, 58, 64, 66, 87, 116, 152, 165, 175, 196, 198, 201, 203, 205-206, 218, 262, 285-286, 288

T

Testimoninos 228-229
Transgender 37-38, 51-52, 54-56

W

Wellness 1, 15, 19, 30, 55, 61, 64, 79, 113, 166, 248, 276
Womanista 86, 94-97, 100, 107, 115-117, 119

Recommended Reference Books

IGI Global's reference books are available in three unique pricing formats:
Print Only, E-Book Only, or Print + E-Book.

Shipping fees may apply.

www.igi-global.com

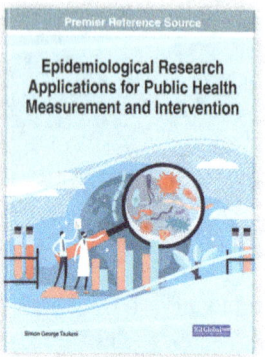

ISBN: 9781799844143
EISBN: 9781799844150
© 2021; 214 pp.
List Price: US$ **295**

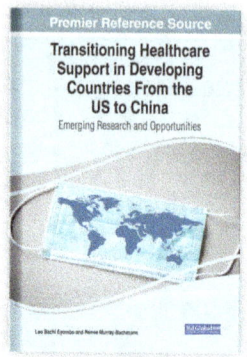

ISBN: 9781799844501
EISBN: 9781799844518
© 2021; 135 pp.
List Price: US$ **245**

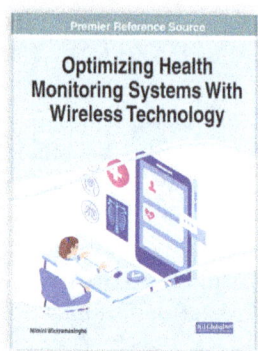

ISBN: 9781522560678
EISBN: 9781522560685
© 2021; 338 pp.
List Price: US$ **265**

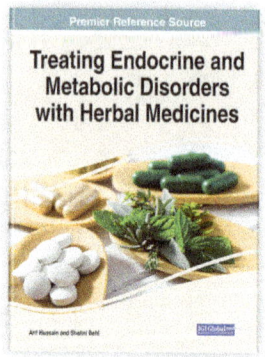

ISBN: 9781799848080
EISBN: 9781799848097
© 2021; 489 pp.
List Price: US$ **295**

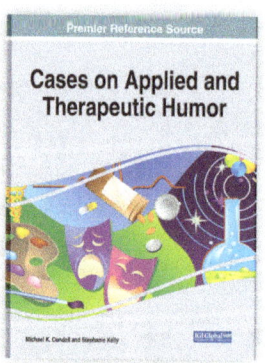

ISBN: 9781799845287
EISBN: 9781799845294
© 2021; 267 pp.
List Price: US$ **255**

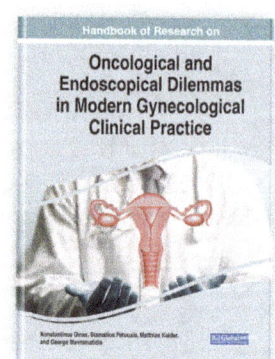

ISBN: 9781799842132
EISBN: 9781799842149
© 2021; 460 pp.
List Price: US$ **385**

Do you want to stay current on the latest research trends, product announcements, news, and special offers?
Join IGI Global's mailing list to receive customized recommendations, exclusive discounts, and more.
Sign up at: **www.igi-global.com/newsletters**.

Publisher of Timely, Peer-Reviewed Inclusive Research Since 1988

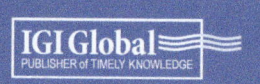

www.igi-global.com   Sign up at www.igi-global.com/newsletters   facebook.com/igiglobal   twitter.com/igiglobal   linkedin.com/igiglobal

Ensure Quality Research is Introduced to the Academic Community

Become an Evaluator for IGI Global Authored Book Projects

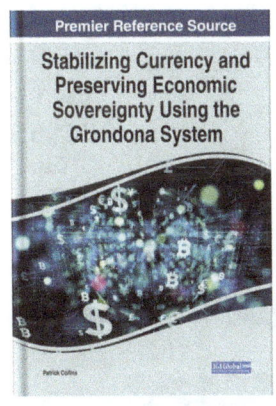
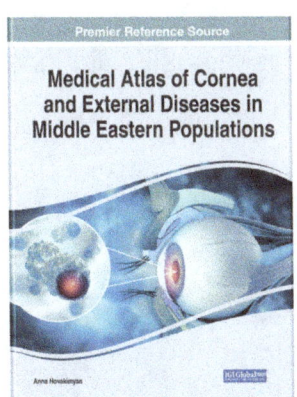
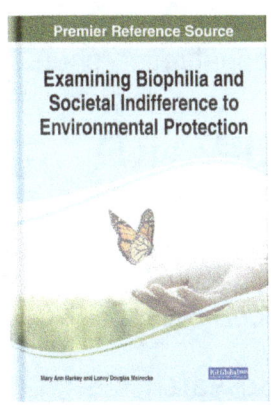
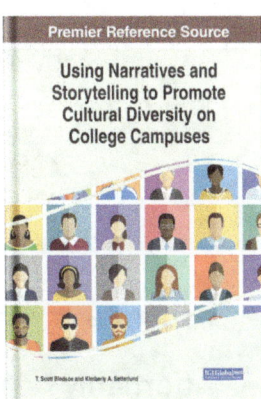

The overall success of an authored book project is dependent on quality and timely manuscript evaluations.

Applications and Inquiries may be sent to:
development@igi-global.com

Applicants must have a doctorate (or equivalent degree) as well as publishing, research, and reviewing experience. Authored Book Evaluators are appointed for one-year terms and are expected to complete at least three evaluations per term. Upon successful completion of this term, evaluators can be considered for an additional term.

If you have a colleague that may be interested in this opportunity, we encourage you to share this information with them.

Easily Identify, Acquire, and Utilize Published Peer-Reviewed Findings in Support of Your Current Research

IGI Global OnDemand

Purchase Individual IGI Global OnDemand Book Chapters and Journal Articles

For More Information:
www.igi-global.com/e-resources/ondemand/

Browse through 150,000+ Articles and Chapters!

Find specific research related to your current studies and projects that have been contributed by international researchers from prestigious institutions, including:

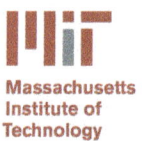 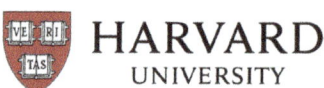 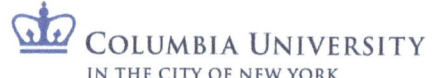 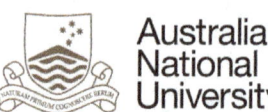

- Accurate and Advanced Search
- Affordably Acquire Research
- Instantly Access Your Content
- Benefit from the InfoSci Platform Features

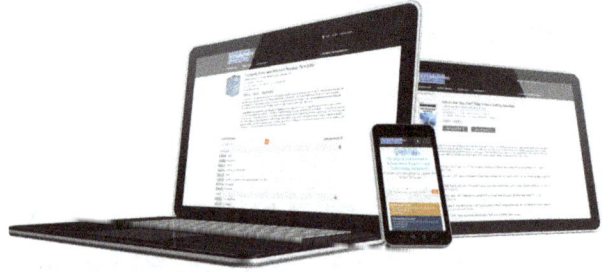

“*It really provides* **an excellent entry into the research literature of the field**. *It presents a manageable number of* **highly relevant sources** *on topics of interest to a wide range of researchers. The sources are* **scholarly, but also accessible** *to 'practitioners'.*”

- Ms. Lisa Stimatz, MLS, University of North Carolina at Chapel Hill, USA

Interested in Additional Savings?

Subscribe to

IGI Global OnDemand 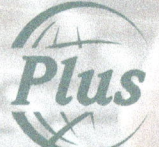 *Plus*

Learn More

Acquire content from over 128,000+ research-focused book chapters and 33,000+ scholarly journal articles for as low as US$ 5 per article/chapter (original retail price for an article/chapter: US$ 37.50).

6,600+ E-BOOKS.
ADVANCED RESEARCH.
INCLUSIVE & ACCESSIBLE.

IGI Global e-Book Collection

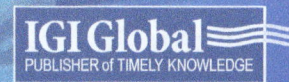

- **Flexible Purchasing Options** (Perpetual, Subscription, EBA, etc.)
- Multi-Year Agreements with **No Price Increases** Guaranteed
- **No Additional Charge** for Multi-User Licensing
- No Maintenance, Hosting, or Archiving Fees
- Transformative **Open Access Options** Available

Request More Information, or Recommend the IGI Global e-Book Collection to Your Institution's Librarian

Among Titles Included in the IGI Global e-Book Collection

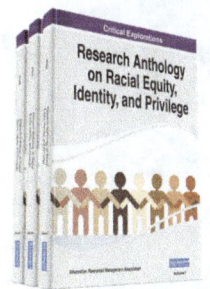

Research Anthology on Racial Equity, Identity, and Privilege (3 Vols.)
EISBN: 9781668445082
Price: US$ 895

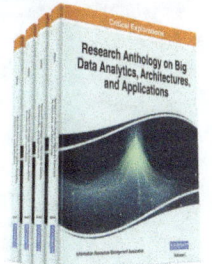

Handbook of Research on Remote Work and Worker Well-Being in the Post-COVID-19 Era
EISBN: 9781799867562
Price: US$ 265

Research Anthology on Big Data Analytics, Architectures, and Applications (4 Vols.)
EISBN: 9781668436639
Price: US$ 1,950

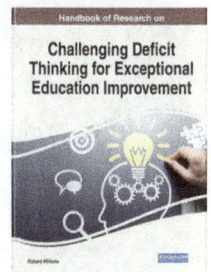

Handbook of Research on Challenging Deficit Thinking for Exceptional Education Improvement
EISBN: 9781799888628
Price: US$ 265

Acquire & Open

When your library acquires an IGI Global e-Book and/or e-Journal Collection, your faculty's published work will be considered for immediate conversion to Open Access *(CC BY License)*, at no additional cost to the library or its faculty *(cost only applies to the e-Collection content being acquired)*, through our popular **Transformative Open Access (Read & Publish) Initiative**.

For More Information or to Request a Free Trial, Contact IGI Global's e-Collections Team: eresources@igi-global.com | 1-866-342-6657 ext. 100 | 717-533-8845 ext. 100

Have Your Work Published and Freely Accessible
Open Access Publishing

With the industry shifting from the more traditional publication models to an open access (OA) publication model, publishers are finding that OA publishing has many benefits that are awarded to authors and editors of published work.

Freely Share Your Research

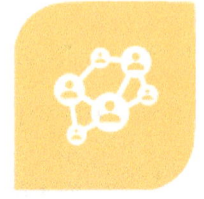
Higher Discoverability & Citation Impact

Rigorous & Expedited Publishing Process

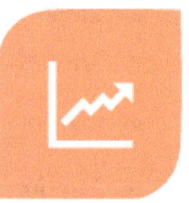
Increased Advancement & Collaboration

Acquire & Open

When your library acquires an IGI Global e-Book and/or e-Journal Collection, your faculty's published work will be considered for immediate conversion to Open Access *(CC BY License)*, at no additional cost to the library or its faculty *(cost only applies to the e-Collection content being acquired)*, through our popular **Transformative Open Access (Read & Publish) Initiative**.

- Provide Up To **100%** OA APC or CPC Funding
- Funding to Convert or Start a Journal to **Platinum OA**
- Support for Funding an **OA Reference Book**

IGI Global publications are found in a number of prestigious indices, including Web of Science™, Scopus®, Compendex, and PsycINFO®. The selection criteria is very strict and to ensure that journals and books are accepted into the major indexes, IGI Global closely monitors publications against the criteria that the indexes provide to publishers.

WEB OF SCIENCE™ **Compendex** **Scopus**®

PsycINFO® **IET Inspec**

Learn More Here:

For Questions, Contact IGI Global's Open Access Team at openaccessadmin@igi-global.com

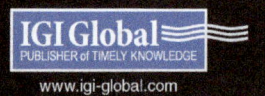

Are You Ready to Publish Your Research

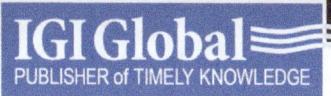

IGI Global offers book authorship and editorship opportunities across 11 subject areas, including business, computer science, education, science and engineering, social sciences, and more!

Benefits of Publishing with IGI Global:

- Free one-on-one editorial and promotional support.
- Expedited publishing timelines that can take your book from start to finish in less than one (1) year.
- Choose from a variety of formats, including Edited and Authored References, Handbooks of Research, Encyclopedias, and Research Insights.
- Utilize IGI Global's eEditorial Discovery® submission system in support of conducting the submission and double-blind peer review process.
- IGI Global maintains a strict adherence to ethical practices due in part to our full membership with the Committee on Publication Ethics (COPE).
- Indexing potential in prestigious indices such as Scopus®, Web of Science™, PsycINFO®, and ERIC – Education Resources Information Center.
- Ability to connect your ORCID iD to your IGI Global publications.
- Earn honorariums and royalties on your full book publications as well as complimentary copies and exclusive discounts.

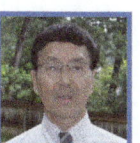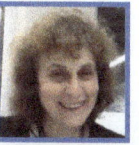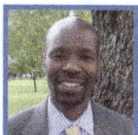
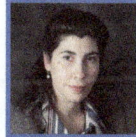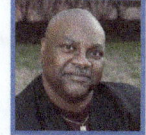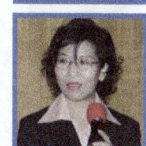
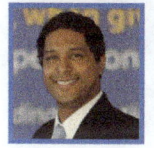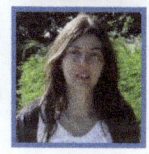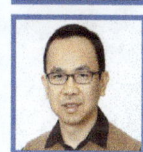

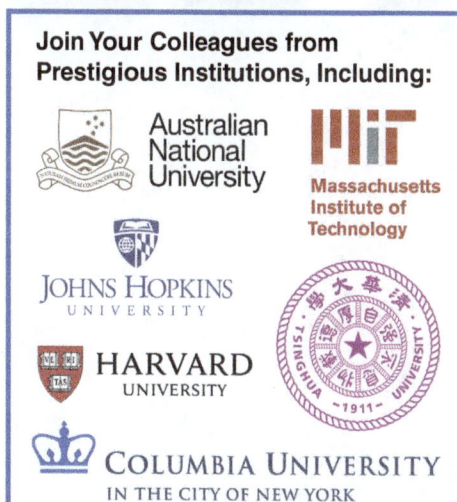

Join Your Colleagues from Prestigious Institutions, Including:
Australian National University, Massachusetts Institute of Technology, Johns Hopkins University, Tsinghua University, Harvard University, Columbia University in the City of New York

Learn More at: www.igi-global.com/publish

or Contact IGI Global's Aquisitions Team at: acquisition@igi-global.com

Printed in the USA
CPSIA information can be obtained
at www.ICGtesting.com
CBHW081459030824
12666CB00005B/224